Infertility, Contraception & Reproductive Endocrinology

Second Edition

Infertility, Contraception & Reproductive Endocrinology

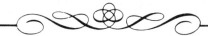

Second Edition

Edited by

Daniel R. Mishell Jr., M.D.
Professor and Chairman, Department of Obstetrics and Gynecology

Val Davajan, M.D.
Professor, Department of Obstetrics and Gynecology

University of Southern California School of Medicine
Los Angeles, California

Medical Economics Books
Oradell, New Jersey 07649

Library of Congress Cataloging in Publication Data

Main entry under title:

Infertility, contraception, and reproductive
  endocrinology.

  Includes bibliographies and index.
  1.Endocrine gynecology.   2. Infertility, Female.
3. Contraception.   I. Mishell, Daniel R.   II. Davajan,
Val, 1934-   .   [DNLM: 1. Contraception.   2. Endocrine
Glands—physiology.   3. Endocrine Glands—physiopathology.
4. Infertility, Female.   5. Reproduction.   WQ   205   R4284]
RG159.I54   1986   618.1   84-27323
ISBN 0-87489-352-6

Design by *A Good Thing Inc.*

Wash drawings by Wesley Bloom

ISBN 0-87489-352-6

Medical Economics Company Inc.
Oradell, New Jersey 07649

Printed in the United States of America

Contents

Contributors

David A. Battin, M.D., Clinical Instructor, Department of Obstetrics and Gynecology, University of Southern California School of Medicine, Los Angeles

Gerald S. Bernstein, Ph.D., M.D., Professor, Department of Obstetrics and Gynecology, University of Southern California School of Medicine, Los Angeles

Paul F. Brenner, M.D., Professor, Department of Obstetrics and Gynecology, University of Southern California School of Medicine, Los Angeles

Val Davajan, M.D., Professor, Department of Obstetrics and Gynecology, University of Southern California School of Medicine, Los Angeles

Gere S. diZerega, M.D., Associate Professor, Department of Obstetrics and Gynecology, University of Southern California School of Medicine, Los Angeles

William E. Gibbons, M.D., Assistant Professor, Department of Obstetrics and Gynecology, University of Southern California School of Medicine, Los Angeles

Uwe Goebelsmann, M.D., Professor, Department of Obstetrics and Gynecology, University of Southern California School of Medicine, Los Angeles

David I. Hoffman, M.D., Assistant Professor, Department of Obstetrics and Gynecology, Northwestern University Medical School, Chicago

Oscar A. Kletzky, M.D., Professor, Department of Obstetrics and Gynecology, University of Southern California School of Medicine, Los Angeles

Rogerio A. Lobo, M.D., Assistant Professor, Department of Obstetrics and Gynecology, University of Southern California School of Medicine, Los Angeles

Charles M. March, M.D., Associate Professor, Department of Obstetrics and Gynecology, University of Southern California School of Medicine, Los Angeles

Richard P. Marrs, M.D., Assistant Professor, Department of Obstetrics and Gynecology, University of Southern California School of Medicine, Los Angeles

Daniel R. Mishell Jr., M.D., Professor and Chairman, Department of Obstetrics and Gynecology, University of Southern California School of Medicine, Los Angeles

Robert M. Nakamura, Ph.D., Associate Professor, Department of Obstetrics and Gynecology, University of Southern California School of Medicine, Los Angeles

John A. Richmond, M.D., Associate Professor, Department of Clinical Radiology, University of Southern California School of Medicine, Los Angeles

Subir Roy, M.D., Associate Professor, Department of Obstetrics and Gynecology, University of Southern California School of Medicine, Los Angeles

Joyce M. Vargyas, M.D., Associate Professor, Department of Obstetrics and Gynecology, University of Southern California School of Medicine, Los Angeles

Preface

The first edition of this book, published in 1979, emphasized recent advances in the field of reproductive biology, particularly gynecologic endocrinology. In the past decade, training programs in obstetrics and gynecology have provided more didactic information as well as clinical training in gynecologic endocrinology, so that physicians in practice today are more knowledgeable about gynecologic endocrinologic diagnostic techniques than they were 10 years ago. However, major obstacles still impede the diagnosis and treatment of couples with infertility. As more women delay childbearing because of career choices or financial reasons, a greater percentage of couples in the US find themselves unable to conceive. Thus, in the second edition of this book, emphasis has been shifted toward the diagnosis and treatment of infertility, although gynecologic endocrinology and contraception are also covered thoroughly.

The second edition continues an important aim of the first: to formulate diagnostic guidelines utilizing only those newly developed laboratory and radiologic tests that are necessary to establish correct diagnoses, thereby avoiding the performance of expensive and frequently unnecessary procedures. Now, as then, our ultimate goal is to describe diagnostic and therapeutic methods simply yet comprehensively. Again we make frequent use of flowcharts to clarify the steps in evaluation of such common presenting symptoms as amenorrhea, galactorrhea, and androgen excess.

We have continued to emphasize the need for objectivity in the application of scientific and clinical knowledge to the practice of reproductive medicine, especially infertility. We present all the available therapies for each condition; where more than one treatment exists, we make specific recommendations to follow in caring for individual patients. The effectiveness and possible side effects of the more recently developed and widely used forms of contraception receive special attention. Again, specific recommendations are made concerning the use of certain contraceptives for particular patients.

We hope that this book will be valuable for both the physician in training and the clinician in practice. To that end, basic information is provided in addition to practical clinical approaches we have found to be successful at the University of Southern California. With the book's shift in emphasis toward infertility, we especially hope it will ease the task of managing patients with reproductive endocrine disorders and infertility problems and increase the proportion of successful results.

We gratefully acknowledge the assistance of our secretaries, who spent many hours typing the original versions and several revisions of each chapter. Special recognition is due Erika Free Wesnousky, who cheerfully devoted much of her time to correcting the printed drafts and proofs as well as coordinating the figures, captions, and tables. Without her invaluable assistance, the second edition of this book could not have been published. We thank her for her extraordinary efforts.

Daniel R. Mishell Jr., M.D.
Val Davajan, M.D.

Part I

Normal Endocrinology

Chapter 1

Reproductive Neuroendocrinology

Oscar A. Kletzky, M.D.
Rogerio A. Lobo, M.D.

The field of neuroendocrinology evolved from the symbiosis of two independent sciences, endocrinology and neurobiology. Endocrinology is the study of hormones secreted into the bloodstream from one organ that have a specific effect on target tissues in other organs. Neurobiology is the study of the biologic effects of nerve cells, which transmit information over long distances by nerve impulses. The classic example of a neurobiologic effect is the release of acetylcholine from the nerve ending into the muscle to produce muscle contractions. The transmission of information from the nerve to the muscle occurs at a point called the synapse. This chemical transmission at the synaptic level occurs in all mammalian peripheral and central nervous systems (CNS).[1]

Neurosecretion is the secretion of a substance by a neuron into the bloodstream. The synthesis and secretion of oxytocin and vasopressin represent examples of neurosecretion.[1] These hormones are produced by the neurons of the supraoptic and paraventricular nuclei of the hypothalamus and are transported along axons into the posterior lobe of the pituitary, which serves as a storage and release station (Figure 1-1). Each molecule of oxytocin and vasopressin circulates bound to a different mole-cule of a protein carrier, called neurophysin. The secretion of pituitary hormones is affected by a variety of environmental and hormonal in-

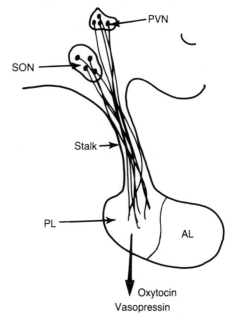

Figure 1-1
Neurosecretion of oxytocin and vasopressin by the hypothalamic supraoptic (SO) and paraventricular (PV) nuclei is released directly into the posterior (neural) lobe of the pituitary gland. AL, anterior lobe; PL, posterior lobe; PVN, paraventricular nucleus; SON, supraoptic nucleus.

fluences acting on the CNS (feedback regulation). The hypothalamus and the pituitary are functionally connected through the portal system.[2] The identification and characterization of neurotransmitters and hypothalamic hormones that control the release of pituitary hormones are discussed in this chapter.

The hypothalamus

The human hypothalamus weighs only about 4 g, but it plays an extremely important role in reproduction and homeostasis (Figure 1-2). The hypothalamic neurons develop during the second and third months of gestation and migrate to their final position to form what will later be the adult hypothalamus. Morphologically, the hypothalamus is divided into three zones: periventricular, medial (rich in cells), and lateral (rich in fibers). Besides its many internuclear connections, the hypothalamus is extensively connected with other areas of the brain via humoral and neural output and input pathways.[3]

Humoral and neural output pathways

The humoral output pathway consists of the magnocellular and the parvicellular systems. The magnocellular secretory system comprises the supraoptic and paraventricular nuclei. Vasopressin and oxytocin are synthesized by the magnocellular nuclei and transported to the posterior pituitary gland, where they are released into the general circulation. It has been reported that vasopressin is secreted mainly by the supraoptic nuclei, whereas oxytocin is secreted predominantly by the paraventricular nuclei.[4]

Hypothalamic inhibiting factors and tropic-releasing hormones are produced in the nuclei of the parvicellular system. In recent years, five hypothalamic hormones that act on the anterior pituitary have been isolated, their chemical structures determined, and synthesized: gonad-otropin-releasing hormone (GnRH), thyrotropin-releasing hormone (TRH), growth hormone release-inhibiting hormone or somatostatin, corticotropin-releasing hormone (CRH), and growth hormone-releasing hormone (GHRH). These hormones are transported by hypothalamic neurons to the median eminence, where they are released into the portal circulation and carried to the anterior pituitary.

Immunohistochemical methods have demonstrated a quantitative difference in the location of GnRH cell bodies among species. In the human and monkey, GnRH cell bodies are easily detected and are concentrated mainly in the arcuate and premammillary nuclei of the medial basal hypothalamus.[5, 6] From these locations, GnRH is transported along axons that terminate

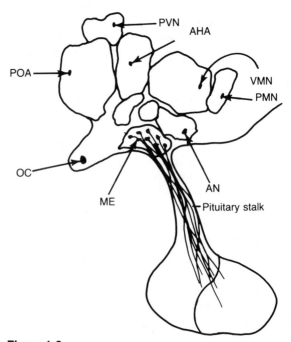

Figure 1-2
Diagrammatic representation of most important hypothalamic nuclei in relation to the pituitary gland. AHA, anterior hypothalamic area; AN, arcuate nucleus; ME, median eminence; OC, optic chiasm; PMN, premammillary nucleus; POA, preoptic area; VMN, ventromedial nucleus.

mainly in the lateral part of the median eminence and in the organum vasculosum of the lamina terminalis (OVLT). In these locations, granules 75 to 90 nm in diameter containing GnRH have been found.[7] TRH-secreting cell bodies have been detected in the dorsomedial nucleus, the perifornical area, and the paraventricular nucleus.[8] The fibers transporting TRH terminate in the medial part of the external layer of the median eminence. Cell bodies containing somatostatin have been identified mainly in the periventricular region of the hypothalamus.[9] Somatostatin has also been found to be secreted by cells in other brain areas and outside the nervous system in such locations as the islets of the pancreas and the intestinal wall. The exact location of cell bodies synthesizing CRH and GnRH is not known.

Neural output channels connect the hypothalamus with other areas of the brain, including the amygdala, hippocampus, septum, thalamus, and pons, forming closed neural circuits.

Humoral and neural input pathways

The input channels are responsible for maintaining a constant flow of information from the external and internal environments into the hypothalamus. This information also follows humoral and neural pathways. The humoral input connection is brought into the hypothalamus through the blood circulation. Peptide and steroid hormones coming into the hypothalamus bind to specific receptors to produce specific effects. Estrogen- and androgen-binding cells are concentrated mainly in the medial preoptic area, medial anterior hypothalamus, ventromedial nucleus, arcuate nucleus, and ventral premammillary nucleus.[10, 11] There these steroids participate in the feedback mechanism involved in controlling gonadotropic secretion from the pituitary. At least in animals, these steroids also affect sexual behavior.

Pituitary hormones may have a direct feedback action on the hypothalamus.[12] It has been reported that pituitary hormone secretion can be influenced by implanting follicle-stimulating hormone (FSH), luteinizing hormone (LH), prolactin (PRL), growth hormone (GH), or adrenocorticotropin (ACTH) into the medial basal hypothalamus. It has been further suggested that hypothalamic releasing hormones may have a direct action on the hypothalamus itself by an ultrashort feedback mechanism.[13] Also, thermoreceptors and osmoreceptors found in the anterior hypothalamus may be involved in regulation of hormone secretion.[14]

The hypothalamus receives information from the same limbic structures (hippocampus, amygdala, and septum) with which it has neural output connections. There are also direct channels to the hypothalamus from the lower brainstem, the thalamus, and the retina. The input from the retina, demonstrated only recently, suggests that the effect of light on the hypothalamus may be a regulatory pathway in controlling some functions of the anterior pituitary.[15]

There is a functional overlap in the hypothalamic regions involved in regulating pituitary function and sexual behavior and those regulating temperature and food and water intake. It is also possible that there are connections among different functional areas such as the regulation of temperature and the control of thyroid-stimulating hormone (TSH) secretion. There may also be a relationship between gonadotropic function and sexual behavior, as well as water intake and vasopressin. Nevertheless, certain hypothalamic areas have predominant involvement in a specific function.

The median eminence

The median eminence, together with the infundibular stalk and the neural lobe of the pituitary, constitutes the neurohypophysis. The pars tuberalis of the anterior lobe of the pituitary covers the base of the hypothalamus and the pituitary stalk. The pars tuberalis is vascularized by the pituitary portal vessels.

The median eminence usually is divided into three areas: the ependymal layer (or zona interna), a subependymal layer (fibrous layer), and a palisade layer (the zona externa). The ependymal layer is formed of cells similar to those found in the region of the third ventricle. However, in this location the ependymal cells are modified and thus are called tanycytes (Figure 1-3).[16] Each tanycyte has numerous microvilli extending throughout the entire width of the median eminence, ending in the capillary plexus in the palisade layer. It has been suggested that these tanycytes carry substances from the third ventricle into the portal circulation.

On its ventral and lateral surfaces, the median eminence is covered by astrocytes, which are specialized glial cells. These cells are replaced by the pericapillaries in the palisade, forming the portal capillaries. An important point to remember is that the capillaries of the median eminence are outside the blood-brain barrier. These capillaries differ from the capillaries present in the brain: Their endothelium is fenestrated and resembles that of capillaries in peripheral tissue. The endothelium of the brain capillaries is not fenestrated. Because of this morphologic difference, certain molecules, especially large ones that cannot cross the brain-blood barrier, will be able to permeate the capillaries of the median eminence.

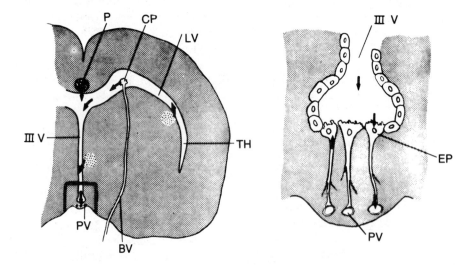

Figure 1-3
Diagrammatic representation of the relationship of the third ventricle and the hypothalamus (rat). The view on the right is an enlargement of the outlined area in the view on the left. III V, third ventricle; P, pineal gland; PV, portal vessel; BV, blood vessel; TH, temporal horn of the ventricle; LV, lateral ventricle; CP, choroid plexus; EP, ependymal cell (tanycyte).

Reproduced, with permission, from Kendall JW, Jacobs JJ, Kramer RM, et al: Studies on the transport of hormones from the cerebrospinal fluid to hypothalamus and pituitary. In Knigge KM, Scott DE, Weindl A (eds): Brain-Endocrine Interaction. Median Eminence: Structure and Function. Proceedings: International Symposium on Brain-Endocrine Interaction, Munich, 1971. Basel, Karger, 1972, p 342.

Normal endocrinology

Portal and pituitary circulation

Elegant studies performed in monkeys have demonstrated a common capillary network for the median eminence, the infundibular stalk, and the neural lobe.[17] Blood is supplied to the neurohypophysis by the superior, middle, and inferior hypophyseal arteries. The adenohypophysis, however, receives no direct arterial supply. Of its blood supply, 80% to 90% is provided by the long portal vessels, while the short vessels provide the remaining 10% to 20%. It has also been demonstrated that most of the return circulation does not go through the cavernous sinus, but through the short portal veins into the neurohypophyseal capillary plexus. In addition, these studies demonstrated a reverse capil-

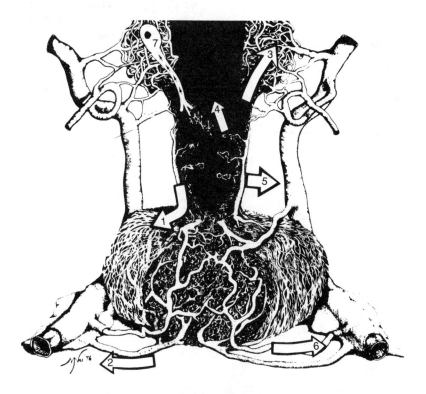

Figure 1-4
In this drawing of a pituitary vascular cast, the posterior of the infundibulum has been removed. The arrows indicate the potential efferent routes from the neurohypophysis: (1) Portal vessels may convey blood to the adenohypophysis; (2) confluent pituitary veins may carry blood to the cavernous sinus; (3) blood may flow from the infundibulum to the hypothalamus via connecting capillaries; (4) tanycytes may transport some substances into the ventricle; (5) substances may leak through the endothelial fenestrations of portal vessels into the subarachnoid space; (6) certain hypophyseal arteries may, under certain conditions, serve as efferent vascular channels; and (7) retrograde axonal flow may carry substances from the neurohypophysis to the hypothalamus. Five of these seven routes are directed toward the brain.

Reproduced, with permission, from Bergland RM, Page RB: Can the pituitary secrete directly to the brain? (Affirmative anatomical evidence). Endocrinology 102:1325, 1978. © 1978, The Endocrine Society.

lary plexus that transports blood from the anterior pituitary into the median eminence or into arteries that supply the medial hypothalamus (Figure 1-4).[17] Therefore, it is conceivable that the hypothalamus and the pituitary can function as an integral unit. It has been suggested that the secretion of pituitary hormones into the hypothalamus could ultimately control, regulate, or modulate the secretion of the same pituitary hormones.

Effects of neurotransmitters on the hypothalamus

The most important neurotransmitters involved in neuroendocrinology are catecholamines (dopamine and norepinephrine), an indolamine (serotonin), and opioids (enkephalin and β-endorphin). Other neurotransmitters include melatonin, acetylcholine, histamine, γ-aminobutyric acid (GABA), substance P, and vasoactive intestinal polypeptide (VIP).[18, 19]

Dopamine

Tyrosine is the precursor of both dopamine and norepinephrine (Figure 1-5). In the neurons of the midbrain, tyrosine is converted into L-dihydroxyphenylalanine (dopa) by the action of the enzyme tyrosine hydroxylase. Dopa is then decarboxylated into dopamine; in this process, pyridoxine (vitamin B) acts as an important coenzyme. Dopamine functions both as a neurotransmitter itself and as the precursor of norepinephrine, another transmitter.

The cell bodies where dopamine is synthesized are located principally in the arcuate nucleus, the periventricular hypothalamic area, and

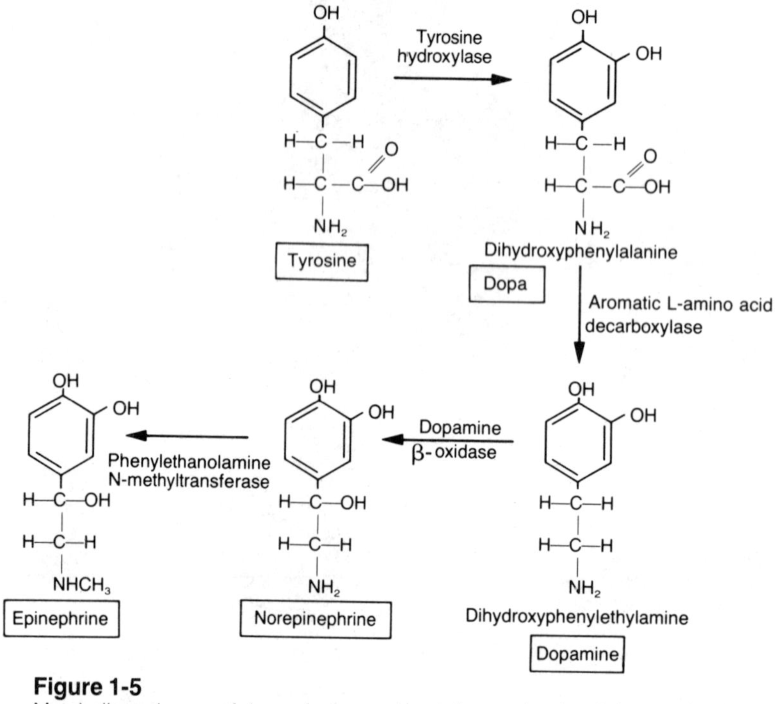

Figure 1-5
Metabolic pathways of dopamine, norepinephrine, and epinephrine synthesis.

the preoptic area. Axon terminals originate in these cell bodies and project into the external layer of the median eminence, the infundibular stalk, and the pituitary. Dopamine does not cross the blood-brain barrier, and therefore the effects of dopamine administered intravenously indicate that it has a direct effect on the median eminence and/or the pituitary.

Intravenous infusion of dopamine for 4 to 6 hours inhibits the secretion of PRL, TSH, and LH, but not FSH, and stimulates growth hormone release.[20] Furthermore, when dopamine infusion was extended to 48 consecutive hours, serum PRL and TSH levels exhibited the greatest degree of inhibition: 80% and 50%, respectively (Figure 1-6).[21] When dopamine infusion was stopped, there was a significant rebound in the release of these hormones.[20,21] This rebound phenomenon suggests that dopamine inhibits the release of TSH and PRL, but synthesis persists. After the infusion was discontinued, both synthesized and stored hormone were released in larger quantities.

Dopamine has a different effect on serum LH and FSH. As Figure 1-7 shows,[21] serum LH was initially inhibited by about 40%. However, despite the continuation of the dopamine infusion, the levels of LH returned to baseline. In these prolonged infusion studies, in contrast to short-term infusion (4 hours), the response of FSH was similar to that of LH: There was an initial mild inhibition (20%), but there was an escape of FSH release despite the continuation of the dopamine infusion.

These results indicate that dopamine has only a temporary direct inhibitory effect on gonadotropin secretion. Thus dopamine seems not to be the most important neurotransmitter controlling the secretion of gonadotropins. Additional experiments indicate that dopamine suppresses the secretion of gonadotropins by inhibiting the release of GnRH through an axon-axon interaction at the median emi-

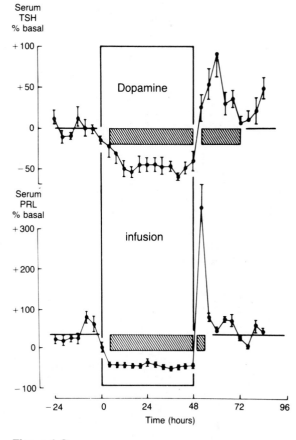

Figure 1-6
Mean (± SE) percentage change from basal levels in serum thyrotropin (TSH) and prolactin (PRL) before, during, and after dopamine administration in six normal male volunteers. Hatched bars indicate values that were significantly different from basal ($P < 0.01$) when compared by two-factor analysis of variance.

Reproduced, with permission, from Kaptein EM, Kletzky OA, Spencer CA, et al: Effects of prolonged dopamine infusion on anterior pituitary function in normal males. J Clin Endocrinol Metab 51:488, 1980. © 1980, The Endocrine Society.

nence.[19] There is also published evidence that the negative feedback produced by estrogens and androgens on gonadotropin secretion may be mediated at least in part by activation of the

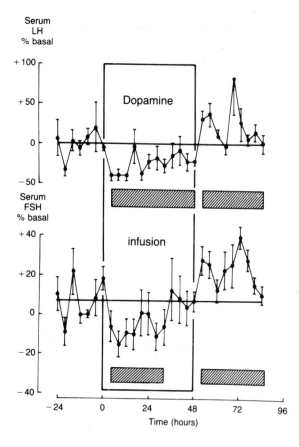

Serum
LH
% basal

Serum
FSH
% basal

Time (hours)

Figure 1-7
Mean (±SE) percentage changes from basal levels in serum LH and FSH before, during, and after dopamine administration in six normal male volunteers. Hatched bars indicate values that were significantly different from basal ($P < 0.01$) when compared by two-factor analysis of variance.

Reproduced, with permission, from Kaptein EM, Kletzky OA, Spencer CA, et al: Effects of prolonged dopamine infusion on anterior pituitary function in normal males. J Clin Endocrinol Metab 51:488, 1980. © 1980, The Endocrine Society.

urine and probably represent CNS dopamine turnover.

Norepinephrine

Unlike the nerve cells that secrete dopamine, norepinephrine nerve cell bodies have not been identified in the hypothalamus. The major source of norepinephrine is neuronal axons arising from the caudal medulla, the pons, and the locus ceruleus, located in the base of the fourth ventricle. In the median eminence, norepinephrine terminals are found mainly within the subependymal layer and within the medial preoptic area. These areas activate GnRH cell bodies and pathways, resulting in the release of gonadotropins.[22] However, it has been demonstrated that norepinephrine systems are not activated in castrated animals.[23] In addition, the norepinephrine-hypothalamic system is known to play a facilitative role in the release of TRH, and it is involved in controlling the regulation of body temperature and the intake of food.[23]

Two major metabolites of norepinephrine can be measured in the urine: 3-methoxy-4-hydroxyphenyl glycol (MHPG), which indirectly reflects the CNS turnover of norepinephrine, and vanillylmandelic acid (VMA), which represents peripheral norepinephrine secretion and metabolism.

Epinephrine

Epinephrine nerve terminals are found in the lateral and ventral portions of the arcuate nucleus and in the subependymal layer of the median eminence. The secretion of epinephrine has little, if any, effect in controlling the synthesis and secretion of hormones involved in the reproductive process.

Serotonin

Serotonin, an indolamine, is produced in cell bodies located in the nucleus raphe dorsalis and medianus and within the raphe nuclei of the

dopamine pathway. The two most important metabolites of dopamine are dihydroxyphenylacetic acid (DOPAC) and homovanillic acid (HVA). Both can be measured in plasma and

10

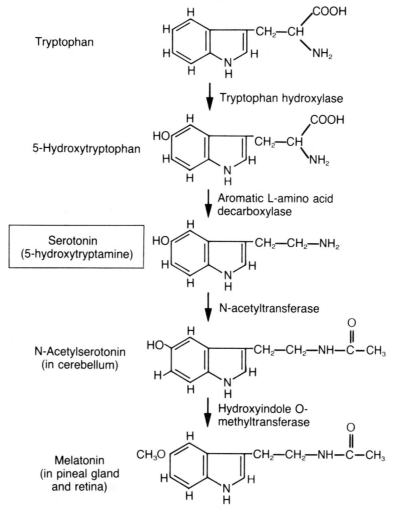

Figure 1-8
Metabolic pathway of serotonin synthesis.

pons. Recently, indolamine cell bodies were also found within the hypothalamus itself.[24] Like the norepinephrine and epinephrine axons, the hypothalamic serotonin axons are located in the lateral hypothalamic area. Tryptophan, the precursor of serotonin (Figure 1-8), is first hydroxylated to 5-hydroxytryptophan and then decarboxylated to serotonin. Its principal metabolite,

5-hydroxyindoleacetic acid (5-HIAA), can be measured in urine.

Serotonin's role in the control of pituitary hormone secretion has recently been described. IV injection of 5-hydroxytryptophan (5-HTP) resulted in a significant increase in serum PRL (Figure 1-9), cortisol (Figure 1-10), and TSH (Figure 1-11) in both men and women.[25] GH in-

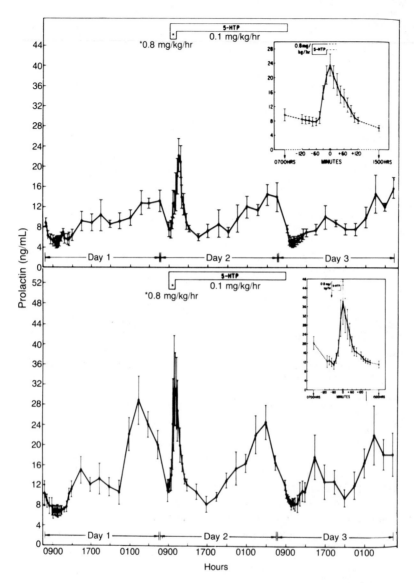

Figure 1-9
Mean (±SE) plasma PRL response to loading and maintenance IV infusions of
5-HTP in normal men (upper panel) and women (lower panel). The insets
represent the data centered around the peak increases.

*Reproduced, with permission, from Mashchak CA, Kletzky OA, Spencer C, et al: Transient
effects of L-5-hydroxytryptophan on pituitary function in men and women. J Clin Endocrinol
Metab 56:170, 1983. © 1983, The Endocrine Society.*

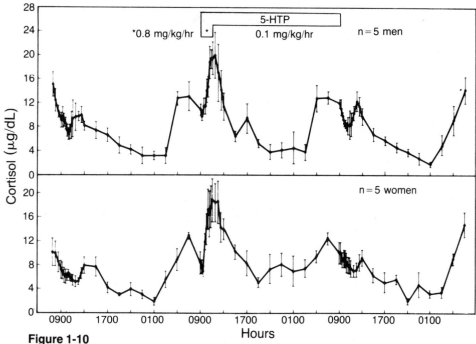

Figure 1-10

Mean (±SE) plasma cortisol response to loading and maintenance IV infusions of 5-HTP in normal men (upper panel) and normal women (lower panel).

creased in men only. However, serum concentrations of LH and FSH were not affected by 5-HTP administration. Repeated administration of IV boluses of 5-HTP to normal men resulted in repeated increments of GH and cortisol, but not of serum PRL (Figure 1-12).[25] This dichotomy of response suggests that serotonin may control the secretion of these hormones by different mechanisms. Two populations of serotonin receptors, 5-HT1 and 5-HT2, have been found in the brain.

In summary, these neurotransmitters are involved in many hypothalamic-pituitary functions. Dopamine, by an inhibitory mechanism, controls the secretion of PRL and, to a lesser degree, the secretion of TSH. Dopamine may inhibit the secretion of LH directly by acting on the pituitary and/or indirectly through a suppressive effect on GnRH secretion. Norepinephrine may have a role in the control of GnRH and TRH secretion at the level of the hypothalamus. Both these hypothalamic hormones stimulate the pituitary to synthesize and release LH, FSH, and TSH. Serotonin stimulates the release of PRL, ACTH, and TSH.

GABA pathways

Immunohistochemical studies have demonstrated a dense concentration of nerve terminals secreting GABA in most hypothalamic nuclei and within the median eminence.[26] The nerve cell bodies of the hypothalamic terminals are located outside the hypothalamus. It has been reported that GABA may exert an inhibitory effect on

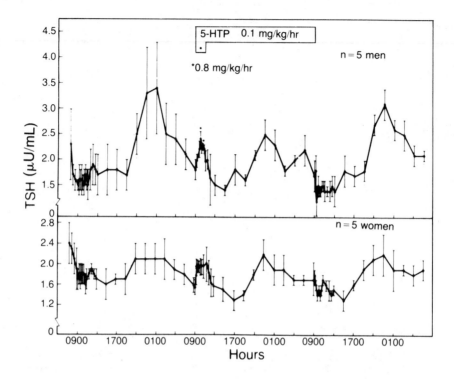

Figure 1-11
Mean ($\pm$ SE) plasma TSH response to loading and maintenance IV infusions of 5-HTP in normal men and women.

Reproduced, with permission, from Mashchak CA, Kletzky OA, Spencer C, et al: Transient effects of L-5-hydroxytryptophan on pituitary function in men and women. J Clin Endocrinol Metab 56:170, 1983. © 1983, The Endocrine Society.

PRL release in humans.[27] The administration of sodium valproate, a drug known to increase endogenous GABA, significantly decreases baseline PRL levels in normal women. The same results were found in hyperprolactinemic subjects who had no evidence of pituitary tumors. However, no significant changes in serum PRL levels were observed when the drug was administered to patients with demonstrable prolactinomas.

Vasoactive intestinal polypeptide (VIP)

Immunohistochemical studies have shown that VIP nerve cell bodies are present mainly in the cortical regions. Nerve terminals transport the synthesized VIP to the suprachiasmatic, medial preoptic, and anterior hypothalamic nuclei.[28] Only a few nerve terminals appear in the median eminence. The intraventricular or IV administration of VIP to rats induced a significant, dose-related increase in plasma PRL.[29] Furthermore, this increase in prolactin could be blunted by the co-administration of either naloxone, an opioid receptor antagonist, or L-dopa, the dopamine precursor. These results suggest that PRL secretion induced by VIP could be activated through an opiate receptor in the CNS and/or by blocking the inhibitory effect of dopamine directly at the pituitary level.

Neurotransmitters' mechanism of action

The effects of these neurotransmitters on the secretion of hypothalamic hormones probably are exerted by different mechanisms. One possible mechanism is through a direct cell-to-cell connection or multisynaptic communication whereby the neurotransmitter is released by the terminal nerve and depolarizes the receptor site on a hypothalamic cell (Figure 1-13). Depolarization results in the release of a specific hormone from the hypothalamic cell. Another conceivable mechanism is direct secretion of the neurotransmitter together with the hypothalamic hormones into the portal vessels, where the former modify the action of the latter hormones on the pituitary cells.

Effects of pharmacologic agents

The specific effects of neurotransmitters on hypothalamic cells can be altered by the systemic administration of certain drugs.[30] Methyldopa and α-methyl-p-tyrosine can block the synthesis of dopamine and norepinephrine by inhibiting tyrosine hydroxylase. Reserpine and chlorpromazine are known to interfere with binding and storage of norepinephrine, dopamine, and serotonin. Tricyclic antidepressants, including imipramine hydrochloride, inhibit the reuptake of neurotransmitters, and propranolol, phentolamine, haloperidol, and cyproheptadine block the receptors at the level of the hypothalamus. The net result of administration of any of these drugs is increased secretion of PRL. As a consequence of hyperprolactinemia or alteration in GnRH-gonadotropin secretion, many women treated with these agents develop galactorrhea and/or oligo-amenorrhea.

Neuromodulators

Prostaglandins

There is a significant body of evidence that deactivation of hypothalamic prostaglandin may be

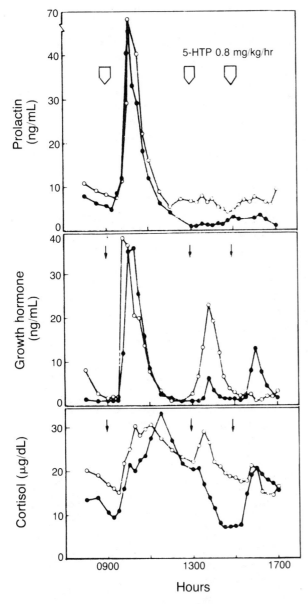

Figure 1-12
Plasma PRL, GH, and cortisol responses to three consecutive doses of 5-HTP in two normal men.

Reproduced, with permission, from Mashchak CA, Kletzky OA, Spencer C, et al: Transient effects of L-5-hydroxytryptophan on pituitary function in men and women. J Clin Endocrinol Metab 56:170, 1983. © 1983, The Endocrine Society.

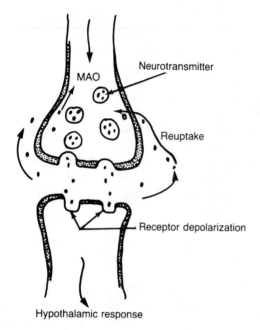

Figure 1-13
A stimulus induces the release of a stored neurotransmitter by exocytosis. Most of it is reuptaken; the rest binds to a specific receptor, resulting in a hypothalamic response.

an obligatory step in modulating the release of GnRH.[31] The administration of prostaglandin E₂ has been shown to induce a significant increase in GnRH levels in the hypothalamic-pituitary portal blood.[32, 33] This stimulatory effect on GnRH can be inhibited by earlier administration of a GnRH antibody. Furthermore, a physiologic role of prostaglandin in regulating or modulating the secretion of GnRH is supported by experiments demonstrating that the midcycle surge in LH can be abolished and, therefore, ovulation can be inhibited in rats by the administration of aspirin or indomethacin, which block the synthesis of prostaglandin.[34]

β-Endorphin

β-Endorphin is derived from the large family of opioid peptides, for which specific receptors in the brain have been identified.[35, 36] One peptide, β-lipoprotein (βLP), contains 91 amino acids.[37] We now know that the opiate family has at least three distinct subgroups. The first is the enkephalin group, pentapeptides equipotent with morphine; the second comprises the endorphins (α, β, γ); the third peptide group is represented by dynorphin, a heptadecapeptide.[35]

Nerve cell bodies containing endorphins are present in the arcuate nucleus, the ventromedial and paraventricular areas, and the premammillary nuclei. Few β-endorphin nerve terminals are found within the hypothalamus.[19] Most of the β-endorphin in the human hypothalamus is found in the region of the arcuate nucleus and the median eminence. Very large amounts of β-endorphin are also present within the pituitary, where the concentration is approximately 1,000 times that of the hypothalamic area.[38] Immunohistochemical studies indicate that β-endorphin and ACTH are localized in the same pituitary cell.[39] β-Endorphin has also been localized in the placenta, pancreas, GI tract, and seminal plasma.

Of the opioid peptides, β-endorphin (βEP) has received the most attention. It contains 31 amino acids and is 5 to 10 times more potent than morphine. The common precursor molecule for this family of endorphins was once thought to be proopiomelanocortin. Selective cleavage by peptidases at various sites would give rise to ACTH, βLP, βEP, or the enkephalins. Recently, however, it has been realized that specific precursors for each of the three major classes of peptides may exist. Because of the necessity for precursor molecules to undergo selective enzymatic cleavage, the quantitative localization of this group of peptides does not necessarily reflect its ability to be released. Therefore, while βEP is plentiful in the pituitary, very small amounts are actually measured in the peripheral circulation.

The stimulatory and inhibitory effects of

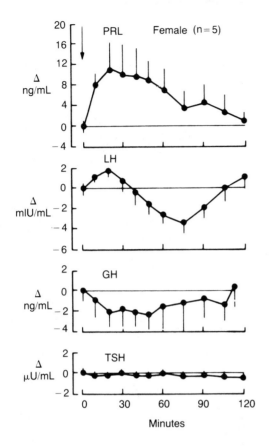

Figure 1-14
Plasma PRL, LH, GH, and TSH response to 2.5-mg IV bolus of β-endorphin in normal women.

Reproduced, with permission, from Reid RL, Hoff JD, Yen SSC, et al: Effects of exogenous β-endorphin on pituitary hormone secretion and its disappearance rate in normal human subjects. J Clin Endocrinol Metab *52:1179, 1981. © 1981, The Endocrine Society.*

peripherally infused βEP on anterior pituitary hormone secretion have been well studied (Figure 1-14).[40] Infusion of βEP in normal men and women causes an increase in serum PRL, but a decrease in LH, while serum GH, cortisol, and TSH levels remain unchanged. However, enkephalin analogs raise PRL as well as GH and TSH and lower LH, FSH, and cortisol. It has been suggested that these hormonal effects of βEP are related to inhibition of catecholamine secretion. This concept agrees with the finding that intraventricular injection of βEP or morphine completely suppressed dopamine release into the portal blood. A pancreatic effect is also evident by increases in insulin, glycogen, and glucose levels after peripheral βEP infusion.[11]

Peripheral measurements of plasma βEP in humans have been difficult to interpret partly because of its low concentration and the cross-reactivity with β-lipotropin (βLPH), but primarily because levels of βEP in the brain and portal vessels do not correlate with those in the circulation. That is, the pituitary and/or peripheral pool of βEP is separate from the pool within the hypothalamus. Peripheral βEP levels reflect, in part, pituitary secretion but also may result from production at non-CNS sites.

Hypoglycemia stimulates βEP secretion in addition to that of βLPH and ACTH. Indeed, βEP may play a role in the regulation of pancreatic α- and β-cell function by the inhibition of islet cell somatostatin. βEP is elevated in obese mice, and large doses of opiate antagonists decrease hyperphagia.

Because of the difficulty of interpreting peripheral plasma βEP levels, investigators have used naloxone, an opiate antagonist, to study the role of βEP and the opiates in reproductive function. Although detailed dose-response studies have not been carried out, it is clear that naloxone infusions of 1 mg/hr or more can stimulate serum LH with no significant changes occurring in serum PRL in the normal follicular phase. Naloxone-stimulated serum LH levels parallel the levels of βEP in the portal blood of rhesus monkeys.[42]

Naloxone studies have suggested that endogenous opioid activity is influenced by the steroid milieu. Serum LH rises following naloxone administration to women in the late follicular and luteal phases, but not in the early follicular phase or during the menopause. This suggests

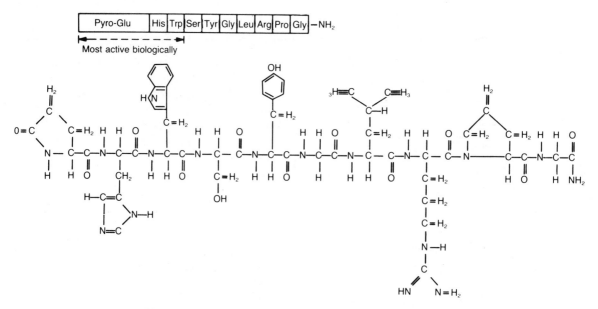

Figure 1-15
Amino acid sequence of gonadotropin-releasing hormone (GnRH).

that estrogen and progesterone exert a positive effect on brain levels of βEP. Further, it has been suggested that the highest levels of βEP in the portal blood occur in the luteal phase of the menstrual cycle.[42] When estrogen and progesterone fall during the late luteal phase, there probably is a fall in βEP.

Recent studies in vitro indicate that βEP directly inhibits GnRH release from human fetal hypothalami.[43] Since βEP affects GnRH release, it has been suggested that βEP may be responsible for the pulsatile changes of LH in the luteal phase of the menstrual cycle (high amplitude, low frequency of pulsation). However, there is some evidence that progesterone may also modulate this LH pulsatility in the luteal phase.

Catecholestrogens

Steroids that resemble both catecholamines and estrogen are called catecholestrogens. These compounds, primarily 2-hydroxyestradiol (2-OH-E_2), 2-hydroxyestrone (2-OH-E_1), and their 3-methyl derivatives, are present in high concentrations in the hypothalamus. Because these catecholestrogen levels exceed those of E_2 and E_1, it has been hypothesized that they may play an important role in neuromodulation of hormones involved in reproduction. The 4-hydroxylated derivatives, also considered to be catecholestrogens, are of less importance. It has been suggested that the catecholestrogens may be derived from the liver as well as the brain.[44]

It has been hypothesized that these compounds exert an important effect on reproduction, because catecholestrogens behave as weak estrogens and play a role in catecholamine metabolism. Catecholestrogens may alter catecholamine function by inhibiting tyrosine hydroxylase and by competing for the enzyme catechol O-methyltransferase. In this way, the production of catecholestrogens may modulate the production and action of catecholamines.

However, a positive feedback role for 2-OH-E_1 or 2-OH-E_2 in LH release has not been

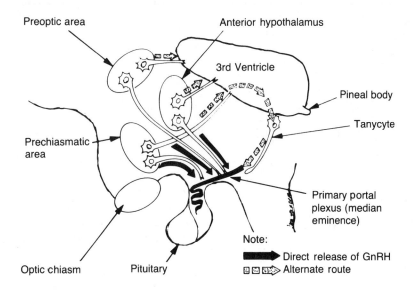

Figure 1-16
Hypothetic alternate pathway of GnRH transport to primary portal vessels.

demonstrated.[45] In estrogen-primed hypogonadal women, a small but significant negative feedback effect on LH has been demonstrated. In these hypogonadal subjects, a constant infusion of 2-OH-E$_1$ caused a decrease in PRL. 2-OH-E$_2$, in contrast, may cause an increase in PRL independent of estrogen priming. Taken together, these data are not convincing enough to indicate that catecholestrogens play a major role in the neuromodulation of reproductive function.

Hypothalamic hormones and their effects on pituitary hormones

Gonadotropin-releasing hormone

The amino acids pyroglutamic acid, histidine, and tryptophan, in addition to the amino-terminal group present in the GnRH molecule, are the most biologically active amino acids (Figure 1-15). Most neurons containing GnRH seem to originate in the hypophysiotropic area of the hypothalamus.[12] In humans and monkeys, GnRH is secreted mainly by the arcuate and premammillary nuclei of the medial hypothalamus.[5, 6] From these nuclei, the axons transport GnRH directly to the external layer of the median eminence. These axons terminate around the capillaries of the primary portal plexus (the tuberoinfundibular system).

An alternative route may exist for the secretion of GnRH, because it has been shown that when GnRH is administered into the third ventricle it is transported into the portal system. Terminal axons from the hypophysiotropic area may transport GnRH into the third ventricle. The tanycytes present in the base of the third ventricle then deliver the GnRH into the primary portal capillary system[46] (Figure 1-16).

Thus, it can be postulated that two different systems for GnRH delivery may function together to stimulate LH and FSH secretion. The tu-

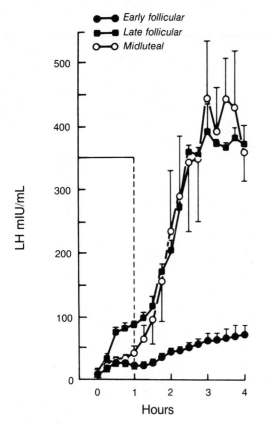

Figure 1-17
Quantitative LH release within first and second pool during GnRH infusion. The dotted line separates the two pools.

Reproduced, with permission, from Hoff JD, Lasley BL, Wang CF, et al: The two pools of pituitary gonadotropin. Regulation during the menstrual cycle. J Clin Endocrinol Metab 44:302, 1977. © 1977, The Endocrine Society.

GnRH can be modulated by dopamine through an inhibitory effect. βEP and prostaglandin also modulate GnRH secretion.

In humans, the administration of GnRH by any route produces a rapid release of LH and FSH from the pituitary. The maximum response for LH occurs at 30 minutes, and for FSH at 60 minutes, following the administration of an IV bolus of GnRH.[47] This initial response represents pituitary sensitivity. Approximately 3 hours after GnRH administration, the levels of LH and FSH return to baseline. The constant infusion of GnRH results in a double pattern of LH increase: an initial peak at 30 minutes followed by a second increase at 90 minutes. These two components (pools) represent the pituitary's release of already synthesized hormone (first pool) and newly synthesized gonadotropin (second pool; Figure 1-17).[48] However, following the initial stimulatory effect, continuous IV administration of GnRH results in a lower gonadotropin response. If the infusion is maintained long enough, gonadotropin secretion is inhibited completely (Figure 1-18), probably because GnRH down-regulates its own receptors.[49]

The natural sequence of the ten amino acids found in the parent molecule of GnRH has been modified to synthesize GnRH analogs.[50] The analog D-Leu6-GnRH has been reported to be up to 9 times more active than the native molecule, and D-Phe6-GnRH and D-Trp6-GnRH 10 to 13 times more potent and longer-acting, in stimulating the release of LH and FSH. In contrast, DES-His2-D-Ala6-DES-Gly10-GnRH ethyl amide, found to inhibit the in vivo and in vitro release of both gonadotropins, is referred to as an analog inhibitor. Because of their antigonadotropic effect, these compounds are being investigated for use as contraceptives. They are also being studied for the treatment of precocious puberty, endometriosis, prostatic cancer, and ovarian causes of hyperandrogenism. In these clinical situations, constant administration

beroinfundibular axons from the hypothalamus could provide a rapid path for the delivery of GnRH to the portal bed, thus providing cyclic control of FSH and LH synthesis and release. This would be superimposed on a continuous low-grade transependymal input of GnRH that would be necessary for maintaining the baseline synthesis and release of FSH and LH secretion (tonic control). We know that the secretion of

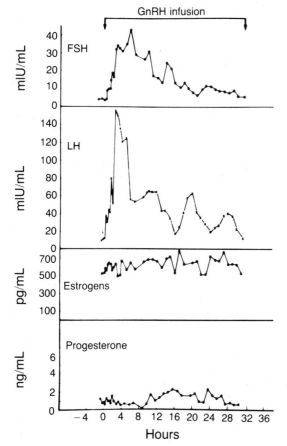

Figure 1-18
Mean serum FSH, LH, estrogen, and progesterone during 30-hour continuous infusions of GnRH at midcycle phase in three normal women.

Reproduced, with permission, from Jewelewicz R, Ferin M, Dyrenfurth I, et al: Long-term LH-RH infusions at various stages of the menstrual cycle in normal women. In Beling CG, Wentz AC (eds): The LH-Releasing Hormone. New York, Masson Publishing, 1980, p 173.

of the GnRH analog down-regulates the GnRH receptors, halting gonadotropin secretion and ovarian stimulation.

Thyrotropin-releasing hormone

TRH, a three-peptide hormone secreted by the hypothalamus, was the first hypothalamic hor-

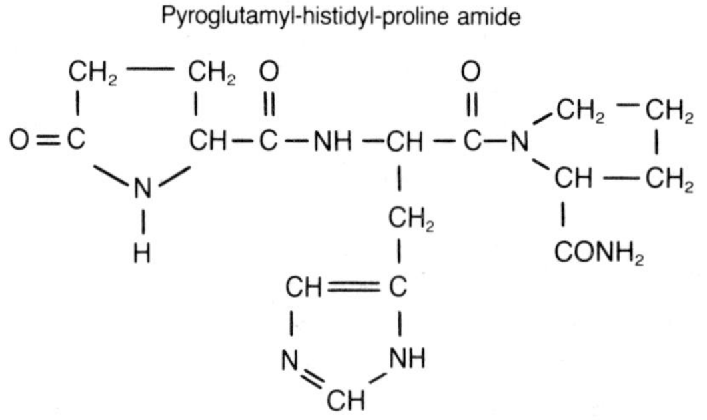

Pyroglutamyl-histidyl-proline amide

Figure 1-19
Sequence of amino acids of thyrotropin-releasing hormone (TRH) molecule.

mone isolated and synthesized[50] (Figure 1-19). TRH is the specific hypothalamic hormone controlling the secretion of TSH, and thereby the secretion of thyroxine. Also, TRH can directly stimulate the pituitary and induce the release of PRL. However, TRH most likely does not play an important role in maintaining physiologic levels of serum PRL.

The constant IV infusion of TRH results in a biphasic pattern of TSH response, reflecting the presence of two pools of TSH.[51] The first is the readily releasable pool of presynthesized TSH; the second represents newly synthesized hormone. They are similar to the two pools of LH released following IV infusion of GnRH. In contrast, the infusion of TRH results in a single significant increase in PRL.

Prolactin release-inhibiting factor

Both in vitro and transplantation studies have firmly established that the secretion of prolactin by the anterior pituitary is controlled mainly by an inhibitory action of the hypothalamus. Furthermore, it has been reported that in situ transection of the pituitary stalk results in increased prolactin secretion from the anterior pituitary. Although an extract of porcine hypothalamus was found to inhibit prolactin release (prolactin release-inhibiting factor, or PIF), its chemical structure has yet to be determined.

Further experiments have demonstrated that dopamine itself has a potent inhibitory effect on PRL release.[50] This effect occurs both in vivo and in vitro. Because dopamine inhibits PRL release, it is widely accepted that dopamine itself is the physiologic inhibitor of PRL by acting directly on the pituitary gland. Dopamine terminals present in the medial palisade of the median eminence are the sites of dopamine release into the primary capillary plexus, to act on the receptors located on the lactotrophs of the anterior pituitary gland.[52] Repeated injections of PRL into rats (induced hyperprolactinemia) increase dopamine turnover in the median eminence.[18, 31] Thus, the clinical observation of hyperprolactinemia associated with reduced LH secretion could be related to the same mechanism. Hyperprolactinemia would increase dopamine turnover and, by a negative modulatory effect, secretion of GnRH would be diminished, resulting in low levels of LH secretion and amenorrhea.

Prolactin-releasing factor

It has been reported that a crude rat hypothalamic extract administered for 5 days to an estrogen-primed female rat induced lactation. These results were interpreted as an indication of a hypothalamic prolactin-releasing factor (PRF).[53] However, such a factor has not yet been isolated. Since it is well established that serotonin stimulates the release of PRL, serotonin may, in fact, be intimately related to the secretion of PRF or may itself be PRF.

Corticotropin-releasing factor

A 41-amino-acid peptide obtained from ovine hypothalami can induce the release of ACTH and β-endorphin from rat pituitary glands.[54] Subsequently, a synthetic replicate of corticotropin-releasing factor (CRF) was found to be effective in stimulating the release of ACTH and cortisol in humans.[55]

Growth hormone-releasing factor

A substance causing acromegaly was recently isolated from two pancreatic tumors.[56] Following the establishment of its amino acid sequence (40 amino acids), growth hormone-releasing factor (GHRF) was synthesized. When GHRF was administered IV to normal subjects and patients with growth hormone deficiency, it selectively stimulated the secretion of growth hormone in both groups. Furthermore, the finding that GHRF can be administered intranasally makes this hormone useful for the treatment of children with growth hormone deficiency.

Somatostatin

Somatostatin is a polypeptide hormone of 14 amino acids with a profound inhibitory effect on GH secretion. This inhibition occurs in normal individuals as well as in patients who have acromegaly and/or diabetes.[57] Administration of somatostatin can blunt the response of TSH, but not that of PRL, to TRH.[58] Somatostatin also lowers the serum concentrations of glucose, insulin, and glucagon.

Synthesis and release of pituitary hormones

The binding of hypothalamic hormones to specific receptors on the pituitary gland induces the synthesis of pituitary hormones[59] (Figure 1-20). Peptide hormones and biogenic amines bind to receptors present on the cell surface, whereas steroids and thyroid hormones penetrate the cell membrane and bind to an intracellular receptor to produce their effects. GnRH is the specific hypothalamic hormone that induces the synthesis and release of LH and FSH. These hormones are synthesized in the ribosomes of

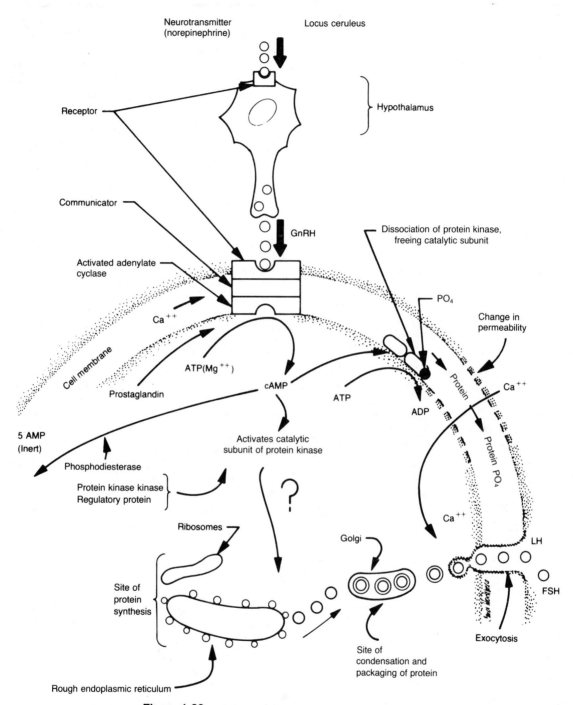

Figure 1-20
Effect of GnRH on the synthesis and release of gonadotropins.

the pituitary cells, transferred to the rough endoplasmic reticulum, and finally move to the Golgi region, where they are condensed and packed into mature granules. Under the stimulatory effect of GnRH, these granules coalesce with the cell membrane, emptying their contents by exocytosis into an adjacent blood vessel.

The binding of GnRH to the gonadotropin cell membrane is facilitated by the action of calcium and prostaglandins. This hormone-receptor complex activates the membrane adenylate cyclase, which in turn converts intracellular adenosine triphosphate (ATP) into the second messenger, cyclic adenosine monophosphate (cyclic AMP). Cyclic AMP then activates the protein kinase by dissociating its regulatory component from the catalytic unit in the cell membrane. The catalytic unit is then phosphorylated by ATP, which, in turn, phosphorylates the membrane protein to change the permeability of the membrane. This change allows calcium to enter the cell. Calcium usually activates the release of the protein hormones without affecting their synthesis. This "stimulus-secretion coupling" is analogous to the conception of "excitation-contraction coupling" in muscle.

It has been shown that for such peptide hormones as PRL, cyclic AMP is not the second messenger. It is possible that after PRL binds to a membrane receptor, the hormonal message is transmitted by a second messenger generated by the receptor. The incubation of PRL with membranes possessing PRL receptors releases a factor that can induce the transcription of β-casein genes.[60] Evidence that hypothalamic hormones exert a dual effect on protein hormone synthesis and release was obtained by studying the changes in synthesis and release of PRL from the pituitary cells of lactating rats. During the first 12 hours after breastfeeding was discontinued, synthesis and storage of PRL continued, while the release of PRL diminished. A rapid involution of the organelles associated with pro-

tein synthesis was observed only after a lag period of 12 hours.

Neurohormones have a stimulatory effect on the release of FSH, LH, and ACTH from the pituitary. In contrast, a balance between the inhibitory and stimulatory effects of the neurohormones on the release of GH, PRL, and TSH appears to be necessary. Of these latter three hormones, PRL is primarily under inhibitory control, whereas GH and TSH are mainly under stimulatory influences. LH and FSH are synthesized and released by the same pituitary cell. In general, LH stimulates the gonads (ovaries and testes), where it induces the synthesis of steroid hormones. In the ovaries, it also participates in follicular development and in the induction of ovulation. FSH regulates the development of both sperm and ova.

Pituitary hormone characteristics

Both LH and FSH are glycoproteins composed of α- and β-polypeptide subunits.[61] Similar characteristics are shared by two other hormones: TSH, secreted by the pituitary, and human chorionic gonadotropin (hCG), secreted by the placenta. These hormones share the same α-subunit characteristics (14,000 daltons). Their specific biologic activity is determined by the β-subunit; however, both subunits need to be combined in order to induce such activity. Each subunit is linked by five disulfide bonds in the α-subunit and six in the β-subunit, with no interchain bonds. The carbohydrate moieties in both subunits are mannose, galactose, fucose, glucosamine, galactosamine, and sialic acid (neuraminic acid). The sialic acid content of each hormone, which varies greatly, is intimately related to its biologic action. LH contains 1 or 2, FSH 5, and hCG 20 residues of sialic acid per molecule. The molecular weight of LH is about 28,000; of

FSH, 33,000; of TSH, 28,000; and of hCG, 35,000. The half-life of LH is about 30 minutes; FSH, 3.9 hours; TSH, 40 minutes; and hCG, 9 hours. Even though both LH and FSH are synthesized by the same cell, FSH does not have a biphasic pattern of secretion following the infusion of GnRH.

The placement of a radiofrequency lesion in the arcuate region of ovariectomized rhesus monkeys resulted in complete abolition of LH and FSH release and estrogen-positive feedback.[62] Constant hourly infusion of GnRH resulted in the restoration of LH and FSH secretion and ovulation. Moreover, administration of

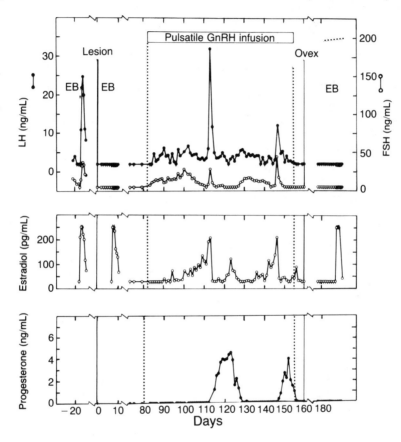

Figure 1-21

Induction of two ovulatory menstrual cycles by the administration of pulsatile GnRH replacement (1 µg/minute for 6 minutes once every hour) in a rhesus monkey with a hypothalamic lesion that had abolished endogenous GnRH secretion. Estradiol benzoate (EB) elicited a gonadotropin response before the placement of the lesion, but not afterward.

Reproduced, with permission, from Knobil E, Plant TM, Wildt L, et al: Control of the rhesus monkey menstrual cycle: Permissive role of hypothalamic gonadotropin-releasing hormone. Science 207:1371-1373, 1980. Copyright 1980 by the American Association for the Advancement of Science.

hourly pulses of 1 µg/min for 6 minutes to pre-pubertal monkeys resulted in ovulatory menstrual cycles (Figure 1-21).[63]

In these experiments, the dose and periodicity of GnRH administration were of utmost importance. If GnRH was administered at a frequency of 2 pulses/hr, instead of 1 pulse/hr, the secretion of gonadotropins was blunted; if it was increased to 5 pulses/hr, secretion was inhibited (Figure 1-22).[62] If the frequency of the pulses was reduced to one every 3 hours, plasma LH concentration diminished whereas FSH increased. Reduction in the dose of GnRH to 0.1 µg/min for 6 minutes, instead of 1 µg, resulted in almost no gonadotropin secretion. Increasing GnRH to 10 µg/min resulted in no LH change from that seen following the 1-µg/min dose, but FSH secretion was suppressed. From these elegant experiments it can be concluded that (1) the arcuate nucleus is the principal center in the hypophysiotropic area of the hypothalamus; (2) an hourly discharge of endogenous GnRH needs to be delivered to the pituitary; and (3) both LH and FSH respond to a single hypothalamic hormone—that is, GnRH.

Before the development of the hypothalamic hypophyseal portal system, the gonadotrophs secrete FSH only; LH release occurs only after the establishment of the portal system.[64] The release of FSH continues to be dominant until puberty, when the normal menstrual cycle is established and LH secretion overtakes that of FSH. With the commencement of the perimenopause, the LH:FSH ratio is again reversed. This preferential inhibition of FSH release during the reproductive age is due to the increasing levels of estradiol. Also, there is evidence that the developing follicle produces a specific substance called inhibin, which preferentially inhibits the secretion of FSH.[65] Thus the secretion of LH and FSH is modulated by one or more ovarian proteins and steroids.

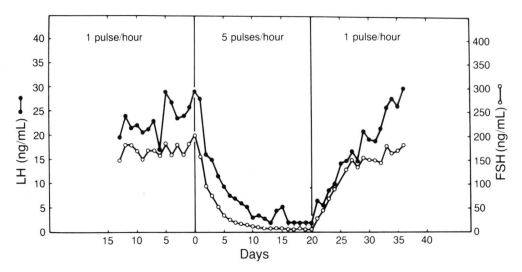

Figure 1-22
Same rhesus monkey preparation as in Figure 1-21. Gonadotropin suppression where GnRH pulse is increased to 5/hour and is restored by returning to the physiologic frequency of 1/hour.

Reproduced, with permission, from Knobil E: The neuroendocrine control of the menstrual cycle. Rec Prog Horm Res 36:53, 1980.

Normal endocrinology

During the early follicular phase, serum LH levels exhibit high-frequency, low-amplitude pulses that diminish during the late follicular phase. That pulses of lower frequency, but higher amplitude, are seen during the luteal phase demonstrates the effects of progesterone or other controlling factors (β-endorphin) on LH pulsatility. In induced or physiologic hypogonadal states, there is an increase in the amplitude and frequency of the pulsatile secretion of pituitary LH and FSH. This increased synthesis and release of both FSH and LH are largely the result of an increase of endogenous GnRH secretion as well as the lack of negative ovarian feedback.

Feedback control of gonadotropin secretion by the ovary

The somewhat complex interplay between ovarian hormonal secretion and the hypothalamic-pituitary axis is not completely understood. Although it is clear that estrogen and progesterone exert the major effects, other steroids, such as androgens, have the potential for influencing the CNS and gonadotropin secretion. Further, several protein substances—particularly inhibin and LH-inhibiting factor—have the ability either to directly inhibit or to modulate the secretion of gonadotropins. Also, these substances may modulate the effect of gonadotropin on the ovaries.

Both estrogen and progesterone exert negative and positive feedback control on GnRH and gonadotropin secretion.[66] Estrogen's positive feedback regulation of gonadotropin secretion is, by necessity, preceded by a negative feedback effect.[67] An injection of estradiol benzoate will induce a decrease in LH in the first 24 hours, followed by a positive surge in LH after approximately 60 hours. Thus a sustained increase of estradiol (above 200 pg/mL) over many hours results in the positive LH surge. More controversial, however, is its anatomic site of action. While studies have indicated that estradiol effects occur only at the level of the pituitary,[62] there is evidence in the intact woman for an integrated hypothalamic site of action as well. That is, while the pituitary alone may be all that is necessary for negative and positive feedback actions, in the intact woman GnRH secretion may also be modulated by estradiol.

Similarly, it has been known for some time that progesterone exerts an inhibitory effect on gonadotropin secretion during the luteal phase. Here the site of action may be at both the hypothalamus and the pituitary. However, a more important role of progesterone may be the augmentation of the midcycle LH and FSH surge.[68] This positive feedback modulation is not a prerequisite for the midcycle LH surge, but its effect appears to be important in assuring a normal LH surge as well as the FSH midcycle peak. A small incremental rise in progesterone (0.5 ng/mL), beginning some 12 hours before the LH surge, may be all that is required for this activity. There is some evidence that brain 5α-reduction of progesterone to dihydroprogesterone may be important in this action.

References

1. Bargmann W, Scharrer E: The site of origin of the hormones of the posterior pituitary. *Am Scientist* 39:255, 1951

2. Harris GH: *Neural Control of the Pituitary Gland.* London, Edward Arnold, 1955

3. Halász B: Functional anatomy of the hypothalamus. In Cox B, Morris ID, Weston AH (eds): *Pharmacology of the Hypothalamus.* Baltimore, University Park Press, 1978, pp 5-30

4. Vandesande F, Dierickz K: Identification of the vasopressin-producing and oxytocin-producing neurons in the hypothalamic magnocellular neurosecretory system of the rat. *Cell Tiss Res* 164:153, 1975

5. Barry J: Immunofluorescence study of LRF neurons in man. *Cell Tiss Res* 181:1, 1977

6. Barry J, Carette B: Immunofluorescence study of LRF neurons in primates. *Cell Tiss Res* 164:163, 1975

7. Goldsmith PC, Ganong WF: Ultrastructural localization of LH-RH in the median eminence of the rat. *Brain Res* 97:181, 1975

8. Hökfelt T, Fuxe K, Johansson O, et al: Distribution of TRH in the central nervous system as revealed with immunohistochemistry. *Eur J Pharmacol* 34:389, 1975

9. Hökfelt T, Efendic S, Johansson O, et al: Immunohistochemical localization of somatostatin (growth hormone release-inhibiting factor) in the guinea-pig brain. *Brain Res* 80:165, 1974

10. Keefer DA, Stumpf WE: Atlas of estrogen-concentrating cells in the central nervous system of the squirrel monkey. *J Comp Neurol* 160:419, 1975

11. Sar M, Stumpf WE: Distribution of androgen-concentrating neurons in rat brain. In Stumpf WE, Grant LD (eds): *Anatomical Neuroendocrinology*. Basel, Karger, 1975, pp 120-133

12. Szentagothai J, Flerke B, Mess B, et al: *Hypothalamic Control of the Anterior Pituitary*. Budapest, Akadémiai Kiadó, 1968, pp 22-109

13. Hyyppä M, Motta M, Martini L: Ultrashort feed-back control of follicle-stimulating hormone-releasing factor secretion. *Neuroendocrinology* 7:227, 1971

14. Cross BA: The hypothalamus in mammalian homeostatis. *Symp Soc Exp Biol* 18:1576, 1964

15. Mason CA, Lincoln DW: Visualization of the retino-hypothalamic projection in the rat by cobalt precipitation. *Cell Tiss Res* 168:117, 1976

16. Kendall JW, Jacobs JJ, Kramer RM, et al: Studies on the transport of hormones from the cerebrospinal fluid to hypothalamus and pituitary. In Knigge KM, Scott DE, Weindl A (eds): *Brain-Endocrine Interaction. Median Eminence: Structure and Function. Proceedings: International Symposium on Brain-Endocrine Interaction, Munich, 1971*. Basel, Karger, 1972, p 342

17. Bergland RM, Page RB: Can the pituitary secrete directly to the brain? (Affirmative anatomical evidence). *Endocrinology* 102:1325, 1978

18. Fuxe K, Ferland L, Anderson K, et al: On the functional role of hypothalamic cathecholamine neurons in control of the secretion of hormones from the anterior pituitary, particularly in the control of LH and PRL secretion. In Scott D (ed): *Brain-Endocrine Interaction, vol 3, Neural Hormones and Reproduction*. Third Intl Symp, Wurzburg, 1977, pp 172-182

19. Fuxe K, Hökfelt T, Anderson K, et al: The transmitters of the hypothalamus. In Cox B, Morris ID, Weston AH (eds): *Pharmacology of the Hypothalamus*. Baltimore, University Park Press, 1978, pp 31-61

20. Leblanc H, Lachelin GCL, Abu-Fadil S, et al: Effects of dopamine infusions on pituitary hormone secretion in humans. *J Clin Endocrinol Metab* 43:668, 1976

21. Kaptein EM, Kletzky OA, Spencer CA, et al: Effects of prolonged dopamine infusion on anterior pituitary function in normal males. *J Clin Endocrinol Metab* 51:488, 1980

22. Sawyer CH: Some recent developments in brain-pituitary-ovarian physiology. *Neuroendocrinology* 17:97, 1975

23. Löfström A, Eneroth P, Gustaffson JA, et al: Effects of E_2 on catecholamine levels and turnover in discrete areas of the median eminence on serum LH, FSH and PRL in ovariectomized female rat. *Endocrinology* 101:1559, 1977

24. Chan-Palav V: Indoleamine neurons and their processes in the normal rat brain and in chronic diet-induced thiamine deficiency demonstrated by uptake of ^{3}H-serotonin. *J Clin Endocrinol Metab* 56:170, 1983

25. Mashchak CA, Kletzky OA, Spencer C, et al: Transient effects of L-5-hydroxytryptophan on pituitary function in men and women. *J Clin Endocrinol Metab* 56:170, 1983

26. Browstein M, Palkovits M, Tappaz M, et al: Effect of surgical isolation of the hypothalamus on its neurotransmitter content. *Brain Res* 117:287, 1976

27. Melis GB, Paoletti AM, Mais V, et al: The effects of the gabaergic drug, sodium valproate, on prolactin secretion in normal and hyperprolactinemic subjects. *J Clin Endocrinol Metab* 54:485, 1982

28. Larson LI, Fahrenkrug J, Schaffalitzky O, et al: Localization of vasoactive intestinal polypeptide (VIP) to central and peripheral neurons. *Proc Nat Acad Sci USA* 73:3197, 1976

29. Kato Y, Iwasaki Y, Iwasaki J, et al: Prolactin release by vasoactive intestinal polypeptide in rats. *Endocrinology* 103:554, 1978

30. Müller EE, Cella S, Locatelli V, et al: Drugs affecting prolactin secretion. In Tolis G, Stefanis C, Mountokalakis T, et al (eds): *Prolactin and Prolactinomas*. New York, Raven Press, 1983, pp 83-103

31. Harms PG, Ojeda SR, McCann SM: Prostaglandin involvement in hypothalamic control of gonadotropin and PRL release. *Science* 181:760, 1973

32. Eskay R, Warberg J, Mical RS, et al: Prostaglandin E_2-induced release of LHRH into hypophyseal portal blood. *Endocrinology* 97:816, 1975

33. Ojeda SR, Wheaton JW, McCann SM: Prostaglandin E_2-induced release of LRH. *Neuroendocrinology* 17:283, 1975

34. Orczyk GP, Behrman HR: Ovulation blockade by aspirin or indomethacin—*in vivo* evidence for a role of prostaglandins in gonadotropin secretion. *Prostaglandins* 1:3, 1972

35. Goldstein A: Endorphins: Physiology and clinical implication. *Ann NY Acad Sci* 311:49, 1978

36. Hughes J, Smith TW, Kosterlitz HW: Identification of two related pentapeptides from the brain with potent opiate activity. *Nature* 258:577, 1975

37. Li CH, Yamashiro D, Tseng LF, et al: Synthesis and analgesic activity of human β-endorphins. *J Med Chem* 20:325, 1977

38. Bloom F, Battenberg E, Rossier J, et al: Endorphins are located in the intermediate and anterior lobes of the pituitary gland, not in the neurohypophysis. *Life Sci* 20:43, 1977

39. Guillemin R, Vargo T, Rossier J, et al: β-endorphin and adrenocorticotropin are secreted concomitantly by the pituitary gland. *Science* 197:1367, 1977

40. Reid RL, Hoff JD, Yen SSC, et al: Effects of exogenous β-endorphin on pituitary hormone secretion and its disappearance rate in normal human subjects. *J Clin Endocrinol Metab* 52:1179, 1981

41. Reid RL, Yen SSC: β-Endorphin stimulates the secretion of insulin and glucagon in humans. *J Clin Endocrinol Metab* 52:592, 1981

42. Wardlaw SL, Thoron L, Frantz AG: Effects of sex steroids on brain β-endorphin. *Brain Res* 245:327, 1982

43. Rasmussen DD, Liu JH, Wolf PL, et al: Endogenous opioid regulation of GnRH release from the human fetal hypothalamus *in vitro. J Clin Endocrinol Metab* 57:881, 1983

44. Fishman J, Nastor B: Brain catecholestrogens: Formation and possible function. *Adv Biosci* 15:123, 1975

45. Adashi EY, Rakoff J, Divers W, et al: The effect of acutely administered 2-hydroxyestrone on the release of gonadotropins and prolactin before and after estrogen priming in hypogonadal women. *Life Sci* 25:2051, 1979

46. Knigge KM, Silverman AJ: Anatomy of the endocrine hypothalamus. In Knobil E, Sawyer WH (eds): *Handbook of Physiology: Endocrinology*, vol 4. Washington, DC, American Physiological Society, 1974, pp 1-32

47. Kletzky OA, Davajan V, Mishell DR Jr, et al: A sequential pituitary stimulation test in normal subjects and in patients with amenorrhea-galactorrhea with pituitary tumors. *J Clin Endocrinol Metab* 45:631, 1977

48. Hoff JD, Lasley BL, Wang CF, et al: The two pools of pituitary gonadotropin. Regulation during the menstrual cycle. *J Clin Endocrinol Metab* 44:302, 1977

49. Jewelewicz R, Ferin M, Dyrenfurth I, et al: Long-term LH-RH infusions at various stages of the menstrual cycle in normal women. In Beling CG, Wentz AC (eds): *The LH-Releasing Hormone.* New York, Masson Publishing, 1980, p 173

50. Schally AV, Coy DH, Armiura A, et al: Hypothalamic peptide hormones and their analogues. In Cox B, Morris ID, Weston AH (eds): *Pharmacology of the Hypothalamus.* Baltimore, University Park Press, 1978, pp 161-206

51. Chan V, Wang C, Yeung RTT: Thyrotropin and PRL responses to 4-hr constant infusion of TRH in normal subjects and patients with pituitary-thyroid disorders. *J Clin Endocrinol Metab* 49:127, 1979

52. MacLeod RM, Lehmeyer JE: Studies on the mechanism of the dopamine-mediated inhibition of PRL secretion. *Endocrinology* 94:1077, 1974

53. Meites J, Clemens JA: Hypothalamic control of prolactin secretion. *Vit Horm* 30:165, 1972

54. Vale W, Spiess J, Rivier C, et al: Characterization of a 41 residue ovine hypothalamic peptide that stimulates secretion of corticotropin and β-endorphin. *Science* 213:1394, 1981

55. Grossman A, Kruseman AC, Perry L, et al: New hypothalamic hormone, CRF, specifically stimulates the release of ACTH and cortisol in man. *Lancet* 1:921, 1982

56. Rivier J, Spiess J, Thorner MD, et al: Characterization of a growth-hormone releasing factor from a human pancreatic islet tumor. *Nature* 300:276, 1982

57. Brazeau P, Vale W, Burgus R, et al: Hypothalamic polypeptide that inhibits the secretion of immunoreactive pituitary growth hormone. *Science* 179:77, 1973

58. Siler TM, Yen SSC, Vale W, et al: Inhibition by somatostatin on the release of TSH induced in man by TRH. *J Clin Endocrinol Metab* 38:742, 1974

59. Conn PM, Smith RG, Rogers DC: Stimulation of pituitary gonadotropin release does not require internalization of GnRH. *J Biol Chem* 256:1098, 1981

60. Djiane J, Houdebine LM, Kelly PA, et al: Down-regulation of PRL receptors and biological effects of PRL in the mammary gland. Evidence for the existence of a PRL second messenger. In Tolis G, Stefanis C, Mountokalakis T, et al (eds): *Prolactin and Prolactinomas.* New York, Raven Press, 1983, pp 29-42

61. Liu WK, Ward DN: The purification and biochemistry of pituitary glycoprotein hormones. *Pharmacol Ther* [B]1:545, 1975

62. Knobil E: The neuroendocrine control of the menstrual cycle. *Rec Prog Horm Res* 36:53, 1980

63. Knobil E, Plant TM, Wildt L, et al: Control of the rhesus monkey menstrual cycle: Permissive role of hypothalamic gonadotropin-releasing hormone. *Science* 207:1371-1373, 1980

64. Pasteels JL, Franchimont P: The production of FSH by cell cultures of fetal pituitary. In Hubinot PO, L'Ermite M, Robyn C (eds): *Progress in Reproductive Biology*, vol 2. New York, S. Karger, 1977, pp 1-11

65. Hoffman JC, Lorenzen JR, Weil T, et al: Selective suppression of the primary surge of FSH in the rat: Further evidence for folliculostatin in porcine follicular fluid. *Endocrinology* 105:200, 1979

66. Chang RJ, Jaffe RB: Progesterone effect on gonadotropin release in women pretreated with estradiol. *J Clin Endocrinol Metab* 47:119, 1978

67. Yen SSC, Tsai CC: The biphasic pattern in the feedback action of ethinyl estradiol on the release of FSH and LH. *J Clin Endocrinol Metab* 33:882, 1971

68. March CM, Goebelsmann U, Mishell DR Jr, et al: Role of estradiol and progesterone in eliciting the midcycle LH and FSH surges. *J Clin Endocrinol Metab* 49:507, 1979

Chapter 2

Mechanisms of Action of Reproductive Hormones

William E. Gibbons, M.D.
David A. Battin, M.D.
Gere S. diZerega, M.D.

Sex steroid and protein hormones act as chemical messengers transporting information to target cells. Hormone receptors located in the target cell facilitate the acceptance and subsequent processing of this information. Therefore, a working knowledge of receptor theory is essential to an understanding of modern reproductive endocrinology.

Receptors are proteins capable of binding a specific hormone ligand for the purpose of eliciting a biologic response. A ligand is a molecule of the hormone that binds to a receptor and produces a specific response. For binding to occur, the structure of the receptor must permit interaction at various sites of the three-dimensional structure of the hormone. Receptors are located only in target tissue cells, although other tissues may contain nonreceptor proteins capable of hormone binding. For example, at any one time, most steroid hormones in the circulation are bound to serum albumin. Other than occupancy and transport, steroid hormone binding to albumin induces no biologic function and, as such, albumin is not a receptor. Receptors for protein

and steroid hormones differ in their cellular location. Protein hormone receptors are located within the plasma membrane of the target cells and are generally linked with other proteins, lipids, or, possibly, prostaglandins. Steroid hormone receptors are located within the cytoplasm of the cell.

Because target cell response is related to the action of a particular hormone, binding between receptor and ligand must be hormone specific. Thus, a specific receptor will bind only a single hormone or, in the case of protein hormones, a single "class" of hormones. For example, estrogen receptors will bind natural estrogens (estradiol, estrone, estriol) and synthetic estrogens (diethylstilbestrol, clomiphene), but will not bind gestagens or androgens at physiologic concentrations. Most protein hormone receptors will bind only a single type of molecule. Because luteinizing hormone (LH) and human chorionic gonadotropin (hCG) have similar structures, receptors for LH will also bind hCG, but they will not bind other protein hormones. Each cell contains a limited number of receptors for their ligands. As a result, receptors become saturated when physiologic amounts of hormone concentrations are present. In contrast, such nonreceptor proteins as albumin can bind pharmacologic levels of hormone. By possessing a limited binding capacity, cells are sensitive to relatively small physiologic changes in hormone concentration.

To induce a specific action, a cell-specific response must follow a receptor-ligand interaction. Protein-receptor binding activates or inhibits the enzyme adenylate cyclase, producing a subsequent change in the concentration of adenosine 3′,5′-cyclic monophosphate (cyclic AMP, cAMP). Steroid-receptor binding initiates a receptor transformation that produces nuclear translocation—that is, movement of the hormone receptor (HR) from the cytoplasm into the nucleus and subsequent DNA transcription.

Characteristics of hormone-receptor binding

The hormone (H) combines with receptor (R) to form hormone-receptor (HR) complexes. The number or concentration of HR complexes, which determines the magnitude of the signal to the cell, depends equally on hormone concentration [H], receptor concentration [R], and affinity [K] with which hormone and receptor interact. For hormone to bind to receptor, some region of the hormone molecule must have a structure that complements a region of the receptor. The fit of the hormone to its specific receptor is described or measured in terms of "affinity." Thus, changes in receptor affinity or changes in receptor concentration are as important as fluctuations in hormone concentration in determining hormone action.

Often, hormones may be present in concentrations of 10^{-9} to 10^{-12} M, whereas the total concentration of the receptors is about 10^{-3} M. Thus, the hormone recognized by the receptor

represents one molecule in one million or even one in a billion. High binding affinity exists between receptors and their ligand, thus allowing for the target cell to respond to low physiologic concentrations of the hormone. This affinity is quantitatively characterized by a constant derived from the law of mass action:

$$H + R \underset{k_d}{\overset{k_a}{\rightleftharpoons}} HR$$

where H is the concentration of free hormone; R, the concentration of unoccupied receptors; HR, the concentration of hormone-receptor complexes; k_a, the rate constant for association; and k_d, the rate constant for dissociation. Thus, the ratio of the rate constants defines the following relationship:

$$K_A = \frac{k_a}{k_d} \quad \text{and} \quad K_D = \frac{1}{K_A}$$

where K_A is the association constant and K_D is the dissociation constant. A large K_A suggests that the direction of the reaction strongly favors the hormone-receptor complex. K_D, the inverse of K_A, is equal to the hormone concentration when half of the receptor sites are occupied. Receptor affinity correlates with physiologic concentration of the hormone. Steroid hormones are present in concentrations of 10^{-10} to 10^{-8} M, and most steroid receptors have a K_D equal to 10^{-9} M. If the affinity of a receptor for its hormone is greater than the physiologic concentration of the hormone, the receptor will always be saturated and, therefore, unable to respond to changes in hormone concentration. Conversely, if receptor affinity is low, receptors will be unable to bind the hormone in sufficient concentrations to induce a biologic effect.

Leydig cells contain approximately 6,000 LH receptors/cell.[1] Mature granulosa cells contain 30,000 LH receptors/cell.[2] Because each target cell contains a limited number of receptors, they may become saturated with physiologic concentrations of hormone. This allows for a maximum cellular response to a low concentration of hormone. Once binding is sufficient for hormone-mediated events, the spare or unoccupied target cell receptors become refractory to additional binding for 12 to 72 hours. The physical mechanism for this change in receptor function is unknown; however, it is a safeguard against perpetual hormonal stimulation.

In summary, receptors are proteins located in target tissue cells and bind specific ligands with high affinity and finite capacity. Following binding, a specific biologic response occurs.

Peptide hormone receptors

The peptide hormones involved in reproductive endocrinology consist of LH, follicle-stimulating hormone (FSH), prolactin, adrenocorticotropic hormone (ACTH), and thyroid-stimulating hormone (TSH). These hormones have high solubility in aqueous (polar) solvents, but have low solubility in lipids (nonpolar solvents). This means that the water-soluble peptide hormones do not readily cross the lipid barrier of the target cell's plasma membrane. Further, protein hormones generally cannot pass through the cell's plasma membrane because of their molecular weight (10,000 to 100,000 daltons) or conformation. Therefore, to allow peptide hormones to control intracellular activity, the target cell receptor, located on the cell surface within the cell membrane, must use a second messenger (usually a cyclic nucleotide) to induce an intracellular effect. The receptor provides a link whereby the extracellular hormone can control intracellular biochemical events.

The binding of a protein hormone to its cell surface receptor activates or inhibits the enzyme adenylate cyclase, producing a subsequent change in intracellular cAMP concentration.

cAMP, which is soluble in the cytoplasm of the cell, activates protein kinase—thus further modifying cellular response. All protein hormones use similar molecules (cAMP or cyclic guanine monophosphate, cGMP) as their second messenger. Because many endocrine cells possess receptors for different protein hormones (LH and FSH by granulosa cells, for example) the expression of a cell's differentiated response to various protein hormones depends on the intracellular processing of this message.

Protein hormone receptors have been isolated by extraction from target tissue cell membranes with detergents. During physical analysis, detergent-solubilized receptors have been found to be asymmetric protein molecules with molecular weights of 200,000 to 300,000 daltons (in contrast to a molecular weight of 30,000 daltons for FSH). Each receptor appears to bind a single molecule of the tissue-specific protein hormone.

Gonadal target tissue cells contain 2,000 to 30,000 membrane receptors per cell. However, hormonal occupancy of only 1% to 5% of these receptors is all that is required for maximal stimulation. The other 95% to 99% function as spares. These spare membrane receptors increase the cell's ability to recognize the protein hormone in its dilute physiologic concentration and prolong the cell's response to hormonal stimulation.

Internalization

After the protein hormone and its receptor bind, the entire complex is brought into the cell membrane, protecting the complex from other interactions. Eventually, receptor proteins (at least in the corpus luteum) are recycled by the cell to appear later within the cell membrane ready to bind a new ligand. However, some of the hormone-receptor complex can be found in the nucleus. This finding raises the question whether protein hormone receptors alter nuclear function.

Adenylate cyclase

Hormone-receptor interaction (Figure 2-1) stimulates adenylate cyclase, a catalyst in the formation of cAMP from adenosine triphosphate (ATP).[3] Adenylate cyclase exists in different relations with receptors that can be interconverted by the actions of the protein hormone and cyclic nucleotides. Guanine nucleotides can influence the formation of cAMP by modifying the activation of adenylate cyclase. We do not know the nature of the physical and functional relationships between hormone receptors and adenylate cyclase in the plasma membrane. However, receptor and/or adenylate cyclase mobility appear to be prerequisites to normal endocrine cell response to hormone binding. The receptor and adenylate cyclase molecules are separate structures that undergo association by lateral diffusion through the cell membrane after the hormone-receptor complex forms. Both receptor and adenylate cyclase diffuse freely within the cell membrane.

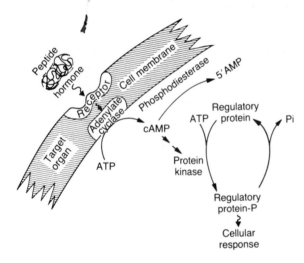

Figure 2-1
The second messenger model of peptide hormone action. The interaction of hormone with receptor leads to activation of membrane-bound adenylate cyclase, resulting in conversion of ATP to cyclic AMP (cAMP). Cyclic AMP then interacts with cyclic AMP-dependent protein kinase, causing activation of the enzyme and phosphorylation of intracellular regulatory protein substrates, using ATP as phosphate donor. Cyclic AMP is inactivated by conversion to 5'-AMP by phosphodiesterase.

Protein kinase

All cAMP actions are thought to be due to its ability to activate cAMP-dependent protein kinases.[3] A "kinase" is an enzyme that phosphorylates its substrate. Protein kinases constitute a subgroup of enzymes that use proteins as their substrates; they transfer a phosphate from ATP to the substrate. Introduction of the phosphate typically modifies the activity of that protein in a specific way, either activating or inactivating it. The effects of the cAMP-dependent protein kinases on their substrates are reversed by phosphoprotein phosphatases, which remove the phosphate by hydrolysis and restore the original activity of the protein. Protein kinases may be soluble and exist within the cytoplasm or may be membrane-bound. In response to cAMP, these enzymes phosphorylate cellular proteins and thereby modify (activate or inactivate) their biologic functions.

The cAMP-dependent protein kinases have a regulatory subunit and a catalytic subunit (Figure 2-2).[4] In the absence of cAMP, the regulatory subunit is bound to the catalytic subunit. cAMP, which is soluble and diffuses within the cell, binds to specific sites on the regulatory subunit; with cAMP bound, the regulatory subunit dissociates from the catalytic unit, and the protein hormone becomes active. Thus, a rise in the concentration of cAMP favors its binding to the regulatory unit. The catalytic subunit of protein kinase is then freed, allowing for its activation of intracellular enzyme systems by the transferring of phosphate. A fall in the concentration of the second messenger favors its dissociation from the regulatory unit, which then reassociates with the catalytic unit, reducing activity. Protein kinase, therefore, acts as a link between the cAMP generated by the hormone and the activation of the biochemical pathway that accounts for the

Normal endocrinology

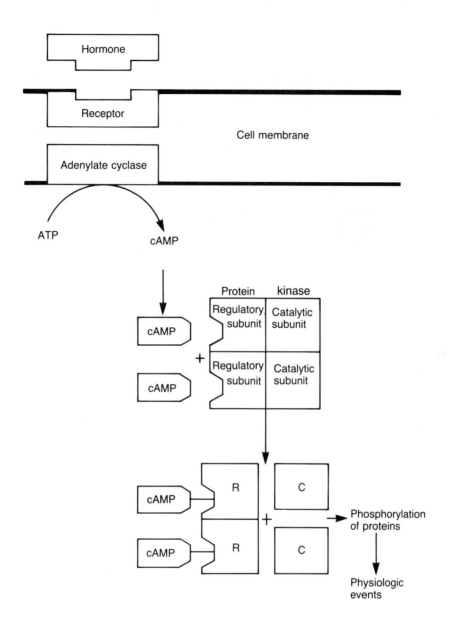

Figure 2-2
Protein hormones induce physiologic events by activating adenylate cyclase, which results in cAMP formation. Cyclic AMP frees the catalytic subunit of protein kinase by binding to the regulatory subunit. The catalytic portion of protein kinase activates enzymatic activity by transferring a phosphate group to the enzyme, which ultimately alters cellular function.

Adapted, with permission, from Speroff LS: How hormones work. Postgraduate Obstetrics and Gynecology, Vol 3, No 6, 1983.

metabolic effects of the hormone.

Besides adenylate cyclase, cAMP, and its kinase system, most cells contain guanylate cyclase, an enzyme that converts GTP to cGMP, as well as protein kinases that are activated specifically by this cyclic nucleotide.[5] cGMP has been implicated as the second messenger for some hormones.

Calcium

Calcium plays a key role in many cellular processes.[6] It is ubiquitous in its free form in extracellular fluids and in bound form within cells. Free Ca^{++} ions in cells, imported from the outside or liberated from intracellular storage sites, are thought to be the active intracellular form of Ca^{++}. When active, Ca^{++} is a soluble, intracellular second messenger similar to cAMP.

The concentration of free Ca^{++} in the extracellular fluid (10^{-7} to 10^{-5} M) is relatively high compared with its concentration inside cells (10^{-9} to 10^{-8} M). In the resting state, the concentration of free Ca^{++} inside cells is kept low by the binding of free Ca^{++} to intracellular binding proteins and by the action of ATPases located within the cell membrane that remove Ca^{++} from inside the cell against an extracellular concentration gradient. Calmodulin, an important intracellular calcium-binding protein, has few or no Ca^{++} ions bound in the resting state. Activation of the cell by hormone-receptor binding sometimes leads to an acute rise in the intracellular concentration of free Ca^{++} (10^{-6} M) derived from the extracellular fluid and/or intracellular storage sites. The increase in Ca^{++} concentration promotes its binding to calmodulin, alters the configuration of calmodulin, and converts it into its active form. It then binds calcium-sensitive proteins, thereby altering such cell activities as hormone secretion, cell division, cell movement, and metabolism.

Methylation

Methylation of membrane lipids has been found to be affected by hormones.[6] This results in modification of hormone action at the target cell. The target cell membrane is composed of a lipid bilayer surrounding a protein core. The distribution of lipids differs on the internal (cytoplasmic) and external side of the membrane. Phosphatidylethanolamine (PE) is more abundant on the inner (cytoplasmic) face, and phosphatidylcholine (PC) is more abundant on the outer (extracellular) face. Two enzymes (methyltransferases) in the plasma membrane can add methyl groups to PE and thereby convert it to PC. This change increases the fluidity of the membrane and facilitates the free movement of receptors and adenylate cyclase in the cell membrane. Because increased methylation of the phospholipids enhances coupling between HR complexes and adenylate cyclase activity, cAMP production is increased. In general, increased fluidity of the membrane enhances coupling between receptor and cyclase, whereas reduction in fluidity diminishes it.

In summary, the interaction of protein hormones and membrane-bound receptors activates membrane-bound adenylate cyclase to produce cAMP. cAMP then interacts with protein kinase in the cytoplasm, causing its activation and subsequent phosphorylation of regulatory protein substrates. Although all of these processes, which are amenable to regulation (both activation and inactivation), account for the biologic effects of protein hormones, protein kinase currently is thought to provide the major specificity for protein hormone action within the cell.

LH and FSH action on the ovary

LH action

Ovarian receptors for LH exist in theca cells, granulosa cells, and the corpus luteum (Figure 2-3).[5] The theca cells contain a relatively con-

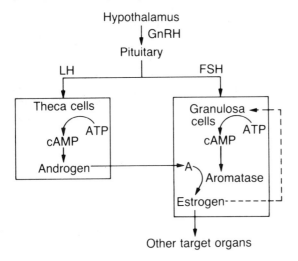

Figure 2-3

Action of gonadotropins on the ovary: LH stimulates the theca cell to synthesize androgen by cyclic AMP (cAMP)-mediated action. FSH stimulates the granulosa cell to activate aromatase via cyclic AMP-mediated action. Aromatase in the granulosa cell converts androgen to estrogen, which is then used by the target organs. Estrogen also stimulates granulosa cell proliferation.

From a concept in Schulster D, Burstein S, Cooke BA (eds): Control of gonadal steroidogenesis by FSH and LH. In Molecular Endocrinology of the Steroid Hormones, *London, John Wiley & Sons, 1976.*

stant number of LH receptors, which are involved primarily with androgen synthesis.[5] The number of LH receptors in granulosa cell membranes depends on the action of estradiol and the specific stimulatory action of FSH.[5] The preantral follicle's granulosa cells contain few LH receptors. As the follicle matures under FSH influence, and as estradiol production increases, the number of LH receptors increases. During the follicular phase of the menstrual cycle, the number of receptors per granulosa cell and the total number of granulosa cells increase in the developing follicle.

The action of LH on ovarian steroidogenesis is primarily to stimulate androgen synthesis by the theca cells and progesterone synthesis by the corpus luteum.[7] The specific action of LH on granulosa cells is unclear at present. In vitro studies using isolated theca cell cultures have shown massive production of androgen after LH stimulation.[3] Addition of LH to slices of corpus luteum markedly increases levels of cAMP and progesterone.[3] The increase in cAMP concentration precedes the increase in progesterone synthesis. These findings are consistent with the role of cAMP as an intracellular mediator of LH action.

Accelerating the conversion of cholesterol to pregnenolone is one action of LH and cAMP on the steroidogenic pathway common to the biosynthesis of all steroids. Just how cAMP speeds this reaction has not been established, but several ways have been proposed (Figure 2-4). There is evidence that cAMP could bring about an increase in (1) the concentration of reduced nicotinamide adenine dinucleotide phosphate (NADPH), the cofactor required for the conversion of cholesterol to pregnenolone; (2) the concentration of cholesterol by activation of the enzyme cholesterol esterase, which catalyzes the formation of cholesterol from cholesterol esters; (3) the transport of cholesterol into the mitochondrion, where it is converted to pregnenolone by side-chain cleavage; (4) the activation of the side-chain cleavage enzyme system; and (5) the transport of an end-product inhibitor, such as pregnenolone, out of the mitochondrion.[3]

LH stimulates a number of other metabolic events in the ovary (ornithine decarboxylase activation, amino acid transport, and RNA synthesis), but they are poorly understood.[2] LH may also play a part in ovulation by stimulating a plasminogen activator that decreases tensile strength of the follicle wall before follicular rupture occurs.[2]

FSH action

Ovarian binding of FSH occurs primarily on granulosa cell membranes (Figure 2-3). FSH stimulates the formation of LH receptors and the activation of the enzymes aromatase and 3-hydroxysteroid dehydrogenase in granulosa cells.[8] Granulosa cells are primarily involved with estrogen production. When isolated in culture, FSH-stimulated granulosa cells produce only small amounts of estrogen. However, when FSH-stimulated granulosa cells are supplied with androgen precursors or are cultured together with theca cells, they produce massive amounts of estrogen.[8]

These results support the two-cell theory of follicular estrogen production (Figure 2-3). This hypothesis proposes that LH acts on the theca cells to produce androgens. The androgens are

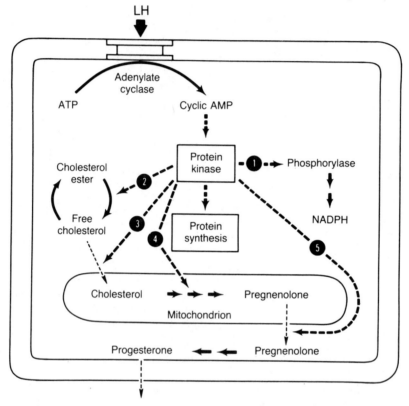

Figure 2-4
Possible sites of action of cyclic AMP on steroidogenesis in a hypothetical gonadal cell. The five heavy broken arrows indicate that cyclic AMP could bring about an increase in (1) the concentration of NADPH, the cofactor required for the conversion of cholesterol to pregnenolone; (2) the concentration of cholesterol by activation of the enzyme cholesterol esterase, which catalyzes the formation of cholesterol from cholesterol ester; (3) the transport of cholesterol into the mitochondrion, where the cholesterol side-chain cleavage enzyme system is located; (4) the activity of the side-chain cleavage enzyme system; (5) the transport of an end-product inhibitor, such as pregnenolone, out of the mitochondrion. Solid arrows indicate biochemical reactions, and light broken arrows indicate transport of a substance through cellular membranes.

Reproduced, with permission, from Marsh JM: The role of cyclic AMP in gonadal steroidogenesis. Biol Reprod 14:30, 1976.

Normal endocrinology

transported from the theca into the granulosa cells. In the granulosa cells, under the influence of FSH, the androgens are converted into estrogens. This latter step is catalyzed by the enzyme aromatase. As estrogen production increases, there is a resultant increase in mitotic activity causing an increase in the number of granulosa cells and in the number of granulosa cell FSH receptors.[8] These events stimulate growth and maturation of the follicle and provide large amounts of estrogen for peripheral use.

Folliculogenesis

Our knowledge of the cyclic changes in peripheral serum LH and FSH concentrations that stimulate follicle growth to produce preovulatory maturation derive from studies of hypophysectomized immature female rats.[5] From these studies, it appears that FSH is dominant in increasing granulosa-cell FSH receptor content. However, estradiol does enhance FSH stimulation of FSH receptors in a dose- and time-related fashion. In the presence of both FSH and estrogen, a marked enhancement of granulosa-cell LH receptors has been reported.[5] This finding suggests that a synergism between FSH and LH may be required for preovulatory follicle maturation.

The effects of LH on follicular development, especially the FSH/estradiol-mediated acquisition of granulosa-cell LH receptors, have recently been determined. LH appears to act directly on granulosa cells to induce luteinization and increase progesterone production, but only if the granulosa cells' have previously been exposed to estradiol and FSH, with resultant increases in LH receptor content and in the granulosa cell's responsivity to LH. Most important, an anovulatory dose of LH or hCG given before appropriate granulosa-cell maturation may not have the desired effect on sequential granulosa-cell maturation, but rather lead to the disruption of preovulatory growth resulting from luteinization and elevated peripheral serum progesterone levels.

In summary, the process of preovulatory follicular maturation requires both steroid and protein hormones. Estradiol and FSH each appear to act on granulosa cells by increasing their own receptors; whereas if FSH is administered after estradiol exposure, it induces the formation of large preantral follicles whose granulosa cells contain both FSH and LH receptors. Further, LH acts synergistically in estradiol-primed preantral follicles to enhance the FSH stimulation of LH receptor. LH, then, can act on these preovulatory follicles to bring about ovulation and luteinization. This action results in reduced levels of estradiol and FSH and LH receptors, and in the secretion of progesterone. Therefore, the initiation of follicular estrogen production and the ability of granulosa cells to respond to estrogen appear to determine whether a follicle can undergo successful preovulatory maturation or, conversely, becomes atretic.

LH-induced prostaglandin action in the ovary

LH can stimulate prostaglandin synthesis in ovarian homogenates, corpus luteum, and follicle cultures through the production of cAMP.[3] However, LH cannot stimulate prostaglandin synthesis in granulosa cells. Prostaglandins appear to be involved in initiating corpus luteum development and in synthesizing progesterone.[6]

During ovulation, prostaglandins play an important role in follicular rupture. Prostaglandin content of preovulatory follicles increases at the time of the gonadotropin surge; follicular rupture and ovulation occur 8 to 16 hours later. If high doses of a prostaglandin synthetase inhibitor (for example, indomethacin) are given systemically, ovulation is blocked despite a normal gonadotropin surge. Prostaglandins may induce rupture of the follicle wall by activating a collagenase-like ovulatory enzyme and stimulating follicular smooth muscle contraction.

LH and FSH action in the testis

LH action

LH binding in the testis occurs on the Leydig cell membrane (Figure 2-5).[1,9] Leydig cells are located in the interstitial tissue of the testis and are responsible for androgen production. Leydig cell membrane receptors for LH isolated by detergent extraction resemble those isolated from ovarian tissue in size, hormone affinity, and hormone specificity. A single LH receptor protein (mol wt 200,000 daltons) binds one LH molecule (mol wt 38,000 daltons) with high affinity ($K_D = 10^{-10}$ M). Each Leydig cell membrane has approximately 6,000 LH receptors.

The second messenger role of cAMP in the testis is well characterized. After LH binds to the membrane receptor, adenylate cyclase activation begins and subsequently the concentration of cytoplasmic cAMP increases. Adenylate cyclase and LH receptors are distinct and separate entities in Leydig cell membranes. Once adenylate cyclase is activated, binding of cAMP to the protein kinase regulatory subunit increases. Only a two- to threefold increase in cytoplasmic cAMP concentration is required for protein kinase activation. Protein kinase dissociates after binding to cAMP, freeing the catalytic subunit to stimulate synthesis and release of androgen.

FSH action

FSH receptors in the testis are located in the Sertoli cells of the seminiferous tubules. In contrast with LH's stimulation of steroidogenesis in the Leydig cell, FSH primarily stimulates protein synthesis in the Sertoli cell. The major protein synthesized and secreted by the Sertoli cell is androgen-binding protein (ABP). ABP is secreted by the Sertoli cell into the testicular fluid within the lumen of the tubules. Because of high androgen affinity ($K_D = 10^{-8}$ M), ABP is able to selectively bind and concentrate testosterone and dihydrotestosterone as they diffuse into the lumen of the tubules from the surrounding blood. Androgens can then be transported by ABP to seminiferous epithelium for germ cell development or to the caput epididymis for spermatocyte maturation. Both processes are believed to require higher androgen levels than are available in the peripheral circulation.

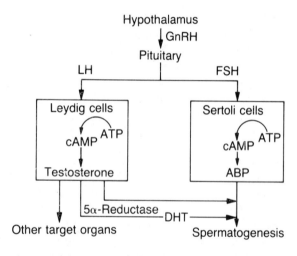

Figure 2-5

Action of gonadotropins on the testis: LH stimulates Leydig cell synthesis of testosterone via cyclic AMP (cAMP)-mediated action. FSH stimulates Sertoli cell synthesis of androgen-binding protein (ABP) via cyclic AMP-mediated action. Testosterone is either used by peripheral tissue or binds to ABP as testosterone or as the metabolite dihydrotestosterone after 5α-reductase metabolism. ABP transports androgen to sites of spermatogenesis.

Reproduced, with permission, from Schulster D, Burstein S, Cooke BA (eds): Molecular Endocrinology of the Steroid Hormones, London, John Wiley & Sons, 1976.

Sex steroid action

Steroid hormones must circulate in the bloodstream bound to proteins or unbound (free).[10] Although it has been thought that only unbound hormones enter the cell, protein-bound steroid hormones may also contribute to intracellular hormone levels. The majority of each hormone in the circulation is bound (60% for aldosterone; more than 99% for thyroxine). In humans, transcortin (corticosteroid-binding globulin, or CBG) has high affinity both for progesterone and for cortisol. The level of CBG is increased by estrogens. Sex hormone-binding globulin (SHBG) binds dihydrotestosterone, testosterone, and estradiol, in order of decreasing affinity. The circulating levels of SHBG are increased by estrogens, obesity, and hyperthyroidism and are reduced in the presence of androgens and hypothyroidism. Thyroid hormones (T_4 and, to a lesser extent, T_3) are bound to thyroid-binding globulin (TBG) and thyroid-binding prealbumin (TBPA). TBG levels are increased by estrogen action and are reduced by testosterone and glucocorticoids.

The role of the serum proteins in the overall action of steroids is incompletely understood. Possibly, they control the release of hormones into tissues. As "free" hormone diffuses into the tissues, its concentration in the serum falls, thus shifting the equilibrium reaction of bound hormone to free hormone. Steroid uptake into the brain increases as serum sex steroid binding decreases.[10] SHBG, testosterone-estradiol-binding globulin (TeBG), and "TeBG-like" serum proteins[11] bind the sex steroids with high affinity ($K_D = 10^{-9}$ to 10^{-8} M). Serum albumin has a relatively low affinity ($K_D = 10^{-6}$ M) for the sex steroids, but is present in such high concentration that it must be considered in serum-binding equilibrium relationships. However, whether serum albumin markedly affects the availability of steroid for target tissues is still controversial.

The degree to which a steroid is bound to serum proteins determines its role in the biologic system. The affinity of a receptor protein for a steroid correlates with the potency of the compound. For instance, the estrogen receptor has a greater affinity for estradiol than for estrone or estriol. Estradiol is the most potent natural estrogen. However, if a potent steroid has a high proportion of its concentration bound to serum proteins, a less potent steroid may be delivered to the tissues in a relatively higher dose and exert a greater effect. 11-Methylethinylestradiol has a greater in vivo uterotropic activity than estradiol, even though the affinity of the estrogen receptor is higher for estradiol.[12] This action results because such substitutions to the basic estrogen structure reduce serum binding and catabolic degradation. Therefore, there is a high plasma concentration of free steroid and a better tissue distribution than for the natural compound, estradiol.

Although protein hormones generally bind to receptors located within the cell's plasma membrane, receptors for steroid hormones are all intracellular. These divisions are not pure, because peptide-hormone complexes are internalized before they stimulate changes in cell response by changing nuclear events. Furthermore, cellular anatomists suggest that all intracellular structures are bound to a three-dimensional cellular matrix and only water and ions may float free. It has been suggested that most intracellular estrogen receptor is also membrane-bound.[13]

The free hormone crosses the cell membrane by simple diffusion (there is evidence that this is not a facilitated or energy-requiring process). The steroid then interacts with the intercellular receptor for that steroid family; for example, estrogen binds to estrogen receptor. Androgens are also capable of binding to the estrogen receptor, at high concentrations, and of translocating the estrogen receptor and completing an estrogen response. Some progestins can bind to certain types of glucocorticoid receptor. Progesterone circulates in the serum bound, in part, to CBG. However, for the most part, the crossover occurs only in nonphysiologic concentrations: Androgens act by binding to androgen receptors, estrogens by binding to estrogen receptors, and so on.

After binding occurs, the receptor-hormone complex is "activated." Activation allows the complex to bind to chromatin acceptor sites in the nucleus. This activation results in a loss of molecular weight and a change in configuration and surface charge. The steroid-binding portion of the receptor may be complexed with a non-steroid-binding component. The stability of this association appears to be governed by the presence of the steroid. In the presence of steroid, the complex becomes less stable, which permits dissociation with resultant nuclear binding.

Once activated, "translocation" of the receptor from the cytoplasmic to the nuclear compartment occurs and allows for chromatin binding. When the receptor-hormone complex has been bound to the chromatin complex, RNA polymerases are then able to "transcribe" the RNA codes for specific proteins in the steroid-sensitive genes. It has been suggested that the progesterone receptor has two subunits, α and β.[14] Each subunit has a binding site for progesterone. The β subunit has a chromatin-binding region that binds to the "acceptor" site of the chromatin on a progesterone-sensitive gene. After binding to the chromatin, a DNA-binding region on the α subunit is exposed, binds to DNA, and initiates transcription.[15] The same investigators subsequently pinpointed the areas of the ovalbumin gene most likely to bind the receptor complex. They suggested that the nuclear matrix, an ultrastructural skeletal component of the nucleus, is the site where the transcriptional events occur.

The "nuclear" messenger RNA sequences synthesized are much larger than the mRNA code that will be used by the ribosomes in the cytoplasmic compartment for "translating" the mRNA code into a new protein. The "nuclear" message must be processed into its final form. This means that all the excess "nonsense" sequences, or "introns," must be removed. This process is critical, because the same nuclear message sequence may be processed differently. If a different cytoplasmic message form results, it will be translated into a different protein. Therefore, post-transcriptional events can also determine how the hormone stimulus will be manifested.[16]

The method by which receptor-mediated events in the nucleus are terminated is not understood. Soon after peak levels of nuclear receptor are observed following the administration of a bolus of hormone, the concentration of measurable nuclear receptor begins to fall. This fall is associated with the first observed levels of messenger RNA, an event that has been referred to as "processing." It is also known that the length of time a ligand-receptor complex remains in the nucleus is often related to the potency of the compound. Therefore, a single injection of estrone or estriol will result in a shorter duration of nuclear occupancy than will an injection of estradiol, thus producing less stimulation of transcriptional events. Using estrogen compounds with very short nuclear occupation times, it has been shown that cytosolic receptor replenishment occurs too rapidly to be explained totally by new receptor synthesis.[17] This means that some recycling of steroid receptor occurs.

Such antiestrogens as tamoxifen or clomiphene citrate act by binding to the estrogen receptor that translocates to the nucleus. The antiestrogen-receptor complex resides in the nucleus for comparatively longer periods than estradiol does, but it initiates and sustains relatively little transcription. As a result, estrogen receptors are depleted without new receptor synthesis, so that the cell cannot sense the presence of estrogen.

Steroid-receptor interactions

Estrogen induces the synthesis of both estrogen and progesterone receptors. However, one way progesterone antagonizes estrogen action is by

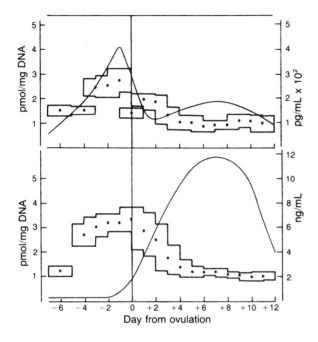

Figure 2-6

Estradiol and progesterone receptors in endometrial cells during the normal menstrual cycle. The concentrations of estradiol receptor (upper panel) and of total progesterone receptor (lower panel) for each day of the cycle were pooled with those of the adjacent days. Each point represents the mean of pooled values. It is surrounded by a rectangle, with its abscissa extending from the preceding to the following day to account for the imprecision of dating and with its ordinate equal to twice the standard error of the mean.

Reproduced, with permission, from Levy C, Robel P, Gautray JP, et al: Estradiol and progesterone receptors in human endometrium: Normal and abnormal menstrual cycles and early pregnancy. Am J Obstet Gynecol 136:647, 1980.

blocking the synthesis of estrogen receptor, which will reduce the levels of cytosolic and nuclear estrogen receptor. Then, because of this reduced synthesis, the levels of progesterone receptor fall. Progestins antagonize estrogen action further by inducing the synthesis of estradiol dehydrogenase, which favors the conversion of the more potent estrogen, estradiol, to es-

trone. Estrone, of course, has a reduced nuclear occupancy. These interactions may, in part, explain the alterations in human endometrial receptors throughout the menstrual cycle (Figure 2-6).[18] Androgens and progesterone also antagonize estrogen action by blocking estrogen stimulation of transcription, but androgens do not block estrogen receptor synthesis.[19]

Two populations of estrogen receptors that differ in their affinity for estradiol have been described in humans.[20] One, the classical estrogen receptor, has a K_D for estradiol of 10^{-10} M; the other, 10^{-9} M. They also have different isoelectric points. The low-affinity population appears to be under the regulation of the high-affinity population. The former is lost after estrogen decreases postmenopausally, whereas the latter remains.[21] A similar effect results from danazol administration, but estrogen replacement therapy results in the reinduction of the low-affinity receptor population.

Peptide steroid-receptor interactions

In the early follicular phase of the menstrual cycle, FSH, via its receptor on the granulosa-cell membrane, induces aromatase activity that results in increasing estrogen concentrations in the granulosa cells of the growing follicle. Estradiol, via its cytosolic receptor, works with FSH to induce the synthesis of a new LH membrane receptor. At the same time, the increasing levels of estradiol are sensitizing the FSH adenylate cyclase system to maintain levels of FSH-stimulated cAMP as levels of FSH decrease. This action is necessary to maintain the growth of the dominant follicle. Follicular estrogen production is a result of the LH-stimulated production of androgens by the theca cells, which provide substrate for granulosa cell aromatization.

References

1. Catt KJ, Dufau ML: Basic concepts of the mechanism of action of peptide hormones. *Biol Reprod* 14:1, 1976

2. Channing CP, Tsafriri A: Mechanism of action of luteinizing hormone and follicle-stimulating hormone on the ovary *in vitro*. *Metabolism Clin Exp* 26:413, 1977

3. Marsh JM: The role of cyclic AMP in gonadal function. *Biol Reprod* 14:30, 1976

4. Speroff LS: How hormones work. *Postgraduate Obstetrics and Gynecology,* Vol 3, No 6, 1983

5. Richards JS, Midgley AR Jr: Protein hormone action: A key to understanding ovarian follicular and luteal cell development. *Biol Reprod* 14:82, 1976

6. Roth J, Grunfeld C: Endocrine systems: Mechanisms of disease, target cells, and receptors. In Williams RH (ed): *Textbook of Endocrinology,* ed 6. Philadelphia, WB Saunders, 1981, p 15

7. Saxena BB, Rathnam P: Mechanism of action of gonadotrophins. In Singhal RL, Thomas JA (eds): *Cellular Mechanisms Modulating Gonadal Hormone Action. Advances in Sex Hormone Research,* vol 2. Baltimore, University Park Press, 1976, p 289

8. Armstrong DT, Dorrington JH: Estrogen biosynthesis in the ovaries and testes. In Thomas JA, Singhal RL (eds): *Regulatory Mechanisms Affecting Gonadal Hormone Action. Advances in Sex Hormone Research,* vol 3. Baltimore, University Park Press, 1977, p 217

9. Dufau ML, Means AR (eds): *Hormone Binding and Target Cell Activation in the Testis.* New York, Plenum Press, 1974

10. Partridge WM: Transport of protein-bound hormones with tissue *in vivo. Endocr Rev* 2:103, 1973

11. O'Brien TJ, Higashi M, Kanasugi H, et al: A plasma/serum estrogen binding protein distinct from testosterone-estradiol binding globulin (TeBG). *J Clin Endocrinol Metab* 54:793, 1982

12. Raynaud JP, Bouton MM, Gallet-Bourguin D, et al: Comparative study of estrogen action. *Mol Pharmacol* 9:520, 1973

13. Szego CM, Pietras RJ: Membrane recognition and effector sites in steroid hormone action. In Litwack G (ed): *Biochemical Actions of Hormones,* vol 3. New York, Academic Press, 1981, p 307

14. O'Malley BW, Schrader WJ: The receptors of steroid hormones. *Sci Am* 234:32, 1976

15. Grody WW, Schrader WT, O'Malley BW: Activation transformation and subunit structure of steroid hormone receptors. *Endocr Rev* 3:141, 1982

16. McCarty KS Jr, McCarty KS Sr: Steroid hormone receptors in the regulation of differentiation. *Am J Pathol* 86:705, 1977

17. Gorski J, Kassis JA: Estrogen receptor replenishment. *J Biol Chem* 256:7378, 1981

18. Levy C, Robel P, Gautray JP: Estradiol and progesterone receptors in human endometrium: Normal and abnormal menstrual cycles and early pregnancy. *Am J Obstet Gynecol* 136:646, 1980

19. Hung TT, Gibbons WE: Evaluation of androgen antagonism of estrogen effect by dihydrotestosterone. *J Steroid Biochem* 19:1513, 1983

20. Gibbons WE, Higashi M, O'Brien TJ: Heterogeneity of estrogen binding proteins in human uterine preparations. *J Steroid Biochem* 19:1291, 1983

21. Gibbons WE, Buttram VC Jr, Besch PK, et al: Estrogen binding proteins in the human post-menopausal uterus. *Am J Obstet Gynecol* 135:799, 1979

Chapter 3

Steroid Hormones

Uwe Goebelsmann, M.D.

Structure and classification

Steroid hormones are lipid-like substances of low molecular weight, ranging from 270 daltons for estrone to 387 daltons for cholesterol. Although insoluble in water, steroids dissolve readily in organic solvents such as ether and chloroform. The skeleton of steroid molecules resembles the structure of cyclopentanoperhydrophenanthrene (Figure 3-1). The steroid nucleus is composed of completely hydrogenated ("perhydro") phenanthrene, a molecule containing three 6-carbon-atom rings (A, B, and C) and the 5-carbon-atom cyclopentane ring (D). While the steroid nucleus resembles the cyclopentanoperhydrophenanthrene molecule, steroid hormone biosynthesis begins with acetate, includes acetylcoenzyme A (acetyl-CoA), mevalonic acid, squalene, and lanosterol as intermediates, and ends with cholesterol, from which all steroid hormones are derived by stepwise degradation.

Many steroid hormones have trivial names such as cortisol, progesterone, testosterone, and estradiol in addition to their systematic scientific names that conform with International Steroid Nomenclature. This nomenclature is based on a generally accepted system of numbering the carbon atoms that form the steroid skeleton. The structures of four common steroids are shown as examples in Figure 3-2.

The following basic facts and rules of nomenclature are most pertinent and deserve at least brief mention. Functional groups that lie above the plane of the steroid molecule are indicated by the Greek letter β (beta) and symbolized by a solid line connecting the carbon atom with that group (such as "—OH" for "β-hydroxy"). Functional groups that lie below the plane of the molecule are indicated by the Greek letter α (alpha) and a dotted line ($\cdots$ OH). The Greek capital letter Δ (delta) indicates a double bond. Cholesterol, pregnenolone, 17-hydroxypregnenolone, and dehydroepiandrosterone (DHEA)

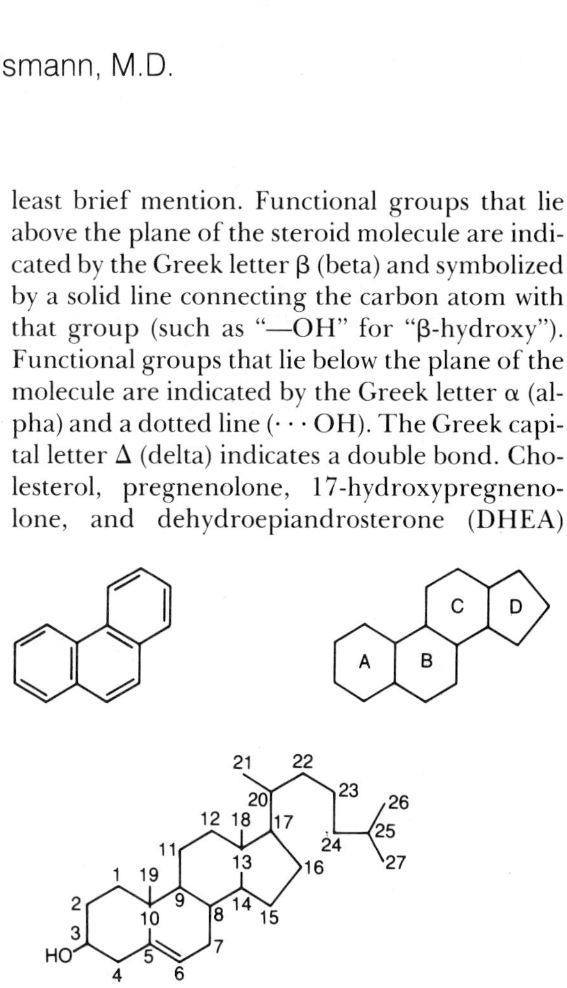

Figure 3-1
Phenanthrene nucleus, top left. Cyclopentanoperhydrophenanthrene nucleus, top right, in which the 6-carbon rings (A, B, and C) resemble the phenanthrene ring system and the 5-carbon ring (D) resembles cyclopentane. Cholesterol, bottom, is the common biosynthetic precursor of steroid hormones. Numbers 1 through 27 indicate the conventional numbering system of carbon atoms of the steroid skeleton.

have a double bond between C-5 and C-6 and are therefore called Δ^5-steroids. Progesterone, all mineralocorticoids and glucocorticoids, 17-hydroxyprogesterone, androstenedione, and testosterone have a double bond between C-4 and C-5 and thus are Δ^4-steroids. Cholesterol, from which progesterone, corticosteroids, androgens, and estrogens are derived by stepwise reduction in carbon atoms, contains 27 carbon atoms (Figure 3-1). Cleavage of its 6-carbon side chain between C-20 and C-22 results in the formation of pregnenolone, with 21 carbon atoms, and isocaproic aldehyde. Mineralocorticoids and glucocorticoids, pregnenolone, progesterone, 17-hydroxypregnenolone, and 17-hydroxyprogesterone have 21 carbon atoms. DHEA, androstenedione, and testosterone ("androgens" or "C_{19} steroids") have 19 carbon atoms. All naturally occurring estrogens have 18 carbon atoms and a phenolic (aromatic) A ring.

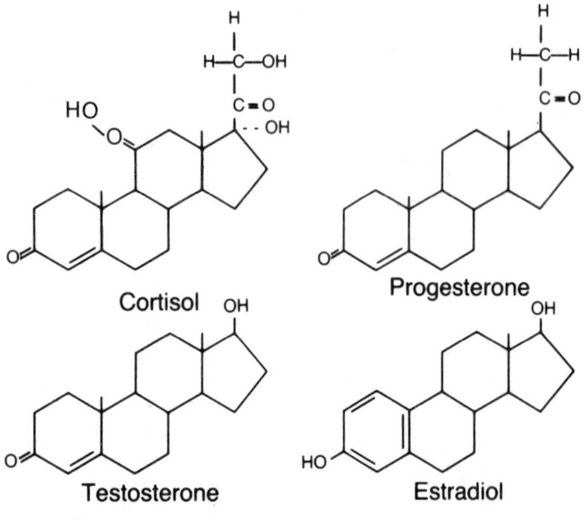

In most naturally occurring adrenal steroids, the 17-hydroxyl group, if present, is in the α configuration (below the plane), while 3-hydroxy and 11-hydroxy groups are in the β configuration (above the plane). The 17-hydroxy group of testosterone and estradiol, essential for androgenic and estrogenic activity, respectively, is in the β configuration.

As outlined in Table 3-1, steroid hormones may be classified according to origin (natural vs synthetic), metabolic stage (agents vs metabolites), or endocrine effect (sex hormones such as androgens, estrogens, and gestagens vs adrenal corticosteroids).

Steroid biosynthesis

Our knowledge of the pathways of ovarian steroid biosynthesis (depicted in Figure 3-3) is largely the result of the pioneering studies of Ryan and his collaborators.[1] Although steroid biosynthesis follows the same pathway in all steroid hormone-producing glands, there are differences among adrenal, ovarian, and testicular steroid biosynthesis. Ovaries and testes, lacking the enzymes 21-hydroxylase, 11β-hydroxylase, and 18-hydroxylase/reductase, are incapable of mineralocorticoid and glucocorticoid hormone formation. The adrenals normally do not convert androstenedione to testosterone or metabolize these androgens to estrone and estradiol. However, adrenal tumors may produce and secrete testosterone and/or estrogens. This suggests that the 17β-reducing enzyme and the aromatizing enzyme system are repressed in the normal adrenal cell. Unlike the ovaries, which secrete little testosterone (about 0.1 mg/day), the testes are most efficient in testosterone production and secretion. Details of placental steroid biosynthesis are presented in Chapter 8.

Cholesterol, the common intermediary for all steroid hormones, is metabolized to pregnen-

Figure 3-2
Examples of the carbon atom numbering system for steroid molecules and the steroid nomenclature for four common steroid hormones: cortisol (11β, 17,20α-trihydroxypregn-4-ene-3,20-dione), progesterone (pregn-4-ene-3,20-dione), testosterone (17β-hydroxyandrost-4-en-3-one), and estradiol (estra-1,3,5(10)-triene-3,17β-diol).

Table 3-1

Classification of natural and synthetic steroid hormones

Androstane C19 Estrane C18 Pregnane C21

Classified by origin	Classified by metabolic stage	Classified by relation to endocrine effect					
		Sex hormones			Corticosteroids		
		Androgens	Estrogens	Gestagens	Glucocorticoids	Mineralocorticoids	
Natural steroid hormones	Agents	Testosterone	Estradiol	Progesterone	Cortisol	Aldosterone	
	Metabolites	Androsterone	Estriol	Pregnanediol	Tetrahydrocortisol		
Synthetic steroid hormones	Agents	Methyltestosterone	Mestranol	Medroxyprogesterone	Prednisolone	Fludrocortisone acetate	
	Metabolites	17α-Methyl-5β-androstane-3α,17β-diol	D-Homoestradiol	6α-Methyl-17α-acetoxy-6β,21-dihydroxy-4-pregnene-3,20-dione	17α,20α,21-Trihydroxy-1,4-pregnadiene-3,11-dione		

Modified from R. Borth: Generic names for steroid hormones and related substances. Contraception 12:373, 1975.

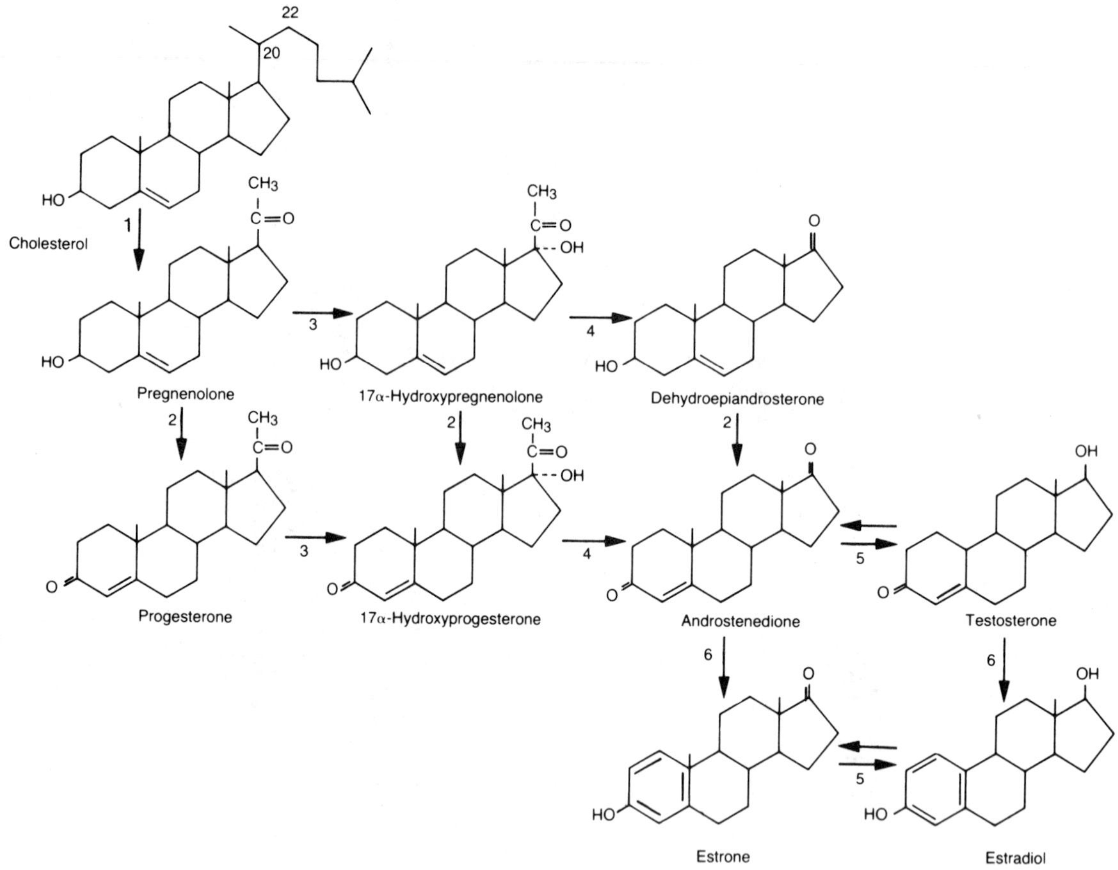

Figure 3-3
Ovarian steroid biosynthetic pathways. The following enzymes are required where indicated: (1) 20-hydroxylase, 22-hydroxylase, and 20,22-desmolase; (2) 3β-ol dehydrogenase and $\Delta^5 \rightarrow \Delta^4$-isomerase; (3) 17α-hydroxylase; (4) 17,20-desmolase; (5) 17β-ol dehydrogenase; and (6) aromatizing enzyme system.

olone by hydroxylation at carbon atoms 20 and 22 and by subsequent cleavage between these two carbon atoms. This step reduces the cholesterol molecule, with 27 carbon atoms, by 6 carbon atoms (isocaproic aldehyde), to form the C_{21} steroid pregnenolone. The conversion of cholesterol to pregnenolone is the rate-limiting step in steroid biosynthesis and is regulated by tropic hormones. In the adrenal, adrenocorticotropic hormone (ACTH) increases the rate of cholesterol to pregnenolone conversion, whereas luteinizing hormone (LH) regulates this step in the ovary and testis. Both tropic hormones act by binding to a cell membrane receptor, activation of adenylate cyclase, and increased conversion of ATP to cyclic AMP (see Chapter 2).

From pregnenolone, steroid hormone biosynthesis proceeds along either of two major pathways: (1) the Δ^5 pathway along 17-hydroxypregnenolone and DHEA or (2) the Δ^4 pathway via progesterone, 17-hydroxyprogesterone, and androstenedione. Conversion of Δ^5 steroids to their Δ^4 counterparts involves two enzymes: 3β-ol dehydrogenase and $\Delta^5 \rightarrow \Delta^4$ isomerase. 17-

Hydroxylation precedes 17,20-desmolase action, which converts the 17-hydroxylated C_{21} steroids to C_{19} steroids ("androgens"). Androstenedione and testosterone undergo 19-hydroxylation, loss of the C_{19} group, and reduction during their conversion to estrone and estradiol, respectively. Because this process results in a phenolic or aromatic A ring, it is also referred to as aromatization.

It is of paramount importance to distinguish between adrenal and gonadal steroid biosynthesis and extraglandular steroid metabolism. The latter entails extraglandular (outside the adrenals and gonads) interconversion of androstenedione and testosterone and of estrone and estradiol. Although testes and ovaries secrete the biologically active 17β-reduced steroids testosterone and estradiol, extragonadal interconversion favors the oxidation of testosterone to androstenedione and of estradiol to estrone. This results in reduction of the activity of the biologically active steroid after it has been secreted by the gonad, and thus is an integral part of steroid metabolism. Also, if large amounts of androstenedione or estrone are secreted abnormally or administered exogenously, substantial quantities of testosterone or estradiol may be produced by peripheral interconversion. In this sense, androstenedione and estrone may be considered prehormones.

The studies of MacDonald and co-workers have shown that androstenedione is peripherally metabolized to estrone,[2] and the rate of extraglandular conversion of androstenedione to estrone appears to increase with advancing age. This extragonadal aromatization converts about 1.3% of the 3 to 4 mg of androstenedione produced each day to some 40 to 50 μg/day of estrone. The extraglandular conversion rate of testosterone to estradiol is much smaller (about 0.1%). Hence the quantitatively most important estrogen produced by extraglandular conversion of androgens is estrone derived from androstenedione. For the most part, this conversion takes place in adipose tissue. Obese women have rates of extragonadal conversion of androstenedione to estrone considerably higher than 1.3% (as high as 7%) and thus produce more estrone. This mechanism may be partly responsible for the higher incidence of endometrial carcinoma among obese women.

Ovarian steroid hormones

In a unique, yet incompletely understood, manner, the ovary combines the gametogenic and endocrine functions essential for reproduction. The integration of ovarian steroid hormone biosynthesis into follicle maturation, ovulation, and corpus luteum function is essential for the following processes: (1) hypothalamic-pituitary feedback control of both morphologic changes and steroid hormone production in the ovary; (2) intraovarian regulation of morphologic and endocrine activity; and (3) timing and support of events associated with fertilization and nidation through the effect of estradiol and/or progesterone on tubal motility and secretion, endometrial stimulation, and the properties of the cervical mucus. Follicle maturation is intimately connected with estradiol biosynthesis and secretion, while the corpus luteum produces both progesterone and estradiol. Normal follicle maturation does not occur without estradiol biosynthesis.

The human ovary synthesizes steroids along the pathways outlined in Figure 3-3. Three major steroid hormones are secreted by the ovary: progesterone, androstenedione, and estradiol. Follicles, corpora lutea, and ovarian stroma all produce steroids along these pathways. However, estradiol is the chief secretory product of the maturing follicle, progesterone that of the corpus luteum, and androstenedione that of the stroma. The relative quantities in which these steroids are secreted by follicles, corpora lutea, and stroma vary according to the morphologic development and state of gonadotropin stimulation of each ovarian subunit. This functional interdependence of germ cells and hormone-producing tissue—arranged in anatomic proximity to facilitate interaction—allows the ovary to regulate the proper sequence of follicle maturation, ovulation, and corpus luteum function through its own hormonal signals.

It has been shown that the ovary secretes not only progesterone, androstenedione, and estradiol but also pregnenolone, 17-hydroxyprogesterone, testosterone, DHEA, and estrone. Daily progesterone production amounts to about 4 mg during the follicular phase and 30 mg during the luteal phase. Follicular phase progesterone production depends more on adrenal than on ovarian progesterone secretion. The pronounced increase in progesterone production after ovulation depends on corpus luteum function. Approximately 10% to 15% of progesterone is metabolized to and excreted as pregnanediol glucuronide. The difference between follicular and luteal phase progesterone secretion is so great that elevated serum progesterone levels and urinary pregnanediol excretion are presumptive evidence of ovulation. The amount of ovarian estradiol secreted daily ranges from 100 to 500 μg. Estradiol secretion is lowest at the onset of menses and peaks before the midcycle LH peak.

It should be noted that estradiol, rather than estrone, is the principal estrogen secreted by the ovary. Outside the ovary, estradiol is readily metabolized to the biologically less active estrone and then to estrone sulfate (Figure 3-4). Circulating estradiol, as well as testosterone, is largely bound to sex hormone-binding globulin (SHBG), while progesterone is bound to corticosteroid-binding globulin (CBG). Estrone sulfate and dehydroepiandrosterone sulfate (DHEA-S) are bound to serum albumin. Estrone sulfate may be converted to estrone and, to a lesser extent, to estradiol (Figure 3-4). Having a relatively long half-life, and being present in plasma in rel-

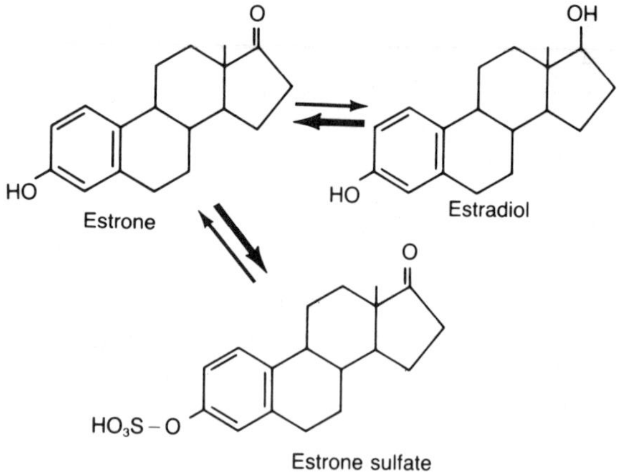

Figure 3-4
Interconversion of the three principal circulating estrogens, favoring the formation of estrone sulfate.

atively large quantities (470 to 890 pg/mL during the follicular and luteal phases of the cycle, respectively), estrone sulfate is quantitatively the most important component of the pool of circulating estrogens. Therefore, measurement of estrone sulfate provides an excellent index of overall estrogen production. Plasma levels, production rates, and metabolic clearance rates of various estrogens, androgens, and progesterone are discussed at the end of this chapter.

The liver converts estradiol and estrone to a large number of estrogen metabolites, of which estriol has been studied most extensively. Estrone, estradiol, and estriol are the so-called "three classical estrogens." These were the first estrogens measured in ether extracts of acid-hydrolyzed urine. Estrogens are conjugated by liver and intestinal mucosa into sulfates, glucuronides, or other conjugates and excreted in the urine. Before radioimmunoassays became available for measuring steroids in blood, urinary estradiol, estriol, and estrone were measured in lieu of serum estradiol and pregnanediol in lieu of serum progesterone. Graphs showing urinary estrogen and pregnanediol excretion during the normal menstrual cycle, in relation to serum

Normal endocrinology

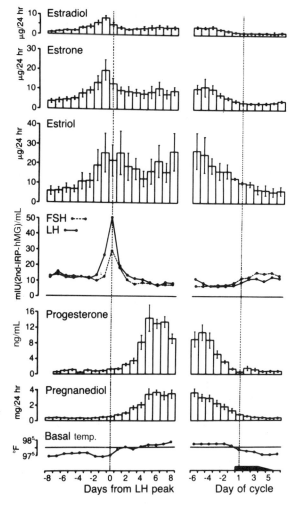

Figure 3-5
Mean serum FSH and LH levels, urinary estrogen and pregnanediol excretion, and basal body temperatures measured daily in five women during an ovulatory menstrual cycle. Bars depict standard errors. Individual results were grouped according to the day of the midcycle LH surge (left) or the first day of menstruation (right) and averaged.

From Goebelsmann U, Midgley AR Jr, Jaffe RB: Regulation of human gonadotropins: VII. Daily individual urinary estrogens, pregnanediol and serum luteinizing and follicle stimulating hormones during the menstrual cycle. J Clin Endocrinol Metab 29:1222, 1969.

The ovaries secrete less than 1 mg of DHEA, 1 to 2 mg of androstenedione, and approximately 0.1 mg of testosterone each day. In addition to the testosterone secreted by the ovaries, peripheral conversion of adrenal and ovarian androstenedione contributes about 0.1 to 0.2 mg to a woman's total daily testosterone production. There is only a minor variation of serum androstenedione and testosterone levels during the menstrual cycle (see Figures 5-7 and 5-8). Serum androstenedione and testosterone concentrations in women average 1.4 ng/mL (range, 0.7 to 3.1) and 0.34 ng/mL (range, 0.15 to 0.55), respectively. Serum DHEA and DHEA-S levels in women (averaging 4.2 ng/mL and 1.78 µg/mL, respectively) depend overwhelmingly on adrenal steroid hormone production. The three C_{19} steroids ("androgens") depicted in Figure 3-6 are excreted, for the most part, as 17-ketosteroids. Testosterone, not a 17-ketosteroid, is metabolized extensively to androstenedione and excreted mainly as androsterone and etiocholanolone (17-ketosteroids). Only a small portion of the testosterone produced is metabolized to testosterone glucuronide and excreted as such in the urine.

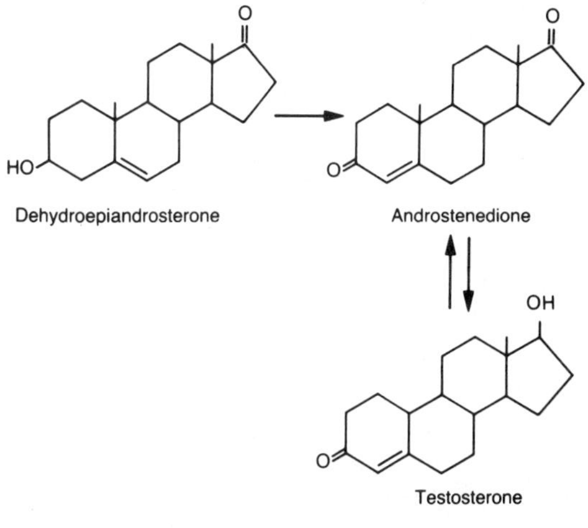

FSH and LH patterns, are presented in Figure 3-5. Almost twice as much conjugated estrone as estradiol, and also as much estriol as the sum of estrone and estradiol, is excreted in the urine.

Figure 3-6
The three principal ovarian C_{19} steroids ("androgens") and their interconversion. With the exception of the hilus cells, ovarian cells produce little testosterone.

Testicular steroid hormones

Testicular steroid hormone production takes place in the Leydig cells under LH stimulation. In male reproductive endocrinology, LH is frequently termed interstitial cell-stimulating hormone (ICSH).

The testis produces steroid hormones via biosynthetic pathways similar to those of the ovary. However, unlike the ovary, the testis secretes large quantities of testosterone and little estradiol. Testosterone originates by the two major routes outlined in Figure 3-7. One pathway entails 17β-reduction of androstenedione, originating from either DHEA or 17-hydroxyprogesterone; the other consists of 17β-reduction of DHEA to androstenediol and subsequent conversion to testosterone by 3β-ol dehydrogenase and $\Delta^5 \rightarrow \Delta^4$-isomerase.

Only relatively small amounts of DHEA, androstenedione, and estrone are secreted by the testis. These 17-oxosteroids are efficiently converted by the Leydig cells to their 17β-reduced counterparts: androstenediol, testosterone, and estradiol. 17β-Hydroxysteroid dehydrogenase is essential for the conversion of androstenedione to testosterone and of DHEA to androstenediol (Figure 3-7).

Hilus cell tumors of the ovary, virilizing adrenal adenomas, and carcinomas also produce and secrete testosterone. The ovaries, however, secrete only 0.1 mg of testosterone per day, compared with the 1 to 2 mg/day of androstenedione. The adrenals secrete mainly DHEA-S, less DHEA and androstenedione, and very little if any testosterone. Thus, with the exception of tumors, the Leydig cell is unique in its capacity to produce testosterone efficiently.

Normal male testosterone production is approximately 6 mg/day. Serum testosterone levels average 4.6 ± 1.6 (SD) ng/mL of male serum and range from 2.5 to 10 ng/mL. Some 92% of the testosterone present in male serum is bound to proteins, largely to SHBG, while the rest circulates in the free (non-SHBG-bound) form. Intratesticular testosterone concentrations are higher than those in plasma. The Sertoli cells, stimulated by FSH and testosterone, produce and secrete androgen-binding protein (ABP) into the seminiferous tubules. This protein binds testosterone. Furthermore, the Sertoli cells metabolize testosterone to estradiol. Outside the testis, testosterone is rapidly converted to androstenedione.

The extragonadal interconversion equilibrium between testosterone and androstenedione favors androstenedione, the biologically less active androgen. As in the female, the major portion of testosterone is converted to androstenedione and further metabolized and excreted as 17-ketosteroids. Only a small fraction is converted to testosterone glucuronide and excreted as such in the urine. Besides undergoing glucosiduronation, testosterone is metabolized in several ways (Figure 3-8): (1) converted to estradiol; (2) partially inactivated to androsterone; (3) totally inactivated to etiocholanolone; and (4) metabolized to androgens of higher androgenicity than that of testosterone. These are 5α-dihydrotestosterone and 5α-androstane-3α,17β-diol. The latter steroid is conjugated to 5α-androstanediol glucuronide, which has been described as an excellent marker of peripheral androgen action in hirsute women (see Chapter 17).

Adrenal steroid hormones

A detailed description of adrenal steroid hormone production is beyond the scope of this chapter; only essential information pertaining to reproductive endocrinology is included.

As outlined in Figure 3-9, the adrenal cortex produces mineralocorticoids, glucocorti-

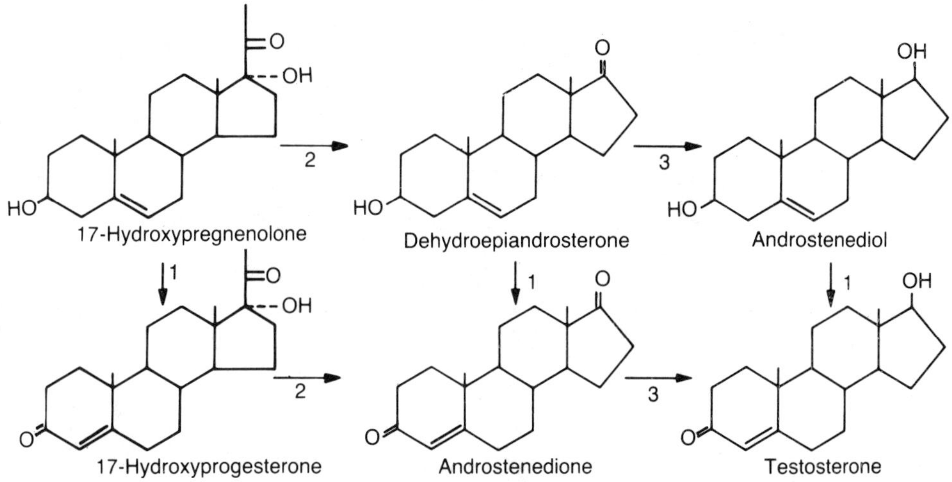

Figure 3-7
Pathways of testicular testosterone biosynthesis involving (1) 3β-ol dehydrogenase/$\Delta^5 \rightarrow \Delta^4$-isomerase, (2) 17,20-desmolase, and (3) 17β-ol dehydrogenase (17β-ol reductase).

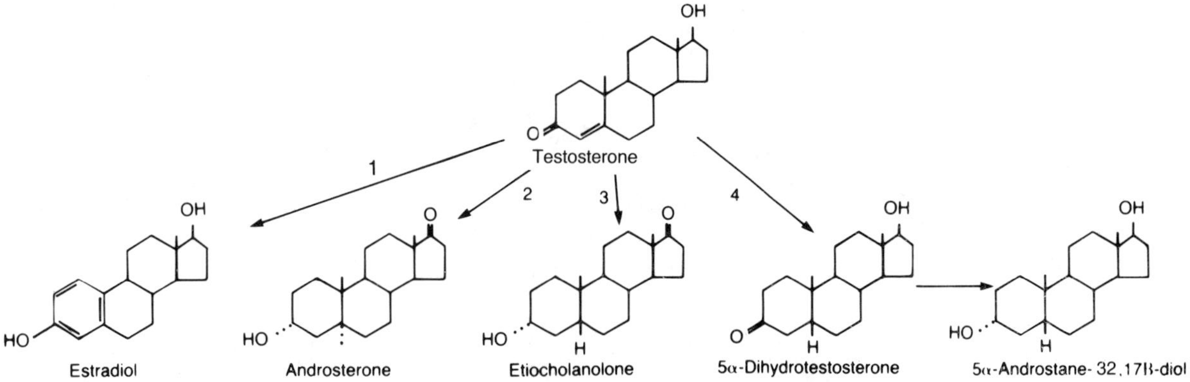

Figure 3-8
Testosterone metabolism to (1) estradiol, (2) androsterone, (3) etiocholanolone, and (4) 5α-dihydrotestosterone and 5α-androstane-3α,17β-diol.

coids, and C_{19} steroids (DHEA-S, DHEA, and androstenedione—but essentially no testosterone). The adrenal cortex uses circulating LDL-cholesterol, which originates in the liver from acetate via acetyl-CoA, mevalonic acid, squalene, and lanosterol. The conversion of cholesterol to pregnenolone, a rate-limiting step for cortisol production, is controlled by ACTH.

Mineralocorticoid biosynthesis consists of 21-hydroxylation of progesterone to 11-deoxy-corticosterone (DOC), which contains mineralo-corticoid activity. DOC undergoes 11β-hydrox-

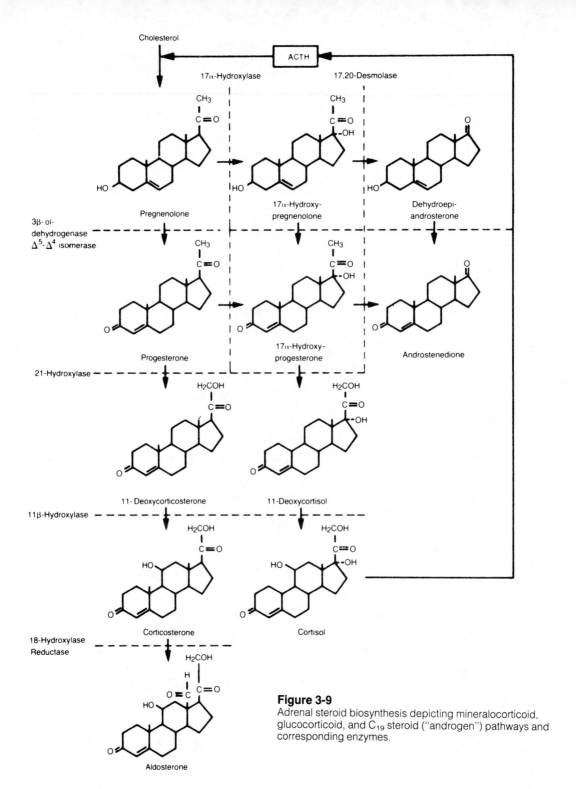

Figure 3-9
Adrenal steroid biosynthesis depicting mineralocorticoid, glucocorticoid, and C_{19} steroid ("androgen") pathways and corresponding enzymes.

Normal endocrinology

ylation to corticosterone (less mineralocorticoid activity than 11-deoxycorticosterone) and is further metabolized to aldosterone. Mineralocorticoids have no hydroxyl group at carbon atom 17. Aldosterone is the principal mineralocorticoid secreted by the adrenal. Its production is regulated by the renin-angiotensin mechanism and is not under direct ACTH control as are DOC, corticosterone, and cortisol. Aldosterone has about 30 times the mineralocorticosteroid activity of deoxycorticosterone. Aldosterone causes sodium retention and potassium loss, the secondary effects of which are increased extracellular fluid volume and rising blood pressure.

Glucocorticoid hormone production includes 17-hydroxylation of progesterone to 17-hydroxyprogesterone, 21-hydroxylation to 11-deoxycortisol (compound S), and 11β-hydroxylation to cortisol (compound F) (Figure 3-9). Cortisol is metabolized to cortisone, which has about 65% of the biologic activity of cortisol. Cortisol and cortisone are reduced to tetrahydrocortisol and tetrahydrocortisone and excreted in urine. Cortisol secretion averages 20 mg/day, that of corticosterone 3 mg/day, and that of aldosterone 0.15 mg/day. Serum cortisol is bound to transcortin, or corticosteroid-binding globulin (CBG).

Corticosteroid hormone production may be assessed by measuring 17-hydroxycorticosteroids or 17-ketogenic steroids in urine. 17-Hydroxycorticosteroids are measured by the Porter-Silber reaction and require the following configuration: a 17-hydroxyl, a keto group in position 20, and a hydroxyl group in position 21. An oxygen function in position 11 is not required. Thus cortisol, cortisone, 11-deoxycortisol, 11-deoxycortisone, and the tetrahydro metabolites of these steroids will be measured as 17-hydroxycorticosteroids (Table 3-2). Normal values are 8 ± 5 and 6 ± 3 mg/24 hr for men and women, respectively. 17-Ketogenic steroids are measured by chemical conversion to 17-ketosteroids, which are measured as such by the Zimmermann reaction. 17-Ketogenic steroids include 17-hydroxycorticosteroids plus other steroids such as pregnanetriol. Hence, the absolute amounts of 17-ketogenic steroid excretion exceed those of 17-hydroxycorticosteroid excretion. 17-Ketogenic steroid excretion averages 15 ± 5 (SD) and 10 ± 5 mg/24 hr in men and women, respectively (Table 3-2).

Besides mineralocorticoid and glucocorticoid hormone production, the adrenal produces C_{19} steroids (DHEA-S, DHEA, and androstenedione), yet virtually no testosterone or estrogen. DHEA-S, DHEA, and androstenedione are excreted as 17-ketosteroids: DHEA, androsterone, and etiocholanolone. The 24-hour urinary excretion of the latter three 17-ketosteroids ranges from 0.5 to 2.7, 0.8 to 4.4, and 1.4 to 5.1 mg/day in men and from 0.02 to 1.7, 0.6 to 3.2, and 0.2 to 2.9 mg/day in women, respectively. The bulk of urinary 17-ketosteroids is of adrenal origin, whereas the ovary contributes less than 1 mg/day of DHEA, 1 to 2 mg/day of androstenedione, and 0.1 mg/day of testosterone. Thus, nearly all urinary 17-ketosteroids, measured by the Zimmermann reaction, represent adrenal C_{19} steroid hormone production and are of no value in assessing ovarian androgen secretion. (For further details, see Chapter 17.)

DHEA-S is secreted by the adrenal in much larger quantities than is DHEA. Plasma or serum DHEA-S concentrations average 1.8 μg/mL and range from 0.5 to 2.8 μg/mL in premenopausal women. Circulating DHEA-S is bound to serum albumin and has a long half-life. Thus, it represents a relatively stable pool of a circulating C_{19} steroid of predominantly adrenal origin.

There is good correlation between plasma DHEA-S and urinary 17-ketosteroids. Plasma DHEA-S measurements assess adrenal C_{19} steroid production more accurately than do urinary 17-ketosteroid determinations, because the latter include the measurement of 11-oxygenated 17-ketosteroids, which include glucocorticosteroid metabolites (Table 3-2). Plasma DHEA-S

Table 3-2
Urinary 17-ketosteroids (17-KS), 17-hydroxycorticosteroids (17-OHCS), and 17-ketogenic steroids (17-KGS)

Test	Chemical reaction	Steroid structure required	Steroids measured	Normal values (mg/24 hr ± SD)
17-KS	Zimmermann reaction		11-Deoxy-17-KS: Dehydroepiandrosterone Androsterone Etiocholanolone 11-Oxy-17-KS: 11-Hydroxyandrosterone 11-Hydroxyetiocholanolone 11-Ketoandrosterone 11-Ketoetiocholanolone	Men: 15 ± 5 Women: 10 ± 5
17-OHCS	Porter-Silber reaction		Only 17,21-dihydroxy-20-ketosteroids: Cortisol Cortisone 11-Deoxycortisol 11-Deoxycortisone Tetrahydro metabolites of the above	Men: 8 ± 5 Women: 6 ± 3
17-KGS	Chemical conversion to 17-ketosteroids, then measurement by Zimmermann reaction		Any 17-hydroxy-20-ketosteroid or 17,20-dihydroxysteroid: Cortisone Cortisol 11-Deoxycortisol 11-Deoxycortisone Tetrahydro metabolites of cortisol, cortisone, 11-deoxycortisol, and 11-deoxycortisone 17-Hydroxyprogesterone Pregnanetriol Cortol Cortolone	Men: 8 ± 5 Women: 6 ± 3

Normal endocrinology

Table 3-3

Plasma concentrations (C), metabolic clearance rates (MCR), and production rates (PR) of androgens, estrogens, and progesterone during menstrual cycle

Steroid hormone	Phase of cycle	Plasma concentration*			Metabolic clearance rate plasma* (L/day)	Production rate (mg/day) (PR = C × MCR)	
		Mean	Range	Units		Mean	Range
Androstenedione	†	1.4	0.7 – 3.1	ng/mL	2,000	2.8	1.4– 6.2
Testosterone	†	0.35	0.15– 0.55	ng/mL	700	0.25	0.1– 0.4
Dehydroepiandrosterone	†	4.2	2.7 – 7.8	ng/mL	1,600	6.7	4.3–12.5
Dehydroepiandrosterone sulfate	†	1.6	0.8 – 3.4	µg/mL	7	11.2	5.6–23.8
Estradiol	Follicular	44	20– 120	pg/mL	1,350	0.059	0.027– 0.162
	Preovulatory	250	150– 600	pg/mL	1,350	0.338	0.203– 0.810
	Luteal	110	40– 300	pg/mL	1,350	0.149	0.054– 0.405
Estrone	Follicular	40		pg/mL	2,200	0.088	
	Preovulatory	170		pg/mL	2,200	0.374	
	Luteal	92		pg/mL	2,200	0.202	
Estrone-sulfate	Follicular	470		pg/mL	146	0.069	
	Luteal	890		pg/mL	146	0.130	
Progesterone	Follicular	0.2	0.06– 0.37	ng/mL	2,300	0.46	0.14– 0.85
	Luteal	8.9	4.3 –19.4	ng/mL	2,300	20.5	9.9–45.0

*These values may vary somewhat depending on investigator and method.
†Unspecified. No major changes during menstrual cycle.

measurements have largely replaced urinary 17-ketosteroid assays for estimating adrenal C_{19} steroid production.

Steroid hormone dynamics

The concentration of a steroid hormone in blood, serum, or plasma depends on its production rate (PR) and metabolic clearance rate (MCR). The PR is defined as the amount of steroid that enters the circulation per unit of time—usually milligrams per day or micrograms per day. It is understood that this definition includes steroids originating from glandular and extraglandular sources as well as steroids secreted as such or derived by extraglandular conversion. The MCR of a steroid is defined as the volume of blood, serum, or plasma that is irreversibly cleared of the steroid per unit of time. Its dimension is liters per day.

The MCR of a steroid is determined by intravenously infusing tracer amounts labeled with tritium or carbon-14 at a constant rate over several hours until a steady blood, serum, or plasma level is reached. This concentration is determined as the amount of unmetabolized tracer per volume of blood, serum, or plasma. The MCR for blood, serum, or plasma is then calculated by dividing the dose of the radioactively labeled steroid administered per unit of time (counts per minute per day) by the tracer concentration in blood, serum, or plasma (counts per minute per liter) according to the formula:

$$MCR = \frac{\text{tracer administered/time}}{\text{tracer concentration}}$$

$$= \frac{\text{cpm/day}}{\text{cpm/liter}}$$

$$= \frac{\text{liters}}{\text{day}}$$

Since radioimmunoassays have become available, the concentration of the endogenous steroid levels (C) is readily determined. When both MCR and C are known, the PR can be determined by multiplying the MCR by C (amount of steroid per liter of blood, serum, or plasma):

$$PR = MCR \times C$$

$$= (\text{liters/day}) \times (\text{amount/liter})$$

$$= \text{amount/day}$$

The following example will clarify this. If the MCR of serum testosterone is found to be 700 L/day in a given premenopausal woman and her serum testosterone concentration is measured as 0.35 μg/L, her testosterone PR is:

$$700 \times 0.35 \text{ μg/day} = 245 \text{ μg/day}$$

Metabolic clearance rates have been determined for most of the clinically important steroid hormones in men and women. The average figures mentioned may be applied to a given patient if the blood, serum, and plasma MCR values for a certain steroid have not been assessed. If the blood, serum, or plasma concentration of the steroid in question has been measured, it is possible to establish that patient's PR for this steroid by applying its average published MCR. If corrections for body surface can be made, the estimated PR most likely will match the patient's true PR quite closely. Normal plasma or serum levels of sex steroids in conjunction with MCRs and PRs have been compiled in Table 3-3.

References

1. Ryan KJ: Biosynthesis and metabolism of ovarian steroids. In Behrman SJ, Kistner RW (eds): *Progress in Infertility*, ed 2. Boston, Little, Brown, 1975, pp 281-297
2. MacDonald PC, Rombaut RP, Siiteri PK: Plasma precursors of estrogen. I. Extent of conversion of plasma Δ^4-androstenedione to estrone in normal males and nonpregnant normal, castrate and adrenalectomized females. *J Clin Endocrinol Metab* 27:1103, 1967

Suggested reading

Eik-Nes KB (ed): *The Androgens of the Testis.* New York, Marcel Dekker, 1970

Freedman MD, Freedman SN (eds): *Introduction to Steroid Biochemistry and Its Clinical Application.* New York, Harper & Row, 1970

Gurpide E, Gandy HM: Dynamics of hormone production and metabolism. In Fuchs F, Klopper A (eds): *Endocrinology of Pregnancy,* ed 3. New York, Harper & Row, 1983

Little AB, Billiar RB: Endocrine disorders. In Romney S, et al (eds): *Gynecology and Obstetrics: The Health Care of Women.* New York, McGraw-Hill, 1980

Yen SSC, Jaffe RB: *Reproductive Endocrinology.* Philadelphia, WB Saunders, 1978

Chapter 4

Measurement of Hormones

Oscar A. Kletzky, M.D.
Robert M. Nakamura, Ph.D.

During the past 30 years, the ability to measure hormones and other substances present in biologic fluids in quantities below the microgram range has opened new horizons in the field of endocrinology. As a result, a new set of terms was created to define these minute quantities. *Nanogram* (10^{-9} g) and *picogram* (10^{-12} g) have replaced *millimicrogram* and *micromicrogram*, respectively. *Femtogram* (10^{-15} g) and *attogram* (10^{-18} g) were defined in anticipation of the development of more sensitive techniques.

The two major methods that made possible the routine measurement of hormones in the nano- and picogram ranges were gas-liquid chromatography–mass spectrometry and radioimmunoassay (RIA). Measurement of hormones had previously been limited to the use of bioassays for gonadotropins and chemical methods for sex steroids in urine (for example, pregnanediol, estrogens, and ketosteroids).

The earliest investigation using bioassay methods dealt with identifying the specific hormonal effect on organs. The organs that responded to the hormone were referred to as target organs (uterus, ovaries, prostate). Once a correlation between a specific hormone and a target organ was established, a dose-response relationship was determined between different amounts of administered hormone present in urine and the growth response of the target organ. The organ specificity and dose-response relationship formed the basis for bioassay methods. A dose-response curve became the standard curve against which an unknown specimen could be measured. To compensate for the wide variations in response, at least five animals per dose were required; and in order to identify a parallel response, a minimum of two dose levels of hormone were necessary.

Chemical methods

The chemical methods for hormone measurement were performed by reaction of specific compounds with steroids to give a color. Three basic steps are necessary before measuring urinary sex steroids: hydrolysis, extraction of the crude hormone, and further purification. Steroid hormones are excreted as conjugates, mainly as glucuronates or sulfates; therefore, acid or enzymatic hydrolysis must first be carried out to remove the glucuronate or sulfate moiety from the steroid itself. Unlike the water-soluble steroid conjugates, steroids themselves are insoluble in water (after hydrolysis) and must first be extracted with organic solvents from the urine hydrolysate. Following evaporation of the organic solvent, the residue of the extract containing the sex steroids is usually purified further by column chromatography on alumina and/or formation of chemical derivatives. Quantitation is then performed using colorimetry, fluorometry, or gas chromatography.

Colorimetry is based on such specific color reactions as the Zimmermann reaction for 17-ketosteroids, the Kober reaction for estrogens, and the sulfuric acid reaction for pregnanediol. Fluorometry, more sensitive than colorimetry, has been used for measurement of estrogens. An example of fluorometry is the Ittrich technique, which has a sensitivity of 1 ng/sample. Gas chromatography combines the techniques of chromatographic separation and quantitation by flame ionization or electron capture, which change the electrical current in proportion to the amount of steroid passing through the detector. These electrical signals are amplified and recorded so that steroids appear as peaks with areas that are proportional to their quantity. For electron capture, the area is proportional to the amount of derivative coupled to the steroid. The sensitivity of this method is similar to that of RIA; however, each sample requires extensive purification and must be assayed individually.

Radioimmunoassay

In 1959, Yalow and Berson developed a method that eventually revolutionized the entire field of endocrinology.[1] They coupled a tracer of radioactive isotopic iodine (^{131}I) to insulin and reacted this ^{131}I-labeled insulin with a specific antibody against insulin. When nonradioactive insulin was found to compete with the tracer, the

method of RIA was developed. In 1963, Greenwood and colleagues developed a method for coupling radioactive iodine to growth hormone that was far superior to any previous method.[2] The coupling was accomplished by using a mild oxidizing agent, Chloramine-T. With minimal damage to the hormone, this method made it possible to bind all proteins with radioactive iodine. A new era of reproductive endocrinology was launched by the development of RIA for LH by Odell and co-workers in 1964, and for estradiol by Abraham in 1968.[3, 4]

RIA requires only a small amount of serum or plasma (1 mL or less), and multiple and frequent sampling therefore has become possible. In contrast with the limited number of assays that could be performed using methods such as gas chromatography and bioassay, it is now possible for one highly trained technician using RIA methodology to measure 100 times as many samples of protein hormones daily—and with greater sensitivity. There is, however, one important difference between RIA and bioassay. RIA measures the hormone concentration based on its immunologic properties, whereas bioassay measures the action of a hormone directly on a target organ. RIA of protein hormones, but not of steroids, has limitations because of the heterogeneity in affinity of binding sites of the different antibodies used, as well as variability in the sources of these antibodies. The clinician should be aware of these limitations. A given hormone value should be evaluated in relation to the range of normal values obtained using the same reagents.

The principle of RIA is based on the competition between labeled and unlabeled antigen for the binding sites on antibodies (Figure 4-1). To quantitate this competition, an antigen (for example, LH) is labeled with a tracer isotope, referred to as the hot antigen; the unlabeled hormone is known as the cold antigen. Tritium (^{3}H) is the isotope most commonly used for the labeling of steroid hormones, and radioactive iodine

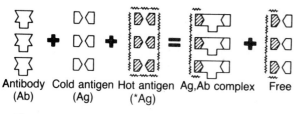

Antibody   Cold antigen   Hot antigen   Ag,Ab complex   Free
(Ab)   (Ag)   (*Ag)

Figure 4-1
Schematic representation of antigen-antibody reaction in radioimmunoassay. For the final analysis, the "free" component must be separated from the Ag,Ab complex.

125 (^{125}I) for the labeling of protein hormones, such as luteinizing hormone (LH), follicle-stimulating hormone (FSH), human chorionic gonadotropin (hCG), thyroid-stimulating hormone (TSH), prolactin (PRL), and growth hormone (GH). However, an increasing number of steroid assays are using ^{125}I-labeled steroids, resulting in more rapid, sensitive, and less expensive determinations. When the hot and cold antigens are incubated with the antibody, the following reaction occurs:

$$Ag\ (cold) + {}^*Ag\ (hot) + Ab \rightleftharpoons Ag^*Ag\ Ab + Ag^*Ag$$

where Ag is the antigen, Ab is the antibody, and Ag*Ag Ab is the antigen-antibody complex. The amount of tracer present in the bound complex is determined with a radioactive analyzer.

Before an unknown specimen can be assayed for the hormone, a standard curve must be constructed using known amounts of the same hormone in several concentrations. With the standard curve, it is then possible to compare the amount of radioactivity present in the known preparation with that of the unknown samples and thus determine the level of hormone present (Figure 4-2).

Antigens

Antigens are proteins or carbohydrates that can induce production of antibodies when injected into animals. Using this definition, only pituitary hormones are antigens, because steroid hormones are haptens and, thus, cannot induce antibody production by themselves. Steroids become antigenic only after a carrier protein is attached to them. The protein most often used for this purpose is bovine serum albumin.

Most hormones involved in reproduction are glycoproteins (LH, FSH, TSH, and hCG) or protein hormones such as GH and PRL. These pituitary and placental (hCG) hormones have been isolated and prepared in relatively pure form. Compared with steroids, they have a much higher molecular weight and have inherent immunogenic properties. Glycoprotein hormones are composed of two nonidentical parts, α- and β-subunits. The α-subunit is species specific and similar in all glycoprotein hormones, whereas the specificity of the hormones is determined by the respective β-subunit. The subunits are composed of specific sequences of amino acids, which are termed peptides. The whole molecule or either of its subunits can induce the formation of specific antibodies when injected into animals.

Antibodies

An injection of a foreign substance (antigen) into an animal will induce the formation of a

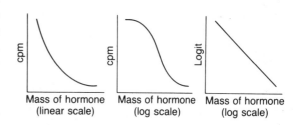

Mass of hormone   Mass of hormone   Mass of hormone
(linear scale)   (log scale)   (log scale)

Figure 4-2
Standard curve using linear scale (left) or log scale (center and right) for the abscissa and linear (left and center) or logit (right) for the ordinate.

specific antibody to the antigen. Antibodies are globulins containing a 3% to 12% carbohydrate moiety produced by the B lymphocytes present in the bone marrow, spleen, lymph nodes, and intestinal lymphoid organs. To obtain a higher titer of antibody and improve its specificity, more than one injection of the antigen is needed. Upon reaching a desirable titer and specificity, the antisera are harvested and stored for future use. Even with the use of highly purified antigen, most antibodies will cross-react against more than one hormone. The specificity of the assay requires the least amount of cross-reactivity of the antibody with similar hormones.

Very recently, the development of monoclonal antibodies has resulted in an important advance in the immunologic measurement of protein hormones. Monoclonal antibodies are a homogeneous population of antibodies that can eliminate the heterogeneity and variability of an antiserum obtained by the regular immunization process. To obtain a monoclonal antibody, it is first necessary to inject the antigen (for example, hCG) into a mouse to induce an immunologic reaction in the spleen (Figure 4-3). Each immunized spleen cell (clone) can produce an antibody of specific characteristics. The most important step in the production of monoclonal antibodies is screening the spleen cells to separate those capable of secreting a single antibody type. When a myeloma cell from the same species is fused with the selected spleen cell, a hybrid or "hybridoma" cell will be produced. This hybridoma will continuously secrete an antibody with the characteristics of that selected spleen cell, because of the immortality of the myeloma cell. A hybridoma cell is able to produce 1,000 similar, specific antibody molecules per second.

A continuous clone line is maintained in culture, becoming a source of homogeneous monoclonal antibody molecules. These antibodies are currently being used in sensitive and specific RIAs of protein hormones (hCG, GH, PRL, etc.). Using monoclonal antibodies, a nonisotopic assay methodology has been developed for the measurement of glycoproteins (hCG, LH, and TSH) in blood and urine. Instead of iodinating the antigen, as in RIA, the antibody is coupled to the enzyme horseradish peroxidase, which replaces the radioactive isotope and consequently is easier, safer, and less expensive than RIA (Figure 4-4). Therefore, instead of using the specific activity of the radiolabeled hormone, the amount of enzyme coupled to the antibody at the end of the procedure is measured by spectrophotometry.

This enzyme-linked immunosorbent assay (ELISA), or "sandwiched" technique, uses a monoclonal antibody against the α-subunit, which is attached to a bead or a plastic tube (Fig-

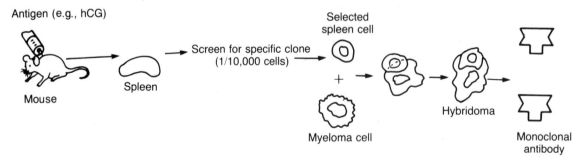

Figure 4-3
Schematic representation of monoclonal antibody production.

Normal endocrinology

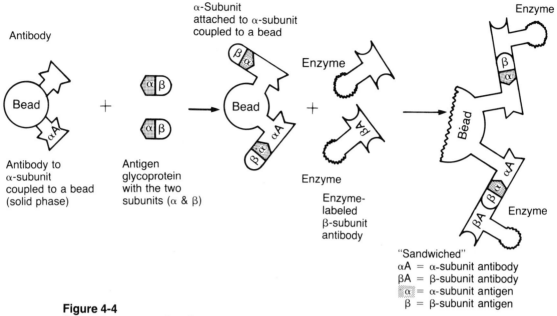

Antibody

Bead

Antibody to
α-subunit
coupled to a bead
(solid phase)

+

Antigen
glycoprotein
with the two
subunits (α & β)

α-Subunit
attached to α-subunit
coupled to a bead

Bead

+

Enzyme

Enzyme

Enzyme-
labeled
β-subunit
antibody

Enzyme

Bead

Enzyme

Enzyme

"Sandwiched"
αA = α-subunit antibody
βA = β-subunit antibody
α = α-subunit antigen
β = β-subunit antigen

Figure 4-4
Schematic representation of enzyme-linked immunosorbent assay (ELISA) or "sandwiched"
technique.

ure 4-4). The α-subunit of the sample to be tested will bind to the α-subunit antibody. The addition of a second monoclonal antibody against the β-subunit coupled to the enzyme will bind to the β-subunit of the hormone present in the patient's serum sample. Following a single washing step, the amount of total hormone present in the unknown sample is read in a spectrophotometer and compared with a standard curve constructed from known amounts of that hormone. An enzymatic assay for α-fetoprotein has been reported by Votila and associates,[5] and for hCG, LH, and TSH by Wada and co-workers.[6] Available enzymatic assays are less sensitive than RIA.

Recently, Lindner's group reported a novel method for the measurement of steroids in serum or unextracted urine samples.[7] In this assay, a chemiluminescent substance (isoluminol) is attached to a monoclonal antibody produced against a steroid. Upon oxidation, after microperoxidase and hydrogen peroxide are added, light is produced. Different concentrations of

steroid produce different amounts of light, which is measured by a luminometer. Using the chemiluminescence-immunoassay (CIA) procedure, progesterone, pregnanediol, estriol, and cortisol have been successfully and accurately measured. The precision and limits of detection of these assays are comparable to those obtained with RIA. ELISA and CIA have the advantages of safety (no radioactive isotope is needed), and CIA is more economical than the other methods.

Bioassay

Assays that combine features of both RIA (immunologic) and bioassay (biologic) properties have been developed. One such method is an in vitro bioassay using a homogenate of testicular tissue as the target organ to LH. This method was first described by DuFau et al.[8] In relation to their concentration, different amounts of LH or hCG will stimulate the production of various amounts of testosterone, which is then measured by RIA. A similar method is being used to measure the effect of FSH on granulosa cell production of estradiol (E_2). The advantage of these bioassays is that only the biologic activity of LH or FSH is measured.

A radioreceptor assay (RRA) for hCG was developed by Haour and co-workers following the characterization of chorionic gonadotropic receptors present in bovine corpus luteum.[9] In this method, the antigen is bound to cell membranes of the target organ, instead of to an antibody. High cost and technical difficulties, such as nonspecific effects of a factor(s) present in serum or urine, remain to be resolved before RRA can become a standard procedure for quantitative measurement of hormones. The only RRA commercially available at present is a qualitative assay for hCG, which has a sensitivity of 200 mIU/mL of hCG. In contrast, a qualitative RIA, using a specific antibody against the β-subunit of hCG, has been developed with a sensitivity as low as 5 mIU/mL.

Standard preparations

A standard is a known preparation that is used by direct comparison to measure the amount of hormone present in an unknown sample. It is essential that the hormone in the standard preparation and that of the unknown samples be immunochemically identical. Steroids used as standards are available as pure chemical preparations; thus, it is possible to express the results of an unknown sample in terms of their mass or weight, such as nanograms or picograms. Furthermore, similar results are obtained in different laboratories and these results are always reported in terms of mass.

Because peptide hormones used as standards are not yet available in pure chemical form, the results on unknown samples should not be expressed in units of mass. To be able to compare results obtained in different laboratories, the use of internationally accepted reference preparations is preferable. Such standard preparations should be characterized by their biologic activity, physicochemical properties, and stability. Because hormone extracts of urine, pituitary, and serum are all used as standards in the RIA of hormones, levels measured in different laboratories often do not agree. Therefore, clinicians should be familiar with the assay characteristics used by the laboratory of their choice.

The results for LH and FSH are usually reported in terms of international units (an international milliunit = 1 mIU/mL of serum). The international unit is the biologic activity contained in a defined weight of an international standard. At present, there is no international standard for FSH and LH; however, an international reference preparation (IRP) is being used as an international standard. Aliquots of the second international reference preparation of human menopausal gonadotropin (2nd IRP-HMG) obtained from extracts of urine from postmenopausal women are used in most laboratories as the standard preparation. This preparation was supplied by the World Health Organization (WHO) and has been assigned a potency of 40 IU of LH and FSH activity per ampule of the second IRP supplied.

Another standard used for LH and FSH assay is LER-907. This preparation is made from a collection of human pituitaries obtained by the National Institutes of Health (NIH), and results are reported as nanograms per milliliter of LER-907. TSH is expressed in terms of microunits per milliliter of a standard provided by WHO, and hCG is expressed in terms of international milliunits per liter of the second international standard for hCG. This standard is a partially purified hCG preparation obtained from urine from women in their first trimester of pregnancy. Since the supply of such standards has been

Normal endocrinology

exhausted, an IRP for hCG has been developed from a highly purified hCG preparation. Although this IRP for hCG is more purified than the previous standard, comparable results using both standards cannot be obtained. In fact, the use of the new IRP renders almost double values of hCG when compared with the second international standards. Because this discrepancy can be confusing for physicians following up patients with hCG-related problems, the results need to be clearly defined in terms of the reference preparation used in the assay. Although WHO has an international reference preparation for PRL, in the US the results are usually expressed in terms of nanograms per milliliter of a highly purified pituitary preparation.

Calculation of normal values

Following the widespread use of RIA and its incorporation into clinical practice, it was necessary to establish the normal range of hormone values in normal individuals. This was especially important in normal ovulatory women, because of the cyclic release of LH, FSH, E_2, and progesterone. It has been customary in biology to calculate the 95% confidence limits for the establishment of the normal distribution of values. Since it was assumed that hormone values throughout the normal menstrual cycle follow a normal distribution, the 95% confidence limit was obtained by adding and subtracting two standard deviations (SD) from the mean value. However, in some instances, the arithmetic mean minus 2 SD gives values either close to zero or actually negative, a biologic impossibility. This point becomes very important when the normal range of such hormones as serum progesterone in the luteal phase of ovulatory women is calculated.

Assuming a normal distribution, we reported that the calculated 95% distribution of progesterone in daily samples obtained in 21 wom-

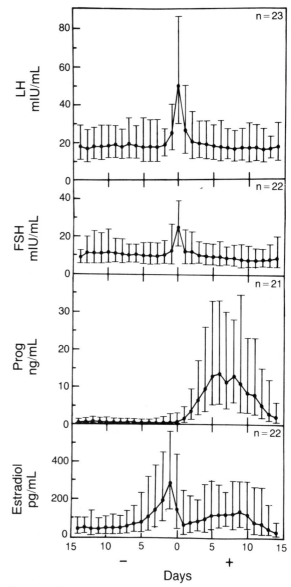

Figure 4-5

Normal menstrual cycle: composite pattern of daily LH, FSH, estradiol, and progesterone in ovulatory cycles. Each point represents the geometric mean value; vertical bars represent 95% confidence limits as determined by log transformation.

Reproduced, with permission, from Kletzky OA, Nakamura RM, Thorneycroft IH, et al: Log normal distribution of gonadotropins and ovarian steroid values in the normal menstrual cycle. Am J Obstet Gynecol 121:688, 1975

Table 4-1
95% confidence limits of hormones used in reproduction

Hormone	Phase of menstrual cycle			
	Follicular	Midcycle	Luteal	Menopause
LH (mIU/mL)	4.0– 20.0	43 –145	3 – 18	>40
FSH (mIU/mL)	3.2– 9.0	10 – 18	3 – 9	>30
PRL (ng/mL)	8.0– 20.0	9 – 22	10 – 30	6 –25
Estradiol (pg/mL)	30 –140	150 –480	50 –250	10 –30
Progesterone (ng/mL)	0.5– 1.0	0.8– 2.0	3.0– 31	0.5– 1.0
Testosterone (ng/dL)	20 – 85	20 – 85	20 – 85	8 –30*
Free testosterone (ng/dL)	1.2– 9.9	1.2– 9.9	1.2– 9.9	3 –13†
DHEA-S (μg/mL)	0.5– 2.8	0.5– 2.8	0.5– 2.8	0.2– 1.5

In oophorectomized women the range is 4–18 ng/dL.
†*In oophorectomized women the range is 1–10 ng/dL.*

en ranged between -0.7 and 24 ng/mL.[10] Although this is a statistical range, it has neither physiologic nor chemical value, because none of the individual values used in the calculation were below 3 ng/mL. In analyzing the rationale concerning the statistical evaluations, we reported that LH, FSH, E_2, and progesterone values in the normal menstrual cycle follow a log-normal rather than a normal or gaussian distribution. Therefore, if the 95% confidence limit is now calculated by adding and subtracting two normal equivalent deviates (NED), rather than 2 SD, from the geometric mean, obtained by a log-transformed method, instead of the arithmetic mean, the interpretation of clinical data is more reliable. The application of this concept to the same serum progesterone values used above gives a normal range between 3 and 31 ng/mL (Figure 4-5).

Considering the variability of results among laboratories, especially in the measurement of peptide hormones, clinicians should use only the values for normal range calculated by the laboratory of their choice. The 95% confidence limits for LH, FSH, PRL, GH, E_2, and progesterone calculated by log-normal distribution for women of different reproductive ages in our laboratory are listed in Table 4-1.

References

1. Yalow RS, Berson SA: Assay of plasma insulin in human subjects by immunological methods. *Nature* 184:1648, 1959

2. Greenwood FC, Hunter WM, Glover JS: The preparation of ^{131}I-labelled human growth hormone of high specific radioactivity. *Biochem J* 89:114, 1963

3. Odell WD, Ross GT, Rayford PL: RIA of luteinizing hormone in human plasma or serum: Physiological studies. *J Clin Invest* 46:248, 1967

4. Abraham GE: Solid-phase radioimmunoassay of estradiol-17β. *J Clin Endocrinol Metab* 29:866, 1969

5. Votila M, Ruoslahti E, Engvall E: Two-site sandwich enzyme immunoassay with monoclonal antibodies to human alpha-fetoprotein. *J Immunol Methods* 42:11, 1981

6. Wada HG, Danish RJ, Baxter SR, et al: Enzyme immunoassay of the glycoprotein tropic hormones—HCG, LH, TSH—with solid-phase antibody specific for the β-subunit. *Clin Chem* 28:1862, 1982

7. Lindner HR, Kohen F, Eshhar Z, et al: Novel assay procedure for assessing ovarian function in women. *J Steroid Biochem* 15:131, 1981

8. DuFau ML, Mendelson R, Catt K: A highly sensitive in-vitro bioassay for LH and HCG: Testosterone production by dispersed Leydig cells. *J Clin Endocrinol Metab* 39:610, 1974

9. Haour F, Saxena BB: Characterization and solubilization of gonadotropin receptor of bovine corpus luteum. *J Biol Chem* 249:2195, 1974

10. Kletzky OA, Nakamura RM, Thorneycroft IH, et al: Log normal distribution of gonadotropins and ovarian steroid values in the normal menstrual cycle. *Am J Obstet Gynecol* 121:688, 1975

Normal endocrinology

Chapter 5
The Menstrual Cycle

Uwe Goebelsmann, M.D.

The hormonal events of the menstrual cycle, which consist of cyclic alterations in gonadotropins, estradiol (E_2), and progesterone (P), are closely related to follicle development and ovulation. Without a thorough understanding of the mechanisms involved in ovarian function and hypothalamic-pituitary feedback regulation, there can be no rational diagnosis and treatment of such menstrual cycle aberrations as anovulation resulting in dysfunctional uterine bleeding, oligomenorrhea, or amenorrhea. This chapter deals with the hormonal events of the menstrual cycle and their regulation as they relate to (1) the ovary as the gametogenic and sex hormone-producing unit, (2) hypothalamic-pituitary control of ovarian function, and (3) temporal and quantitative aspects of gonadotropin and sex hormone levels throughout the normal menstrual cycle. These values can be used as references to compare with hormonal aberrations discussed in later chapters.

The ovary

Integration of follicle development and steroid production

The ovary combines two important functions: gametogenesis and sex hormone production. The integration of ovarian steroid hormone biosynthesis and secretion with follicle maturation, ovulation, and corpus luteum function is essential for (1) the intraovarian control of morphologic and hormonal activity, (2) hypothalamic-pituitary feedback control of gonadotropin release, which, in turn, regulates morphologic changes and steroid hormone production in the ovary, and (3) timing and support of events associated with fertilization and nidation through the effects of E_2 and/or P on tubal motility and secretion, endometrial proliferation, and the properties of the cervical mucus.

The functional interdependence of germ cells and hormone-producing cells, arranged in close anatomic proximity, allows the ovary to regulate the proper sequence of follicle maturation, ovulation, and corpus luteum formation, function, and regression through its own hormonal signals. The state of follicle maturation is indicated by the amount of E_2 secretion; circulating levels of P in conjunction with E_2 reflect corpus luteum function.

The hypothalamus and anterior pituitary regulate the sequence and extent of these morphologic and endocrine events in the ovary through the secretion of gonadotropin-releasing hormone (GnRH) and gonadotropins, respectively. Both gonadotropins act synergistically, although follicle-stimulating hormone (FSH) primarily stimulates follicle growth whereas luteinizing hormone (LH) mainly affects gonadal steroid biosynthesis. The ovary synthesizes a number of sex steroids along the biosynthetic pathways outlined in Chapter 3. However, only three steroid hormones are secreted by the ovary in physiologically important quantities: P, androstenedione (A), and E_2.

Since the pioneering in vitro studies of Ryan and collaborators in the late 1950s and early 1960s,[1] it has been known that ovarian stroma and theca cells produce primarily androgens, foremost A, that E_2 is quantitatively the most important steroid hormone of the granulosa cells and an indicator of follicle maturation, and that P is the characteristic product of the corpus luteum. The balance of ovarian steroid hormone production—that is, the total amounts of A, E_2, and P produced and secreted by the ovaries—depends on the number and developmental stages of ovarian follicles, as well as on gonadotropin stimulation at any given time. The number of granulosa cells increases dramatically as the primordial follicle develops to a primary (preantral), then to an antral, and finally to a mature preovulatory follicle. Parallel with the increasing number and functional state of granulosa cells, ovarian E_2 production and secretion increase.

Animal studies have shown that steroid hormones within the ovary play an important regulatory role in follicle growth and atresia. Estrogen administration, for example, stimulates preantral follicle growth, reduces follicle atresia, and enhances ovarian FSH uptake in hypophysectomized immature rats.[2] When the biologic effects of estrogens are neutralized in these animals and exogenous gonadotropins are administered, follicle growth is inhibited and follicle atresia is enhanced. Animal studies have shown that testosterone (T) reduces preantral follicle growth and increases follicle atresia.[2] These data have been interpreted by Ross et al as "indicating that local concentrations of estrogens and possibly androgens determine whether a given follicle grows or becomes atretic." Ross and co-workers concluded that gonadotropins are essential for follicle maturation and that estrogens mediate the ovarian effects of gonadotropic stimulation.[3]

In recent years, the two-cell, two-gonadotropin concept of ovarian follicle maturation and E_2 production has gained general acceptance. LH stimulates the conversion of cholesterol to A and T in theca cells that have LH receptors via the ATP/cyclic AMP mechanism. The granulosa cells contain FSH receptors and, stimulated by FSH, convert the A and T that is being synthesized by the theca cells to estrone (E_1) and E_2.[4] This FSH-stimulated and cyclic AMP-mediated increase in the aromatization of A and T to E_1, but primarily to E_2, has several effects: The E_2 thus generated (1) induces additional granulosa cell FSH receptors, (2) stimulates granulosa cell mitoses and thereby further increases the number of granulosa cells, and (3) enhances the content of E_2 in the antral fluid and raises circulating E_2 concentrations.

The E_2-mediated induction of FSH receptors and reduplication of granulosa cells further enhances follicle development. This mechanism provides a positive FSH-E_2 feedback response within the granulosa cells. It functions as an amplifier system by which (1) a cohort of developing follicles is able selectively to undergo rapid development and (2) a single follicle may proceed toward maturation and ovulation ahead of all other follicles within this cohort. The latter follicle is also called the dominant follicle. Additional factors are operative in this amazing array of events—during which the dominant follicle is recruited, matures, produces a fertilizable oocyte, and turns into a functioning corpus luteum. These factors include gonadotropin control of ovarian steroidogenic and morphologic events, and vascularization of theca and granulosa cells, as well as nonsteroidal ovarian substances that modulate follicle development.

Follicle maturation, ovulation, and corpus luteum formation

Follicle maturation

This process starts from an undeveloped state: that of the primordial follicle. This follicle is an oocyte that, still in the diplotene stage of its first meiotic division since it was initiated during fetal life, is covered by a single layer of granulosa cells. Primordial follicles develop into primary (preantral) follicles consisting of an oocyte covered by multiple granulosa cell layers. Such development proceeds even in the absence of gonadotropin stimulation—for example, during childhood, pregnancy, or oral contraceptive medication. The primary follicles that develop under these circumstances do not produce significant amounts of E_2 and end in atresia. For advanced follicle development, both gonadotropins and ovarian steroid hormone production are required. Women with 17-hydroxylase deficiency, for instance, who fail to produce estrogens despite the presence of follicles and elevated serum gonadotropins, neither will have normal follicle development nor will ovulate.

During its progress to the preantral stage, the oocyte enlarges and surrounds itself with the zona pellucida while the granulosa cells multiply and form several cell layers around the oocyte. Theca cells develop from the neighboring stroma, separated from the granulosa cells by the basement membrane. FSH interacts with its receptors on the granulosa cells of the preantral follicle and stimulates aromatization of androgens, which originate in the theca cells, producing primarily E_2. FSH initiates E_2 production in granulosa cells and also augments the number of granulosa cell FSH receptors. In conjunction with the E_2 produced by granulosa cells, through conversion of theca cell-derived precursors, FSH enhances the mitotic activity of the granulosa cells. Consequently, the number of granulosa cells increases rapidly and the number of FSH receptors enlarges both with the growing number of granulosa cells and with the number of FSH receptors per granulosa cell. The androgens necessary for aromatization to the estrogens involved in this process are provided by the surrounding theca cells. In an abnormally high androgen milieu within the ovary, such as that encountered in many patients with polycystic ovarian syndrome, the FSH-stimulated conversion of androgens to estrogens and normal follicle development through FSH/estrogen-mediated granulosa cell proliferation are inhibited. Follicle atresia results.

As the preantral follicle proliferates under the combined effects of FSH and E_2, follicular fluid accumulates, forming the so-called antrum, whereby the follicle advances from the preantral to the antral stage. Follicular fluid contains both steroids and gonadotropins.[5] It provides a reservoir of potentially stimulatory and inhibitory factors for the oocyte and its surrounding granulosa cells. The combination of follicular fluid FSH and E_2 favors follicle maturation to the preovulatory state, whereas intrafollicular androgens and LH inhibit further granulosa cell mitosis. Enhanced by E_2, FSH induces LH receptors on granulosa cells. The midcycle rise of LH provides enough LH to react with these receptors, halt granulosa cell proliferation, and initiate P production. The appearance of LH in follicular fluid and its interaction with granulosa cell LH receptors are physiologic happenings at midcycle. The progressive enlargement of the antral cavity parallels both follicle maturation and E_2 production. It is easily detected by ultrasonography using a high-resolution sector scanner. Ultrasound is most valuable for assessing follicle development. Table 5-1 presents plasma FSH, LH, and E_2 levels corresponding to dominant follicle diameters measured with ultrasound.[6]

Recent research has focused on the mechanism of follicle selection. In the beginning of

Table 5-1
Endocrine and ultrasonic predictors of ovulation

Days to ovulation	FSH (mIU/mL)	LH (mIU/mL)	Estradiol (pg/mL)	Follicle diameter (mm)
7	5.9	11.9	98	8.9
5	4.8	11.7	118	13.4
4	4.5	11.3	129	14.4
3	4.1	10.4	174	17.4
2	4.0	12.6	221	18.1
1	4.9	24.1	290	20.9
0	7.7	42.6	256	24.6

The data represent means of data obtained in 14 women with normal ovulatory cycles. From Bryce RL, Shuter B, Sinosich MJ, et al: The value of ultrasound, gonadotropin and estradiol measurements for precise ovulation prediction. Fertil Steril 37:42, 1982. Reproduced with permission of the publisher, The American Fertility Society.

each cycle, circulating FSH and, to a lesser degree, LH levels rise and initiate the proliferation of a cohort of follicles. Follicle development is associated with a rise in ovarian E_2 secretion. By cycle days 5 to 7, the ovary bearing the dominant follicle, which is destined to ovulate and to become the next corpus luteum, secretes more E_2 than the contralateral ovary.[7] This is interpreted as indicating that the dominant follicle has been selected by cycle days 5 to 7.

The dominant follicle produces rapidly increasing quantities of E_2, which accomplish a variety of objectives: E_2 (1) enhances the number of granulosa cells and density of FSH receptors for further rapid proliferation, despite declining concentrations of circulating FSH; (2) decreases circulating FSH levels through an amazingly sensitive negative feedback mechanism; and (3) stops the development of other follicles within the cohort of proliferating follicles by lowering circulating FSH concentrations. The last occurs because all developing follicles, except the dominant one, have fewer granulosa cells, lower granulosa cell FSH receptor density, and lower intrafollicular E_2 levels than the dominant one. When the decreasing FSH levels become inadequate, they become atretic.

The tremendously increased sensitivity of the dominant follicle to FSH, resulting from the FSH-E_2 amplifier effect characteristic of granulosa cell function, allows the dominant follicle to continue its development to the preovulatory state. This proceeds despite the E_2-mediated decline in circulating FSH during the second half of the follicular phase. Other factors are also involved. The theca cells of the dominant follicle begin to become vascularized by the seventh day of the cycle.[7] Two days later, the theca cell apparatus of the dominant follicle is twice as vascularized as that of other antral follicles. This feature allows the former much better access to the dwindling levels of circulating FSH.

Ovulation

The fully developed preovulatory follicle is approximately 20 mm in diameter. Multiple layers of granulosa cells line the antral side of the basement membrane, and a cumulus of granulosa cells surrounds the oocyte covered by its zona pellucida. The surrounding theca cell apparatus is fully vascularized by now. The preovulatory follicle produces rapidly increasing amounts of E_2, which account for about 80% of the approximately 500 µg of E_2 produced each day during the preovulatory phase. The remainder of E_2 is produced by the other developing follicles as well as by peripheral conversion from T and E_1. The peak E_2 production is reached about 24 hours (range, 17 to 32 hours) before ovulation.[8]

In response to rising plasma E_2 levels, LH secretion increases as outlined above. This rise in LH starts a rise in P production by the dominant follicle through interaction with the LH receptors at the granulosa cells. Circulating P levels are substantially increased above those achieved in the follicular phase. In conjunction with the rise in E_2, the small but significant increase in circulating P, which occurs 12 to 24 hours before ovulation, elicits a rapid and marked surge in LH secretion and evokes the accompanying midcycle FSH peak.[9] It is possible to predict the day of the midcycle LH peak by measuring the marked midcycle rise in serum P levels or urinary pregnanediol glucuronide excretion that occurs before the crest of the LH surge.[10] Thus, the preovulatory follicle, when ready, provides its own signal—a continued and pronounced rise in E_2, followed by a small but significant increase in P, which produces the midcycle LH/FSH peak by positive feedback mechanisms. The latter rise initiates ovulation.

The actual events of ovulation—rupture of the follicle and extrusion of the oocyte surrounded by the cumulus of granulosa cells—occur about 16 hours after the crest of the LH peak, according to results of a multicenter World Health Organization (WHO) study,[11] and about 10 to 12 hours after the LH peak, as estimated by in vitro fertilization studies.[6] Both groups of investigators agree that ovulation takes place about 32 hours after the initial rise of the midcycle LH surge. These midcycle alterations in circulating or urinary LH levels appear to be the most predictive hormonal indicators that the maturing follicle is about to ovulate.

The midcycle LH surge evokes ovulation by (1) stimulating prostaglandin (PG) synthesis and (2) initiating completion of the first meiotic division of the oocyte. The LH surge also causes a decrease in E_2 production. LH effects luteinization of granulosa cells and increases P biosynthesis. These LH-induced and cyclic AMP-mediated hormonal events override the inhibiting influence of nonsteroidal substances on oocyte maturation and luteinization. Such products have recently been shown to be present in antral fluid and, in contradistinction to follicular inhibition, to act within the follicle rather than centrally by influencing gonadotropin secretion.[12]

Both PGF and PGE rise as a result of the LH surge. These increases have been shown to be necessary for follicle rupture.[13] This event was blocked in rats and rabbits by administering indomethacin and by inhibition of PG synthesis.[14] Furthermore, LH induces the production of proteolytic enzymes (collagenases). These and PGF and PGE generated in the preovulatory follicle are essential for follicle rupture and extrusion of the oocyte. FSH rises concomitantly with the midcycle LH surge. This increase in FSH appears to stimulate the production of a plasminogen activator that converts plasminogen to the proteolytic enzyme plasmin.[15] The latter appears to allow the cumulus to become detached from the parietal granulosa cells and extrude readily at the time of follicle rupture. Finally, it is thought that the short midcycle FSH burst may be of importance for the conversion of the granulosa cells of the ovulating follicle into a properly functioning and hormonally competent corpus luteum.

Corpus luteum formation

Follicle rupture is associated with a loss of follicular fluid and extrusion of the oocyte. The follicle wall, consisting of the parietal granulosa cells, basement membrane, and theca cells, loses its stabilizing tension and becomes convoluted. The granulosa and surrounding cells become luteinized. They take up lipids and lutein pigment, which confers their typical yellow appearance. Whereas the theca cells of the dominant follicle become vascularized during the second half of the follicular phase, vascularization of the granulosa cells begins after ovulation, with the formation of the corpus luteum. The latter produces P in amounts of about 20 mg/24 hr and, in addition, secretes E_2.

P and E_2 production increases from the early postovulatory phase to reach peak levels during the midluteal phase and decline toward the end of the menstrual cycle. The biosynthesis of P by the corpus luteum requires continued LH stimulation.[16] The corpus luteum produces more than 80% of all the P generated during the luteal phase of the cycle by both the ovaries and the adrenals. The production and secretion of P by the corpus luteum reflect its functional state. A poorly developed corpus luteum, likely the result of inappropriate follicle maturation, produces inadequate quantities of P. Thus, measurement of circulating P or of its urinary metabolite, pregnanediol glucuronide, provides evidence for the existence and quality of the corpus luteum.

Within the ovary, P suppresses follicle maturation locally. diZerega and Hodgen observed in primates that ovulation in the subsequent cycle will occur in the ovary that secretes less P than the contralateral one. This finding indicates that intraovarian P concentrations negatively affect follicle maturation and recruitment of the next dominant follicle.[17] Also, the combined secretion of P and E_2 results in decreased FSH and LH secretion via negative feedback mechanisms, eliminating the central gonadotropic stimulus for follicle development. The pulsatile pattern of circulating LH persists during the luteal phase, but LH pulses become less frequent and lower in amplitude.[18] Irrespective of decreasing LH stimulation, the life span of the corpus luteum appears limited and the corpus luteum seems to progressively lose sensitivity to LH stimulation. Furthermore, there is evidence that through its E_2 production the corpus luteum exerts a certain degree of luteolytic ac-

tion. It remains to be established whether this luteolytic effect of E_2, which has been substantiated in vivo and in vitro,[19] acts by reducing LH receptors or LH receptor binding, and/or is mediated by prostaglandins.

Only the rapidly rising levels of circulating human chorionic gonadotropin (hCG), which become detectable 8 days after the midcycle LH peak, are capable of rescuing the corpus luteum from its otherwise inevitable fate of regression and involution. But, despite the logarithmic rise in circulating hCG, P secretion by the corpus luteum remains limited and its hormone production actually declines well before hCG levels peak at 9 to 10 weeks' gestation. When corpus luteum function ceases at the end of the menstrual cycle, the decline in circulating P and E_2 results in a rise of FSH and LH.[3] The latter rise initiates renewed follicle development and recruitment of a new dominant follicle within the cohort of developing follicles.

Hypothalamic-pituitary regulation of ovarian function

Cyclic ovarian function depends on appropriately timed and quantitated secretion of both FSH and LH by the anterior pituitary gland in response to hypothalamic GnRH. Release of the latter by the hypothalamus and, in turn, FSH and LH secretion by the anterior pituitary in response to GnRH are modulated by E_2 and P reaching these centers. Hypothalamic-pituitary-ovarian feedback mechanisms consist of (1) FSH and LH secretion during the early follicular phase in response to low serum E_2 and P levels, after the preceding corpus luteum ceases to function (negative feedback response); (2) reduced FSH secretion during the mid- to late follicular phase, in response to rising E_2 produced by maturing follicles (negative feedback response); (3) the midcycle rise of LH, in response to the preovulatory E_2 surge initiating ovulation and corpus luteum function (positive feedback response); and (4) reduced FSH and LH secretion during the luteal phase, in response to E_2 and P secreted by the corpus luteum (negative feedback response).

Hypothalamic-pituitary regulation of ovarian cyclicity, however, is governed not only by steroid hormones, signaling the functional state of the ovary, but also by neural stimuli from extrahypothalamic parts of the central nervous system (CNS), mediating input from the external as well as internal environment through bioaminergic neurons. For example, it is known that stress or profound weight loss can cause amenorrhea. Thus, the hypothalamus functions as an integration center for both neural and hormonal signals, which are then translated into GnRH secretion.

GnRH reaches the anterior pituitary gland via the blood traveling through the hypothalamic-pituitary portal vessels. Unlike the posterior pituitary, the anterior pituitary has no neuronal connections to the brain. Its only line of communication consists of the hypothalamic-pituitary portal vessels. The superior hypophyseal artery supplies a system of capillaries within the hypothalamus that represents the proximal part of the portal system. When these tributaries reach the anterior pituitary, they form a secondary vascular plexus before they leave the anterior pituitary as veins. Pituitary FSH and LH secretion is modulated in response to blood-borne GnRH as well as E_2 and P. Hypothalamic-pituitary regulation of ovarian function is outlined below.

Hypothalamic GnRH secretion

The hypothalamus regulates gonadotropin secretion via GnRH, a decapeptide. Axons of GnRH neurosecretory cells, whose cell bodies are located in the basal hypothalamus, terminate around the capillaries within the median eminence, which make up the primary vascular plexus of the pituitary portal vessels. These carry GnRH, as well as the other well-known hypo-

physiotropic hormones, to the pituicytes. GnRH can be measured by radioimmunoassay (RIA). However, current RIA methods are not sensitive enough to quantitate the minute concentrations of GnRH present in peripheral plasma.

Studies that describe GnRH levels in peripheral plasma appear to indicate a tendency for a midcycle rise. However, peripheral plasma levels of GnRH do not seem to be of too much importance. Because GnRH travels in the portal blood from the hypothalamus to the anterior pituitary, where it exerts its biologic function, portal blood levels are of much greater physiologic importance than peripheral levels. Neill and co-workers measured GnRH in pituitary stalk (portal) blood of rhesus monkeys and found that mean GnRH levels rose from approximately 10 to 30 pg/mL during the follicular phase to about 40 to 300 pg/mL at the time of the preovulatory LH surge, and also after ovariectomy, when LH was elevated as well.[20] These data show a high correlation between pituitary stalk (portal) plasma concentrations of GnRH and peripheral plasma LH levels. They indicate that both positive and negative feedback mechanisms are mediated, in part, by hypothalamic GnRH secretion in response to changing E_2 and P levels.

GnRH is secreted episodically. A prerequisite for normal hypothalamic-pituitary control of cyclic ovarian function, via GnRH-mediated FSH and LH secretion, is that GnRH is released in pulses of appropriate frequency and amplitude. Constant GnRH secretion causes downregulation of the gonadotrophs, most likely through internalization of their GnRH receptors. Down-regulation of the gonadotrophs results in complete absence of LH and FSH secretion and, therefore, in lack of follicle development as well as ovarian steroid hormone production, manifest clinically as amenorrhea.

Leyendecker and co-workers pioneered the periodic IV administration of GnRH to women with hypothalamic amenorrhea.[21] By giving 15- or 20-μg pulses of GnRH every 90 minutes by a portable pump, these authors were able to produce follicle development and ovulation. Based on these data, it was presumed that GnRH pulse frequency in humans is about one pulse every 90 minutes. In a more recent study, Reame and collaborators measured plasma LH and FSH levels every 10 to 20 minutes for 12 to 24 hours at 7-day intervals during the same ovulatory cycle in eight volunteers.[22] They established that the LH pulse frequency averages 12 to 24 pulses per 12 hours during the follicular phase and only eight pulses per 12 hours during the luteal phase. As LH pulses are synchronous with the episodes of GnRH release, it can be concluded that the GnRH pulse frequency in women is about one pulse every hour during the follicular phase and approximately one pulse every 90 minutes during the luteal phase of the cycle. Recently, Filicori and co-workers demonstrated that pulses further decrease in frequency during the late luteal phase.[18]

The generation of GnRH pulses takes place in the arcuate nucleus (Figure 5-1). For cyclic ovarian function, this most important hypothalamic nucleus contains the bodies of GnRH-producing neurons, which deliver GnRH along their axons (the tubero-infundibular tract) to the capillaries of the portal system. GnRH pulse frequency and amplitude are modulated by dopamine and norepinephrine. These catecholamines are generated, in part, within the arcuate nucleus or reach the arcuate nucleus from other hypothalamic or suprahypothalamic centers via neuronal pathways.

Dopamine suppresses and norepinephrine stimulates GnRH pulse activity. These catecholamines are modulated by β-endorphins as well as by catecholestrogens. β-Endorphin appears to enhance the inhibitory effect of dopamine on GnRH pulsatile activity. In a dose- and time-dependent manner, circulating E_2 and P levels influence catecholestrogen, β-endorphin, norepinephrine, and dopamine levels via the long-loop feedback (Figure 5-1). In this way, sex hormone

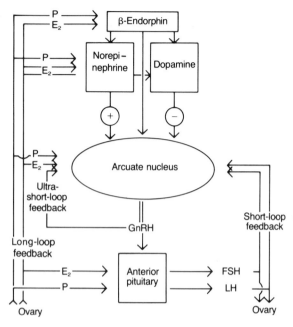

Figure 5-1
Regulation of pulsatile hypothalamic GnRH secretion.

levels regulate the frequency and amplitude of GnRH pulses generated by the arcuate nucleus. GnRH itself, through so-called ultrashort-loop feedback, influences its own secretion. By stimulating pituitary FSH and LH secretion, which inhibits hypothalamic GnRH secretion via the so-called short-loop feedback, GnRH further modulates its own secretion.

Pituitary FSH and LH secretion

The basophilic gonadotropin-producing cells, the so-called gonadotrophs, of the anterior gland synthesize and episodically secrete FSH and LH in response to GnRH pulses. The response of the gonadotrophs to GnRH is modulated by E_2 and P. FSH and LH are glycoproteins that, like hCG and thyroid-stimulating hormone (TSH), contain a common α-subunit of approximately 90 amino acids, but different β-subunits. Both subunits are linked by disulfide bridges. The β-subunits of all three gonadotropins, as well as of TSH, differ in amino acid and carbohydrate contents, thus providing specificity for each of these four hormones. The α-subunits of these hormones appear to be more abundant than the β-subunits. Synthesis of the β-subunits therefore appears to be the rate-limiting step in the production of these hormones.

FSH and LH can be measured in serum (plasma) or urine by RIAs as well as by bioassays. Before RIAs were available, FSH and LH were measured by bioassays: FSH was determined by the Steelman-Pohley ovarian weight augmentation assay in hypophysectomized rats; LH was quantitated by the ovarian ascorbic acid depletion assay. The modern bioassay of LH uses Leydig cell cultures. The endpoint of this LH bioassay is T formation, which is readily quantitated by a specific steroid RIA. Serum (plasma) FSH and LH are most commonly measured by RIAs. Levels are reported either as international milliunits per milliliter, which refer to international reference preparations as standards, or as nanograms per milliliter, utilizing an internationally accepted reference preparation as standard.

It must be emphasized that neither FSH nor LH is a homogeneous molecule. The pituitary secretes different FSH and LH molecules. This fact is readily observed when aliquots of serial serum or urine specimens from the same subject are submitted for both bioassay and RIA: Radioimmunoassayable FSH or LH levels may differ substantially from their bioassay-determined concentrations.[23] The immuno-to-bioassay ratios also may vary among different samples from the same subject. Circulating LH and FSH have different half-lives. The half-life of radioimmunoassayable LH has been reported to be about 20 minutes, whereas the half-life of the initial disappearance phase of radioimmunoassayable FSH has been quoted as 3.9 hours. Both LH and FSH are secreted episodically in response to GnRH pulses. Because of its shorter half-life, the episodic fluctuations of serum LH are much more pronounced than those of FSH.

By infusing submaximal doses of GnRH for several hours to women at various stages of the menstrual cycle, Yen and collaborators established the concept of two functioning pools of pituitary gonadotropins: (1) a pool of acutely releasable LH and FSH, which they equated with the sensitivity of the gonadotrophs, and (2) a second pool of gonadotropins, which becomes releasable after repeated GnRH stimulation.[24] The latter pool is considered to represent pituitary gonadotropin reserve. The combined size of both pituitary sensitivity (pool 1) and reserve (pool 2) has been termed the functional capacity of the gonadotrophs. GnRH induces synthesis (pool 2) and release (pool 1) of gonadotropins. Its positive effects on the gonadotrophs are amplified by the high (preovulatory) levels of circulating E_2.

Negative and positive feedback

Two principal feedback mechanisms are essential for the appropriate coordination of both the endocrine and morphologic events of the menstrual cycle, as well as for the initiation of a subsequent cycle: (1) negative and (2) positive feedback. Negative feedback consists of suppression of FSH and LH secretion in response to elevated E_2 and P levels and, conversely, increased FSH and LH secretion in response to decreasing or low E_2 and P concentrations. Estradiol appears to inhibit mainly FSH secretion, whereas P, in combination with E_2, seems to reduce both LH and FSH secretion. Negative feedback response is observed during the follicular and luteal phases. Positive feedback entails a stimulatory effect of progressively rising E_2 levels (which exceed a certain threshold before circulating P concentrations increase) upon LH secretion. This phenomenon is observed in response to the preovulatory E_2 surge. It may also be elicited by exogenous E_2 administered so that a marked serum E_2 rise is achieved over a few days.

In the past, the pattern of gonadotropin secretion during the menstrual cycle has been described as consisting of a "tonic" and a "cyclic" mode. "Tonic" gonadotropin secretion referred to FSH and LH secretion in the follicular and luteal phases; "cyclic" secretion was used to describe the midcycle LH/FSH surge. Although hypothalamic centers apparently responsible for tonic and cyclic gonadotropin secretion have been identified in the rat hypothalamus, no such centers have been found in primates. Hypothalamic lesions in humans abolish both tonic and cyclic gonadotropin secretion. Furthermore, LH and FSH are secreted episodically throughout the menstrual cycle, although their pulse frequencies and amplitudes vary. Hence the terms "tonic" and "cyclic" convey little information. Knobil has suggested the term "tonic secretion" be replaced by "basal secretion," in contradistinction to the midcycle LH and FSH surge.[25] More appropriately, one should refer instead to mechanisms of negative and positive hypothalamic-pituitary-ovarian feedback response.

Negative feedback control is known to undergo changes in its sensitivity to sex steroids during fetal and neonatal life and to reach a very sensitive "set point" prior to age 2. Before initiation of puberty, the negative feedback operates at a low set point of sex hormone levels. Puberty is triggered by a readjustment of negative feedback control to operate at a higher set point of steroid concentrations. Positive feedback control matures during puberty.

Estradiol is most effective in evoking a negative feedback response with regard to FSH release. If circulating E_2 levels fall, FSH secretion rises promptly. This is observed at the onset of menstruation, when the corpus luteum ceases to secrete E_2 and P. Conversely, serum FSH levels decline during the second half of the follicular phase, when the dominant follicle secretes increasing amounts of E_2, as well as during the luteal phase. Granulosa cells produce and secrete inhibin, a nonsteroidal substance that suppresses FSH secretion and may be responsible, in part, for the preovulatory decline in circulating

FSH. The effect of circulating E_2 on LH secretion is complex: Circulating E_2 below a certain level and/or of limited duration activates a negative LH feedback response. Furthermore, concomitant elevation of E_2 and P during the luteal phase results in decreased LH secretion. However, when circulating E_2 levels rise beyond a critical threshold of approximately 200 pg/mL, and are maintained at this level or above for at least 2 days, LH secretion increases in a positive feedback response. The latter is the primary stimulus for the midcycle LH surge.

To study the roles of E_2 and P in eliciting the midcycle LH/FSH surge (positive feedback response) in humans, March et al conducted the following experiments.[9] Parous women of reproductive age who had undergone hysterectomy and bilateral salpingo-oophorectomy for benign disease received subdermal implants of 25-mg E_2 pellets at gonadectomy and every 6 months thereafter. Their serum E_2 levels were 60 to 125 pg/mL (midfollicular phase), and serum LH and FSH levels remained in the normal to borderline elevated range. These women received IM injections of gradually increasing amounts of E_2 benzoate alone and in combination with P administered via release from intravaginal P-impregnated polysiloxane rings. When only E_2 benzoate was injected, increasing serum E_2 levels mimicking the preovulatory E_2 peak were followed by a marked surge in LH, but not in FSH (Figure 5-2). When P was administered after serum E_2 levels had already risen to preovulatory concentrations, the LH surge occurred earlier, was more pronounced, and was accompanied by a rise in FSH. However, when both E_2 benzoate and P were administered simultaneously, and serum P levels rose before serum E_2 concentrations had increased to preovulatory levels, no LH or FSH surge occurred (Figure 5-2).

Similar results were obtained by other investigators.[26] These data allow the conclusion that E_2 is the primary signal for the positive

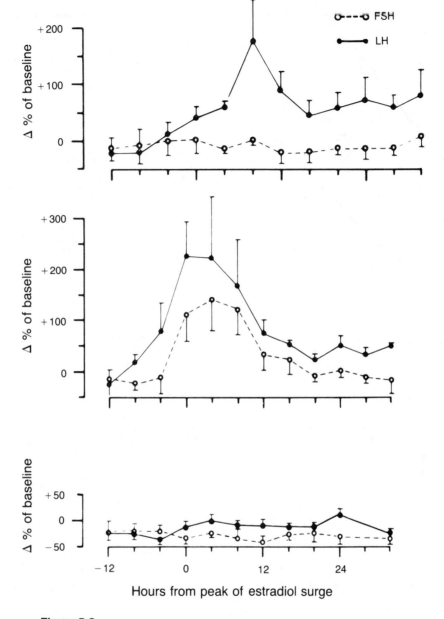

Figure 5-2
FSH and LH response to rising serum estradiol (E₂) levels comparable to the midcycle E₂ peak alone (top panel) following IM E₂ administration in three oophorectomized women; when serum progesterone (P) rises 36 hours after E₂ has begun to rise (middle panel); and when P rises concomitantly with E₂ (bottom panel).

Adapted from March CM, Goebelsmann U, Nakamura RM, et al: Roles of estradiol and progesterone in eliciting the midcycle luteinizing hormone and follicle-stimulating hormone surges. J Clin Endocrinol Metab 49:507, 1979.

feedback response at midcycle. However, as shown in monkeys and humans, it requires a certain strength and duration. Furthermore, the positive feedback response can be blocked or facilitated by P: If circulating P levels rise before a critical level of E_2 has been reached and maintained for a certain length of time, positive feedback is inhibited. However, if P levels rise moderately, after the rise in circulating E_2 has achieved preovulatory concentrations, the E_2-mediated release of LH is accelerated and a concomitant FSH peak is evoked.[9]

This concept of positive feedback is supported by the study of Thorneycroft and coworkers, who conducted frequent measurements of serum E_2, P, LH, and FSH in periovulatory women (Figure 5-3).[27] These data indicate that a rise of serum P precedes the midcycle LH and FSH surge, whereas serum E_2 levels fall when the LH peak is achieved.

The sites of E_2 and P action that elicit both negative and positive feedback have been the subject of numerous studies. Research in monkeys with hypothalamic lesions suggested that both negative and positive gonadotropin feedback functions could be maintained if GnRH pulses were administered to compensate for the lack of endogenous GnRH pulsatile activity,[25] but could not be maintained without GnRH. These data led to the conclusion that GnRH plays only a permissive, albeit mandatory, role, whereas negative and positive feedback responses occur primarily in the pituitary.

E_2 and P are known to change the pulsatile activity of GnRH (1) through direct effects on the neurons of the arcuate nucleus, the GnRH pulse generator, (2) through effects on norepinephrine and dopamine neuronal activity stimulating and inhibiting GnRH pulsatile activity, respectively, and (3) via effects on catecholestrogen and β-endorphin mechanisms that modulate norepinephrine and dopamine activity. Evidence has been presented that the rate and amplitude of GnRH pulses vary under the

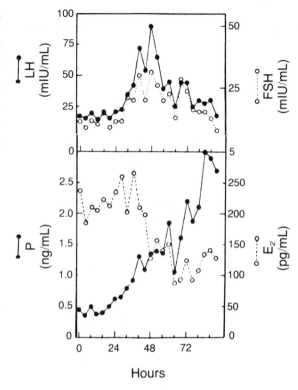

Figure 5-3
Serum FSH, LH, estradiol (E_2), and progesterone (P) around midcycle.

From Thorneycroft IH, Sribyatta B, Tom WK, et al: Measurement of serum LH, FSH, progesterone, 17-hydroxyprogesterone, and estradiol-17β levels at 4-hour intervals during the periovulatory phase of the menstrual cycle. J Clin Endocrinol Metab 39:754, 1974.

influence of E_2 and P. This indicates that these steroids exert an important effect on negative and positive feedback responses via hypothalamic centers.

The recent work of Filicori and associates showed that the frequency of LH pulses closely correlated with GnRH pulsatile activity progressively decreases during the luteal phase in a manner that appears to correlate with the duration of exposure to luteal phase serum P concentrations.[18] It slows down from a rate of one pulse every 60 to 90 minutes, during the follicular

Normal endocrinology

phase, to one pulse every 99, 162, and 173 minutes, during the early, mid-, and late luteal phases, respectively. Furthermore, primate studies indicate that the combined elevation of circulating E_2 and P raises hypothalamic levels of β-endorphin. The latter is known to decrease GnRH pulsatile activity, either by reducing norepinephrine activity or by increasing dopamine activity. Therefore, one must conclude that negative and positive feedback occurs through E_2- and P-mediated effects at both the pituitary and the hypothalamic level. Many facets of the interplay of sex hormones, gonadotropins, GnRH, bioamines, catecholestrogens, β-endorphin, and perhaps other substances that regulate hypothalamic-pituitary-ovarian feedback still remain to be elucidated.

Quantitative and temporal aspects of hormonal alterations throughout the cycle

Quantitative aspects

Before highly sensitive RIA techniques for the measurement of hormones in plasma or serum became available, gonadotropins and steroid hormones were measured in urine by bioassays and physicochemical methods. Urine extracts were purified and subjected to bioassay (FSH, LH, estrogen) or colorimetry (estrogens, pregnanediol) for quantitation. Whereas urinary FSH and LH excretion amount to approximately 1 to 10 IU/24 hr, serum or plasma levels range from 1 or 2 to 100 mIU/mL. With the development of specific RIAs, it became possible to measure FSH and LH directly in serum or plasma. The patterns of serum FSH and LH measured by RIA daily during the menstrual cycle are similar to those obtained by measuring urinary FSH and LH by bioassay. The midcycle serum LH peak coincides with a simultaneous urinary LH

surge. Instead of the short and much smaller concomitant elevation of serum FSH, however, a modest rise in urinary FSH occurs 2 days after the midcycle LH peak (Figure 5-4).[23] This discrepancy can be explained, in part, by the differences in the short half-life of LH (approximately 20 minutes) and the much longer half-life of FSH (about 3.9 hours).

In 1955, Brown developed a colorimetric method for the determination of the three "classical" urinary estrogens: E_1, E_2, and E_3.[28] Urinary excretion of all three estrogens (measured fluorometrically) is lowest during the early follicular phase, rises toward midcycle, peaks before or at the midcycle LH peak, decreases thereafter, and rises again in the luteal phase. This luteal phase increase in E_2 is smaller, but of longer duration, than the preovulatory E_2 peak. The amount of estrogen excreted decreases before menstruation. The major estrogen secreted by the ovary is E_2. It is metabolized to E_1 and E_3 by the liver. Of these three estrogens, E_3 is biologically the least active and is excreted in the greatest amount. Estradiol is the most potent estrogen and is excreted in the least amount. The peak excretion of all three estrogens combined totals 50 to 75 μg/24 hr at midcycle.

Progesterone is the product of the corpus luteum. Before it was possible to measure serum P by RIA, measurement of its major metabolite, pregnanediol (PD), in urine was used as an indicator of ovulation. When determined by gas chromatography, urinary PD excretion averages 0.4 mg/24 hr (consistently less than 0.9 mg/24 hr) during the follicular phase and begins to rise concomitantly with the midcycle LH peak. It reaches mean luteal phase levels of 3 to 4 mg/24 hr (consistently more than 1 mg/24 hr). The subject-to-subject variation of urinary PD excretion is considerably less than that of estrogen excretion. The level of PD increases about tenfold from the follicular phase to the luteal phase. For these reasons, a single PD determination during the luteal phase may be used to provide pre-

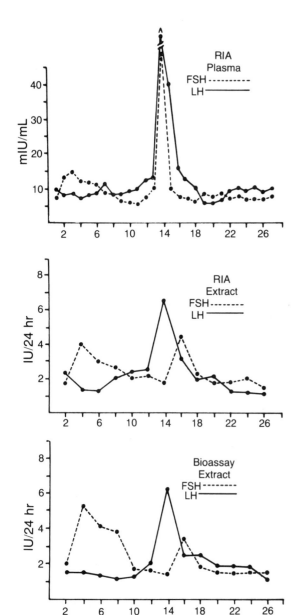

Figure 5-4
Serum FSH and LH measured by radioimmunoassay (RIA) and urinary FSH and LH measured by RIA as well as by bioassay through an entire ovulatory menstrual cycle.

From Stevens VC: Comparison of FSH and LH patterns in plasma, urine and urinary extracts during the menstrual cycle. J Clin Endocrinol Metab 29:904, 1969.

sumptive evidence as to whether or not ovulation has occurred.

More recently, specific RIAs have been developed for the direct measurement of urinary pregnanediol 3-glucuronide (PD-3G), without hydrolysis and extraction.[10] As shown in Figure 5-5, both total 24-hour and overnight urinary PD-3G facilitate convenient detection of ovulation and assessment of corpus luteum function. Such tests can be carried out in a few minutes and require only a special spectrophotometer, rather than the instruments for measuring radioactivity that are needed to conduct RIAs. Ongoing research in this field promises the availability of an enzyme-mediated color reaction, which is the endpoint of a direct immunoassay for urinary PD-3G. Available as a simple kit, this test may be used to detect ovulation within minutes in the office or even at home.

With the development of specific RIAs in the late 1960s and early 1970s, it became possible to measure sex hormones in serum or plasma. Estradiol, P, and 17-hydroxyprogesterone (17-OHP) have all been measured during many menstrual cycles.[29] As depicted in Figure 5-6, serum E_2 concentrations rise from less than 50 pg/mL, in the early follicular phase, to a midcycle (preovulatory) peak ranging from 200 to 500 pg/mL. Concentrations fall rapidly thereafter and rise again to a smaller, but broader, luteal phase serum E_2 peak of about 100 to 150 pg/mL. Progesterone levels are well below 1 ng/mL during the follicular phase, begin to rise at the onset of the midcycle LH surge, and reach about 10 to 20 ng/mL during the luteal phase peak, which parallels that of serum E_2. Israel and co-workers reported that a single serum P level above 3 ng/mL obtained between 11 and 4 days before the onset of the next menstruation could be considered presumptive evidence that ovulation has occurred.[30] However, serum P measurements in cycles that resulted in normal pregnancies indicate that a normally functioning corpus luteum produces midluteal serum P concentrations of at

Normal endocrinology

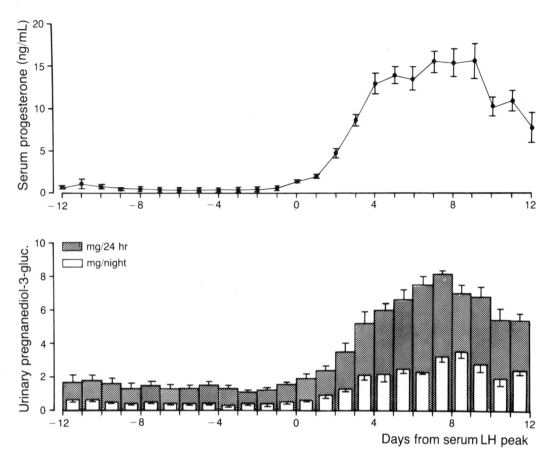

Figure 5-5
Means and standard errors of daily 8:00 AM serum progesterone concentrations and 24-hour (8:00 AM to 8:00 AM) and overnight urinary excretion of radioimmunoassayable pregnanediol 3-glucuronide in seven women during an entire menstrual cycle. The data obtained in individual subjects were grouped according to the day of the midcycle LH peak and averaged.

Reproduced, with permission, from Stanczyk FZ, Miyakawa I, Goebelsmann U: Direct radioimmunoassay of urinary estrogen and pregnanediol glucuronides during the menstrual cycle. Am J Obstet Gynecol 137:443, 1980.

least 8 to 10 ng/mL (depending on the particular RIA used).[31]

Although a single serum P measurement during the midluteal phase can be used as presumptive evidence of ovulation, a low serum P level (<8 μg/mL) may either be indicative of inadequate corpus luteum function or represent a nadir in circulating P at the time of blood drawing. Filicori and collaborators have shown in their frequent sampling studies of circulating LH and P that luteal phase serum P levels may vary considerably in response to episodic LH secretion.[18] The latter study casts doubt on the diagnostic value of a single serum P measurement if this happens to be low. Overnight urinary PD-3G measurements allow one to circumvent the uncertainty associated with episodic variation in serum P levels. During the follicular phase, over-

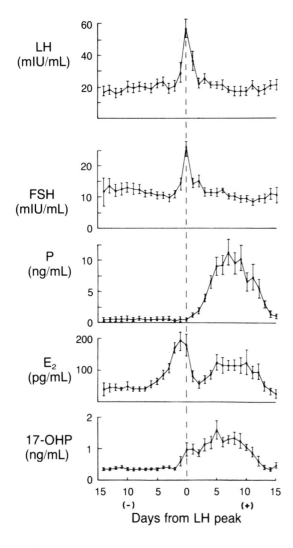

LH (mIU/mL)

FSH (mIU/mL)

P (ng/mL)

E₂ (pg/mL)

17-OHP (ng/mL)

Days from LH peak

Figure 5-6
Means and standard errors of serum LH, FSH, progesterone (P), estradiol (E₂), and 17-hydroxyprogesterone (17-OHP) measured in nine women daily during an entire ovulatory menstrual cycle. Individual daily results were grouped according to the day of the midcycle LH peak and averaged.

From Thorneycroft IH, Mishell DR Jr, Stone SC, et al: The relation of serum 17-hydroxyprogesterone and estradiol-17β levels during the human menstrual cycle. Am J Obstet Gynecol 111:947, 1971.

night urinary PD-3G excretion remains well below 1 mg. It exceeds 2 mg during the midluteal phase.[10]

Levels of 17-hydroxyprogesterone average less than 0.5 ng/mL during the follicular phase and begin to rise at the same time as the initial rise of the midcycle LH surge.[27,29] Serum 17-OHP levels reach a luteal phase peak of 1 to 2 ng/mL, which coincides with the serum P peak. Circulating 17-OHP does not appear to be involved in negative or positive gonadotropin feedback. Although luteal phase 17-OHP levels exceed follicular phase concentrations, 17-OHP is not used clinically as presumptive evidence of ovulation. The serum levels of all three steroids (E₂, P, and 17-OHP) begin to decrease 4 to 6 days before the onset of menstruation.

Statistically analyzed, serum concentrations of LH, FSH, P, and E₂ follow a log-normal rather than a normal distribution; that is, the spread of values above the mean is greater than that below the mean.[32] For this reason, 95% confidence limits calculated by rankit or probit analysis (taking the log-normal distribution into account) represent a more appropriate reference scheme for clinical interpretation of laboratory results for most hormones than do calculated standard deviations.

In addition to LH, FSH, E₂, 17-OHP, and P, many other hormones have been measured in plasma or serum throughout the menstrual cycle. Serum concentrations of both A and T (Figures 5-7 and 5-8) exhibit only small changes during the menstrual cycle. When the means of daily serum A and T levels of six to eight women were measured throughout their menstrual cycles, levels of both androgens appeared to be higher during the follicular phase than during the second half of the luteal phase.[33,34] It is well known that under normal circumstances neither serum A levels nor serum T levels play a significant role in the regulation of the menstrual cycle. One should also consider the fact that serum levels of steroid hormones depend not only on

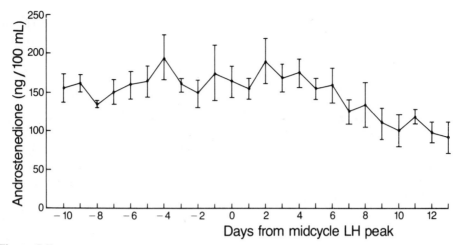

Figure 5-7
Means and standard errors of serum androstenedione concentrations measured in six women daily during an entire ovulatory menstrual cycle. Individual daily results were grouped according to the day of the preovulatory serum estradiol peak and averaged.

From Ribeiro WO, Mishell DR Jr, Thorneycroft IH: Comparison of the patterns of androstenedione, progesterone, and estradiol during the human menstrual cycle. Am J Obstet Gynecol 119:1026, 1974.

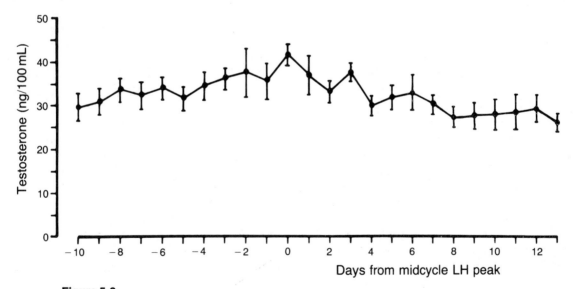

Figure 5-8
Means and standard errors of serum testosterone concentrations measured daily in eight women during an entire ovulatory menstrual cycle. Individual daily results were grouped according to the day of the midcycle LH peak and averaged.

From Goebelsmann U, Arce JJ, Thorneycroft IH, et al: Serum testosterone concentrations in women throughout the menstrual cycle and following hCG administration. Am J Obstet Gynecol 119:445, 1974.

their rate of secretion but also on their metabolic clearance rate. These are explained and listed in Chapter 3.

Temporal relationship of gonadotropins and steroid hormones

The patterns of FSH, LH, and sex hormones measured in urine or serum during numerous menstrual cycles (Figures 5-3 to 5-6) not only convey normal values but also exemplify temporal and causal relationships. The hormonal patterns are consistent with the following concept of the menstrual cycle: During the early follicular phase, the ovary secretes only small quantities of E_2 and P. In response to negative feedback, FSH and LH secretion is increased to stimulate follicle development. As a cohort of follicles matures, E_2 is consequently secreted in steadily increasing amounts. FSH secretion falls in response to rising E_2 concentrations—again an example of negative feedback. The final stage of follicle maturation is associated with the preovulatory E_2 peak. Rapidly rising serum E_2 levels, in turn, cause a further decrease in FSH secretion and initiate the midcycle LH surge.

Frequent hormone assays performed near midcycle provide detailed information about the sequence of hormonal events (Figure 5-3): The preovulatory E_2 peak is clearly the first hormonal event. Serum LH levels rise in response to increasing serum E_2. This midcycle LH surge is accompanied by a small rise in circulating FSH. When LH reaches the crest of its midcycle surge, serum E_2 levels have already fallen. Concomitant with the initiation of the LH surge, but distinctly before the crest of the midcycle LH peak, there is a rise of serum P and 17-OHP. The midcycle LH surge appears to initiate the decrease in E_2 secretion and further increase in serum P. Corpus luteum function is reflected by the relatively broad luteal phase peak of serum P and E_2 and of urinary estrogen (E_1, E_2, E_3) and PD excretion. Luteal phase P and E_2 levels suppress gonadotropin secretion by negative feedback ac-

tion. However, episodic LH secretion still occurs and is required for corpus luteum function. But despite continued LH secretion, the life span of the corpus luteum is limited. As soon as the corpus luteum begins to regress, serum P and E_2 levels start to decrease gradually. On the day before the onset of menstruation, serum FSH and LH rise again in response to decreasing E_2 and P levels. This initiates the development of another cohort of follicles, out of which the next dominant follicle will be recruited during the subsequent cycle.

This sequence of events may be interrupted if (1) the ovum is fertilized and, following implantation, hCG from the trophoblast maintains the corpus luteum, thereby overriding hypothalamic-pituitary control of ovarian function; (2) the ovary is depleted of stimulatable follicles; or (3) the hypothalamus and/or pituitary fail to provide appropriate gonadotropin response either secondary to external or internal environmental stimuli or because of pathology within the hypothalamus and/or anterior pituitary.

Those readers who are interested in the levels of other steroid or protein hormones in plasma (serum) or urine throughout the menstrual cycle are referred to the extensive review by Diczfalusy and Landgren.[35] What follows is a brief summary of these patterns.

Among the protein hormones listed, serum TSH levels do not exhibit cyclic changes, while both adrenocorticotropin (ACTH) and growth hormone (GH) appear to show a periovulatory peak. There is no consensus as to serum PRL patterns during the menstrual cycle. Some investigators have reported no change; others have found higher PRL levels during the luteal phase. Steroid hormones that are metabolites of P, 17-OHP, or E_2 obviously will exhibit cyclic (circatrigintan) changes correlated with those of the parent hormone. Serum levels of 20α-dihydroprogesterone, a substantial portion of which originates from peripheral conversion of P, follow the cyclic pattern of serum P. The 20α-dihydroprogesterone levels, however, are three to five times lower and appear to peak somewhat earlier than those of P.

The cyclic pattern of urinary pregnanetriol, a metabolite of 17-OHP, is characterized by a rise at the time of ovulation and elevated levels throughout the luteal phase similar to those of 17-OHP (see Figure 5-6). The circatrigintan variations of serum E_1, E_1 sulfate, and E_2 3-sulfate, the principal circulating metabolites of E_2, closely follow those of serum E_2. The ratio of serum E_2 to serum E_1 concentrations varies throughout the cycle: It is highest during the immediate preovulatory phase, when the production of E_2 increases rapidly, and lowest at the time of menstruation.

Those steroid hormones that do not appear to affect the regulation of the menstrual cycle and their metabolites exhibit less pronounced or no cyclic changes. While pregnenolone, 17-hydroxypregnenolone, and dehydroepiandrosterone all exhibit a marked circadian variation, only pregnenolone shows a limited but sharp rise during the luteal phase. The levels of cortisol, corticosterone, and aldosterone show a marked circadian variation, as well as an increase during the luteal phase. The small portions of circulating P and estrogens that are secreted by the adrenals, or result from the peripheral conversion of adrenal androgens, are subject to the circadian rhythm of adrenal steroids. However, adrenal contribution of sex hormones is comparatively small and overshadowed by ovarian steroid hormone secretion, which does not follow a circadian rhythm.

References

1. Ryan KJ, Smith OW: Biogenesis of steroid hormones in the human ovary. *Rec Prog Horm Res* 21:367, 1965

2. Richards JS: Hormonal control of ovarian follicular development: A 1978 perspective. *Rec Prog Horm Res* 35:343, 1979

3. Ross GT, Cagrille CM, Lipsett MB, et al: Pituitary and gonadal hormones in women during spontaneous and induced ovulatory cycles. *Rec Prog Horm Res* 26:1, 1970

4. Hillier SG, van den Boogaard AMJ, Reichert LE, et al: Intraovarian sex steroid hormone interactions and the regulation of follicular maturation: Aromatization of androgens by human granulosa cells *in vitro. J Clin Endocrinol Metab* 50:640, 1980

5. McNatty KP, Smith DM, Makris A, et al: The microenvironment of the human antral follicle: Interrelationships among the steroid levels in antral fluid, the population of granulosa cells, and the status of the oocyte *in vivo* and *in vitro. J Clin Endocrinol Metab* 49:851, 1979

6. Bryce RL, Shuter B, Sinosich MJ, et al: The value of ultrasound, gonadotropin and estradiol measurements for precise ovulation prediction. *Fertil Steril* 37:42, 1982

7. diZerega GS, Hodgen GD: Folliculogenesis in the primate ovarian cycle. *Endocr Rev* 2:27, 1981

8. Hackeloer BJ, Fleming R, Robinson HP, et al: Correlation of ultrasonic and endocrinologic assessment of human follicular development. *Am J Obstet Gynecol* 135:12, 1979

9. March CM, Goebelsmann U, Nakamura RM, et al: Roles of estradiol and progesterone in eliciting the midcycle luteinizing hormone and follicle-stimulating hormone surges. *J Clin Endocrinol Metab* 49:507, 1979

10. Stanczyk FZ, Miyakawa I, Goebelsmann U: Direct radioimmunoassay of urinary estrogen and pregnanediol glucuronides during the menstrual cycle. *Am J Obstet Gynecol* 137:443, 1980

11. World Health Organization Task Force Investigators: Temporal relationships between ovulation and defined changes in the concentration of plasma estradiol-17β, luteinizing hormone, follicle-stimulating hormone, and progesterone. *Am J Obstet Gynecol* 138:383, 1980

12. diZerega GS, Goebelsmann U, Nakamura RM: Identification of protein(s) secreted by the preovulatory ovary which suppresses the follicle response to gonadotropins. *J Clin Endocrinol Metab* 54:1091, 1982

13. LeMaire WJ, Leidner R, Marsh JM: Pre- and postovulatory changes in the concentration of prostaglandins in rat Graafian follicles. *Prostaglandins* 9:221, 1975

14. O'Grady JP, Caldwell BV, Auletta FJ, et al: The effects of an inhibitor of prostaglandin synthesis (indomethacin) on ovulation, pregnancy, and pseudopregnancy in the rabbit. *Prostaglandins* 1:97, 1972

15. Beers W, Strickland S: Studies on the role of plasminogen activator in ovulation. *J Biol Chemistry* 251:5694, 1976

16. Vande Wiele RL, Bogumil J, Dyrenfurth I, et al: Mechanisms regulating the menstrual cycle in women. *Rec Prog Horm Res* 26:63, 1970

17. diZerega GS, Hodgen GD: The interovarian progesterone gradient: A spatial and temporal regulator of folliculogenesis in the primate ovarian cycle. *J Clin Endocrinol Metab* 54:495, 1982

18. Filicori M, Butler JP, Crowley WF: Neuroendocrine regulation of the corpus luteum in the human. Evidence for pulsatile progesterone secretion. *J Clin Invest* 73:1638, 1984

19. Karsch FJ, Sutton GP: An intra-ovarian site for the luteolytic action of estrogen in the rhesus monkey. *Endocrinology* 98:553, 1976

20. Neill JD, Patton JM, Dailey RA, et al: Luteinizing hormone releasing hormone (LHRH) in pituitary stalk blood of rhesus monkeys: Relationship to level of LH release. *Endocrinology* 101:430, 1977

21. Leyendecker G, Wildt L, Hansmann M: Pregnancies following chronic intermittent (pulsatile) administration of GnRH by means of a portable pump ("Zyklomat")— A new approach to the treatment of infertility in hypothalamic amenorrhea. *J Clin Endocrinol Metab* 51:1214, 1980

22. Reame N, Sauder SE, Kelch RP, et al: Pulsatile gonadotropin secretion during the human menstrual cycle: Evidence for altered frequency of gonadotropin-releasing hormone secretion. *J Clin Endocrinol Metab* 59:328, 1984

23. Stevens VC: Comparison of FSH and LH patterns in plasma, urine and urinary extracts during the menstrual cycle. *J Clin Endocrinol Metab* 29:904, 1969

24. Yen SSC: The human menstrual cycle. In Yen SSC, Jaffe RB (eds): *Reproductive Endocrinology*. Philadelphia, WB Saunders, 1978, p 126

25. Knobil E: The neuroendocrine control of the menstrual cycle. *Rec Prog Horm Res* 36:53, 1980

26. Chang RJ, Jaffe RB: Progesterone effects on gonadotropin release in women pretreated with estradiol. *J Clin Endocrinol Metab* 47:119, 1978

27. Thorneycroft IH, Sribyatta B, Tom WK, et al: Measurement of serum LH, FSH, progesterone, 17-hydroxyprogesterone, and estradiol-17β levels at 4-hour intervals during the periovulatory phase of the menstrual cycle. *J Clin Endocrinol Metab* 39:754, 1974

28. Brown JB: Urinary excretion of oestrogen during the menstrual cycle. *Lancet* 1:320, 1955

29. Thorneycroft IH, Mishell DR Jr, Stone SC, et al: The relation of serum 17-hydroxyprogesterone and estradiol-17β levels during the human menstrual cycle. *Am J Obstet Gynecol* 111:947, 1971

30. Israel R, Mishell DR Jr, Stone SC, et al: Single luteal phase serum progesterone assay as an indicator of ovulation. *Am J Obstet Gynecol* 112:1043, 1972

31. Hull MGR, Savage PE, Bromham DR, et al: The value of a single serum progesterone measurement in the midluteal phase as a criterion of a potentially fertile cycle ("ovulation") derived from treated and untreated conception cycles. *Fertil Steril* 37:355, 1982

32. Kletzky OA, Nakamura RM, Thorneycroft IH: Log normal distribution of gonadotropins and ovarian steroid values in the normal menstrual cycle. *Am J Obstet Gynecol* 121:688, 1975

33. Ribeiro WO, Mishell DR Jr, Thorneycroft IH: Comparison of the patterns of androstenedione, progesterone, and estradiol during the human menstrual cycle. *Am J Obstet Gynecol* 119:1026, 1974

34. Goebelsmann U, Arce JJ, Thorneycroft IH, et al: Serum testosterone concentrations in women throughout the menstrual cycle and following hCG administration. *Am J Obstet Gynecol* 119:445, 1974

35. Diczfalusy E, Landgren BM: Hormonal changes in the menstrual cycle. In Diczfalusy E, Diczfalusy A (eds): *Regulation of Human Fertility*. Copenhagen, Scriptor, 1977, pp 21-71

Suggested reading

Abraham GE: Ovarian and adrenal contribution to peripheral androgens during the menstrual cycle. *J Clin Endocrinol Metab* 39:340, 1974

Abraham GE, Maroulis GB, Marshall JR: Evaluation of ovulation and corpus luteum function using measurements of plasma progesterone. *Obstet Gynecol* 44:522, 1974

Auletta FJ, Agins H, Scommegna A: Prostaglandin F mediation of the inhibitory effect of estrogen on the corpus luteum of the rhesus monkey. *Endocrinology* 103:1183, 1978

Channing CP, Schaerf FW, Anderson LD, et al: Ovarian follicular and luteal physiology. In Greep RO (ed): *Reproductive Physiology III* (International Review of Physiology), vol 22, chap 3. Baltimore, University Park Press, 1980, p 117

Fritz MA, Speroff L: The endocrinology of the menstrual cycle: The interaction of folliculogenesis and neuroendocrine mechanisms. *Fertil Steril* 38:509, 1982

Goebelsmann U, Midgley AR Jr, Jaffe RB: Regulation of human gonadotropins. VII. Daily individual urinary estrogens, pregnanediol and serum luteinizing and follicle stimulating hormones during the menstrual cycle. *J Clin Endocrinol Metab* 29:1222, 1969

McNatty KP, Makris A, DeGrazia C, et al: The production of progesterone, androgens, and estrogens by granulosa cells, thecal tissue, and stromal tissue from human ovaries *in vitro. J Clin Endocrinol Metab* 49:687, 1979

Midgley AR, Jaffe RB: Regulation of human gonadotropins. IV. Correlation of serum concentrations of follicle-stimulating and luteinizing hormones during the menstrual cycle. *J Clin Endocrinol Metab* 28:1699, 1968

Mishell DR Jr, Nakamura RM, Crosignani PG, et al: Serum gonadotropin and steroid patterns during the normal menstrual cycle in women. *Am J Obstet Gynecol* 111:60, 1971

Moghissi KS, Syner FN, Evans TN: A composite picture of the menstrual cycle. *Am J Obstet Gynecol* 114:405, 1972

Pauerstein CJ, Eddy CA, Croxatto HD, et al: Temporal relationships of estrogen, progesterone, and luteinizing hormone levels to ovulation in women and infrahuman primates. *Am J Obstet Gynecol* 130:876, 1978

Ryan KJ: Biosynthesis and metabolism of ovarian steroids. In Behrman SJ, Kistner RW (eds): *Progress in Infertility*, ed 2. Boston, Little, Brown and Company, 1975

Terasawa E, Rodriguez-Sierra JF, Dierschke J, et al: Positive feedback effect of progesterone on luteinizing hormone (LH) release in cyclic female rhesus monkeys: LH response occurs in two phases. *J Clin Endocrinol Metab* 51:1245, 1980

Young JR, Jaffe RB: Strength-duration characteristics of estrogen effects on gonadotropin response to gonadotropin-releasing hormone in women. II. Effects of varying concentrations of estradiol. *J Clin Endocrinol Metab* 42:432, 1976

Zeleznik AJ, Schuler HM, Reichert LE: Gonadotropin-binding sites in the rhesus monkey ovary: Role of the vasculature in the selective distribution of human chorionic gonadotropin to the preovulatory follicle. *Endocrinology* 109:356, 1981

Chapter 6

The Endometrium in the Menstrual Cycle

Charles M. March, M.D.

Variability of the normal menstrual cycle

Patterns of menstruation vary considerably, even though most women claim to have "regular" menstrual cycles of "about 28 days." Figure 6-1 shows the distributions of menstrual intervals reported in 10 studies. The wide variations represent differences in the populations studied. The solid lines represent studies that mainly reported the intervals of adult women, whereas many young and postpubertal females were included in the studies graphed as broken lines.

Treloar and his associates analyzed 275,947 menstrual intervals recorded by more than 2,700 women over extended periods—the longest being 29 years.[1] This study, whose population was mainly University of Minnesota graduates, probably contains the most accurately reported menstrual cycle data. The greatest variation in interval length occurred in the postmenarcheal and premenopausal years. The transitions to and from the comparative irregularity of the postmenarcheal and premenopausal years to the "regularity" of the middle years

occurred smoothly over 7 to 8 years. Three years after the menarche, the range of menstrual intervals for 90% of the recorded cycles was 20.4 to 47.7 days. Following menarché, individual differences in the mean length of the menstrual cycle, the amount and variation of cycle length, and the duration of the transition from irregular to regular length were very pronounced.

Three years before menopause, 90% of the recorded intervals were between 16.2 and 54.7 days (Figure 6-2). At the extremes of the reproductive years, there is a higher incidence of long intervals than of short intervals, although both can occur. This trend toward longer intervals is more marked in the premenopausal than in the postmenarcheal years.

Less variation in interval occurred in women who were 20 to 40 years old. In this group, 90% of the menstrual intervals ranged from 22.1 to 32.0 days. Among all subjects studied, the least variation in menstrual interval occurred at age 36, when the median standard deviation of menstrual intervals was 1.83 days. However, even in this group, the range for 98% of the cycles varied between 20 and 43 days, and the standard deviation for 98% of the intervals

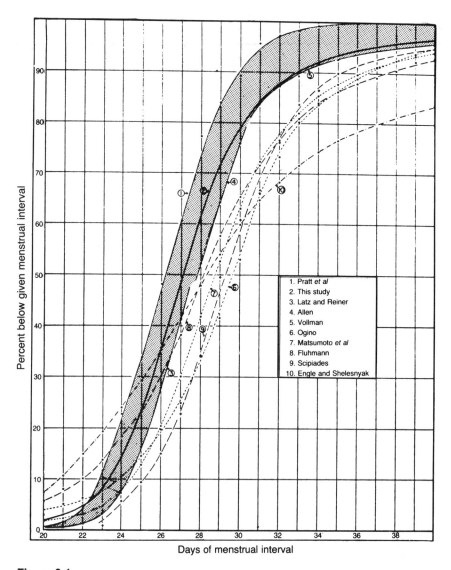

Figure 6-1
Distribution curves of menstrual intervals from 10 published series reviewed by Treloar and co-workers. The shaded area represents the boundaries for menstrual intervals from another 10 studies. For the references cited in the figure, refer to the original report by Treloar et al.

From Treloar AE, Boynton RE, Behn BG, et al: Variation of the human menstrual cycle through reproductive life. Int J Fertil *12:77, 1967.*

was 9.9 days. Figure 6-3 shows the distribution of the standard deviations of menstrual intervals throughout life.

To understand the general trend in variation in bleeding intervals, Treloar and associates constructed curves representing the "average

Normal endocrinology

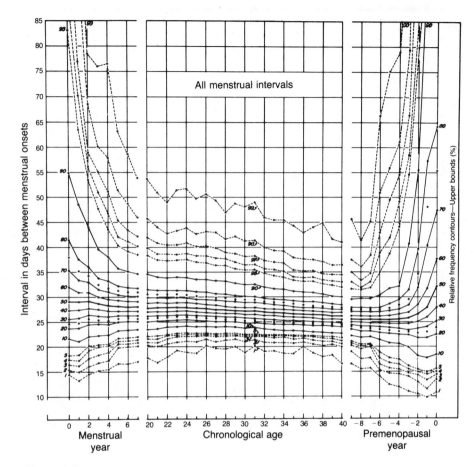

Figure 6-2
Contours for the frequency distribution of all menstrual intervals in the three zones of menstrual life.

From Treloar AE, Boynton RE, Behn BG, et al: Variation of the human menstrual cycle through reproductive life. Int J Fertil *12:77, 1967.*

woman" at each age (Figure 6-4). For example, at age 20 the range for the central 90% of intervals is 13 days (23.5 to 36.5 days). Means and standard deviations for menstrual intervals at selected ages are listed in Table 6-1.

Vollman recorded 21,499 menstrual intervals of 592 women over 20 years. According to Hartman, Vollman found that only two-thirds of these cycles lasted 25 to 31 days. In his most regular patient, only 136 of 225 cycles (60%) were between 27 and 29 days (Figure 6-5).[2]

A number of conclusions may be drawn from these menstrual interval data compiled by numerous investigators. On average, women menstruate periodically for 36 to 37 years, but Fraenkel's dictum, "The only regularity in the menstrual cycle is its irregularity," remains unchallenged. Even between ages 20 and 40, the so-called "mature" years of the hypothalamic-pituitary-ovarian-endometrial axis, variation is considerable. There is no justification for the common belief that women normally vary in

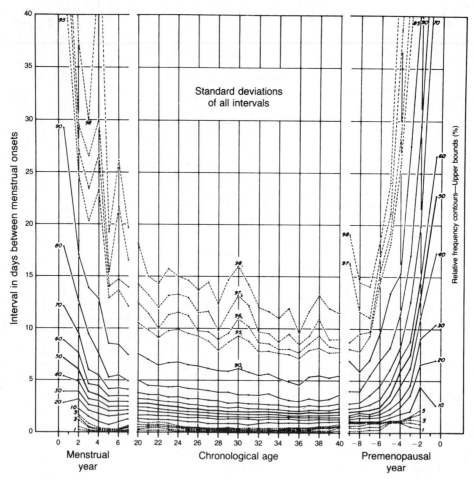

Figure 6-3

Contours for the distribution of standard deviations of menstrual intervals for all person-years of experience.

From Treloar AE, Boynton RE, Behn BG, et al: Variation of the human menstrual cycle through reproductive life. Int J Fertil *12:77, 1967.*

menstrual interval about a standard value of 28 days—a 28-day interval being, somehow, common to all. Each woman has her own mean and variability, both of which change with age. Only one of the 2,702 women studied by Treloar and associates had cycles of 28 days for 1 year. There was a continual decrease in menstrual interval from menarche to approximately 8 years before

menopause, when the median interval was 25.5 days. The median interval then increased rapidly, reaching the maximum length just before menopause.

Within this framework, the following broad guidelines for normal uterine bleeding hold: cycle length, 28 ± 7 days; duration of flow, 4 ± 2 days; blood loss, 40 ± 20 mL. Patterns vary

Table 6-1
Means and standard deviations for menstrual intervals
at selected ages

Age	Mean (days)	Standard deviation (days)
2 years postmenarche	32.20	6.38
20 years	30.09	3.94
25 years	29.84	3.45
30 years	29.30	3.16
35 years	28.22	2.67
40 years	27.26	2.83
3 years premenopause	33.20	14.24

From Treloar AE, Boynton RE, Behn BG, et al.: Variation of the human menstrual cycle through reproductive life. Int J Fertil *12:77, 1967.*

from cycle to cycle in the same woman. However, during the middle years, these variations usually are no more than ±2 days from her mean duration of flow. The variability of cycle length is greatest during the 5 to 7 postmenarcheal years and the 6 to 8 years before menopause. The frequency distribution of menstrual intervals during these two transition zones, times when anovulation is common, are mirror images. These variations include a pattern of both long and short menstrual intervals. Extreme variations in menstrual patterns are discussed in Chapter 19.

Histology of the endometrium

The role of the endometrium in conception has not been thoroughly elucidated. The endometrium is involved in reproductive phenomena such as sperm transport from the cervix to the oviducts, nourishment of the blastocyst before and after implantation, removal of the zona pellucida from the fertilized ovum, and attachment and implantation of the blastocyst.

Advances in radioimmunoassay have made detailed analysis of the hormonal fluctuations in the normal menstrual cycle possible. The anatomic changes occurring during the cycle are concurrent with, and reflect, the changes in the circulating levels of estrogens and progesterone. Although absolute correlation does not always occur, Good and Moyer, using castrated monkeys, found that inadequate amounts of estrogen and progesterone caused glandular and stromal hypoplasia.[3] Reduced estrogen or excessive progesterone resulted in glandular hypoplasia but excessive stromal development. Excessive estrogen or insufficient progesterone produced excessive glandular development and stromal insufficiency. Administration of excessive amounts of both hormones caused glandular involution and excessive stromal maturation.

In most women, correlation between the histology of the endometrium and the hormonal patterns, as described by Noyes and associates,[4] represents the only investigation performed (Figure 6-6). Our current knowledge of endometrial physiology is, in fact, limited. A number of patients with unexplained infertility may have abnormal endometrial physiology that is morphologically undetectable.

Menstrual phase

The endometrium has three layers. The stratum compactum, the uppermost layer, consists of hypertrophied stromal cells and the necks of the uterine glands. The stratum spongiosum, the middle zone, consists predominantly of tortuous, dilated glands with very little stroma. To-

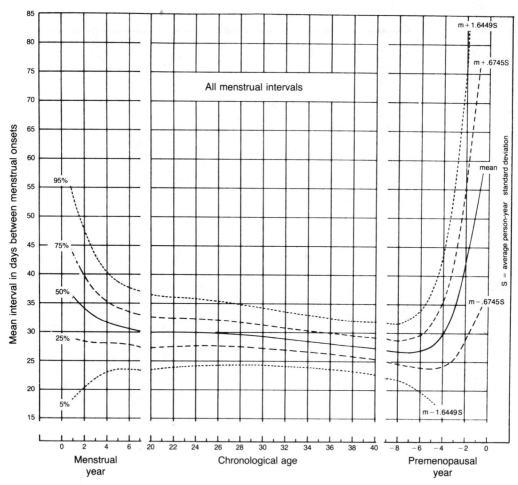

Figure 6-4
Normal curve contours for the distribution of menstrual intervals in the three zones of menstrual life.

From Treloar AE, Boynton RE, Behn BG, et al: Variation of the human menstrual cycle through reproductive life. Int J Fertil *12:77, 1967.*

gether the stratum compactum and stratum spongiosum make up the stratum functionale. The stratum basale is adjacent to the muscularis and often penetrates it. It is made up of glands and dense, compact stroma.

Desquamation occurs irregularly (segmentally) throughout the endometrium. In the cornual recesses and in the isthmus, destruction is minimal. The key to identifying early or mid-menstrual endometrium is the finding of both desquamating endometrium and some intact late secretory endometrium. Although desquamation can continue until the third day of the cycle, regeneration begins as early as 36 hours after the onset of menstruation. This reparative process lasts until the fifth day and occurs only in areas where the secretory spongiosum has been denuded from the underlying stratum ba-

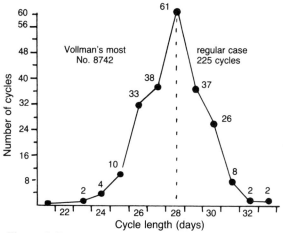

Figure 6-5
Frequency distribution of cycle lengths of Vollman's "most regular" subject.

From Hartman CG: The irregularity of the menstrual cycle. In Hartman CG (ed): Science and the Safe Period. Huntington, New York, Robert E. Krieger Publishing Co, 1972, p 128.

mainly of the basal layer. Throughout the cycle, the histology of the stratum basale remains relatively constant, consisting of inactive stroma and small, straight glands. All the changes occur in the surface layer, or stratum functionale. The scanty surface epithelium and the collapsed, narrow crypts or glands are lined by cuboidal cells. The stroma is dense and compact.

During the proliferative phase, under the influence of estrogen, there is marked proliferation of epithelial and stromal cells. Mitotic figures are abundant. Initially, the stroma becomes dense. Glycogenesis is a critical activity in the proliferative phase, and glycogen storage begins on approximately day 10. The glands subse-

sale. Regeneration begins from the exposed ends of basal glands and from the intact edges of epithelium in the cornual and isthmic regions.[5] Stromal cells do not participate in this repair and remain inactive until surface reepithelialization has been completed.

The reparative process occurs during the period when circulating estrogen levels are low, and is unaccompanied by such estrogen-dependent changes as mitosis and ciliogenesis. Therefore, it has been postulated that endometrial regeneration occurs in response to tissue loss rather than hormonal influence. The changes in endometrial histology are most marked in the upper fundus. The glands and stroma of the lower uterine segment respond inadequately to hormonal stimuli. Consequently, the histologic pattern is chronologically behind that of the uterine fundus.

Proliferative phase

Immediately after the cessation of menses, the endometrium is 1 to 2 mm thick and consists

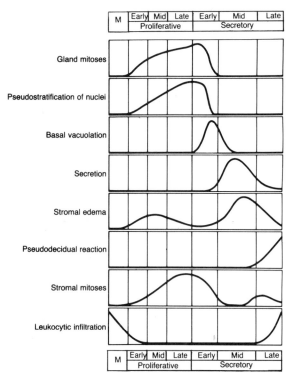

Figure 6-6
Patterns of histologic changes throughout the menstrual cycle.

Modified from Noyes RW, Hertig AT, Rock J: Dating the endometrial biopsy. Fertil Steril 1:3, 1950.

quently become increasingly long and tortuous. Maximal pseudostratification of glandular cells occurs just before ovulation. As glycogen storage increases in the glandular epithelium, migration of the nuclei toward the surface begins. At this time, columnar cells compose the surface epithelium.

Secretory phase

Within 48 to 72 hours following ovulation, glycogen-rich subnuclear vacuoles appear in the cells of the glands (Figure 6-7). The subnuclear vacuoles are the first indication of progestation-al effect. Without the synergistic effect of estrogen and progesterone, glycogen does not accumulate. Under the influence of continued progesterone stimulation, the vacuoles begin to ascend from their subnuclear location toward the gland lumina and become supranuclear. The glycogen content increases as endometrial histology matures. Glycogen storage peaks between days 16 and 20, reaching 15 times the level during the proliferative phase (Figure 6-8).

Blood vessel and glandular tortuosity increases to a maximum, as does secretory activity (Figure 6-9). The stroma becomes edematous

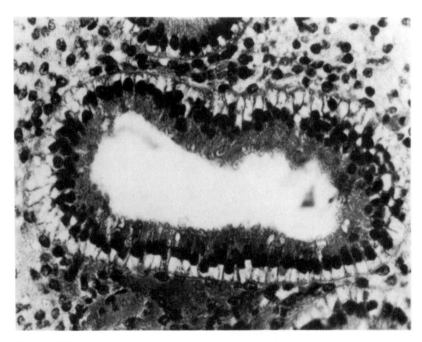

Figure 6-7
Subnuclear vacuoles lining the base of an endometrial gland 2 to 3 days after ovulation (×500, reduced by 22%).

Normal endocrinology

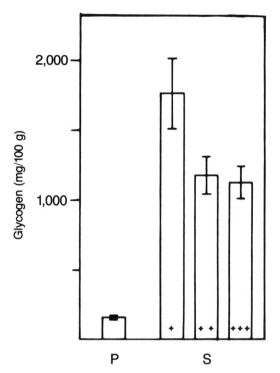

Figure 6-8
Glycogen concentration of the endometrium during the proliferative (P), early secretory (S+), mid-secretory (S++), and premenstrual (S+++) phases. The values given are means ± SE.

Reproduced, with permission, from Milwidsky A, Palti Z, Gutman A: Glycogen metabolism of the human endometrium. J Clin Endocrinol Metab *51:765, 1980. © 1980, The Endocrine Society.*

and more vascular. Stromal cells and their nuclei enlarge, providing a pseudodecidual reaction (Figure 6-10). Endometrial height progresses to 5 to 6 mm.

In the middle of the secretory phase (6 to 7 days after ovulation), the endometrium is best prepared for implantation. Glycogenolysis is maximal at this time. Under the influence of phosphorylase, glycogen is broken down to glucose to provide for the nutritional needs of the free-floating blastocyst. Phosphorylase activity is stimulated by progesterone and reaches twice the level seen in the proliferative phase (Figure

6-11). However, recent data by Milwidsky and co-workers suggest that the active form of this enzyme is not increased in the luteal phase, and that the major enzymatic change during the luteal phase is the almost 20-fold increase in the activity of glycogen synthetase phosphatase (Figure 6-12).[6]

At the end of the secretory phase, the maximal endometrial response to ovarian sex steroids has occurred. The premenstrual exhausted glands begin to collapse and fragment. Marked infiltration with polymorphonuclear and mononuclear leukocytes occurs (Figure 6-13). Autolysis begins. Throughout the secretory phase, there is progressive accumulation of a specific protein, progestogen-dependent endometrial protein (PEP).[7] The levels of PEP, which continue to rise during very early pregnancy, correlate with serum progesterone levels. The specific purpose of PEP and its relation to fertility are unknown.

Endometrial biopsy

At any stage of the secretory phase, the endometrium may be examined histologically to provide presumptive evidence of ovulation; however, a biopsy performed 1 or 2 days before menstruation begins may be used not only to document ovulation but also to assess the adequacy of the luteal phase. At this time, almost all ovarian steroid production has occurred and the endometrium has been stimulated maximally. If only a single piece of tissue is removed from the anterior uterine fundal wall, there need be little concern about possible damage to a recently implanted blastocyst.

A single, long, steady aspiration technique should be used, beginning from the top of the uterine fundus, where the hormonal response is highest. A 2-mm Novak curette will provide an adequate sample with minimal discomfort for

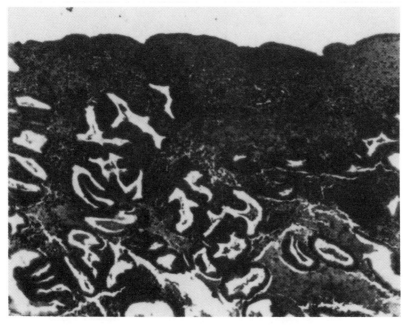

Figure 6-9
Maximal secretory activity characteristic of 7 to 8 days after ovulation
(×90, reduced by 22%).

the patient. A 10-mL syringe should be attached to the curette to provide gentle aspiration during endometrial sampling. If biopsy is delayed until the onset of bleeding, the risk of interrupting an early gestation will not be substantially reduced, and interpreting biopsies obtained at this time is difficult.

Both surface epithelium and glands and stroma are needed to interpret the pattern. Proper interpretation of a biopsy performed for endometrial dating requires knowledge of the first day of the next menstrual period, because of the variable length of the follicular phase of the cycle. Correlation with the date of the thermogenic basal body temperature (BBT) shift is also helpful. The diagnosis should be made according to the most advanced portion of tissue obtained. Using the criteria of Noyes and coworkers, experienced pathologists will agree on the same day 25% of the time, and within 2 days 80% of the time.[8]

Theories of menstruation

Menstruation is bleeding that occurs concurrently with the shedding of a secretory endometrium. The prerequisites of menstruation include the series of hormonal events discussed in the preceding chapter, and a properly nourished endometrium capable of responding to the cyclic ebb and flow of ovarian sex steroids.

The characteristics of normal and abnormal uterine bleeding are:

- Premenstrual ischemia followed by dilation of the coiled arteries of the endometrium
- Simultaneous desquamation and regeneration of the endometrium
- Endometrial shedding during normal ovulatory cycles, during anovulatory states, and after the administration of natural and synthetic sex steroids.

Multiple theories have been advanced to explain the etiology of menstruation. The most valid of these are discussed below.

Estrogen deprivation

Estrogen is responsible for the growth and development of endometrial glands, stroma, vasculature, and ground substance. Acute withdrawal or moderate reduction of estrogen levels will lead to endometrial shedding. Castration and the cessation of estrogen administration are examples of acute withdrawal, whereas the postovulatory decline in serum estradiol concentration is an example of a moderate decrease. However, maintaining the same level of estrogen for a long time may also produce uterine bleeding (for example, following estradiol pellet implantation in the castrated or postmenopausal wom-

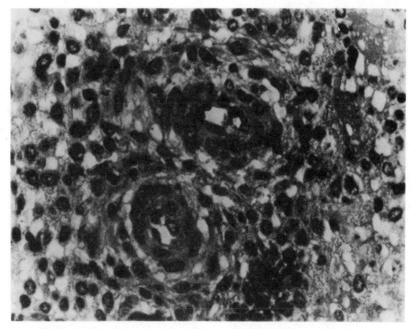

Figure 6-10
Pseudodecidual reaction around spiral arterioles 9 to 10 days after ovulation (×500, reduced by 22%).

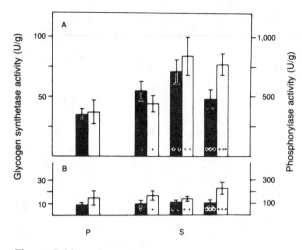

Figure 6-11
Activity of GS and phosphorylase during the phases of the menstrual cycle. ■, GS activity; □, phosphorylase activity; A, total activity; B, activity of *a* forms of GS and phosphorylase. Values given are means ± SE.

Reproduced, with permission, from Milwidsky A, Palti Z, Gutman A: Glycogen metabolism of the human endometrium. J Clin Endocrinol Metab 51:765, 1980. © 1980, The Endocrine Society.

an), and acute withdrawal of estrogen may not cause bleeding (for example, in postmenopausal women receiving estrogen therapy for 3 or 4 weeks). Progesterone administration usually will prevent the bleeding associated with acute estrogen withdrawal. Although estrogen deprivation explains some of the mechanisms associated with menstruation, it does not explain them all.

Progesterone deprivation

Progesterone also has an effect on endometrial glands, stroma, and vasculature. Regression of the corpus luteum and withdrawal of progesterone, even if estrogen administration is continued, will cause endometrial shedding. However, progesterone deprivation can only partially explain menstruation, because endometrial bleeding can occur in the absence of progesterone. Also, a prerequisite for progesterone-stimulated

withdrawal bleeding is an endometrium that has been adequately prepared by estrogen.

Inadequate lymphatic drainage

The accumulation of endometrial catabolites secondary to poor lymphatic drainage might cause breakdown of the endometrium and result in menstruation. The normal premenstrual events of stromal edema and vascular stasis lead to spiral arteriolar constriction. This initiates the accumulation of metabolites and subsequent endometrial breakdown. Only a well-developed lymphatic system could clear these catabolites and prevent menstruation. This theory, though attractive, remains unproven, because of a lack

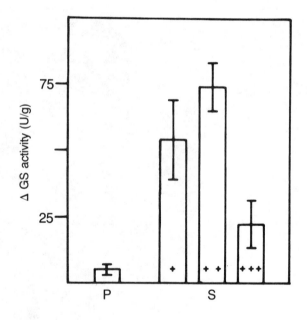

Figure 6-12
Activity of GS phosphatase during the phases of the menstrual cycle. Phosphatase activity is defined as the change in GS activity after incubation of the enzyme preparation for 60 minutes at 20°C. Values are means ± SE.

Reproduced, with permission, from Milwidsky A, Palti Z, Gutman A: Glycogen metabolism of the human endometrium. J Clin Endocrinol Metab 51:765, 1980. © 1980, The Endocrine Society.

Normal endocrinology

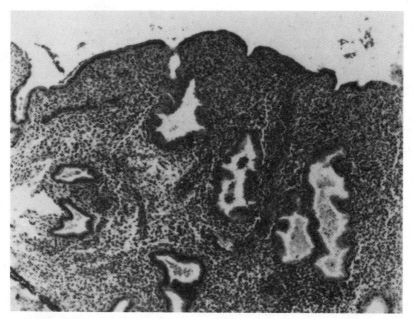

Figure 6-13
Glandular exhaustion and leukocyte infiltration 12 to 13 days after ovulation (×90, reduced by 22%).

of techniques adequate to identify and study endometrial and uterine lymphatic channels.

Depolymerization of endometrial ground substance

The integrity of the developing endometrium is maintained by an interlacing network of collagen bundles amid ground substance. The latter is composed primarily of condensed and polymerized acid mucopolysaccharides (AMPS). AMPS synthesis ceases after progesterone secretion begins, and a slow depolymerization process increases vascular permeability. Endometrial nutrition is maintained despite the increasing density of the luteal phase stroma. Unless progesterone production is maintained, this increased permeability leads to the release of hydrolytic enzymes and subsequent menstruation.

Endometrial "toxins"

Lysosomal enzymes, endometrial catabolites, and prostaglandins can induce endometrial desquamation. Prostaglandins, especially prostaglandin $F_{2\alpha}$ ($PGF_{2\alpha}$), affect the endometrium. The concentration of $PGF_{2\alpha}$ rises sharply throughout the menstrual cycle and is greatest during menses.[9] The potent vasoconstrictive properties of $PGF_{2\alpha}$ initiate myometrial contraction and spiral arteriolar constriction, leading to necrosis and desquamation. Levels of NAD^+-dependent 15-hydroxyprostaglandin dehydrogenase (PGDH) peak during the luteal phase and continue to rise if pregnancy occurs.[10] The levels of this enzyme, which catalyzes the conversion of prostaglandins to inactive 15-keto products, correlate with serum progesterone levels. If pregnancy does not occur, serum progesterone levels and those of PGDH (located primarily in the glandular epithelium) fall. The decrease in PGDH activity would favor a rise in prostaglandin activity and subsequent menstruation. Normal prostaglandin accumulation is not seen in women who have estrogen-induced breakthrough bleeding.[11] Alkaline phosphatase and peroxidase levels have also been shown to rise during the luteal phase.[12]

Acting in concert, all these factors and others still unknown are responsible for normal menstruation. The production, diffusion, and metabolism of ovarian steroids, and their binding to and influence on endometrial receptor sites, coupled with local and systemic factors, are responsible for normal cyclicity and minor variations as well as for extremes beyond the norm.

References

1. Treloar AE, Boynton RE, Behn BG, et al: Variation of the human menstrual cycle through reproductive life. *Int J Fertil* 12:77, 1967

2. Hartman CG: The irregularity of the menstrual cycle. In *Science and the Safe Period*. Huntington, New York, Robert E Krieger Publishing Co, 1972

3. Good RG, Moyer DL: Estrogen-progesterone relationships in the development of secretory endometrium. *Fertil Steril* 19:37, 1968

4. Noyes RW, Hertig AT, Rock J: Dating the endometrial biopsy. *Fertil Steril* 1:3, 1950

5. Ferenczy A: Studies on the cytodynamics of human endometrial regeneration. *Am J Obstet Gynecol* 124:64, 1976

6. Milwidsky A, Palti Z, Gutman A: Glycogen metabolism of the human endometrium. *J Clin Endocrinol Metab* 51:765, 1980

7. Joshe SG, Henriques ES, Smith RA, et al: Progestogen-dependent endometrial protein in women. Tissue concentration in relation to developmental stage and to serum hormone levels. *Am J Obstet Gynecol* 138:113, 1980

8. Noyes RW, Homan JO: Accuracy of endometrial dating. *Fertil Steril* 4:504, 1954

9. Maathuis JB, Kelly RW: Concentrations of prostaglandins $F_{2\alpha}$ and E_2 in the endometrium throughout the human menstrual cycle, after the administration of clomiphene or an oestrogen-progestogen pill and in early pregnancy. *J Endocrinol* 77:361, 1978

10. Casey ML, Hemsell DL, MacDonald PC, et al: NAD^+-dependent 15-hydroxyprostaglandin dehydrogenase activity in the human endometrium. *Prostaglandins* 19:115, 1980

11. Smith SK, Abel MH, Kelly RW, et al: The synthesis of prostaglandins from persistent proliferative endometrium. *J Clin Endocrinol Metab* 55:284, 1982

12. Holinka CF, Gurpide E: Peroxidase activity in glands and stroma of human endometrium. *Am J Obstet Gynecol* 138:599, 1980

Suggested reading

Israel R, Mishell DR Jr, Labudovich M: Mechanisms of normal and dysfunctional uterine bleeding. *Clin Obstet Gynecol* 13:386, 1970

Nogales-Ortiz F, Puerta J, Nogales FF Jr: The normal menstrual cycle. *Obstet Gynecol* 51:259, 1978

Normal endocrinology

Chapter 7

Oocytes
From Development to Fertilization

Richard P. Marrs, M.D.

Among mammals, the development and release of an oocyte during the reproductive cycle is all-important for replication of the species. The interest that has been generated by the procedure of removing oocytes from the follicle, fertilization in an extracorporeal environment, and replacement of a developing embryo into the uterus emphasizes the necessity of understanding the genesis of the oocyte and its ability to undergo fertilization.

The term oogenesis refers to the production of the female germ cell. This process begins in embryonic life with the development of the fetus in utero. It is thought that within 4 weeks of conception, primordial germ cells migrate from the yolk sac epithelium to the genital ridges, where sexual differentiation begins at approximately 7 weeks' gestation.[1-3] The germ cells, or oogonia, that form in the genital ridges are mitotically active in the differentiating ovary. Oogonia actually form between the second and seventh months of fetal life. Because these primordial germ cells are extremely active mitotically, cell division occurs during gestation. This process increases the number of germ cells in each ovary during fetal life. After mitosis is completed, an oogonium is formed. These cells then begin the process of meiosis. Once meiotic division begins, no further proliferation or rep-

lication of the oogonia can occur.[4] These structures are then called primary oocytes. All female mammals initiate their reproductive life with a definite number of primary oocytes, which are used throughout the reproductive life span. These oocytes either undergo maturation and complete meiotic division, so that they can be released and fertilized, or undergo atresia and are resorbed.[5]

Meiosis

Oogonia that no longer are involved in mitotic activity enter the prophase of the first meiotic division. At that point, these structures are called primary oocytes. The prophase of meiosis I can be divided into four separate stages: leptotene, zygotene, pachytene, and diplotene (Figure 7-1).[3] The nucleus of the leptotene oocyte contains 46 chromosomal threads, or 23 pairs of chromosomes. During the zygotene stage of prophase of meiosis I, the maternal and paternal threads associate in pairs, forming synapses. If the primary oocyte is viewed during the pachytene stage, it does not appear that there are 23 pairs of threaded chromosomes, because the threads are so tight that even with electron microscopy there

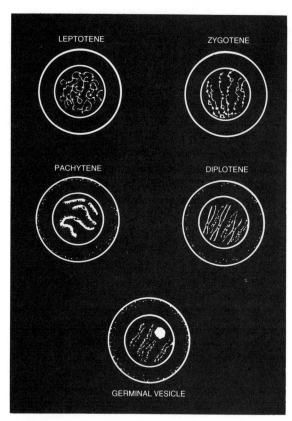

Figure 7-1
Stages of meiotic development in the primary oocyte.

Reproduced, with permission, from Shea BF, Baker RD, Latour JPA: Oogenesis, folliculogenesis and maturation of follicular oocytes. In Hafez ES (ed): Human Ovulation: Mechanisms, Prediction, Detection, and Induction. *New York, Elsevier-North Holland, 1979.*

appear to be only 23 chromosomes present. However, meiotic division has not yet reduced the primary oocyte to a 23-chromosome cell. As the diplotene stage approaches, the chromatids separate and the separate chromosome threads can be viewed. Within the ovary of the mammalian fetus, primary oocytes in all four stages of prophase of meiosis I may be seen.[5, 6]

Immediately before birth, the primary oocytes reach the diplotene stage. They remain quiescent in this stage until gonadotropin stimu-

lation occurs during the reproductive cycle. This stage of meiotic arrest is commonly called germinal vesicle stage development. During human in vitro fertilization, it has become commonplace to see oocytes recovered from partially stimulated ovarian follicles in the germinal vesicle, or diplotene, stage of meiosis.[7] The first meiotic division is completed only after gonadotropin stimulation of the primary oocyte. Luteinizing hormone (LH) and follicle-stimulating hormone (FSH) change the primary oocyte into the Graafian follicle. The LH-induced completion of metaphase II of meiosis begins approximately 36 hours before full maturation and release of the fertilizable oocyte from the ovary. At the same time, germinal vesicle breakdown occurs and extrusion of the first polar body takes place.[5]

Development of the follicle

In the human female, the development of the mature ovarian follicle is regulated by the hypothalamic-pituitary axis. This complex hormonal interrelationship is discussed in Chapter 1. However, it is important to understand not only the process of folliculogenesis, but also the process of maturation of the oocyte before its release. Gonadotropins are involved primarily in the initial stimulation and selection of follicles during the early part of the menstrual cycle. diZerega and Hodgen have reported that, in the primate, FSH release early in the menstrual cycle is necessary for selection of primary ovarian follicles that undergo changes necessary for maturation of a single dominant follicle.[8]

Many changes occur in the primordial follicle early in the cycle, after gonadotropin stimulation appears. Before gonadotropin exposure, the follicle is a small structure containing an oocyte surrounded by flattened epithelial cells. After initial stimulation by gonadotropins (primarily FSH), there is expansion of follicular cells

Normal endocrinology

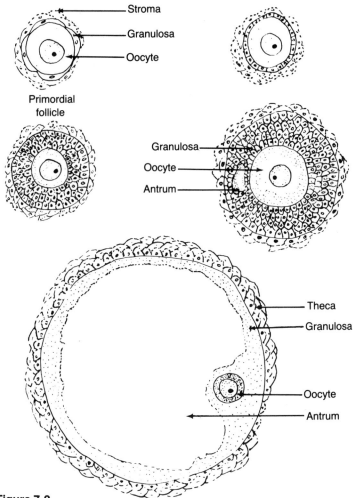

Figure 7-2
Changes occurring during follicular maturation.

Reproduced, with permission, from Shea BF, Baker RD, Latour JPA: Oogenesis, folliculogenesis and maturation of follicular oocytes. In Hafez ES (ed): Human Ovulation: Mechanisms, Prediction, Detection, and Induction. *New York, Elsevier-North Holland, 1979.*

and increased fluid secretion that initially will form an antrum. Further stimulation by FSH causes growth of the follicle and differentiation of the granulosa and theca cell structures (Figure 7-2).

FSH secretion initially stimulates the follicular cells (granulosa cells) to generate receptors for FSH and LH. The result is production and secretion of estradiol. The estrogen production has a positive feedback influence on the hypothalamus and pituitary. As further secretion of FSH and subsequently LH occurs, the dominant follicle increases in size as it approaches maturation. The maturing follicle is very dependent on fluctuations in gonadotropins (primarily LH) when ovulation becomes imminent. Midcycle LH release not only triggers a chain of events within the follicle and the follicular fluid, but also initiates the completion of the first meiotic division of the oocyte before oocyte release.

Once stimulation by LH occurs, nuclear changes begin to occur within the ooplasm. The oocyte has been maintained at nuclear arrest, or the germinal vesicle stage, since fetal life; once midcycle LH secretion occurs, germinal vesicle breakdown takes place and metaphase I of meiosis is completed. As further stimulus and nuclear changes take place, at the completion of this maturational stage, the oocyte enters metaphase II of the first meiotic division. At this stage, the oocyte is characterized by the appearance of the first polar body (Figure 7-3). The oocyte will remain at this maturational stage until penetration by spermatozoa occurs. Then completion of meiosis takes place.

Other follicles that have been stimulated, but do not reach dominant follicle status, undergo atresia. Not all oocytes will be selected to mature and be released at the time of ovulation. In fact, the vast majority of oocytes generated by mitosis during fetal development undergo atresia. It is commonly accepted that atresia can occur at three different stages in the process of oogenesis: during the mitotic production of oogonia, at the pachytene stage, or in the diplotene stage.

It has been estimated that in the human female, at 2 months of fetal life, there are approximately 600,000 oogonia. By 5 to 6 months of gestation, this number is increased to almost 7 million germ cells in both ovaries. At term gestation, the number of oogonia is approximately 10 million, but probably only 1 million will ultimately be viable. It is also estimated that within 7 or 8 years after birth, only 300,000 to 500,000 of these primary oocytes will be capable of responding to gonadotropin stimulation.[1]

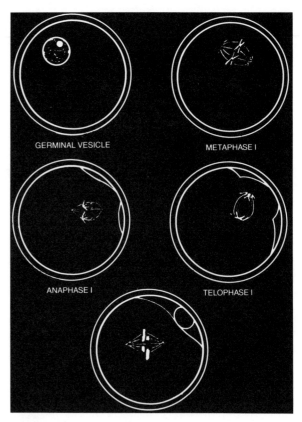

Figure 7-3
Stages of oocyte maturation after midcycle gonadotropin exposure.

Reproduced, with permission, from Shea BF, Baker RD, Latour JPA: Oogenesis, folliculogenesis and maturation of follicular oocytes. In Hafez ES (ed): Human Ovulation: Mechanisms, Prediction, Detection, and Induction. New York, Elsevier-North Holland, 1979.

A mucopolysaccharide coat around the ooplasm, the zona pellucida, forms early in the process of follicular development.[9] The zona pellucida, an extremely important structure, provides species specificity to the oocyte. With an intact zona pellucida, only spermatozoa from the same species can penetrate and fertilize the oocyte. Underlying the zona pellucida on the surface of the ooplasm is the vitelline membrane. As the oocyte matures, cortical granules

Normal endocrinology

form in this membrane. Once the oocyte is fully mature, and after ovulation occurs, the cortical granules play an important role in normal fertilization. Cortical granule formation, which can be visualized by electron microscopy, is the mechanism that limits penetration of the zona pellucida to a single sperm (Figure 7-4).[10] Through a complex set of interactions, once the zona pellucida has been penetrated by a sperm cell and fusion with the vitelline membrane occurs, the cortical granules are released and block further sperm penetration of the zona pellucida. Therefore, as the follicle develops, successful development of the oocyte within it is important for the ultimate outcome of fertilization.

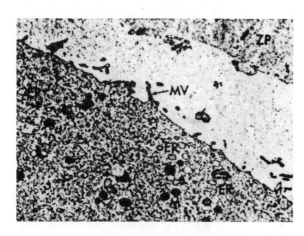

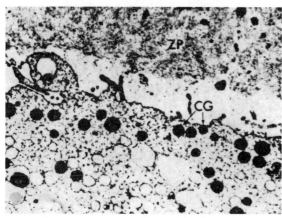

Figure 7-4
Electron micrographs of cortical granule (CG) formation. ZP, zona pellucida; MV, vitelline membrane; ER, endoplasmic reticulum; M, mitochondria.

Fertilization

After the oocyte matures and is released from the preovulatory follicle as a metaphase II oocyte, if interaction with sperm takes place, the surrounding covering of the oocyte is penetrated by a single sperm. After the vitelline and sperm membranes fuse, decondensation of the sperm head occurs and the chromatin material within it is released. The results of this process can be viewed in vitro by visualizing the formation of male and female pronuclei (Figure 7-5) and extrusion of the second polar body. Within hours, syngamy, or fusion of the male and female pronuclei, takes place. This is the pairing of the maternal and paternal chromosomal components to form a 46-chromosome cell. Within 24 to 27 hours after fertilization, two-cell embryonic development, or the first cleavage division, occurs (Figure 7-6). Then cleavage division proceeds at a fairly consistent rate until the blastocyst develops approximately 100 hours after fertilization (Figure 7-7). Thereafter, hatching from the zona pellucida, with formation of the trophoblastic plate, occurs, and implantation or nidation in the uterine cavity follows.

Edwards's observations of growth rates of human embryos cultured in vitro (Table 7-1) correlate well with reports from Croxatto and co-workers concerning embryo migration in the human reproductive tract.[11, 12] The latter data suggest that the fertilized oocyte is maintained within the tubal environment for the first 72 hours following ovulation, during which time it grows to 8 to 16 cells; it then completes embry-

Table 7-1
Stages of human embryo development in vitro

Stage	Time (hr) after insemination, earliest observation
2 cells	26
4 cells	38
8 cells	46
16 cells	68
Morula	100
Blastocyst	120

From Edwards RG (ed): Conception in the Human Female. *New York, Academic Press, 1980.*

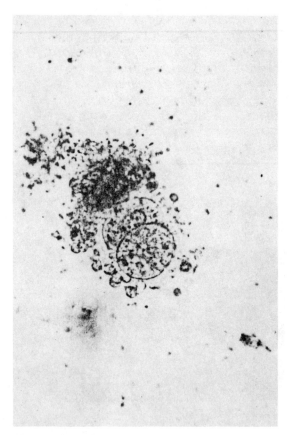

Figure 7-6
Human two-cell embryo 32 hours after insemination in vitro.

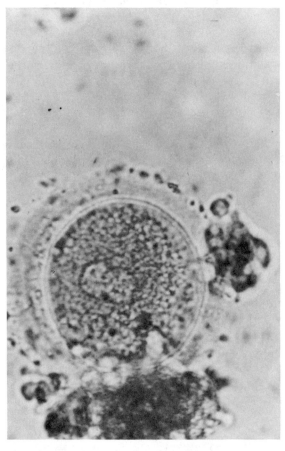

Figure 7-5
Human oocyte with appearance of male and female pronuclei, 16 hours after sperm exposure.

onic cleavage and development inside the uterine cavity during the next 72 hours, at which time implantation occurs. The stage of cleavage seen in the embryos Croxatto's group recovered correlates well with growth profiles reported by Edwards. This finding supports the time sequence for embryo migration and implantation.

Even though it is now possible to recover oocytes from maturing follicles in the human, it is still difficult to successfully mature oocytes recovered from the ovary by in vitro techniques. New methods of stimulation are being attempted in order to produce a larger cohort of maturing follicles and therefore collect larger numbers of mature oocytes. The interovarian and intrafollicular events that take place before either ovulation or oocyte collection are extremely important in determining the ultimate quality of the oocyte itself. Abnormal fertilization—that is, polyspermia (Figure 7-8)—may be an event that occurs when oocytes are exposed to spermatozoa before full maturational development. As our knowledge of germ cell maturational events grows, more and more research is being performed on in vivo, as well as in vitro, maturation of human oocytes.

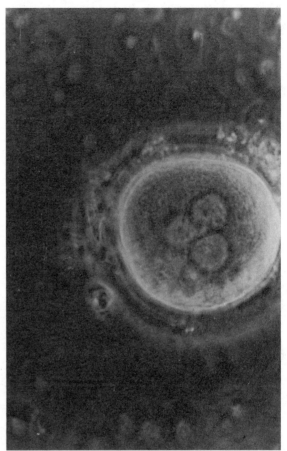

Figure 7-8
Human oocyte with three pronuclei, 16 hours after insemination in vitro.

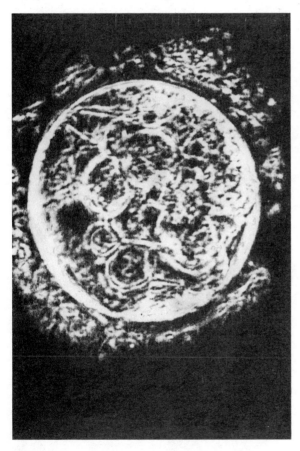

Figure 7-7
Human blastocyst 120 hours after fertilization in vitro.

References

1. Baker TG: The quantitative and cytological study of germ cells in human ovaries. *Proc Roy Soc* 158:417, 1963

2. Baker TG: Gametogenesis. *Acta Endocrinol Suppl* 166:18, 1971

3. Shea BF, Baker RD, Latour JPA: Oogenesis, folliculogenesis and maturation of follicular oocytes. In Hafez ES (ed): *Human Ovulation: Mechanisms, Prediction, Detection, and Induction.* New York, Elsevier-North Holland, 1979

4. Young WC: Mammalian ovary. In Young WC (ed): *Sex and Internal Secretions.* Baltimore, Williams & Wilkins, 1961

5. Edwards RG: Meiosis in ovarian oocytes of adult mammals. *Nature* 196:446, 1962

6. Greep RO: Cytology, histochemistry and ultrastructure of the adult ovary. In Grady HG, Smith DE (eds): *The Ovary.* Baltimore, Williams & Wilkins, 1963

7. Marrs RP, Sato H, Yee B, et al: Effect of variation of *in vitro* culture techniques upon oocyte fertilization and embryo development in human *in vitro* fertilization procedures. *Fertil Steril* 41:519, 1984

8. diZerega G, Hodgen GD: Folliculogenesis in the primate cycle. *Endocr Rev* 2:27, 1981

9. Chiquoine AD: The development of the zona pellucida of the mammalian ovum. *Am J Anat* 106:149, 1960

10. Lopata A, Sathananthan AH, McBain JC, et al: The ultrastructure of the preovulatory human egg fertilized in vitro. *Fertil Steril* 33:12, 1980

11. Edwards RG: The cleaving embryo and the blastocyst. In Edwards RG (ed): *Conception in the Human Female.* New York, Academic Press, 1980, p 687

12. Croxatto HB, Díaz S, Fuentealba B, et al: Studies on the duration of egg transport in the human oviduct. I. The time interval between ovulation and egg recovery from the uterus in normal women. *Fertil Steril* 23:447, 1972

Chapter 8

Endocrinology of Pregnancy

Uwe Goebelsmann, M.D.

Gestation is associated with profound hormonal and metabolic alterations in the mother. These changes facilitate the establishment and maintenance of pregnancy, fetal growth and development, and postpartum lactation. The hormonal changes that the pregnant woman undergoes benefit mainly the fetus, whose metabolic needs vary greatly during gestation. Maternal endocrine and metabolic alterations must adapt to these changing fetal requirements. In this chapter, the maternal hormonal alterations during gestation, the endocrinology of the fetus and placenta, and the hormones involved in the maintenance of pregnancy and initiation of labor will be discussed. Maternal, fetal, and placental endocrinology are intimately related; however, to deal with this complex subject concisely, maternal and fetal changes will be discussed separately.

Maternal endocrine alterations in pregnancy

Hypothalamic-pituitary-ovarian function

The earliest hormonal signal of pregnancy is the appearance of human chorionic gonadotropin (hCG). As the blastocyst implants into the endometrium, and the trophoblast cells gain access to the endometrial capillaries, hCG becomes detectable in the maternal circulation on day 8 or 9 after ovulation (Figure 8-1).[1] The rapidly rising hCG levels, doubling every 1.7 to 2 days, maintain corpus luteum function to assure ovarian estradiol (E_2) and progesterone (P) production until the trophoblast can provide sufficient amounts of E_2 and P to sustain pregnancy.[2]

Stimulated by hCG, the corpus luteum of pregnancy produces E_2 and P in the absence of stimulation by luteinizing hormone (LH) and follicle-stimulating hormone (FSH). The normal hypothalamic-pituitary-ovarian feedback is interrupted during pregnancy. The LH/FSH-independent production of ever-increasing quantities of E_2 and P, first by the corpus luteum of pregnancy, and soon thereafter by the placenta, results via negative feedback mechanisms in a decrease in the frequency and amplitude of hypothalamic gonadotropin-releasing hormone (GnRH) output and a lack of pituitary responsiveness to GnRH (Figure 8-2).[3] The pituitary remains insensitive to GnRH during pregnancy and regains sensitivity shortly after delivery. Thus, there is a virtual absence of LH and FSH in the maternal circulation during pregnancy.

Stimulated by hCG, the corpus luteum of pregnancy continues to produce E_2 and P (Figure 8-3).[4] For the first weeks of gestation, the es-

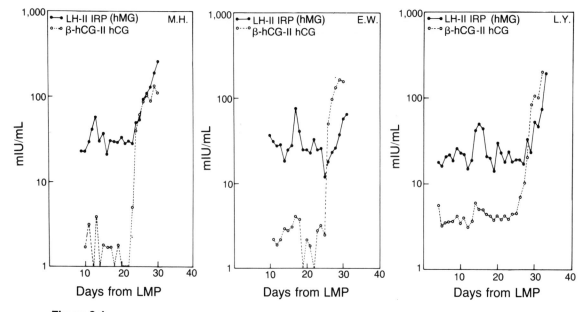

Figure 8-1
Daily determinations of hCG by unspecific (LH/hCG) and specific (β-hCG) radioimmunoassay during three conception cycles.

From Mishell DR Jr, Nakamura RM, Barberia JM, et al: Initial detection of human chorionic gonadotropin in serum in normal human gestation. Am J Obstet Gynecol 118:990, 1974.

tablishment and maintenance of pregnancy depend on this essential corpus luteum function. It has been shown that oophorectomy, resulting in the loss of the corpus luteum of pregnancy, leads to abortion if carried out before 7 weeks' gestation.[5] Thereafter, the trophoblast is capable of supplying sufficient amounts of E_2 and P to maintain pregnancy without a functioning corpus luteum.

Progesterone replacement therapy is indicated whenever the corpus luteum of pregnancy is removed surgically before completion of the seventh week of gestation. A daily IM injection of 100 mg of progesterone in oil or a 100-mg progesterone suppository inserted into the vagina every 12 hours constitutes adequate P replacement. Although circulating maternal E_2 levels rise progressively in early gestation, there

is no need to replace E_2 if the corpus luteum is removed before 7 weeks' gestation.

The decline in corpus luteum function becomes evident when one compares serum 17-hydroxyprogesterone (17-OHP) with E_2 and P levels during the first trimester. As shown in Figure 8-3, serum E_2 and P levels continue to rise progressively, whereas 17-OHP levels begin to fall at 5 weeks' gestation. In early pregnancy, 17-OHP is derived solely from the corpus luteum, whereas E_2 and P originate from both the corpus luteum and the placenta. Hence, the decline in circulating 17-OHP is biochemical evidence of decreasing corpus luteum function. This decline in function cannot be detected when either E_2 or P is measured, because these hormones are produced in increasing quantities as the placenta grows while corpus luteum function is fading.

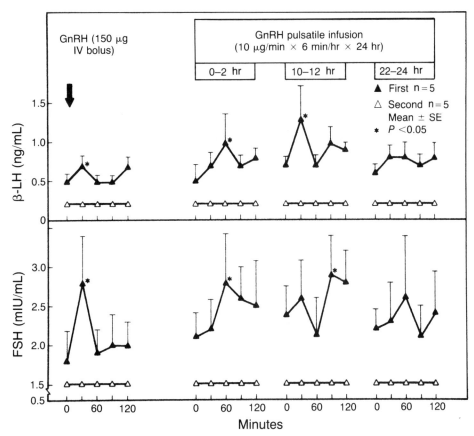

Figure 8-2
Plasma β-LH and FSH response following the initial GnRH stimulation test and pulsatile infusion in women during the first (▲) and second (△) trimesters of pregnancy following 10-day priming with GnRH Asterisks indicate significant increase ($P < 0.05$) above baseline.

Reproduced, with permission, from Shoupe D, Kletzky OA: Priming with GnRH restores gonadotropin secretion during first but not second trimester of pregnancy. Am J Obstet Gynecol 150:460, 1984.

The rise in E_2 has a marked effect on hepatic protein synthesis and pituitary prolactin (PRL)-producing cells (lactotrophs) in early gestation.

Adrenocortical function

Maternal total plasma cortisol levels are elevated in pregnancy because of an elevation in corticosteroid-binding globulin (CBG), or transcortin. The liver increases CBG synthesis in response to increased E_2 levels. Although the major rise in total plasma cortisol (up to threefold) is caused by an increase in CBG-binding cortisol, plasma free cortisol is elevated to about twice its pre-pregnancy levels. Because of increased binding to CBG, the metabolic clearance rate (MCR) of cortisol is decreased in pregnant women, whereas the production rate (PR) is essentially unchanged. Similarly, the urinary excretion of cor-

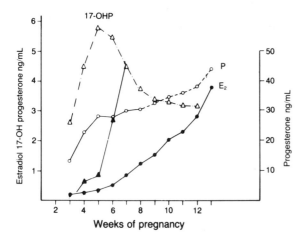

Figure 8-3
Mean plasma concentrations of progesterone (P),
17-hydroxyprogesterone (17-OHP), and estradiol (E_2)
during the first 12 weeks of gestation, indicating the
transition from steroid biosynthesis by the corpus luteum
to that by the placenta.

*Modified, with permission, from Tulchinsky D, Hobel CJ: Plasma
human chorionic gonadotropin, estrone, estradiol, estriol,
progesterone, and 17α-hydroxyprogesterone in human pregnancy.
III. Early normal pregnancy. Am J Obstet Gynecol 117:884, 1973.*

tisol metabolites remains unchanged during
pregnancy. However, urinary free cortisol excretion is increased during pregnancy. The placenta does not produce gluco- or mineralocorticoids, and maternal ACTH levels are essentially
unaltered. The diurnal variations of plasma
ACTH and cortisol persist during pregnancy.

Maternal mineralocorticosteroid metabolism is altered. Aldosterone production, controlled by the renin-angiotensin mechanism
(Figure 8-4),[6] and excretion are increased during pregnancy. The rise in E_2 raises hepatic angiotensinogen formation. In addition, plasma
renin activity and angiotensin II increase. These
alterations cause a rise in aldosterone production, a six-to twentyfold increase in plasma aldo-

sterone levels, and an increase in aldosterone excretion during pregnancy. The marked rise in
circulating P, through its antagonistic effect,
counteracts the effect of the increased aldosterone levels on the kidneys. Besides aldosterone,
circulating 11-deoxycorticosterone (DOC) is elevated up to sixfold during pregnancy.

The concentrations of dehydroepiandrosterone (DHEA) and, in particular, dehydroepiandrosterone sulfate (DHEA-S) in blood decrease during pregnancy, the latter to about
50% to 33% of prepregnancy levels. This decrease is caused by placental clearance and hepatic metabolism. Serum testosterone concentrations, however, rise approximately threefold
above prepregnancy levels, because of the estrogen-induced increase in hepatic sex hormone-
binding globulin (SHBG) production. The result is a marked increase in SHBG-bound
testosterone and a concomitant decrease in the
MCR of testosterone. Unlike testosterone, serum androstenedione concentrations rise only
slightly during pregnancy. Androstenedione,
which is not bound to SHBG, is not affected by
rising SHBG levels.

Cushing's syndrome occurs very rarely during pregnancy. When it does occur, it is likely to
be caused by an adrenal tumor (adenoma or carcinoma), which demands immediate diagnosis
and surgical therapy. Patients with adrenal insufficiency, primary or secondary, who are on
replacement therapy, will require the same
amounts of glucocorticoid therapy they received
before becoming pregnant. For delivery, vaginal
or by cesarean section, additional cortisol must
be given as would be done for other forms of
surgical stress.

Thyroid function

Because the kidneys excrete more iodine during
pregnancy, the pool of extrathyroidal iodine is
reduced. Hence, the maternal thyroid gland has
to make a greater effort to trap iodine. Mild enlargement of the thyroid gland during pregnan-

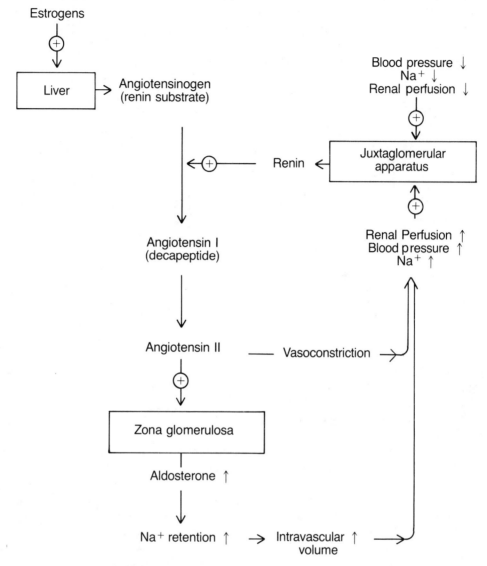

Figure 8-4
Schematic representation of the renin-angiotensin mechanism.

cy, therefore, is not abnormal. The estrogen-mediated increase in hepatic thyroxine-binding globulin (TBG) production causes increased TBG levels, a rise in TBG-bound thyroxine (T_4) and triiodothyronine (T_3), and a decrease in the resin uptake of iodinated T_3. Serum TBG com-petes with the resin for T_3 in T_3 resin uptake tests. Circulating levels of non-TBG-bound T_4 and T_3 (that is, free T_4 and T_3), the biologically active thyroid hormones, remain unchanged. However, the basal metabolic rate is increased during pregnancy, because it measures oxygen consumption, which in pregnancy is the sum of maternal and fetal oxygen consumption.

With regard to placental permeability of hormones and drugs related to thyroid function, thyroid-stimulating hormone (TSH, a glycoprotein hormone) does not cross the placenta. The thyroid hormones T_4 and T_3, which are small but hydrophilic, cross the placenta very sparingly. But long-acting thyroid stimulator (LATS), as well as immunoglobulin, iodine, propylthiouracil (PTU), and propranolol, do cross the placenta readily. The transplacental passage of thyroid-related hormones and agents should be kept in mind when dealing with thyroid disorders during pregnancy. Hyperthyroidism is not uncommon, with one to two cases occurring in 1,000 pregnancies. Also, the risk of thyroid storm during labor is increased in hyperthyroid patients. Hypothyroidism, however, is rarely encountered during pregnancy.[7]

Parathyroid function

Parathyroid hormone (PTH) regulates the metabolism of calcium, which is most important for fetal bone development (Figure 8-5).[8] Maternal calcium uptake must increase during pregnancy to supply the fetus with the calcium it needs. The levels of active vitamin D (1,25-dihydroxyvitamin D, 1,25-$(OH)_2D$), which stimulate the absorption of calcium from the gut, are increased in maternal but lower in fetal blood, raising calcium absorption by the mother. PTH may be slightly elevated in pregnant women, but calcitonin (CT) is not. Total maternal serum calcium is decreased because of a decrease in serum albumin, but the serum concentration of ionized calcium (Ca^{++}), the biologically active form of circulating calcium, remains unchanged. While calcium and phosphate ions do cross the placenta readily, the protein hormones PTH and CT do not traverse the placental barrier. In the fetus, PTH is decreased until term, whereas the concentration of Ca^{++} is increased.

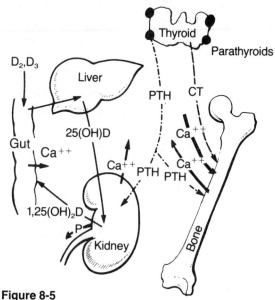

Figure 8-5

Sites of action of regulators of calcium metabolism. PTH, parathyroid hormone; CT, calcitonin; D_2, D_3, vitamins D_2 and D_3; Ca^{++}, calcium; P, phosphorus; 1,25$(OH)_2D$, 1,25-dihydroxyvitamin D; 25(OH)D, 25-hydroxyvitamin D.

Reproduced, with permission, from Furth ED: Thyroid and parathyroid hormone function in pregnancy. In Fuchs F, Klopper A (eds): Endocrinology of Pregnancy, *ed 3. Philadelphia, Harper & Row, 1983, p 176.*

Growth hormone and prolactin

Maternal serum (plasma) human growth hormone (hGH) concentrations in the fasting state, in all trimesters, are similar to those found in nonpregnant women.[9] However, pituitary hGH secretion in response to stimuli such as hypoglycemia or arginine infusion is altered. The hGH response to provocative tests is enhanced during the first half and blunted during the second half of gestation. It has been postulated that the increase in circulating E_2 is the cause of the augmented hGH response during the first half of pregnancy. The metabolic effects of the relatively large concentrations of circulating human placental lactogen (hPL) during the second half of gestation may contribute to the decreased hGH response to provocative stimuli.[10]

Normal endocrinology

Maternal serum PRL concentrations begin to rise during the first trimester, concomitant with the increase in circulating E_2, and continue to climb until term, when they are about 10 times as high as in the nonpregnant state (Figure 8-6).[11] The diurnal changes of circulating PRL, characterized by a nocturnal, sleep-cycle-dependent rise, continue during pregnancy. The sleep-associated pattern of PRL secretion proceeds in a manner analogous to that in the nonpregnant state, but at a higher set point. The rise in serum PRL levels during gestation is caused by the marked increase in circulating E_2, and is related to the hypertrophy and hyperplasia of PRL-producing cells (the so-called lactotrophs) in the anterior pituitary gland. Despite the continued rise in serum PRL levels until term, lactation is inhibited. This inhibition appears to be due to the effect of E_2 on the mammary glands.

Serum PRL concentrations exhibit astonish-ing changes during labor and delivery. PRL levels decline during labor and begin to rise before delivery, with a marked PRL peak immediately after delivery (Figure 8-7).[12] Basal PRL levels decrease postpartum and return to about pre-pregnancy levels within 3 weeks. During lactation, suckling stimulates episodic PRL secretion. The suckling-induced periodic release of PRL maintains lactation.

Placental and fetal endocrinology

Placental polypeptide hormones

Human chorionic gonadotropin (hCG)
Pregnancy can continue after implantation only if menstruation is prevented through continuation of estrogen and progesterone secretion by the corpus luteum. The latter, therefore, has to

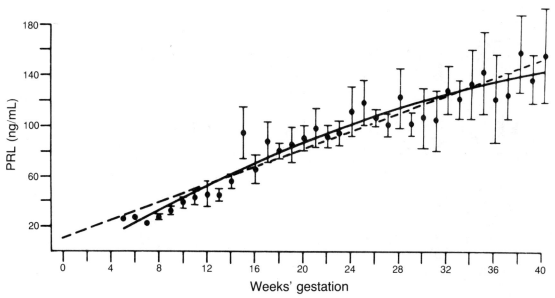

Figure 8-6
Serum prolactin (PRL) concentrations (±SE) during pregnancy.

Reproduced, with permission, from Rigg LA, Lein A, Yen SSC: The pattern of increase in circulating prolactin levels during human gestation. Am J Obstet Gynecol 129:454, 1977.

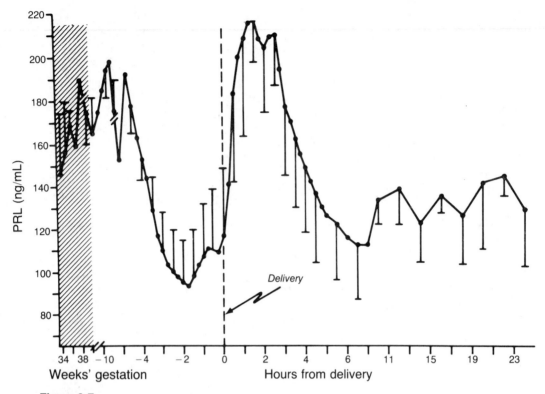

Figure 8-7
Serum prolactin (PRL) concentrations (±SE) during labor, delivery, and the immediate postpartum period.

Reproduced, with permission, from Rigg LA, Yen SSC: Multiphasic prolactin secretion during parturition in humans. Am J Obstet Gynecol 128:215, 1977.

be maintained beyond its usual life span through an LH-like hormone. Such hormonal stimulus must come before the corpus luteum ceases to function 2 weeks after ovulation, but cannot arise before fertilization or perhaps implantation. Furthermore, this hormonal stimulus, logically, should come from the trophoblast, because it is the life-support system of the embryo. This hormone is hCG, which is produced by the trophoblast and detectable as early as 8 days following ovulation (Figure 8-1). When the trophoblast has established its own progesterone and estradiol production, the corpus luteum becomes unnecessary. Thus, it becomes obvious

why hCG is the protein hormone of early gestation and has little apparent function in mid- and late pregnancy.

hCG is a glycoprotein with a molecular weight of 36,700 daltons. Its polypeptide portion accounts for about 70% of its molecular weight, and its carbohydrate portion, which appears to be essential for its biologic activity, for approximately 30%. hCG shares immunologic and biologic properties with LH. Like FSH, LH, and TSH, hCG consists of an α- and a β-subunit of molecular weight 14,500 and 22,200 daltons, respectively. While the α-subunit is common to these four tropic glycoproteins, the β-subunit is specific to each. The α-subunit of hCG, with its 92 amino acids, is virtually identical with that of the other three glycoproteins (FSH, LH, and TSH). The β-subunit, containing 145 amino acids, is specific for hCG. The development of specific antisera against the β-subunit of hCG has facilitated specific measurement of hCG—that is, with little or no cross-reaction with LH. Immunofluorescent techniques have localized hCG in syncytiotrophoblastic cells, where it is thought to be synthesized. Normal placental tissue, intrauterine or extrauterine, as well as hydatidiform moles, choriocarcinomas, and, at times, even nonendocrine tumors of the lung, adrenal gland, or liver, produce hCG.

The action of hCG biologically is similar to that of LH. It causes luteinization of ovarian follicular and interstitial cells, induction of ovulation of a mature follicle, stimulation of Leydig cells, and augmentation of progesterone (ovary) and testosterone (testis) biosynthesis. Compared with LH, hCG has a stronger luteotropic action, which may be due to its longer half-life and/or higher affinity for LH/hCG receptors. hCG exerts its biologic effect (increasing steroid biosynthesis by augmenting the conversion of cholesterol to pregnenolone) via activation of adenylate cyclase and increase of adenosine cyclic 3′,5′-monophosphate (cyclic AMP, cAMP).

It has been calculated that ovulation occurs approximately 16 hours (range, 9.5 to 23 hours) after the peak of the midcycle LH surge and that implantation occurs as early as 6 days after the presumed time of ovulation. It appears that hCG becomes detectable in maternal serum soon after implantation has occurred. Using a radioimmunoassay for hCG that could not distinguish between hCG and LH, it was found that hCG levels began to rise above luteal-phase LH levels approximately 11 days after the midcycle LH peak, but as early as day 8 in 5.3% of cycles (Figure 8-1).[1,13] With a radioimmunoassay system using an antiserum against the β-subunit of hCG, it is possible to measure hCG specifical-

ly. Using this assay, β-hCG can be detected 8 to 9 days after the LH peak (Figure 8-1). Thus, there is evidence that hCG is secreted by the trophoblast into the peripheral serum soon after implantation. It is thought that the trophoblast cells produce hCG at the time of, and even prior to, implantation on day 5 or 6 after ovulation. However, hCG from the trophoblast appears to enter the circulation in substantial amounts only after the trophoblast has begun to reach the endometrial (decidual) capillaries.[14]

hCG levels rise very rapidly following implantation, doubling every 1.7 to 2.0 days and reaching a serum concentration of 100 mIU/mL around 14 days after ovulation (Table 8-1). Peak levels occur at approximately 9 to 10 weeks' gestation and average about 40,000 to 60,000 mIU/mL (Figure 8-8).[15] hCG then falls to much lower levels, approximately 10,000 mIU/mL, and remains low for the remainder of pregnancy. The apparent rise in serum hCG levels during the third trimester, found with less specific

Table 8-1
Mean plasma hCG concentrations and 95% confidence limits in 19 women during the second and third weeks after ovulation

Day following midcycle LH peak	Mean plasma hCG (mIU/mL)	95% confidence limit (mIU/mL)
8	<2.0	—
9	2.8	1.4– 5.3
10	5.0	1.9– 13.1
11	16.5	8 – 35
12	34	20 – 59
13	55	33 – 91
14	89	57 – 140
15	159	100 – 252
16	260	156 – 433
17	443	276 – 706
18	700	473 –1,033
19	933	626 –1,394
20	1,399	973 –1,998

From Lenton EA, Neal LM, Sulaiman R: Plasma concentrations of human chorionic gonadotropin from the time of implantation until the second week of pregnancy. Fertil Steril 37:773, 1982.

radioimmunoassays, is not observed with highly specific radioimmunoassays that use a β-hCG-specific antiserum (Figure 8-8).

Besides the immunologic pregnancy tests, other sensitive radiologic assays are available for the detection and quantitation of hCG in blood or urine. The radioimmunoassays depend on the competition of endogenous hCG with radioactive hCG for a limited amount of anti-hCG antibodies. The radioreceptor assays use the competition of endogenous hCG with radioactive hCG for a limited amount of LH/hCG binding sites in a preparation of cell membrane receptors for LH and hCG obtained from bovine corpora lutea. Radioreceptor assays are fast, sensitive, and relatively simple to perform, but do not discriminate between LH and hCG.

The β-subunit-specific radioimmunoassays permit the specific measurement of hCG; that is, without interference by LH. Sensitive radioimmunoassays can detect as little as 1 mIU/mL of hCG, and radioreceptor assays can measure 5 mIU/mL of hCG. By the first missed menstrual period, hCG levels are so much higher than serum LH concentrations during the menstrual cycle that the LH cross-reactivity of hCG should not lead to false-positive tests. To avoid a falsely positive radioreceptor assay pregnancy test, the sensitivity of commercially available radioreceptor assay kits has been reduced to 150 mIU/mL. At very low hCG titers, radioreceptor assays may be subject to nonspecific interference by plasma proteins. This may lead to the spurious detection of circulating hCG during the first few days

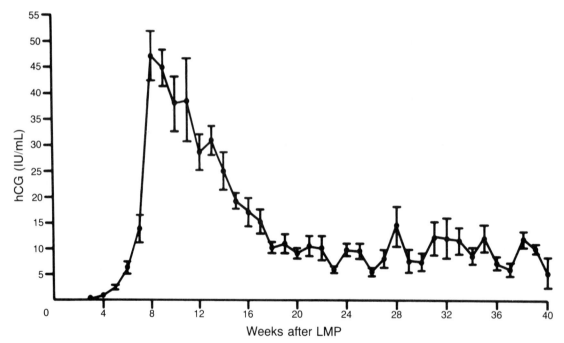

Figure 8-8
Mean serum hCG concentrations (±SE) throughout normal pregnancy measured by a radioimmunoassay specific for β-hCG.

Reproduced, with permission, from Braunstein GD, Rasor J, Adler D, et al: Serum human chorionic gonadotropin levels throughout normal pregnancy. Am J Obstet Gynecol 126:678, 1976.

Normal endocrinology

after fertilization. Claims that radioreceptor assays could detect a pregnancy as early as 4 to 6 days after conception (before implantation occurs) are incorrect.

The principal clinical application of hCG assays is testing for pregnancies and trophoblastic disease. The least sensitive pregnancy tests are slide tests, which can be performed within 2 minutes (Table 8-2). Using latex particle agglutination inhibition as the principle, these tests require 500 to 800 mIU of hCG per milliliter of urine before they become positive. Thus, these slide tests become reasonably reliable during the sixth week after the last menstrual period (LMP). More sensitive are the tube latex and hemagglutination inhibition tests, which require some 150 to 200 mIU of hCG per milliliter of urine to become positive and therefore can be used during the fifth week after the LMP. These tube tests have been improved considerably by incorporating β-hCG-specific antibodies, allowing the detection of as little as 150 mIU of hCG per milliliter of urine (Table 8-2). Thus, pregnancies can be detected during the fifth week after the LMP. The latter test can be performed within 1 or $1\frac{1}{2}$ hours in the emergency room. Some 80% to 90% of all women with ectopic pregnancies who have lower β-hCG levels than those encountered in normal pregnancies will have positive pregnancy tests when their urine is tested with these highly sensitive and specific latex or hemagglutination inhibition tube tests (Table 8-2).[16]

Most recently, enzyme-linked immunosorbent assays (ELISA) have been developed for measuring β-hCG in urine. These assays use highly specific monoclonal anti-α-hCG and anti-β-hCG antibodies. The endpoint of these tube assays is a color reaction initiated by an enzyme linked to a specific antibody. The sensitivity of these assays is 50 mIU/mL of hCG (Table 8-2).

Much more sensitive than the above urinary hCG-agglutination inhibition slide and tube assays, as well as the recent ELISA tests, are the radioimmunoassays for β-hCG. The latter detect as little as 1 mIU of hCG per milliliter of serum or urine, but use radioiodinated hCG and require a gamma counter. Hence they cannot be used in the emergency room. These β-hCG assays are most useful for detecting very early or chronic ectopic pregnancies, when following patients with serial quantitative β-hCG levels to predict pregnancy outcome in threatened abortion, or when dealing with patients who have trophoblastic disease.

Quantitative measurement of hCG in early pregnancy has been shown to have predictive value for the outcome of pregnancy. In a retrospective study, Mishell and Davajan published data indicating that women with threatened abortion between 55 and 110 days' gestation have a very poor prognosis if their urinary hCG levels are less than 10,000 mIU/mL, but are most likely to carry their pregnancies to term if urinary hCG concentrations equal or exceed 20,000 mIU/mL.[17] Similarly, Nygren and co-workers showed that serum β-hCG concentrations above 20,000 mIU/mL were usually associated with good outcome and β-hCG levels below 10,000 mIU/mL associated with bad outcome, in women with threatened abortion (Figure 8-9).[18] The latter authors found that neither serum progesterone nor serum estradiol concentration was as good a predictor of outcome as hCG in threatened abortion. Single or serial serum hCG measurements allow one to predict the outcome of threatened abortion in the large majority of instances. However, careful ultrasonography, using the vastly improved modern scanners available, appears to be more practical than β-hCG radioimmunoassay in assessing the status and probable outcome of an early pregnancy complicated by threatened abortion.

Also of clinical interest is the disappearance of hCG from serum and urine following first- and second-trimester abortion, as well as after term delivery. Studies in humans indicate a half-life of circulating hCG of 12 to 36 hours. The

Table 8-2
Various urinary pregnancy tests

Test	Type	Antibody	Sensitivity (mIU/mL hCG)	Approximate time required	% positive results in 108 ectopic pregnancies
Tandem-Visual hCG® (Hybritech)	Enzyme-linked immunosorbent	Monoclonal mouse anti-α-hCG and anti-β-hCG	50	1 hr	90 (97/108)
Mod EI® (Monoclonal Antibodies)	Enzyme-linked immunosorbent	Monoclonal mouse anti-α-hCG and anti-β-hCG	50	1 hr 15 min	90 (97/108)
Sensitex® (Roche)	Latex agglutination inhibition tube test	Goat anti-β-hCG	250	90 min	85 (92/108)
UCG-Beta Stat® (Wampole)	Hemagglutination inhibition tube test	Rabbit anti-β-hCG	200	1 hr	85 (92/108)
β-Neocept® (Organon)	Hemagglutination inhibition tube test	Rabbit anti-β-hCG	150	1 hr	82 (88/108)
Sensi Slide® (Roche)	Latex agglutination inhibition slide test	Goat anti-β-hCG	800	5 min	61 (66/108)
UCG-Beta Slide® (Wampole)	Latex agglutination inhibition slide test	Rabbit anti-β-hCG	500	5 min	51 (54/108)
Serum β-hCG	β-hCG-specific radioimmunoassay	Rabbit anti-β-hCG	1.5	48 hr	99 (107/108)

Sensitivity, time of performance, and percentage of positive results in patients with ectopic pregnancies are compared with those of the β-hCG-specific radio-immunoassay for serum hCG. From Barnes RB, Roy S, Yee B, et al: Sensitivity of urinary pregnancy tests in surgically proven ectopic pregnancies. J Reprod Med, in press.

Normal endocrinology

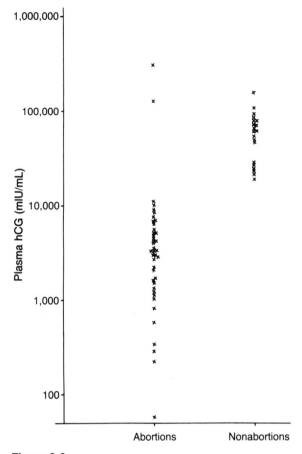

Figure 8-9
Plasma hCG concentrations in women with threatened abortion divided according to outcome.

From Nygren K-G, Johansson EDB, Wide L: Evaluation of the prognosis of threatened abortion from the peripheral plasma levels of progesterone, estradiol, and human chorionic gonadotropin. Am J Obstet Gynecol 116:916, 1973.

going first-trimester suction curettage had undetectable serum hCG levels within 38 days (mean) following the procedure, whereas women following second-trimester prostaglandin-induced abortion or hysterectomy cleared their circulating hCG within 27 and 40 days, respectively. If second-trimester abortion/hysterectomy was performed with minimal uterine manipulation, and using early ligation of uterine blood vessels to minimize deportation of trophoblast tissue, serum hCG levels were undetectable within 14 days.[19] The data illustrated in Figure 8-10 indicate that a pregnancy test detecting 150 mIU/mL of hCG in serum or urine may be positive for 2 weeks following termination of a normal first-trimester pregnancy.[19] If a patient's 24-hour urine approximates 1,000 mL, the serum hCG concentration (in international mil-

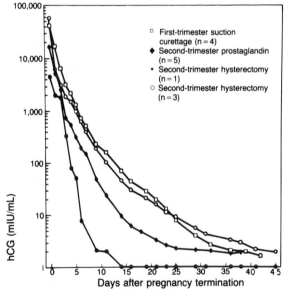

Figure 8-10
Disappearance of hCG (average serum concentrations of hCG) following various modes of pregnancy termination.

Reproduced, with permission, from Marrs RP, Kletzky OA, Howard WF, et al: Disappearance of human chorionic gonadotropin and resumption of ovulation following abortion. Am J Obstet Gynecol 135:731, 1979.

half-lives of the α- and β-subunits, however, are much shorter: 6 and 11 minutes, respectively. As circulating hCG levels are much lower at term than during the first and early second trimesters, hCG drops rapidly to undetectable levels following delivery at term. Marrs and co-workers showed that the rate of hCG disappearance from the circulation depends on the timing and mode of pregnancy termination. Patients under-

liunits per milliliter) roughly approximates the urinary hCG level (in international milliunits per milliliter or international units per liter).

Surveillance of patients with serial serum β-hCG determinations following evacuation of molar pregnancies is of paramount importance for the recognition and early treatment of persistent or metastatic trophoblastic disease.[20] Figure 8-11 represents the normal disappearance of serum hCG following evacuation of molar

pregnancies.[20] It is noteworthy that patients with gestational trophoblastic disease commonly, but not always, have considerably higher hCG levels (>100,000 mIU/mL) than women with uncomplicated pregnancies. Although multiple gestation is associated with elevated hCG levels, hCG titers continue to rise in molar pregnancy. This is in contrast to normal singleton or twin pregnancies, where hCG levels characteristically decline after their peak at 9 to 10 weeks' gestation. Serial specific β-hCG determinations are essential for the postevacuation follow-up of all molar pregnancies. Any marked deviation in the decline of serial hCG titers from the pattern depicted in Figure 8-11 signals possible recurrent or persistent trophoblastic disease and indicates that appropriate therapy must be started.

hCG is important physiologically, because it maintains steroidogenesis in the corpus luteum through its luteotropic effect. If a constant amount of exogenous hCG is injected into women daily, or three times weekly, beginning in the first half of the luteal phase of the cycle, the onset of menses can be delayed for about 2 weeks. The hCG injections have to begin 10 days after ovulation to prevent degeneration of the corpus luteum. Daily measurements of hCG during normal pregnancies indicate that during the first few days after implantation, levels of this hormone are no higher than normal luteal-phase levels of LH. However, these relatively low levels of hCG are sufficient to prevent degeneration of the corpus luteum, because hCG is biologically more active than LH. The corpus luteum contains specific receptors with high affinity for hCG.

Besides its role of maintaining and stimulating steroid production by the corpus luteum, hCG also appears to promote fetoplacental-unit steroidogenesis. hCG has been shown to enhance placental conversion of cholesterol to pregnenolone and progesterone in vitro. Also, hCG has been found to stimulate fetal adrenal DHEA-S synthesis. The fetal testis has specific

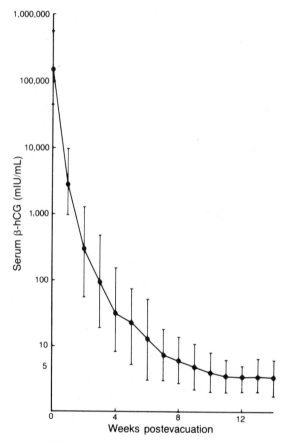

Figure 8-11
Normal decline (means ± 2 SD) of serum hCG following evacuation of molar pregnancies.

Reproduced, with permission, from Morrow CP, Kletzky OA, DiSaia PJ, et al: Clinical and laboratory correlates of molar pregnancy and trophoblastic disease. Am J Obstet Gynecol 128:424, 1977.

Normal endocrinology

binding sites for hCG, and the hormone stimulates testosterone production in the fetal testis during early pregnancy.[21] Fetal serum testosterone levels and Leydig cell proliferation reach a peak around 15 to 17 weeks' gestation; that is, after serum hCG concentrations have peaked (Figure 8-12).[21] Finally, hCG appears to possess some thyrotropic activity, which, on an equimolar basis, amounts to approximately 0.025% of that of TSH.

Human placental lactogen (hPL)

hPL has also been called chorionic growth hormone prolactin and human chorionic somatomammotropin (hCS). Chemically, hPL is a single-chain polypeptide of 191 amino acids with two disulfide bridges and a molecular weight of 21,000 to 23,000. Immunologically, hPL is closely related to, but still distinct from, growth hormone. The source of hPL is the trophoblast: It has been localized by immunofluorescent tech-

nique in syncytiotrophoblast cells and is thought to be synthesized by the syncytiotrophoblast.

When measured by radioimmunoassay, hPL becomes detectable at 5 to 6 weeks' gestation. Serum hPL levels rise gradually, from approximately 0.1 μg/mL between 7 and 10 weeks to a plateau ranging from 6 to 8 μg/mL between 34 weeks and term.[22] Unlike hCG, serum hPL levels rise concomitantly with placental weight (Figure 8-13).[22] The concentration of hPL in placental tissue is constant throughout gestation. Very little hPL is found in the fetal compartment. Although hPL is produced by the trophoblast, most of it is secreted into the maternal compartment to effect metabolic changes in the mother that benefit the fetus. Its half-life is about 12 minutes and its metabolic clearance rate 175 L/day. hPL disappears rapidly from the blood following delivery of the placenta. At term, the daily production of hPL averages 1 to 2 g/day.

hPL has been found to have lactogenic, luteotropic, and growth-hormone-like activities in experimental animals. In rabbits, hPL stimulates milk production. In the human, however, hPL is no longer present in plasma when lactation is established, and is not lactogenic. It has luteotropic action in rats, but has not been shown to have this activity in humans. Serum hPL levels are very low in early gestation (Figure 8-13). Its growth-hormone-like effect appears to be responsible for the maternal glucose-sparing effect noted in pregnancy. hPL causes mobilization of free fatty acids from maternal fat depots, shifting glucose toward the growing fetus. Against insulin, hPL exerts an antagonistic effect. Its administration will provoke a diabetic glucose tolerance test (GTT) in those nonpregnant women who showed abnormal GTT curves during a previous pregnancy. Therefore, hPL is one of the diabetogenic factors of pregnancy. Its levels are highest during the last 4 weeks of gestation, when the fetus needs the largest quantities of glucose (Figure 8-13).

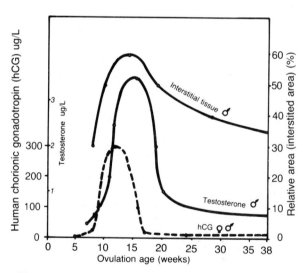

Figure 8-12
Fetal circulating hCG and testosterone levels as well as Leydig cell development.

Reproduced, with permission, from Pellinemi LJ, Dym M: The fetal gonad and sexual differentiation. In Tulchinsky D, Ryan KJ (eds): Maternal-Fetal Endocrinology. Philadelphia, WB Saunders, 1980, p 262.

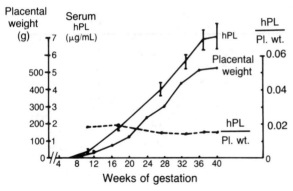

Figure 8-13
Serum concentrations of human placental lactogen (hPL) during pregnancy in relation to placental weight.

Reproduced, with permission, from Selenkow HA, Saxena BN, Dana CL, et al: Measurement and pathophysiologic significance of human placental lactogen. In Pecile A, Finzi C (eds): The Foeto-Placental Unit. Amsterdam, Excerpta Medica Foundation, 1969, p 340.

In pregnancies complicated by hypertension and intrauterine growth retardation, hPL has been used as a diagnostic adjunct. The levels reflect placental size, rather than fetal status itself.[22] Levels below 4 µg/mL after 30 weeks' gestation are considered to reflect fetal jeopardy.[23] However, based upon hPL levels alone, it is difficult to decide when to deliver such patients electively. hPL is of little or no value in pregnancies complicated by diabetes. Essentially a test of placental size and function, hPL fails to herald the relatively sudden fetal demise in a diabetic mother, who usually has a larger-than-average placenta and, therefore, higher hPL levels. Because of widely available antepartum fetal heart rate testing and ultrasonography, hPL assays today are infrequently used to monitor pregnancies complicated by intrauterine growth retardation or prolonged gestation.

Other protein hormones and substances of the trophoblast
It has been reported that the placenta also produces human chorionic thyrotropin (hCT),

ACTH, β-lipotropin, β-endorphin, various releasing factors, enzymes, and proteins. So far, the physiologic significance of these substances is unknown.

Although hCT was first detected in 1955, its physiologic role in normal pregnancies remains to be defined. This hormone appears to be a glycoprotein of molecular weight 28,000 and to differ from hCG. It is well known that thyrotropic activity is increased in many patients who have gestational trophoblastic disease.[24] The latter has been attributed to the intrinsic thyrotropic activity of the hCG molecule. However, hCT contains only 0.025% of the thyrotropic activity of TSH. Therefore, it is unlikely that hCT is solely responsible for the increase in thyroid activity observed in many patients with gestational trophoblastic disease. Both β-endorphin and β-lipotropin have been detected in human placental tissue. Most recently, Liotta and co-workers have provided data indicating that cultured human placental cells produce β-endorphin.[25] Analogous to the pituitary, the placental β-endorphin-like peptide is derived from a larger precursor molecule, pro-opiomelanocortin, by post-translational proteolytic cleavage. In this context, it appears plausible that the placenta produces ACTH. The presence of such a human chorionic corticotropin (hCC) has been described by several groups of investigators. Furthermore, recent research indicates that the placenta produces human chorionic luteinizing hormone-releasing factor (hCLRF) and thyrotropin-releasing factor (hCTRF). These factors appear to be indistinguishable from their hypothalamic counterparts (LRF or GnRH and TRF, respectively).

The placenta is known to produce and secrete such proteolytic enzymes as oxytocinase and heat-stable alkaline phosphatase. In addition, the placenta synthesizes and secretes pregnancy-specific β_1-glycoprotein (PSβG), which becomes detectable in maternal blood 7 to 14

Normal endocrinology

days after implantation.[26] Its circulating levels rise until term. PSβG is also produced by various tumors and therefore may be used as a tumor marker. Besides PSβG, the placenta appears to produce two other proteins that have been detected in maternal blood: pregnancy-associated plasma proteins A and B (PAPP-A, PAPP-B). Their physiologic role and that of PSβG remain to be established.

Fetoplacental steroid hormones

During the first 5 or 6 weeks after fertilization, the corpus luteum is the principal source of progesterone and estradiol. The trophoblast is too small to produce these steroids in amounts sufficient to maintain pregnancy. At 7 to 8 weeks' gestation, however, the trophoblast begins to secrete substantial quantities of steroid hormones, which meet the requirements for pregnancy maintenance without any ovarian contribution.[5] Clinically, surgical removal of the corpus luteum after 7 weeks' gestation does not cause abortion.

Placental steroid biosynthesis generally proceeds along the same biosynthetic pathways that operate in ovaries and testes. However, there are several important differences between placental and gonadal steroid biosynthesis. The placenta is considered an incomplete endocrine organ, because it lacks some enzymes necessary for steroid biosynthesis. These are present in the ovaries and testes. For this reason, placental steroid hormone production depends on maternal and/or fetal steroid precursors. Placenta and fetus collaborate, as the so-called fetoplacental unit, in producing large quantities of steroid hormones during human gestation. Numerous steroid biosynthetic pathways in the fetoplacental unit have been described. Only the quantitatively most important pathways are reviewed here: progesterone, androgen, estradiol and estrone, and estriol biosynthesis and metabolism by the placenta and the fetoplacental unit.

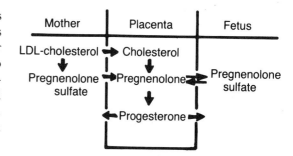

Figure 8-14
Placental progesterone biosynthesis.

Reproduced, with permission, from Goebelsmann U: Protein and steroid hormones in pregnancy. J Reprod Med 23:166, 1979.

Placental progesterone production

Maternal low-density lipoprotein (LDL) cholesterol is the principal precursor of placental progesterone (Figure 8-14).[27] As maternal LDL cholesterol is abundantly available, the amount of progesterone produced by the placenta depends on placental size and perfusion. Also, maternal and fetal pregnenolone sulfate is converted by the placenta to pregnenolone and progesterone. Pregnenolone is an intermediate in the conversion of cholesterol to progesterone.[27]

Maternal serum (plasma) progesterone concentrations rise progressively throughout gestation from an apparent nadir at 9 weeks' gestation to a plateau at approximately 36 weeks (Figure 8-15).[28] Serum progesterone levels, by and large, parallel placental weight during gestation. Hence, they could serve as an indicator of placental size and perfusion. During the last month of gestation, serum progesterone concentrations (C) average about 150 ng/mL, whereas the MCR of progesterone is approximately 2,000 L/day. By using these figures and the formula PR = MCR × C, the daily production rate (PR) for progesterone is calculated as 300 mg/day.

Unlike the adrenals, ovaries, or testes, the placenta does not metabolize progesterone to

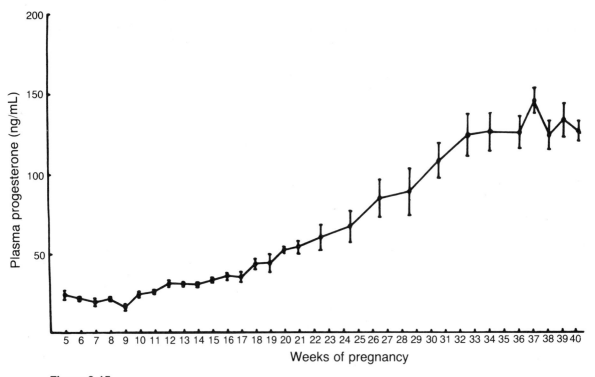

Figure 8-15
Plasma progesterone concentrations (±SE) during uncomplicated pregnancies.

From Johansson EDB: Plasma levels of progesterone in pregnancy measured by a rapid competitive protein binding technique. Acta Endocrinol (Kbh) 61:607, 1969.

17-hydroxyprogesterone, nor 17-hydroxyprogesterone to androstenedione; that is, the placenta lacks both 17-hydroxylase and 17,20-desmolase activity. It secretes progesterone into both the maternal and fetal circulation. Umbilical venous blood levels of progesterone exceed those of umbilical arterial blood (Table 8-3). The high progesterone concentrations in retroplacental (intervillous) blood are thought to be responsible for the finding that myometrial progesterone concentrations (150 ng/g) are highest in that part of the uterus to which the placenta is attached.[29] The myometrium contains progesterone receptors. Progesterone decreases uterine sensitivity to oxytocic stimuli, and thus counteracts the initiation of labor and propagation of

uterine contractions. Progesterone received its name because of this action.

Progesterone is metabolized both in the mother and in the fetus. In the fetus, progesterone is metabolized to corticosteroids. The most important maternal progesterone metabolite is pregnanediol. The conversion rate of progesterone to pregnanediol is on the order of 10% to 15%, whether or not pregnancy exists. Pregnanediol is excreted as the 3α-glucuronide in the urine. The level of urinary pregnanediol excretion rises during pregnancy and parallels that of serum progesterone.

In contrast with serum progesterone levels, 17-hydroxyprogesterone concentrations at midpregnancy (1.5 to 3.2 ng/mL) are not substantial-

Normal endocrinology

Table 8-3
Mean plasma progesterone concentrations ($\pm$SE) in five patients undergoing elective cesarean section at term

Location	Progesterone concentration (ng/mL)
Maternal peripheral vein	174 $\pm$ 37
Retroplacental space	886 $\pm$ 162
Umbilical artery	318 $\pm$ 39
Umbilical vein	440 $\pm$ 69

Compiled from data published by Tulchinsky D, Okada DM: Hormones in human pregnancy. IV. Plasma progesterone. Am J Obstet Gynecol 121:293, 1975.

ly higher than those observed during the luteal phase of the menstrual cycle. This finding is consistent with the lack of 17-hydroxylase activity in the placenta. The marked rise in levels of 17-hydroxyprogesterone after 35 weeks' gestation is largely due to production of 17-hydroxypregnenolone and 17-hydroxyprogesterone by the fetal adrenals.[30] Although the placenta does not convert progesterone to 17-hydroxyprogesterone, it metabolizes fetal 17-hydroxypregnenolone to 17-hydroxyprogesterone.

Placental androgen metabolism

As outlined above, the placenta does not metabolize pregnenolone and progesterone to their 17-hydroxylated metabolites, and neither 17-hydroxypregnenolone nor 17-hydroxyprogesterone undergoes 17,20-desmolase action to become C_{19} steroids ("androgens"). Hence, there is no conversion of pregnenolone or progesterone to DHEA, androstenedione, or testosterone. However, the placenta extracts DHEA-S from the maternal and fetal circulation and converts it to DHEA. The placenta hydrolyzes steroid sulfates quite readily, whereas the fetus sulfurylates steroids extensively. Containing 3β-ol dehydrogenase and $\Delta^5 \rightarrow \Delta^4$-isomerase activity, the placenta converts DHEA to androstenedione and testosterone, most of which is converted into estrone and estradiol rather than released into the circulation.

Since the placenta does not convert progesterone to androstenedione and testosterone and rapidly converts androstenedione and testosterone to estrone and estradiol (Figure 8-16),[27] the fetus is protected against exposure to androgens that might virilize a female. Maternal serum testosterone levels rise approximately two- to threefold during pregnancy and decrease postpartum. The rise in serum testosterone is explained largely by an increase in SHBG. During pregnancy, about 99% of serum testosterone is

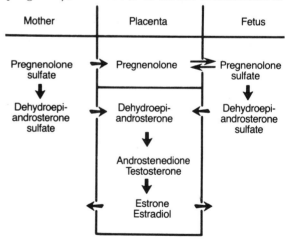

Figure 8-16
Placental estrone and estradiol biosynthesis from maternal and fetal precursors.

Reproduced, with permission, from Goebelsmann U: Protein and steroid hormones in pregnancy. J Reprod Med 23:166, 1979.

bound to this globulin. As the placenta converts androgens readily to estrogens, maternal serum testosterone levels may increase considerably before intrauterine virilization of the female fetus takes place. It has not been reported at which levels of serum testosterone virilization may occur. Marked increases (exceeding 4 ng/mL) in serum testosterone during pregnancy caused by tumors (luteomas and other testosterone-producing ovarian or adrenal tumors), however, may result in virilization of the female fetus. Recently, testosterone levels > 4 ng/mL in association with a theca-lutein cyst were reported not to result in virilization of the fetus.[31]

In comparison with androstenedione and testosterone concentrations, maternal serum levels of DHEA-S and DHEA decrease during pregnancy—DHEA-S by 50%.[32] DHEA originates from the adrenal predominantly as the sulfate and, because steroid sulfates are bound to serum albumin, circulates mainly as the sulfate. Placental extraction of DHEA-S and DHEA from the maternal circulation accounts for increased metabolic clearance of DHEA-S and DHEA as the placenta grows. In the absence of pregnancy, the MCR of DHEA-S is 7 L/day; at term in normal pregnancies it is 30 L/day. In toxemia of pregnancy, however, because of decreased placental size and perfusion, it is only 8 to 17 L/day. Thus, during pregnancy, the MCR of DHEA-S is a function and indicator of placental size and perfusion.

Fetoplacental estradiol and estrone production

As outlined in Figure 8-16, the placenta converts androstenedione and testosterone into estrone and estradiol. This conversion entails hydroxylation at carbon atom 19 (C-19), and C-19 removal and conversion into a steroid with a phenolic A ring. The latter conversion is termed "aromatization," because the resulting estrogens are, chemically speaking, aromatic compounds. The conversion of androstenedione and testosterone to estrone and estradiol provides necessary estrogens and prevents an increase in androgens that otherwise might cause virilization of a female fetus. The placenta is not capable of "aromatizing" such 19-norsteroids as norethindrone, which are well known to have the ability to effect virilization in utero and cause female pseudohermaphroditism. It is possible that this action of 19-norsteroids is brought about by inhibition of placental microsomal enzymes involved in the conversion of androgens to estrogens.

In late pregnancy, the placenta produces estrone and estradiol from approximately equal amounts of maternal and fetal DHEA-S, the C_{19} steroid precursor most abundantly available to the placenta. Placental estrone and estradiol production depends only partially on the availability of a fetal precursor, and, therefore, estradiol or estrone measurement is not an ideal test of fetal status.

The placenta does not metabolize estrone or estradiol further. Being unable to 16-hydroxylate, the placenta cannot form estriol from estrone or estradiol. Estrone and estradiol are secreted by the placenta into both the maternal and fetal circulations. The fetus inactivates the biologically active estradiol by hydroxylating the steroid molecule, as well as by sulfurylating it to the 3-sulfate. It is thought that such nonsteroidal estrogens as diethylstilbestrol may not be inactivated as efficiently as are the naturally occurring estrogens. Thus they may affect the fetus adversely by inhibiting Müllerian duct regression. The placenta cleaves estrogen sulfates. The resulting unconjugated estrogens traverse the placenta to the maternal compartment more readily than estrogen sulfates.

Maternal serum levels of estradiol rise throughout pregnancy until term, reaching a mean level of 16 ng/mL (Figure 8-17).[33] Serum estradiol is largely bound to SHBG. The maternal liver metabolizes and conjugates estrone and estradiol. Part of the metabolites is converted to

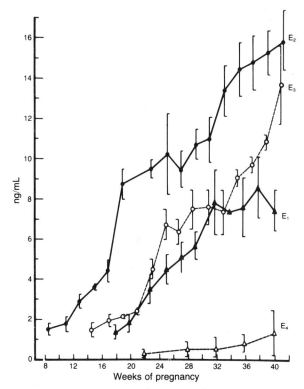

Figure 8-17
Mean plasma concentrations (±SE) of unconjugated estrone (E_1), estradiol (E_2), estriol (E_3), and estetrol (E_4) in pregnant women.

Reproduced, with permission, from Levitz M, Young BK: Estrogens in pregnancy. Vitamins Horm 35:109, 1977.

estriol. Maternal urinary estrone and estradiol excretion increases 100-fold from preovulatory values to term. Urinary estriol excretion, however, increases 1,000-fold over this period. This leads to the conclusion that 90% of the maternal urinary estriol does not originate in estrone and estradiol.

Fetoplacental estriol production

Biosynthetic collaboration of the fetus and the placenta is required to synthesize the large quantities of estriol produced and excreted during human pregnancy. The fetal adrenal secretes DHEA-S, which is converted by the fetal liver to 16-OH-DHEA-S. This is the principal fetal contribution to estriol biosynthesis. In the placenta, 16-OH-DHEA-S is hydrolyzed by sulfatase to 16-OH-DHEA. The placenta converts 16-OH-DHEA to 16-OH-androstenedione and 16-OH-testosterone, and aromatizes these compounds to 16-OH-estrone and 16-OH-estradiol (that is, estriol). This is analogous to the conversion of DHEA to androstenedione and testosterone and their subsequent metabolism to estrone and estradiol. Thus, both the fetus and the placenta play a mandatory role in the biosynthesis of estriol (Figure 8-18).[27]

In the absence of fetal ACTH stimulation, little or no fetal adrenal DHEA-S is produced. This situation is found in congenital absence of the pituitary gland, frequently in anencephalic fetuses, and in cases in which corticosteroids given the mother cross the placenta and suppress fetal ACTH secretion. Very rarely, a fetus may lack 16-hydroxylase activity. In this instance, estrone and estradiol are normal, but there is very low estriol formation. Placental sulfatase deficiency, however, prevents cleavage of DHEA-S as well as 16-OH-DHEA-S.[34] This leads to greatly decreased placental levels of estrone and estradiol, as well as greatly decreased estriol formation. Lack of estradiol appears to cause delayed onset of labor, which may lead to postmaturity and/or intrauterine death unless labor is induced or cesarean section is performed.[35]

The placenta secretes estriol into the maternal as well as the fetal circulation. In the fetus, estriol is predominantly sulfurylated, but is also converted into glucosiduronates. Unconjugated estriol crosses the placenta most readily. In the mother, estriol is metabolized almost entirely into four major conjugates, whereas its steroid moiety remains unchanged. Ninety percent of the estriol produced is excreted in the urine.

Approximately 90% to 92% of maternal plasma estriol is conjugated, and only 8% to 10%

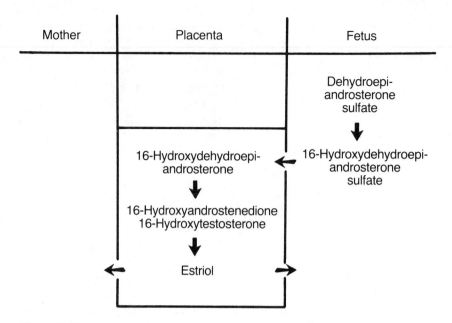

Figure 8-18
Principal pathway of fetoplacental estriol biosynthesis.

Reproduced, with permission, from Goebelsmann U: Protein and steroid hormones in pregnancy.
J Reprod Med 23:166, 1979.

is unconjugated ("free") estriol. Estriol 3-sulfate and estriol 3-sulfate 16-glucosiduronate, which bind to serum albumin, make up about 60% of circulating estriol. Estriol 16-glucosiduronate and estriol 3-glucosiduronate account for more than 90% of urinary estriol conjugates. Unconjugated plasma estriol concentrations at term average approximately 18 ng/mL, while total plasma estriol levels are about 220 ng/mL. Urinary estriol excretion at term averages 45 mg/24 hr.[33]

Plasma or urinary estriol levels serve as an indicator of fetal well-being in pregnancies complicated by diabetes mellitus, prolonged gestation ("postmaturity"), and intrauterine growth retardation, whether maternal hypertension is present or not. Besides estriol, plasma (serum) and urinary estetrol levels have been measured to assess fetal status in utero. Estetrol is distinguished from estriol by a fourth hydroxyl group at C-15. 15α-Hydroxylation takes place in the fe-

tal liver. Therefore, estetrol production is overwhelmingly of fetoplacental origin. It was postulated that estetrol production would reflect fetal status more accurately than estriol. However, clinical experience has shown that plasma estetrol measurements are no more useful than estriol assays. Also, plasma estetrol concentrations at term (1.2 ng/mL) are much lower than unconjugated plasma estriol levels.[33]

Figure 8-17 depicts mean plasma estrone, estradiol, estriol, and estetrol levels during pregnancy. Circulating estradiol levels are higher than estriol levels, because estradiol is bound to SHBG; plasma estetrol levels are much lower than those of the other three estrogens. Because of its low levels in the presence of much higher estrone, estradiol, and estriol concentrations, plasma estetrol is a difficult hormone to measure, and its measurement has remained, for the most part, a research tool.

Fetal endocrinology

Fetal ACTH and adrenal function

The primordia of both the adrenal cortex and the gonads originate in proximity to each other. By 6 weeks' gestation (that is, 4 weeks after conception), the adrenocortical primordium can be recognized histologically. At 8 weeks, the adrenal cortex has a discernible inner "fetal" and outer "definitive" zone. The developing fetal adrenal already contains chromaffin cells for the formation of the adrenal medulla. The fetal zone enlarges substantially during fetal life and involutes after delivery. The entire fetal zone has disappeared from the adrenal when the child is 1 year old. The relatively large size of the fetal adrenal, which at 16 weeks' gestation equals as much as 0.5% of the entire fetal volume, is largely due to the mass of the fetal zone, which comprises 80% of the entire adrenal.[36]

The fetal adrenal is capable of synthesizing steroids de novo from acetate and of metabolizing circulating LDL cholesterol, pregnenolone, and progesterone along the well-established pathways to cortisol and DHEA-S. It is remarkable that fetal 3β-ol-dehydrogenase activity—necessary to convert pregnenolone, 17-hydroxypregnenolone, and DHEA to progesterone, 17-hydroxyprogesterone, and androstenedione, respectively—is rather low. This may be due, in part, to the high estrogen milieu in the fetus. During the first half of pregnancy, hCG affects the ultrastructure of the fetal zone, suggesting a stimulatory effect.[37] This finding is consistent with the clinical observation that anencephalic fetuses lacking ACTH maintain normal adrenal development during the first half of pregnancy, when sufficient amounts of hCG enter the fetal compartment.

During the second half of pregnancy, fetal ACTH is the principal tropic hormone of the fetal adrenal. Fetal ACTH is necessary for fetal cortisol and adrenal androgen production. Anencephaly and congenital pituitary hypoplasia or aplasia (a rare disorder) result in adrenal hypoplasia, as is evident by low fetoplacental estriol production. When the mother receives large doses of corticosteroids, a certain portion crosses the placenta and suppresses fetal ACTH secretion. The latter leads to a decrease in fetal DHEA-S and, consequently, in fetoplacental estriol synthesis. Fetal plasma ACTH levels are highest during midgestation and decline noticeably during the last trimester. This decrease in fetal plasma ACTH could be due, in part, to increasing sensitivity of the maturing hypothalamic-pituitary centers to circulating cortisol. Or the reason may be an increase in the sensitivity of the adrenocortical cells to ACTH.

Maternal corticosteroid therapy affects both fetal ACTH levels and adrenocortical steroidogenesis. Maternal cortisol crosses the placenta. However, on its transplacental passage, cortisol is converted to the biologically less active cortisone. Similarly, relatively little maternal prednisone is found in the fetal compartment. Dexamethasone and betamethasone, however, which are transferred across the placenta more effectively, are subject to less placental and fetal metabolism than cortisol and prednisone. Thus, for the purpose of treating the fetus with glucocorticosteroids, betamethasone or dexamethasone should be used. For maternal glucocorticoid therapy, however, one should prescribe cortisol.

Fetal gonadotropins and gonadal function

The testes develop much earlier than the ovaries. Leydig cells appear at 7 weeks' gestation and, under hCG stimulation, produce rapidly increasing amounts of testosterone, which is required for the development of the male internal and external genitalia. Male fetal testosterone levels and Leydig cell numbers peak at 15 to 17 weeks.[21] At midgestation, fetal plasma testosterone levels fall and Leydig cells noticeably regress. By this time, hCG levels have fallen from their peak at 9 to 10 weeks' gestation to relatively low levels. Fetal testosterone production, under hCG stimulation during the first and early second trimesters, is regulated by fetal gonadotropins during the second half of gestation. Fetal testosterone appears to influence fetal LH and FSH secretion through negative feedback via the hypothalamus and pituitary. The fact that male fetal plasma FSH and LH levels, on the average, are lower than female fetal gonadotropin concentrations supports this contention. The clinical experience that male fetal hypopituitarism results in a micropenis at birth is proof that fetal gonadotropins are necessary for fetal testosterone production after midpregnancy.[38] Furthermore, male fetal plasma testosterone, which reaches male pubertal levels, affects the hypothalamus, where it is metabolized, in part, to estradiol (E_2).

FSH and LH can be detected in fetal pituitaries by 10 weeks' gestation.[39] Both gonadotropins are present in higher concentrations in the pituitary in female than in male fetuses. Also, fetal pituitary gonadotropin contents peak earlier in females than in males. Similarly, plasma FSH and LH levels are higher, and peak earlier, in female than in male fetuses.[39] In both sexes, plasma gonadotropins peak during the second trimester. Whereas hCG stimulates Leydig cell testosterone production in male fetuses beginning at 7 weeks, fetal FSH and LH are necessary to initiate follicle development in female fetuses. Primary follicles develop at 20 to 25 weeks' gestation when plasma FSH and LH (in that order)

levels culminate. That fetal FSH and LH are necessary for gonadal development is evident from the clinical observation that anencephalic fetuses have small ovaries. Follicle development proceeds throughout the third trimester with some Graafian follicle development by approximately 28 weeks and an increase in Graafian follicles by 35 weeks.

Fetal gonadal function is reflected in amniotic fluid sex hormone levels. At 15 to 17 weeks' gestation, amniotic fluid testosterone and androstenedione levels in women bearing male fetuses are substantially higher than in those bearing female fetuses. Amniotic fluid testosterone concentrations, in contrast with androstenedione levels, show essentially no overlap between sexes. However, amniotic fluid estradiol concentrations at midpregnancy are significantly higher in women carrying female fetuses (see Table 8-4).[40]

Fetal thyroid function

The thyroid gland can be detected at 9 weeks' gestation. Between 1 and 2 weeks later, thyroid hormone synthesis is demonstrable. The pituitary begins to develop at 7 weeks, when Rathke's pouch, from which it originates, establishes contact with the infundibulum. TSH can be identified at 12 weeks' pregnancy. The hypothalamic nuclei develop between 35 and 100 days after conception in the ventral portion of the diencephalon, forming the hypothalamus.

Table 8-4
Mean amniotic fluid concentrations ($\pm$SE) of androstenedione (A), testosterone (T), estrone (E_1), and estradiol (E_2) at midgestation

Fetal sex	A (pg/mL)	T (pg/mL)	E_1 (pg/mL)	E_2 (pg/mL)
Male	1,024 $\pm$ 53	224 $\pm$ 11	353 $\pm$ 38	64 $\pm$ 4
Female	668 $\pm$ 39	39 $\pm$ 2	331 $\pm$ 28	96 $\pm$ 8

Compiled from data published by Robinson JD, Judd HL, Young PE, et al: Amniotic fluid androgens and estrogens at midgestation. J Clin Endocrinol Metab 45:755, 1977.

Normal endocrinology

TSH-releasing hormone (TRH), as well as GnRH, is present by 8 to 10 weeks. Last to be completed in the hypothalamic-pituitary-thyroid feedback system is the portal system. The capillaries, constituting the proximal or hypothalamic portion of the hypothalamic-pituitary portal circulation, can be recognized at 15 to 16 weeks. The system is fully developed anatomically by 30 to 35 weeks.[21]

Fetal pituitary TSH content is low until 16 to 18 weeks and plasma TSH levels are relatively low up to 20 weeks' gestation. At this time, TSH levels begin to rise. Fetal circulating T_4 levels rise rapidly between 20 and 30 weeks and more slowly thereafter. After 30 weeks, fetal plasma TSH levels fall as free T_4 concentrations rise, indicating activation of the feedback that matures between midpregnancy and 1 month of life. The fetus converts T_4 primarily to reverse T_3 (rT_3), the α-monodeiodinated metabolite. As soon as the baby is born, there is a dramatic shift from α- to β-monodeiodination. This results in metabolism of T_4 to T_3 instead of rT_3. At birth, neonatal TSH levels rise most dramatically within hours, reaching 80 to 90 μU/mL—the highest levels ever achieved under physiologic conditions in life. This initiates a rapid rise in neonatal plasma T_4 and T_3, which is followed by a subsequent decline in plasma TSH. The premature infant is incapable of responding with such a pronounced rise in TSH, T_4, and T_3 when delivered into the cold world. Ill preemies have an even lower TSH, T_4, and T_3 rise. Hence, maintenance of body temperature through increased cell metabolism is a serious problem for the premature infant.

Fetal prolactin

Levels of fetal plasma PRL, which is of fetal pituitary origin, remain relatively low until the end of the second trimester. At this time, PRL levels begin to rise, first slowly and then exponentially, paralleling the pronounced rise in fetal plasma estradiol (E_2) levels.[41] In anencephalic fetuses, PRL is the only fetal pituitary hormone present in normal concentrations. The anterior pituitary is present but smaller in anencephalics. At term, umbilical venous PRL levels exceed maternal venous PRL concentrations. In infants, however, plasma PRL levels are very low. They begin to rise in girls in conjunction with the pubertal rise in circulating E_2 levels.

The highest PRL concentrations are found in amniotic fluid. PRL levels in amniotic fluid rise during pregnancy to reach a peak at 16 weeks and then plateau until 28 weeks, after which they decline (Figure 8-19).[42] Amniotic fluid PRL is thought to originate in the decidua. When a pregnant woman receives bromocriptine, fetal plasma PRL levels are suppressed, but amniotic fluid PRL concentrations remain unaffected. Bromocriptine passes the placenta and has the same effect on the fetus as it has on the mother. It decreases pituitary PRL release. That amniotic fluid PRL levels remain unaffected by bromocriptine indicates that it is of neither maternal nor fetal pituitary origin. However, amniotic fluid PRL might arise in the placenta as well.

Roles of hormones in pregnancy maintenance and initiation of labor

Maintenance of pregnancy

Elaboration of large amounts of estrogens and progesterone by the fetus and/or placenta is unique to the human species. Although their physiologic role is still incompletely understood, one may reasonably presume that these profound endocrine changes are in the interest of pregnancy maintenance. At term, however, physiology requires that the uterus expel the fetus at the appropriate time, reversing its quiescence into an active state that leads to timely delivery without undue trauma. It would be logical to hypothesize that the fetus is somehow involved in initiating labor at the appropriate point in gestation.

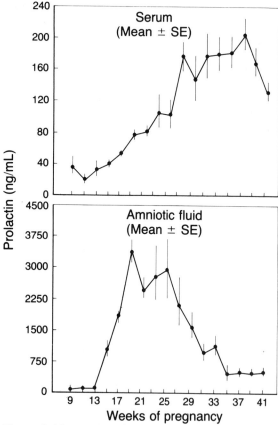

Figure 8-19
Mean prolactin levels (±SE) in serum and amniotic fluid throughout normal gestation.

Reproduced, with permission, from Kletzky OA, Rossman F, Bertolli SI, et al: Dynamics of human chorionic gonadotropin, prolactin and growth hormone in serum and amniotic fluid throughout normal human pregnancy. Am J Obstet Gynecol, in press.

Both estradiol and progesterone are involved in pregnancy maintenance. The approximately 100-fold rise in estradiol production, between the preovulatory estradiol peak and term pregnancy, stimulates uterine growth. During pregnancy, the uterus increases tenfold in weight and 500-fold in volume, largely by hypertrophy of existing myometrial cells. Besides this estrogen-mediated action, the stretching effect of the growing products of conception provides another stimulus for myometrial growth and uterine expansion. Besides stimulating myometrial hypertrophy, estradiol increases uteroplacental blood flow. It should be noted that in contrast with its otherwise weak estrogenic activity, estriol appears to be almost as effective as estradiol in increasing uterine blood flow.

In addition to this uterotropic effect, estradiol increases hepatic protein synthesis. Plasma CBG, SHBG, and TBG concentrations all increase markedly during pregnancy. CBG binds both corticosteroids and progesterone, whereas SHBG binds testosterone and, to a lesser extent, estradiol. As protein-bound hormones are neither as readily taken up by tissue receptors nor as rapidly metabolized as unbound ("free") hormones, binding proteins modify both the physiologic effects and the half-lives of hormones. Also, the rise in estradiol during pregnancy stimulates angiotensinogen (renin substrate) production and results in increasing aldosterone production. At the hypothalamic and pituitary levels, the markedly elevated concentrations of estradiol, in conjunction with rising progesterone levels, effect FSH and LH suppression.

Progesterone has been found to block cellular immune responses to foreign (fetal) antigens. Thus it may play a role in preventing maternal rejection of the trophoblast.[43] Animal experiments have shown that progesterone can inhibit T-lymphocyte responses that mediate xenogenic graft rejection.

Studies in rats and rabbits, notably those of Csapo and Pulkkinen,[5] have shown that progesterone renders the uterus unresponsive to oxytocic stimuli. But massive doses of exogenous progesterone or progestins have been ineffective in preventing uterine contractions in women. Estradiol, in turn, has been shown to enhance uterine muscle excitability. States of low fetoplacental estrogen production, such as anencephaly and placental sulfatase deficiency, often are associated with prolonged gestation and inadequate uterine contractility. Multiple modes

Normal endocrinology

of action by which estradiol and progesterone influence uterine activity have been elucidated: effects on membrane potentials and Ca^{++} flux; gap junctions that permit the organized spread of action potentials from fiber to fiber to facilitate a concerted and mechanically effective uterine contraction; β-adrenergic receptor density; and prostaglandin synthesis.[44]

Recent studies have shown that myometrial cells produce prostacyclin (PGI_2), which relaxes the uterine muscle. Relaxin, which originates in the corpus luteum (of the cycle and of pregnancy) and—quite likely—locally in decidua and myometrium, has been shown to stimulate myometrial prostacyclin synthesis.[45] Relaxin levels are particularly high during early pregnancy. It is conceivable that this product of the corpus luteum is as important as progesterone in maintaining pregnancy during the first trimester.[45] It is of interest, however, that cortisol inhibits myometrial prostacyclin synthesis, thus diminishing one of the primary factors that maintain uterine quiescence. It is well known that labor, through the pain and stress associated with it, increases maternal ACTH, β-endorphin, and cortisol levels. This rise in maternal plasma cortisol may further stimulate uterine contractions by inhibiting myometrial prostacyclin synthesis.[46]

Initiation of labor

The sequence of hormonal events that lead to labor is well established in sheep.[47] The ovine fetus initiates its delivery itself, by increased cortisol production. The rise in cortisol causes a decrease in placental progesterone and increase in estradiol production through increased 17-hydroxylase, 17,20-desmolase, and aromatase activity. This alteration of placental progesterone and estradiol production, favoring the latter steroid hormone, stimulates the production of prostaglandins PGE_2 and $PGF_{2\alpha}$. These cause uterine contractions and effect delivery of the lamb. If the ovine fetus is hypophysectomized or adrenalectomized, these changes do not occur.

But ACTH or cortisol administration will result in uterine contractions in sheep.

The hormonal mechanisms that initiate human labor are not well identified. The principal agents that actually cause uterine contractions appear to be the same as in other mammalian species: prostaglandins PGE_2 and $PGF_{2\alpha}$. However, the chain of events that lead to PGE_2 and $PGF_{2\alpha}$ synthesis in humans remains to be fully elucidated. Although oxytocin causes uterine contractions, it seems to play a minor role in the initiation of labor. It appears to be of greater importance during the second and, particularly, the third stage of labor. Many investigators have searched for a possible decrease in placental progesterone and increase in estradiol production before the onset of labor in women.

However, the majority of researchers have not found such a change in circulatory progesterone and estradiol levels. Despite these negative findings, there could still be an absolute or relative decrease in progesterone and/or increase in estradiol levels in target tissues.

Casey and collaborators established the hypothesis that a relative decrease in fetal membrane progesterone levels would result in the release of phospholipase A_2 from lysosomes.[48] This enzyme then would cleave arachidonic acid from phospholipids, and the labor would initiate prostaglandin synthesis in fetal membranes and decidua. PGE_2 and $PGF_{2\alpha}$ thus synthesized would then cause cervical ripening and uterine contractions. This hypothesis is consistent with the well-known clinical experience that "stripping" of the membranes, as well as amnionitis, a destabilization of the fetal membrane-decidual-myometrial unit, often results in uterine contractions. More recently, Casey et al have presented data that indicate the human fetus excretes a proteinaceous substance, pisseaktis, in its urine.[49] This stimulates prostaglandin synthesis in cultured human amnion as well as endometrial stromal cells (the equivalent of the decidua of pregnancy). This as yet unidentified substance apparently stimulates prostaglandin synthetase activity. It remains to be established which mechanism(s), if any, regulate(s) the production and/or excretion of the above substance by the fetal kidney. If this hypothesis proves to be correct, we will know that the human fetus is capable of determining its time of delivery.

References

1. Mishell DR Jr, Nakamura RM, Barberia JM, et al: Initial detection of human chorionic gonadotropin in serum in normal human gestation. *Am J Obstet Gynecol* 118:990, 1974

2. Mishell DR Jr, Thorneycroft IH, Nagata Y, et al: Serum gonadotropin and steroid patterns in early pregnancy. *Am J Obstet Gynecol* 117:631, 1973

3. Shoupe D, Kletzky OA: Priming with GnRH restores gonadotropin secretion during first but not second trimester of pregnancy. *Am J Obstet Gynecol* 150:460, 1984

4. Tulchinsky D, Hobel CJ: Plasma human chorionic gonadotropin, estrone, estradiol, estriol, progesterone, and 17α-hydroxyprogesterone in human pregnancy. III. Early normal pregnancy. *Am J Obstet Gynecol* 117:884, 1973

5. Csapo AI, Pulkkinen M: Indispensability of the human corpus luteum in the maintenance of early pregnancy. Luteectomy evidence. *Obstet Gynecol Surv* 33:69, 1978

6. Gibson M, Tulchinsky D: The maternal adrenal. In Tulchinsky D, Ryan KJ (eds): *Maternal-Fetal Endocrinology.* Philadelphia, WB Saunders, 1980, p 129

7. Fisher DA: Maternal-fetal thyroid function in pregnancy. *Clinics Perinatol* 10:615, 1983

8. Furth ED: Thyroid and parathyroid hormone function in pregnancy. In Fuchs F, Klopper A (eds): *Endocrinology of Pregnancy,* ed 3. Philadelphia, Harper & Row, 1983, p 176

9. Yen SSC, Samaan N, Pearson OH: Growth hormone levels in pregnancy. *J Clin Endocrinol Metab* 27:1341, 1967

10. Yen SSC, Vela P, Tsai CC: Impairment of growth hormone secretion in response to hypoglycemia during early and late pregnancy. *J Clin Endocrinol Metab* 31:29, 1970

11. Rigg LA, Lein A, Yen SSC: The pattern of increase in circulating prolactin levels during human gestation. *Am J Obstet Gynecol* 129:454, 1977

12. Rigg LA, Yen SSC: Multiphasic prolactin secretion during parturition in humans. *Am J Obstet Gynecol* 128:215, 1977

13. Lenton EA, Neal LM, Sulaiman R: Plasma concentrations of human chorionic gonadotropin from the time of implantation until the second week of pregnancy. *Fertil Steril* 37:773, 1982

14. Catt KJ, Dufau ML, Vaitukaitis JL: Appearance of hCG in pregnancy plasma following the initiation of implantation of the blastocyst. *J Clin Endocrinol Metab* 40:537, 1975

15. Braunstein GD, Rasor J, Adler D, et al: Serum human chorionic gonadotropin levels throughout normal pregnancy. *Am J Obstet Gynecol* 126:678, 1976

16. Barnes RB, Roy S, Yee B, et al: Sensitivity of urinary pregnancy tests in surgically proven ectopic pregnancies. *J Reprod Med,* in press

17. Mishell DR Jr, Davajan V: Quantitative immunologic assay of hCG in normal and abnormal pregnancy. *Am J Obstet Gynecol* 96:231, 1966

18. Nygren K-G, Johansson EDB, Wide L: Evaluation of the prognosis of threatened abortion from the peripheral plasma levels of progesterone, estradiol, and human chorionic gonadotropin. *Am J Obstet Gynecol* 116:916, 1973

19. Marrs RP, Kletzky OA, Howard WF, et al: Disappearance of human chorionic gonadotropin and resumption of ovulation following abortion. *Am J Obstet Gynecol* 135:731, 1979

20. Morrow CP, Kletzky OA, DiSaia PJ, et al: Clinical and laboratory correlates of molar pregnancy and trophoblastic disease. *Am J Obstet Gynecol* 128:424, 1977

21. Pellinemi LJ, Dym M: The fetal gonad and sexual differentiation. In Tulchinsky D, Ryan KJ (eds): *Maternal-Fetal Endocrinology.* Philadelphia, WB Saunders, 1980, pp 252-280

22. Selenkow HA, Saxena BN, Dana CL, et al: Measurement and pathophysiologic significance of human placental lactogen. In Pecile A, Finzi C (eds): *The Foeto-Placental Unit.* Amsterdam, Excerpta Medica Foundation, 1969, p 340

23. Spellacy WN, Teoh ES, Buhi WC: Human chorionic somatomammotropin (hCS) levels prior to fetal death in high-risk pregnancies. *Obstet Gynecol* 35:685, 1970

24. Odell WD, Bates RW, Rislin RS: Increased thyroid function without clinical hypothyroidism in patients with choriocarcinoma. *J Clin Endocrinol Metab* 23:658, 1963

25. Liotta AS, Houghton R, Krieger D: Identification of a β-endorphin-like peptide in cultured placental cells. *Nature* 295:593, 1982

26. Grudzinskas JG, Lenton EA, Gordon YB, et al: Circulating levels of pregnancy specific β_1 glycoprotein in early pregnancy. *Br J Obstet Gynecol* 84:740, 1977

27. Goebelsmann U: Protein and steroid hormones in pregnancy. *J Reprod Med* 23:166, 1979

28. Johansson EDB: Plasma levels of progesterone in pregnancy measured by a rapid competitive protein binding technique. *Acta Endocrinol (Kbh)* 61:607, 1969

29. Tulchinsky D, Okada DM: Hormones in human pregnancy: IV. Plasma progesterone. *Am J Obstet Gynecol* 121:293, 1975

30. Tulchinsky D, Hobel CJ, Yeager E, et al: Plasma estrone, estradiol, estriol, progesterone, and 17-

hydroxyprogesterone in human pregnancy: I. Normal pregnancy. *Am J Obstet Gynecol* 112:1095, 1972

31. Berger NG, Repke JT, Woodruff JD: Markedly elevated serum testosterone in pregnancy without fetal virilization. *Obstet Gynecol* 63:260, 1984

32. Nieschlag E, Walk T, Schindler AE: Dehydroepiandrosterone (DHA) and DHA-sulfate during pregnancy in maternal blood. *Horm Metab Res* 6:170, 1974

33. Levitz M, Young BK: Estrogens in pregnancy. *Vitamins Horm* 35:109, 1977

34. France JT, Liggins GC: Placental sulfatase deficiency. *J Clin Endocrinol Metab* 29:138, 1969

35. France JT, Seddon RJ, Liggins GC: A study of a pregnancy with low estrogen production due to placental sulfatase deficiency. *J Clin Endocrinol Metab* 36:1, 1973

36. Jaffe RB: The endocrinology of pregnancy. In Yen SSC, Jaffe RB (eds): *Reproductive Endocrinology*. Philadelphia, WB Saunders, 1978, p 521

37. Serón-Ferré M, Lawrence CC, Jaffe RB: Role of hCG in regulation of the fetal zone of the human fetal adrenal gland. *J Clin Endocrinol Metab* 46:834, 1978

38. Lee PA, Mazur T, Danish R, et al: Micropenis. I. Criteria, etiologies and classification. *Johns Hopkins Med J* 146:156, 1980

39. Kaplan SL, Grumbach MM: The ontogenesis of human foetal hormones. II. Luteinizing hormone (LH) and follicle-stimulating hormone (FSH). *Acta Endocrinol* 81:808, 1976

40. Robinson JD, Judd HL, Young PE, et al: Amniotic fluid androgens and estrogens at midgestation. *J Clin Endocrinol Metab* 45:755, 1977

41. Winters AJ, Colston C, McDonald PC, et al: Fetal plasma prolactin levels. *J Clin Endocrinol Metab* 41:626, 1975

42. Kletzky OA, Rossman F, Bertolli SI, et al: Dynamics of human chorionic gonadotropin, prolactin and growth hormone in serum and amniotic fluid throughout normal human pregnancy. *Am J Obstet Gynecol*, in press

43. Siiteri PK, Febres F, Clemens LE: Progesterone and maintenance of pregnancy: Is progesterone nature's immunosuppressant? *Ann NY Acad Sci* 286:384, 1977

44. Toro KI, Csapo AI: The effects of progesterone, prostaglandin $F_{2\alpha}$ and oxytocin on the calcium-activation of the uterus. *Prostaglandins* 12:253, 1976

45. Weiss G: Relaxin. *Clin Perinatol* 10:641, 1983

46. Thorburn GD, Challis JRG: Endocrine control of parturition. *Physiol Rev* 59:863, 1979

47. Liggins GC, Fairclough RG, Grieves SA, et al: The mechanism of initiation of parturition in the ewe. *Recent Prog Horm Res* 29:111, 1973

48. Casey ML, Winkel CA, Porter JC, et al: Endocrine regulation of the initiation and maintenance of parturition. *Clin Perinatol* 10:709, 1983

49. Casey ML, McDonald PC, Mitchell PC: Stimulation of prostaglandin E_2 production in amnion cells in culture by a substance(s) in human fetal urine. *Biochem Biophys Res Commun* 114:1056, 1985

Suggested reading

Diczfalusy E: Steroid metabolism in the foeto-placental unit. In Pecile A, Finzi C (eds): *The Foeto-Placental Unit*. Amsterdam, Excerpta Medica Foundation, 1969, p 65

Goebelsmann U: Hormonal assessment of pregnancy. In Sciarra JJ (ed): *Gynecology and Obstetrics*, vol 3. Philadelphia, Harper & Row, 1983

Josimovich JB: Placental protein hormones in pregnancy. *Clin Obstet Gynecol* 16:46, 1973

Little AM, Billiar RB: Endocrine disorders. In Romney SL, Gray MJ, Little AB, et al (eds): *Gynecology and Obstetrics: The Health Care of Women*. New York, McGraw-Hill, 1980, pp 373-420

Marrs RP, Mishell DR Jr: Placental tropic hormones. *Clin Obstet Gynecol* 23:721, 1980

Stark RI, Frantz AG: ACTH-β-endorphin in pregnancy. *Clin Perinatol* 10:653, 1983

Chapter 9

Endocrinology of Lactation and the Puerperium

Daniel R. Mishell Jr., M.D.
Richard P. Marrs, M.D.

Only recently have studies been performed that provide a basic understanding of the endocrinologic alterations occurring during the puerperium, as well as of the mechanism whereby lactation interferes with the postpartum resumption of ovulation. The relatively recent development of a radioimmunoassay for measuring prolactin in humans has been of great assistance in providing such knowledge. In many countries, breast-feeding is the principal source of infant nutrition; therefore, an understanding of the endocrine mechanisms involved in lactation is of great importance.

Hormones influencing the breast

At least seven hormones directly influence the structure and function of the human breast: insulin, hydrocortisone, thyroxine, estradiol, progesterone, prolactin, and oxytocin. Actually, the number is much higher because many related compounds (for example, triiodothyronine, other steroidal and nonsteroidal estrogens, and synthetic progestins) may also affect the breast. For convenience, however, the following discussion is limited to the first seven hormones named.

Two hormones that are sometimes called "lactogenic" will not be considered in any detail. Growth hormone (GH), which is secreted by the pituitary, and human placental lactogen (hPL), which is produced by the placenta, have very similar amino acid sequences. They are lactogenic in some animals, but in humans their primary influence is on maternal carbohydrate metabolism. Neither GH nor hPL has been shown to have an important physiologic influence on the human breast.

Insulin, hydrocortisone, and thyroxine

The roles of insulin, hydrocortisone, and thyroxine have been inferred primarily from in vitro and animal studies. Although a deficiency of any of these hormones usually prevents lactation, a detailed understanding of their function in humans is lacking. They appear to exert permissive and relatively nonspecific effects on mammary gland cells.

These three hormones are involved with the maintenance of protein synthesis in all cells.

This function differs from that of prolactin, which appears to be unnecessary for generalized protein synthesis. Prolactin initiates specific lactogenic activity in normally functioning mammary alveolar cells.

Estradiol, progesterone, and prolactin

Estradiol, progesterone, and prolactin each have specific breast effects that are manifested during different stages of the reproductive cycle. At puberty, under the influence of rising estradiol levels, the breasts begin to assume their adult size and configuration. The changes consist primarily in the growth of fatty and connective tissue between and within the 15 to 20 lobes that make up each breast. The nipples and the areolae also enlarge and become darkly pigmented. There is some development of the mammary ducts within each lobe, but this limited growth contributes little to the overall size of the breast. The ducts terminate in small buds without the alveoli. This entire process can be produced in hypoestrogenic women by exogenous administration of estrogen alone, without progesterone.

With the onset of ovulation, some women experience cyclic premenstrual breast discomfort, or mastodynia. The exact cause of this symptom is unknown, but presumably it is related to vascular and lymphatic changes. Although progesterone has been shown to stimulate devel-

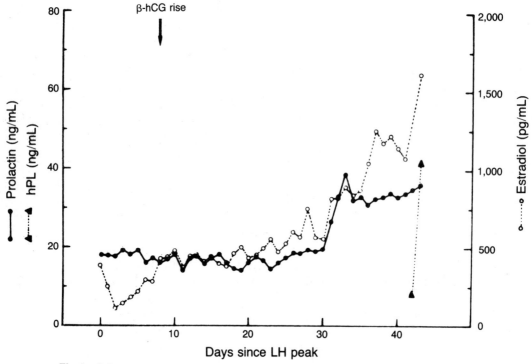

Figure 9-1
Measurement of prolactin, human placental lactogen, and estradiol in serum samples obtained daily. The day of initial detection of β-hCG is indicated by the downward arrow.

From Barberia JM, Abu-Fadil S, Kletzky OA, et al: Serum prolactin patterns in early human gestation. Am J Obstet Gynecol 121:1107, 1975.

opment of mammary gland acini, there is disagreement among pathologists as to whether the breast undergoes cyclic alveolar histologic changes analogous to those of the endometrium.

During pregnancy, the circulating levels of estradiol and progesterone increase by ten- to 100-fold at term. Also, there is a marked increase in circulating prolactin levels. Mean serum prolactin levels increase fivefold during the first trimester, with a subsequent doubling in each succeeding trimester.[1] The increase in prolactin is probably stimulated by the increase in estrogen secretion in pregnancy. Circulating prolactin levels begin to increase early in pregnancy when endogenous estrogen levels increase (Figure 9-1),[2] and there is an excellent correlation between the levels of these two hormones throughout gestation (Figure 9-2).[3] Morphologically, the breast undergoes striking alterations during the gestational period. Beginning in the second trimester, a true alveolar system appears for the first time. Both the ductal and acinar elements hypertrophy, and the alveoli become distended with secretion. This secretory material, colostrum, can sometimes be expressed in small amounts during pregnancy. Most women, however, do not lactate before delivery, even though the anatomic preparation for lactation has occurred and all the required hormones are present in high concentrations.

True lactation does not occur during pregnancy because estradiol inhibits prolactin-receptor interaction in the alveolar cells. Estradiol thus affects the breast in contradictory ways: It has a tropic effect on breast development and mammary gland structure, but an inhibitory effect on lactation. Lactation does not begin postpartum until circulating estradiol has been cleared to levels at or lower than those usually found during the early follicular phase of the menstrual cycle (20 to 40 pg/mL).

Usually, maternal estradiol levels are low enough to permit lactation by the second or third day postpartum. Relieved of this steroidal

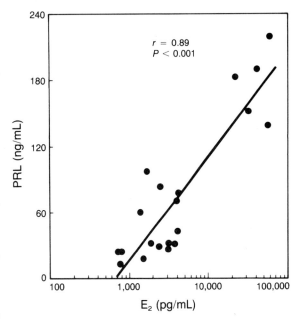

Figure 9-2
Correlation between plasma PRL and E_2 values during first, second, and third trimesters of pregnancy.

Reproduced, with permission, from Kletzky OA, Marrs RP, Howard WF, et al: Prolactin synthesis and release during pregnancy and puerperium. Am J Obstet Gynecol 136:545, 1980.

inhibition, mammary gland function becomes dependent on prolactin and oxytocin, both of which are secreted in response to the suckling stimulus, but by different mechanisms.

Oxytocin

Breast stimulation results in the release of oxytocin by the posterior pituitary. Unlike the secretion of prolactin, this response is a classic neurohormonal conditioned reflex that may be elicited by such visual stimuli as playing with the infant and is inhibited by various kinds of stress. Oxytocin causes contraction of the myoepithelial cells that partially surround the alveoli, resulting in the expulsion or "letdown" of milk. Oxytocin also causes uterine contractions that are often symptomatic and that may reduce postpartum blood loss.

Effects of prolactin on lactation

Prolactin appears to be the primary stimulus of lactogenesis, acting directly on the alveolar secretory cells. The hormone does not enter its target cells, but rather exerts its effect through binding to specific cell membrane receptors.

Noel and colleagues have shown that in a group of women studied between 1 and 6 weeks postpartum, baseline plasma prolactin levels were elevated and markedly increased within 10 minutes after suckling.[4] Levels rose steadily until 10 minutes after the end of the 30-minute suckling period, at which time they started to decline steadily, and reached prenursing levels about 3 hours after the beginning of the nursing period (Figure 9-3).[4] In a group of nursing

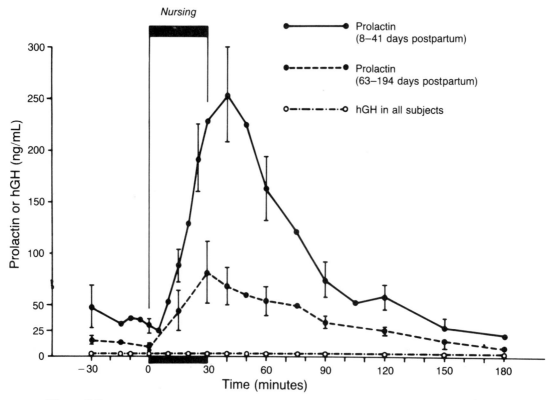

Figure 9-3
Plasma prolactin and growth hormone concentrations during nursing in postpartum women. Twelve studies were performed on eight women between 8 and 41 days postpartum, and six studies were performed on six women between 63 and 194 days postpartum. Vertical lines indicate standard errors of the mean. Growth hormone, shown at the bottom, did not rise with suckling.

Reproduced, with permission, from Noel GL, Suh HK, Frantz AG: Prolactin release during nursing and breast stimulation in postpartum and nonpostpartum subjects. J Clin Endocrinol Metab 38:413, 1974. © 1974 The Endocrine Society.

Normal endocrinology

women studied by these same investigators 2 to 7 months postpartum, baseline prolactin levels were lower, in the normal range. They increased to a much lesser extent, reached maximum levels about 30 minutes after nursing began, and declined to prenursing levels within 2 hours. There was much individual variation in prolactin levels among the subjects studied in both groups. These investigators determined that the mechanism of activation of prolactin release is tactile stimulation of the breast and nipple area.

This effect is similar to, but much more marked than, that which occurs after breast and nipple stimulation in the nonpregnant woman.

In a group of women who played with their infants for 30 minutes before breast contact, milk letdown, brought about by oxytocin release, occurred within 5 minutes of seeing or holding the infant, but prolactin levels did not rise until after the start of nursing (Figure 9-4).[4] The pattern of prolactin response and amount of increase were similar among a group of lactat-

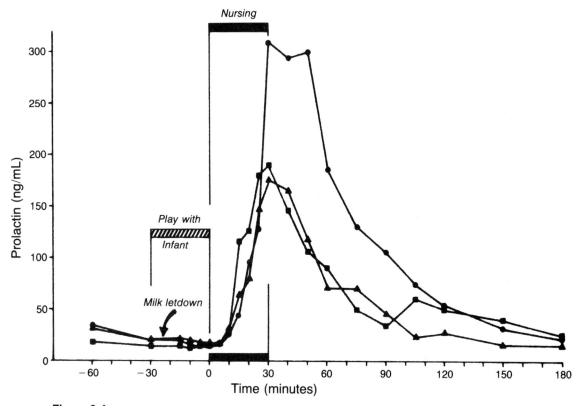

Figure 9-4
Plasma prolactin concentrations during anticipation of nursing and actual nursing in three women who were between 22 and 26 days postpartum. The women played with their infants for 30 minutes before suckling began; milk letdown occurred in each case 25 and 30 minutes before suckling.

Reproduced, with permission, from Noel GL, Suh HK, Frantz AG: Prolactin release during nursing and breast stimulation in postpartum and nonpostpartum subjects. J Clin Endocrinol Metab 38:413, 1974. © 1974 The Endocrine Society.

ing women whose breast milk was expressed for 30 minutes with a breast pump (Figure 9-5).[4] Thus, prolactin release is stimulated by mechanical, not psychological, factors. It has been shown that oxytocin does not stimulate the release of prolactin.

Battin and colleagues recently performed a longitudinal study of eight women whose infants were exclusively breast-fed for the first 6 months after birth. Prolactin levels were measured before and at four intervals during the 2 hours after nursing began on five different days from 10 to 180 days postpartum.[5] Both mean baseline and peak prolactin levels declined during this period, but the mean baseline prolactin levels at 6 months were still elevated above normal (44 ng/mL; Figure 9-6).[5] The percentage of maximum increase of prolactin levels over baseline remained relatively constant during the study period. The increase was about 120% 10 days postpartum and about 130% 6 months postpartum (Figure 9-7).[5] Again, as has been reported

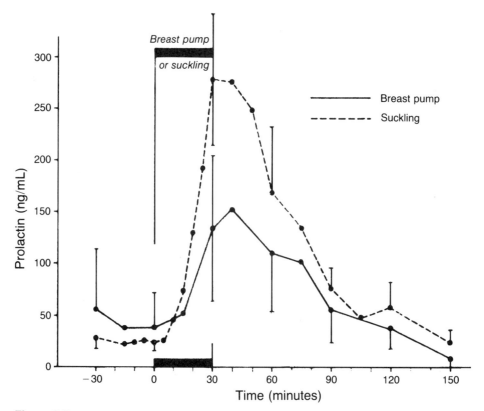

Figure 9-5
Comparison of the effects of breast pump with suckling on plasma prolactin in three women. Mean days postpartum during suckling study, 24; mean days postpartum during breast pump study, 60. Vertical lines represent standard errors of the mean.

Reproduced, with permission, from Noel GL, Suh HK, Frantz AG: Prolactin release during nursing and breast stimulation in postpartum and nonpostpartum subjects. J Clin Endocrinol Metab 38:413, 1974. © 1974 The Endocrine Society.

Normal endocrinology

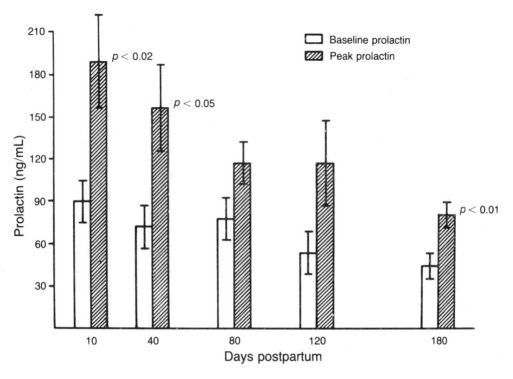

Figure 9-6
Comparison of baseline and peak serum prolactin levels post-suckling in all subjects during the first 180 days postpartum (means ± SE).

From Battin DA, Marrs RP, Fleiss PM, et al: The effects of suckling on serum prolactin, LH, FSH, and estradiol during prolonged lactation. Obstet Gynecol 65:785, 1985. Reprinted with permission from The American College of Obstetricians and Gynecologists.

in other studies, there was marked variability among subjects in the magnitude and time of the peak prolactin level after suckling began.

Tyson and colleagues measured serial prolactin levels in a group of nursing women and also found a variable prolactin response. There was a correlation between the duration and frequency of each nursing event and the prolactin increment as well as milk yield. These investigators stated that the amount of prolactin increase was related to the intensity of the infant's suckling (that is, activity during nursing), whereas the milk yield was unrelated to the amount of PRL increment.[6] Delvoye and associates reported that in a population of central African women, whose lactation is prolonged for up to 2 years after delivery and mothers breast-feed on demand, baseline prolactin levels remained elevated until 15 months postpartum.[7] A similar finding was reported by Gross and Eastman in a group of urban Australian women who breast-fed their babies on demand for more than 1 year.[8] In their study, baseline prolactin levels remained elevated for 15 months postpartum. In both these studies, only a slight increase or no increase of prolactin levels occurred after suckling beyond 6 months postpartum (Figure 9-8).[8]

Ovarian function during the puerperium

It is well established that the resumption of menstruation, as well as ovulation, is delayed after parturition in mothers who breast-feed their infants, compared with nonlactating women. It is also established that the time of return of ovulation is related to the frequency as well as the total duration of breast-feeding. In certain societies where infants breast-feed on demand for as long as 2 years after delivery, the incidence of amenorrhea and lack of conception remains high for a similar interval.

Cronin evaluated basal body temperature curves and menstrual calendars of a group of nursing and nonnursing women.[9] He found that among 93 nonnursing mothers, the mean time of first ovulation was about $10\frac{1}{2}$ weeks after delivery; about 30% had ovulated between 4 and 8 weeks postpartum; 60% had ovulated by 14 weeks postpartum; and 80% had ovulated by 16 weeks postpartum. About 5% of these non-

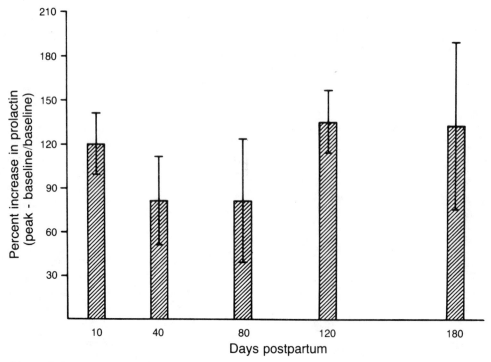

Figure 9-7
Percentage increase of peak serum prolactin after suckling over baseline in all subjects during the first 180 days postpartum (means ± SE, no statistical difference between groups).

From Battin DA, Marrs RP, Fleiss PM, et al: The effects of suckling on serum prolactin, LH, FSH, and estradiol during prolonged lactation. Obstet Gynecol 65:785, 1985. Reprinted with permission from The American College of Obstetricians and Gynecologists.

Normal endocrinology

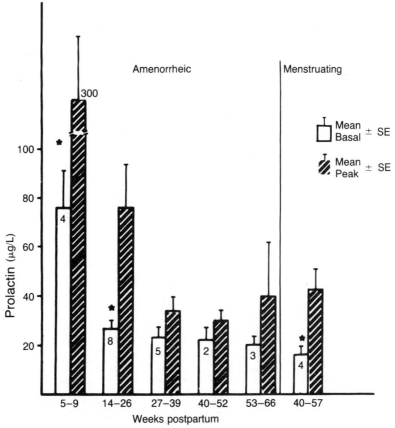

Figure 9-8
Mean concentration of serum prolactin before and after suckling in amenorrheic breast-feeding women during 5 to 66 weeks postpartum and in menstruating breast-feeding women. The number of women in each group is indicated in the open column. Values are expressed as means ± SE. The level of prolactin after suckling was significantly different (*$P < 0.05$) from the base level before suckling at 5 to 9 weeks and 14 to 26 weeks in amenorrheic women and menstruating women, but was not significantly different at other times.

Reproduced, with permission, from Gross BA, Eastman CJ: Prolactin secretion during prolonged lactational amenorrhoea. Aust NZ J Obstet Gynaecol 19:95, 1979.

nursing mothers ovulated between 4 and 6 weeks postpartum, as determined by a rise in basal temperature for 10 or more days. The earliest day of ovulation was 27 days postpartum.

Perez and colleagues performed a similar study in Chile and, in addition to evaluating menstrual calendars and basal temperatures, performed vaginal cytology, cervical mucus examinations, and endometrial biopsies. In their study, only 30 women did not nurse, and their mean time of return of ovulation was 49 days, with the earliest being 36 days. Women who stopped nursing after 2 weeks had a similar rapid return of ovulation.[10] In Cronin's study, all but one of the five women who ovulated before 6 weeks did so before their first menses. Overall, about one-third of the nonlactators ovulated before their first menses. In agreement with the reports of Salber and co-workers and Tietze, who found that the median duration of postpartum amenorrhea in nonnursing women was about 8 weeks,[11,12] the mean time for the return of menstruation in the nonlactators in Cronin's study was 60 days postpartum. About half of these women had resumed menses by 8 weeks, and 90% by 12 weeks postpartum. This finding agrees with the results of Berman and colleagues, who studied nonnursing Eskimo women.[13] They found that 84% had resumed menstruating by the end of the second postpartum

month and all had menstruated by the end of the third month. In each of these studies, the resumption of ovulation as well as menstruation was delayed in women who nursed, provided they had nursed for at least 4 weeks. The delay in onset of ovulation as well as menstruation was directly related to the duration of breast-feeding (Table 9-1).[10]

There was less chance of ovulating when the total daily duration and frequency of nursing was greater. In Perez and colleagues' study, only one full nursing mother (no supplemental feeding) ovulated before the end of the ninth postpartum week, and the chance of ovulating before 10 weeks postpartum in fully nursing mothers was less than 1%.[10] However, even if full nursing continued, the chance of ovulating increased to 17% by 12 weeks postpartum and to

Table 9-1
Predicted time for first ovulation and menstrual onset in relation to total lactation length

Length of lactation (months)	Predicted mean time of first menstrual onset (months)	Predicted mean time of first ovulation (months)
0	1.5	1.3
1	2.1	2.0
2	2.7	2.6
3	3.3	3.3
4	3.9	3.9
5	4.5	4.6
6	5.1	5.2
7	5.7	5.9
8	6.3	6.5
9	6.9	7.2
10	7.5	7.8
11	8.1	8.5
12	8.7	9.1
13	9.3	9.8
14	9.9	10.4
15	10.5	11.1
16	11.1	11.7
17	11.7	12.4
18	12.3	13.0

Adapted from Perez A, Vela P, Masnick GS, et al: First ovulation after childbirth: The effect of breast-feeding. Am J Obstet Gynecol 114:1041, 1972.

Normal endocrinology

Table 9-2
Probability of ovulation not occurring within specified number of weeks

	Probability (SE)			
Type of exposure	6 weeks	9 weeks	12 weeks	18 weeks
1. Full nursing	1.00 (±0.000)	0.99 (±0.004)	0.83 (±0.017)	0.64 (±0.025)
2. Continuation of nursing (whether partial or full)	0.99 (±0.002)	0.96 (±0.005)	0.76 (±0.014)	0.60 (±0.018)
3. Nursing 8 weeks or less	0.91 (±0.011)	0.47 (±0.026)	0.10 (±0.016)	0.01 (±0.003)
4. Nursing 4 weeks or less	0.86 (±0.023)	0.11 (±0.024)	0.005 (±0.003)	

Adapted from Perez A, Vela P, Masnick GS, et al: First ovulation after childbirth: The effect of breast-feeding. Am J Obstet Gynecol 114:1041, 1972.

36% by 18 weeks postpartum (Table 9-2).[10] Two of these women conceived while fully nursing. When supplemental feeding is introduced, or nursing is discontinued before 8 weeks postpartum, the chance of ovulation increases. Thus, lactation usually will provide protection against conception for at least 10 weeks, provided that absolutely no supplemental feeding is used and the mother continues to breast-feed her infant.

Berman and colleagues performed a study of the effect of breast-feeding on postpartum menstrual patterns and pregnancy in a group of Eskimo women who nursed their babies on demand, usually every 2 to 3 hours for as long as 3 years, with a median duration of nursing of 7 months.[13] Supplemental feeding was usually begun when the infant was approximately 6 months of age. With the use of life-table analyses, the probability of menstruating was calculated for the women who nursed their infants as well as a group who did not nurse. As seen in Table 9-3, 84% of the nonnursing women had resumed menstruating by the end of the second postpartum month and all had menstruated by the end of the third month. The nursing mothers, however, had only about a 50% chance of resuming menstruation by the end of the tenth postpartum month.[13]

The Berman data agree with a study by Potter and co-workers of nursing women in India who had an 11-month median delay of menstruation.[14] Of the group who remained amenorrheic while nursing, 58% resumed menstruation during the first month, and 95% by the end of the second month, after discontinuing nursing. In general, in this and other studies, the mean duration of amenorrhea was about 75% of the mean duration of nursing. In the Berman study, menstrual cycle length after the resumption of menstruation was more irregular in women who continued to nurse than in nonlactators. The intervals between the first and second and be-

Table 9-3
Probability of first postpartum menstrual flow occurring by end of month by group

Month	Nursing women	Nonnursing women
1	0.03	0.32
2	0.09	0.84
3	0.15	1.00
4	0.25	
5	0.30	
6	0.35	
7	0.39	
8	0.44	
9	0.47	
10	0.51	
11	0.54	
12	0.57	
Total women: 214		

Adapted from Berman ML, Hanson K, Hellman IL: Effect of breast-feeding on postpartum menstruation, ovulation, and pregnancy in Alaskan Eskimos. Am J Obstet Gynecol 114:524, 1972.

tween the second and third postpartum menses were substantially prolonged in nursing mothers compared with non-breast-feeders.

None of the women in the Berman study used any form of contraception. When the probability of becoming pregnant was calculated, it was found to be significantly higher in all months beyond the first postpartum month for nonnursing women than for nursing women, independent of age. Although 3.7% of the nonnursing women conceived in the second postpartum month, no pregnancies occurred in the first 4 months postpartum in the women who breast-fed their babies every 2 to 3 hours day and night (Table 9-4).[13] This finding is in agreement with that of Perez et al, who found that ovulation did not occur before 10 weeks postpartum in women who breast-fed their infants without supplemental feedings. Berman's group calculated that at the end of 1 year, only about 20% of fully nursing women would be expected to conceive. In contrast, 50% of nonnursing mothers using no contraception would be expected to conceive within 7 months, and 80% within 10 months, after delivery. These rates indicate that there is about a 3-month delay in mean conception rates in nonlactating postpartum women compared with a group of nonpostpartum ovulating women who are not practicing contraception.

Only three of 116 nursing women (2.6%) studied by Berman's group conceived before their first menstruation while nursing. This incidence, in agreement with figures published in other reports, reinforces the belief that the first menstruation in nursing women is usually not preceded by ovulation. In the study by Perez and co-workers, first menstruation tended to precede ovulation when lactation was long, but the reverse occurred in women who nursed for only a short period. In Cronin's study, where the duration of nursing was short, about one-fourth of the lactating women had evidence of ovulation before their first postpartum menstruation. The mean time of conception after first postpartum menstruation in women using no other form of contraception in this and other studies is about 2 to 3 months for nonnursing women and 2 to 4 months for nursing women.

The reason lactation inhibits the onset of ovulation postpartum has not been completely elucidated. Short suggested that the act of suckling itself inhibits GnRH release.[15] Others have proposed that the elevated prolactin levels produced by suckling directly inhibit ovulation. Delvoye and co-workers found that in long-term lactational amenorrhea, basal serum prolactin levels were significantly higher in a group of amenorrheic nursing mothers than they were in menstruating nursing mothers.[7] The duration of amenorrhea was correlated with the degree of hyperprolactinemia and the return to normal prolactin levels correlated positively with the resumption of menstruation (Figure 9-9).[7]

In the Battin study of eight nursing women, four resumed menses during the first 6 months postpartum and four did not.[5] The basal and af-

Table 9-4
Postpartum conception rates

Month	Cumulative percentage pregnancy at end of month	
	Nursing women (%)	Nonnursing women (%)
1	0	0
2	0	3.7
3	0	9.4
6	1.4	42.3
9	9.7	72.5
12	23.0	83.7
15	33.8	85.7
18	54.2	89.6
21	66.7	91.5
24	87.2	91.5
Total women:	253	55

Adapted from Berman ML, Hanson K, Hellman IL: Effect of breast-feeding on postpartum menstruation, ovulation, and pregnancy in Alaskan Eskimos. Am J Obstet Gynecol 114:524, 1972.

Normal endocrinology

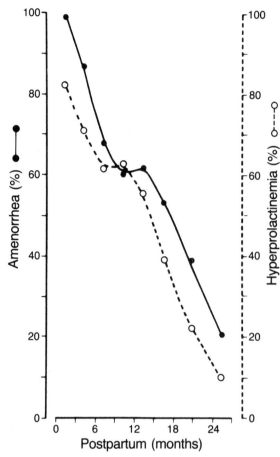

Figure 9-9
Incidence of amenorrhea and of hyperprolactinemia (i.e., serum prolactin higher than 600 μU/mL or 25 ng/mL) in 465 nursing mothers investigated during the first 2 postpartum years.

Reproduced, with permission, from Delvoye P, Demaegd M, Uwayitu-Nyampeta, et al: Serum prolactin, gonadotropins, and estradiol in menstruating and amenorrheic mothers during two years' lactation. Am J Obstet Gynecol 130:635, 1978.

Although estradiol levels were significantly higher in the group who began menses, there was no significant difference in FSH or LH levels. These results are similar to the findings of Delvoye and co-workers, who also obtained only sporadic gonadotropin measurements.[7] Tyson and associates performed frequent sampling of LH and PRL for 10 hours in a group of women who were nursing and then weaned their infants.[6] They found an indirect correlation between integrated mean prolactin levels and integrated mean LH levels. As PRL fell, LH rose, indicating that elevated PRL levels interfere with episodic but not necessarily with basal LH release. In a study by Marrs et al performed in postabortal women (first and second trimesters), the decline of PRL appeared to correlate with the resumption of LH secretory activity,[16] thus supporting the postpartum findings of Tyson and associates.

In a longitudinal study of breast-feeding women, McNeilly and co-workers found that basal mean prolactin levels correlated well with both suckling frequency and total suckling duration.[17] Each of these measurements, which have been found to be important in maintaining elevated PRL levels during lactation, correlated indirectly with the introduction of supplementary feeding. When the data were centered around the time of introduction of supplementary feeding, it was found that supplementing was associated with a rapid decrease in the duration of suckling, a decline in the basal prolactin level, and a resumption of follicle development (as determined by an increase of urinary estrogen secretion above 10 μg/24 hr) as well as by a resumption of ovulation 6 weeks later (as determined by an increase in urinary pregnanediol levels above 1 mg/24 hr) (Figure 9-11).[17] Because both PRL and suckling activity declined before resumption of ovarian activity, no conclusions could be made concerning the relative importance of each of these factors in preventing the return of ovarian steroidogenesis.

ter-suckling peak prolactin (PRL) levels were significantly lower in the menstruating group than in the amenorrheic group, although there was no significant difference in the suckling frequency between the two groups (Figure 9-10).[5]

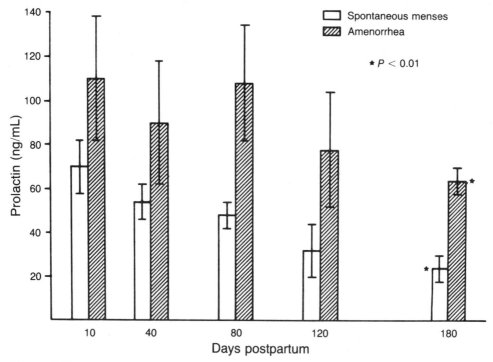

Figure 9-10
Comparison of baseline serum prolactin levels in subjects with spontaneous menses vs subjects with amenorrhea during the first 180 days postpartum (means ± SE).

From Battin DA, Marrs RP, Fleiss PM, et al: The effects of suckling on serum prolactin, LH, FSH, and estradiol during prolonged lactation. Obstet Gynecol 65:785, 1985. Reprinted with permission from The American College of Obstetricians and Gynecologists.

Nevertheless, when PRL levels were centered around the time of increase of urinary estrogen above 10 μg/24 hr, it was found that PRL levels were significantly elevated until 1 week before resumption of ovarian activity. These levels reached normal nonpregnant levels 5 weeks after the resumption of ovarian activity. When PRL levels were centered about presumed resumption of ovulation (pregnanediol > 1 mg/24 hr), it was found they declined significantly 3 weeks before the resumption of ovulation and reached normal levels about the time ovulation resumed.

Theoretical considerations concerning the mechanisms of inhibition of the hypothalamic-pituitary ovarian axis during lactation are conflicting, because factual information is limited. Andreassen and Tyson showed that during the early puerperium (less than 30 days postpartum), the ovary has the ability to respond to exogenous gonadotropin stimulation.[18] When menopausal gonadotropins were administered to lactating or nonlactating postpartum women, there was a prompt increase in both estradiol and progesterone; however, during this same interval, no gonadotropin response was seen af-

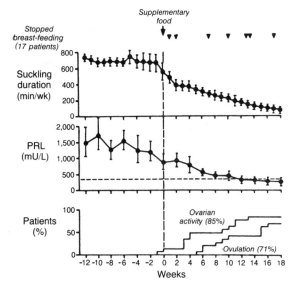

Figure 9-11
Relationships among the introduction of supplementary food and mean (±SE) suckling duration, serum prolactin, and the percentage of women with ovarian activity or ovulation, in 14 women. The arrowheads at the top indicate when individual women stopped breast-feeding.

Reproduced, with permission, from McNeilly AS, Howie PW, Houston MJ: Relationship of feeding patterns, prolactin, and resumption of ovulation postpartum. In Zatuchni GI, Labbok MH, Sciarra JJ (eds): Research Frontiers in Fertility Regulation. *Hagerstown, MD, Harper & Row, 1981, p 102.*

ter administration of GnRH. This finding indicates a lack of pituitary but not ovarian responsiveness in the early puerperium.

This pituitary insensitivity may be a result of prolonged steroid suppression during gestation or other endocrinologic factors during the puerperium. Even though estradiol and progesterone concentrations rapidly decrease to very low levels following delivery, the hypothalamic-pituitary axis appears to be extremely sensitive to the negative feedback effects of these low levels of estradiol. This effect is similar to that seen before the onset of puberty. Such sensitivity to

negative feedback was nicely demonstrated by Baird and co-workers in lactating and nonlactating women who were given estradiol benzoate at 7, 30, and 100 days postpartum.[19] In contrast with what occurred in cycling women—that is, an initial decrease followed by substantial release of LH and FSH—no gonadotropin response was seen at the seventh day. However, at 30 and 100 days postpartum, the nonlactating group had a normal negative and positive gonadotropin response, whereas the lactating group had only a negative feedback effect, which was significantly greater than that seen with the nonlactating women (Figure 9-12).[19] These data may indicate that the effect of suckling itself, or possibly the elevated PRL concentrations produced by suckling, may suppress the role of positive estrogen feedback on the hypothalamic-pituitary axis.

These differences in LH response in lactating women may be due to factors other than the direct effect of PRL. Several reports have shown conflicting data on PRL levels in menstruating or amenorrheic breast-feeding women. In our own studies, performed on women undergoing pregnancy termination during the first or second trimester, elevated PRL levels appeared to be correlated with suppression of β-LH activity.[16] When PRL fell into a normal range, there was an increase in β-LH (Figure 9-13).[16] Rolland and Schellenkens also found that in postpartum women elevated prolactin levels had a negative influence on LH release.[20] However, when these investigators administered bromocriptine (2-bromo-α-ergocryptine), PRL fell rapidly and LH secretion returned earlier than in the lactating women.

These studies suggest that PRL may have a direct effect on ovarian responsiveness. However, in a recent unpublished study at our institution, postpartum women who received bromocriptine, 2.5 mg twice a day for 15 days beginning the day of delivery, were still found to lack a gonadotropin response to GnRH stimula-

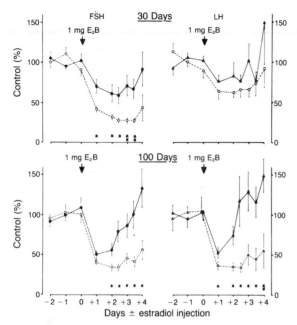

Figure 9-12
The concentration of FSH and LH in plasma of 14 women before and after the IM injection of 1 mg estradiol benzoate (E_2B) at 30 and 100 days postpartum. The results have been expressed as a percentage of the mean basal values before the injection. Each point represents the mean ± SE of seven women. The significance of the difference between lactating (– – –) and nonlactating (——) groups was determined by Student's t-test ($*P < 0.05$; $**P < 0.01$).

Reproduced, with permission, from Baird DT, McNeilly AS, Sawers RS, et al: Failure of estrogen-induced discharge of luteinizing hormone in lactating women. J Clin Endocrinol Metab 49:500, 1979. © 1979, The Endocrine Society.

tion at 5, 10, and 15 days postpartum. Their response was similar to that observed in nonlactating controls as well as in women who were lactating. Thus, it appears that women treated with bromocriptine postpartum for lactation suppression will not resume ovulation sooner than nontreated patients. These findings support the contention that PRL may play only a minor role in curtailing gonadotropin release in the immediate puerperium. A direct inhibitory effect of PRL at the level of the granulosa cell, curbing estradiol production, has been postulat-

ed. But this mechanism for preventing resumption of cyclic ovarian activity is unlikely, because ovulatory activity can be induced by exogenous gonadotropin stimulation during the early postpartum period (less than 14 days).

To understand the endocrine relationships during the puerperium, one must also take into account endorphin activity. Hoffman and coworkers found that β-endorphins increase during gestation.[21] Endorphin release has been shown to have a negative effect on GnRH secretion, which is probably mediated by a dopaminergic pathway.[22] These two findings suggest that throughout gestation, as well as the puerperium, elevated endorphins decrease GnRH and thus decrease gonadotropin stores or secretory activity. Even though gonadotropins are measurable and steroid concentrations are low, cyclic ovarian activity is not present. Moreover, in another recent report, individuals with hyperprolactinemia demonstrated opioid inhibition of LH release.[23] This finding supports a theory that elevated PRL may act synergistically with elevated endorphin to suppress hypothalamic-pituitary-ovarian interactions during the puerperium. These isolated studies are provocative, but offer no definitive explanation of why nursing women have a delay in the resumption of ovulation postpartum. We still don't know how suckling and/or elevated prolactin levels inhibit resumption of cyclic ovarian activity. Studies are now under way in an attempt to identify the mechanism to explain this phenomenon.

Suppression of postpartum lactation

Use of exogenous agents for the suppression of puerperal breast engorgement and lactation is controversial. Inhibition of lactation is usually accomplished either by hormonal inhibition with estrogens, alone or in combination with androgens, by administration of bromocriptine, or by mechanical compression of the breasts with or without fluid restriction.

Postpartum breast engorgement and lactation normally begin 40 to 72 hours after delivery and persist for at least 1 week in the absence of nursing. During this period, the symptoms may be treated by such measures as breast binders, ice packs, and analgesics. The degree to which hormonal preparations have been found to be superior to these means and to placebos varies among the different studies, depending on the study population, experimental design, and specific drugs evaluated.

The conclusion of most prospective studies has been that long-acting parenteral estrogen preparations effectively prevent symptoms, without rebound engorgement, in about 80% of patients. This rate is substantially higher than that obtained when placebos are used. For example, Morris and associates, in a randomized double-blind study, compared the effects of a testosterone enanthate-estradiol valerate combination (Deladumone) with a placebo.[24] The results indicated that the hormonal preparation was significantly more effective than the placebo in preventing lactation, engorgement, and discomfort when evaluated on the third, fourth, and fifth postpartum days. Similar results were obtained by questionnaire 14 days postpartum. At the 6-week examination, the placebo- and drug-treated groups were indistinguishable in terms of breast and uterine involution, lochia, and resumption of menses. Varga and associates found, in a double-blind randomized trial, that oral diethylstilbestrol suppressed postpartum lactation to a significantly greater extent than a placebo.[25]

A problem with nearly all randomized studies of lactation inhibition comparing drugs and placebos is the failure to use breast binders in the placebo group. In a double-blind, placebo-controlled study performed by Schwartz and as-

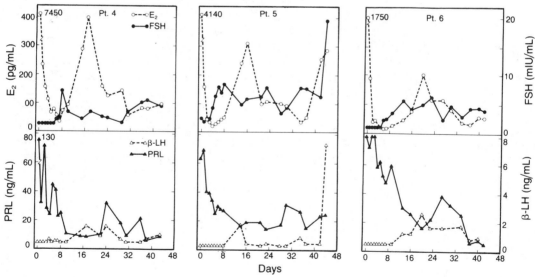

Figure 9-13
Hormonal patterns after second-trimester pregnancy termination.

Reproduced, with permission, from Marrs RP, Kletzky OA, Mishell DR Jr: A separate mechanism of gonadotropin recovery after pregnancy termination. J Clin Endocrinol Metab *52:545, 1981.* © *1981, The Endocrine Society.*

sociates, all patients were fitted with a tight bra soon after delivery.[26] On the third and fourth postpartum days, patients treated with any of the three estrogens used in the trial, chlorotrianisene (TACE), diethylstilbestrol, and Deladumone, had significantly less breast tenderness and evidence of lactation than the placebo group (Table 9-5).[26] About half of all patients had continued or rebound breast engorgement after leaving the hospital; the differences among the four groups were not significant (Table 9-6).[26] The results of this study indicate that estrogen therapy is superior to breast binding alone in suppressing postpartum breast tenderness and lactation during the first few postpartum days, but this improvement is not sustained during the next few weeks.

The efficacy of estrogenic drugs must be weighed against their risks and side effects. The most important of these is their reported association with venous thrombosis and thromboembolism. Retrospective studies have suggested such a relationship, but the actual incidence of thrombosis in estrogen-treated puerperas is unknown. Although the incidence may be presumed to be low, estrogens should not be administered to patients with a history of thrombosis or thromboembolism. Carcinoma of the breast, active hepatic disease, operative delivery, obesity, and age greater than 35 are also contraindications. Uterine subinvolution and endometrial hyperstimulation have been reported to occur more frequently with estrogen therapy, but the addition of an androgen to the estrogenic agent appears to prevent these effects.

In summary, long-acting estrogen-androgen preparations are effective in preventing puerperal breast engorgement, lactation, and discomfort in about 80% of patients. Their use carries very low risk in most cases. Nevertheless, their use is not mandatory and in most patients the symptoms of breast engorgement may be relieved by nonhormonal methods.

In an attempt to avoid the risks of estrogen use, mainly that of thromboembolism, other drugs have been given to suppress postpartum lactation. Clomiphene citrate, a weak estrogen, has been reported by Zuckerman and Carmel to inhibit lactation effectively in a dose of 100 mg/day for 5 days.[27] But the most widely used nonestrogenic substance to inhibit lactation is the dopamine agonist bromocriptine. This drug effectively reduces serum PRL levels in both puerperal and nonpuerperal women and has been used extensively in the treatment of nonpuerperal galactorrhea. Several studies have shown that bromocriptine prevents puerperal lactation as well as suppressing lactation once it has been established.

Varga and associates compared the use of bromocriptine with that of diethylstilbestrol and a placebo in a random double-blind study.[25] They found that bromocriptine, 5 mg twice a day for the first 6 days after delivery and then 5 mg/day for 3 additional days, suppressed postpartum lactation as effectively as diethylstilbes-

Table 9-5
Incidence of breast tenderness and lactation on third postpartum day

Clinical findings	Placebo (n = 83)	Chlorotrianisene (TACE) (n = 85)	Diethylstilbestrol (n = 89)	Deladumone (n = 89)	P
Breast tenderness (history)	35	9	3	3	<0.005
Breast tenderness (exam)	23	6	2	2	<0.005
Lactation	19	5	7	6	<0.05
No. of patients: 346					

Adapted from Schwartz DJ, Evans PC, Garcia L-R, et al: A clinical study of lactation suppression. Obstet Gynecol 42:599, 1973.

Normal endocrinology

Table 9-6
Follow-up examinations of same patients in Table 9-5

Follow-up findings (5 weeks postpartum)	Placebo (n = 67)	Chlorotrianisene (TACE) (n = 62)	Diethylstilbestrol (n = 64)	Deladumone (n = 67)	P
Breast engorgement	35	32	30	27	NS
Lactation	6	5	9	7	NS
Mean number of days of vaginal bleeding after delivery	15.6	18.3	15.5	18.8	<0.05
No. of patients: 260					

Adapted from Schwartz DJ, Evans PC, Garcia L-R, et al: A clinical study of lactation suppression. Obstet Gynecol 42:599, 1973.

trol and to a significantly greater degree than the placebo. Furthermore, there was less rebound mammary engorgement with bromocriptine than with diethylstilbestrol.

Rolland and Schellenkens compared bromocriptine with a placebo in a randomized double-blind study.[20] Therapy with bromocriptine was significantly more effective than with the placebo in terms of inhibition of mild secretion, engorgement, and pain. These authors recommended that a dosage of 2.5 mg twice a day be used for 2 weeks, followed by 2.5 mg once a day for an additional week. Therapy of shorter duration did not prevent a rebound phenomenon. These authors stated that bromocriptine's lactation-inhibiting effect was better than the combination of hormonal and mechanical treatment previously used in their clinic. With this drug, they were also able to suppress lactation in women who had established full mammary activity.

The recommended dosage of bromocriptine to prevent puerperal lactation is now 2.5 mg one to three times a day. The usual dosage is 2.5 mg twice a day for 2 weeks. Clinical studies have shown that about 30% of women treated with this drug postpartum developed significantly lowered systolic and diastolic blood pressure. For this reason, the first dosage of bromocriptine should not be administered until after vital signs are stabilized and no earlier than 4 hours after delivery. Blood pressure should be monitored during the first few hours of treatment.

Other side effects reported include dizziness, headache, nausea and vomiting, fainting, and syncope. Each of these effects occurred in fewer than 10% of treated patients. Rebound breast enlargement after therapy was discontinued occurred in about 30% of patients, but usually was not severe. Tapering the dosage by administration of one tablet a day for a third week may reduce the symptoms of rebound enlargement.

It has been established that serotonin stimulates release of prolactin from the pituitary. A serotonin antagonist, 8β-[(carbobenzoxyamino)-methyl]-1,6-dimethyl-10α-ergoline (metergoline), has also been investigated for use in preventing puerperal lactation. Delitala and associates administered metergoline in a dosage of 4 mg twice a day for 5 days after delivery. They found this drug inhibited milk secretion, prevented mammary engorgement, and lowered PRL levels in all patients treated.[28] Rebound phenomena were rare. Crosignani and associates administered metergoline in a dosage of 4 mg tid for 5 days to a group of 30 postpartum women.[29] This short course of therapy was extremely effective in preventing lactation if administered from the first postpartum day. The incidence of rebound lactation and breast engorgement was very low, and no side effects were observed. Serum PRL levels progressively declined at a gradual rate, in contrast with the rapid fall observed with bromocriptine. This finding indicates that these two agents probably have different mechanisms of action in inhibiting prolactin synthesis and/or release. Metergoline is not approved for use in the US.

In summary, either bromocriptine, estrogenic preparations, or breast binders and ice bags may be used to prevent immediate postpartum lactation and pain. Estrogenic formulations should not be given to women with such risk factors as a past history of thrombosis or thromboembolism, operative delivery, obesity, carcinoma of the breast, active hepatic disease, and age greater than 35.

References

1. Jacobs LS, Daughaday WH: Physiologic regulation of prolactin secretion in man. In Josimovich JB, Reynolds M, Cobo E (eds): *Lactogenic Hormones, Fetal Nutrition, and Lactation.* New York, John Wiley & Sons, 1974, pp 351-377

2. Barberia JM, Abu-Fadil S, Kletzky OA, et al: Serum prolactin patterns in early human gestation. *Am J Obstet Gynecol* 121:1107, 1975

3. Kletzky OA, Marrs RP, Howard WF, et al: Prolactin synthesis and release during pregnancy and puerperium. *Am J Obstet Gynecol* 136:545, 1980

4. Noel GL, Suh HK, Frantz AG: Prolactin release during nursing and breast stimulation in postpartum and nonpostpartum subjects. *J Clin Endocrinol Metab* 38:413, 1974

5. Battin DA, Marrs RP, Fleiss PM, et al: The effects of suckling on serum prolactin, LH, FSH, and estradiol during prolonged lactation. *Obstet Gynecol* 65:785, 1985.

6. Tyson JE, Carter NJ, Andreassen B, et al: Nursing-mediated prolactin and luteinizing hormone secretion during puerperal lactation. *Fertil Steril* 30:154, 1978

7. Delvoye P, Demaegd M, Uwayitu-Nyampeta, et al: Serum prolactin, gonadotropins, and estradiol in menstruating and amenorrheic mothers during two years' lactation. *Am J Obstet Gynecol* 130:635, 1978

8. Gross BA, Eastman CJ: Prolactin secretion during prolonged lactational amenorrhoea. *Aust NZ J Obstet Gynaecol* 19:95, 1979

9. Cronin TJ: Influence of lactation upon ovulation. *Lancet* 2:422, 1968

10. Perez A, Vela P, Masnick GS, et al: First ovulation after childbirth: The effect of breast-feeding. *Am J Obstet Gynecol* 114:1041, 1972

11. Salber EJ, Feinleib M, MacMahon B: The duration of postpartum amenorrhea. *Am J Epidemiol* 82:347, 1965

12. Tietze C: Fertility after discontinuation of intrauterine and oral contraception. *Int J Fertil* 13:385, 1968

13. Berman ML, Hanson K, Hellman IL: Effect of breast-feeding on postpartum menstruation, ovulation, and pregnancy in Alaskan Eskimos. *Am J Obstet Gynecol* 114:524, 1972

14. Potter RG, New ML, Wyon JB: Applications of field studies to research on the physiology of human reproduction: Lactation and its effects upon birth intervals in 11 Punjab villages, India. *J Chron Dis* 18:1125, 1965

15. Short RV: Lactation—the central control of reproduction. In *Breast-feeding and the Mother.* Ciba Foundation Symposium 45, Amsterdam, Elsevier, Excerpta Medica, North Holland, 1976, p 73

16. Marrs RP, Kletzky OA, Mishell DR Jr: A separate mechanism of gonadotropin recovery after pregnancy termination. *J Clin Endocrinol Metab* 52:545, 1981

17. McNeilly AS, Howie PW, Houston MJ: Relationship of feeding patterns, prolactin, and resumption of ovulation postpartum. In Zatuchni GI, Labbok MH, Sciarra JJ (eds): *Research Frontiers in Fertility Regulation.* Hagerstown, MD, Harper & Row, 1981, p 102

18. Andreassen B, Tyson JE: Role of the hypothalamic-pituitary-ovarian axis in puerperal infertility. *J Clin Endocrinol Metab* 42:1114, 1976

19. Baird DT, McNeilly AS, Sawers RS, et al: Failure of estrogen-induced discharge of luteinizing hormone in lactating women. *J Clin Endocrinol Metab* 49:500, 1979

20. Rolland R, Schellenkens L: A new approach to the inhibition of puerperal lactation. *J Obstet Gynaecol Br Commonw* 80:945, 1973

21. Hoffman DI, Abboud TK, Haase HR, et al: Plasma β-endorphin concentrations prior to and during pregnancy, in labor, and after delivery. *Am J Obstet Gynecol* 150:492, 1984

22. Ropert JF, Quigley ME, Yen SSC: Endogenous opiates modulate pulsatile luteinizing hormone release in humans. *J Clin Endocrinol Metab* 52:583, 1981

23. Quigley ME, Sheehan KL, Casper RF, et al: Evidence for an increased opioid inhibition of luteinizing hormone secretion in hyperprolactinemic patients with pituitary microadenomas. *J Clin Endocrinol Metab* 50:427, 1980

24. Morris JA, Creasy RK, Hohe PT: Inhibition of puerperal lactation. Double-blind comparison of chlorotrianisene, testosterone enanthate with estradiol valerate and placebo. *Obstet Gynecol* 36:107, 1970

25. Varga L, Lutterbeck PM, Pryor JS, et al: Suppression of puerperal lactation with an ergot alkaloid: A double-blind study. *Br Med J* 2:743, 1972

26. Schwartz DJ, Evans PC, Garcia L-R, et al: A clinical study of lactation suppression. *Obstet Gynecol* 42:599, 1973

27. Zuckerman H, Carmel S: The inhibition of lactation by clomiphene. *J Obstet Gynaecol Br Commonw* 80:822, 1973

28. Delitala G, Masala A, Alagna S, et al: Metergoline in the inhibition of puerperal lactation. *Br Med J* 1:744, 1977

29. Crosignani PG, Lombroso GC, Caccamo A: Suppression of puerperal lactation by metergoline. *Obstet Gynecol* 51:113, 1978

Normal endocrinology

Chapter 10

Puberty

Subir Roy, M.D.
Paul F. Brenner, M.D.

During puberty the secondary sex characteristics appear, skeletal growth accelerates, behavior and attitudes change, and the capacity for fertility is realized. These events result from the production of adult levels of sex steroids by the gonads and the achievement of full maturation of gametogenic function.

In 1969, Marshall and Tanner defined five stages of breast maturation and pubic hair development (Figure 10-1; Tables 10-1 and 10-2).[1] Some investigators have combined the breast and pubic hair developmental stages and denoted them as Tanner stages 1 through 5 (T1–T5) or pubertal stages 1 through 5 (P1–P5). Because breast and pubic hair development are not always correlated, we will use the original Marshall and Tanner classification.

Marshall and Tanner also reported the mean age of the sequence of events for puberty in a population of Anglo-Saxon girls.[1] They found considerable variation from one individual to another in the duration of a particular pubertal stage as well as in the total time for all the clinical events of female puberty. Some girls pass through all stages within 18 months; others may take 5 years or longer (Table 10-3).[1] Marshall and Tanner also observed mean time intervals of initial breast budding (B2) to peak height velocity (PHV), to menarche (M), to complete pubic hair development (PH5), and to complete breast development (B5) (Table 10-4).[1]

Marshall and Tanner's data indicate that initial breast development is usually the earliest of the events of puberty and menarche the latest.[1] The initial pubic hair growth usually occurs after initial breast budding, but the last stage of hair growth is completed more rapidly than breast development. Peak height velocity (the rapid linear growth phase) immediately precedes menarche and is reached soon after breast budding occurs. The peak height velocity, which decreases just before menarche, is followed by completion of pubic hair development and

Table 10-1
Classification of breast growth

B 1	Prepubertal: elevation of papilla only
B 2	Breast budding
B 3	Enlargement of breasts with glandular tissue, without separation of breast contours
B 4	Secondary mound formed by areola
B 5	Single contour of breast and areola

Table 10-2
Classification of pubic hair growth

PH 1	Prepubertal: no pubic hair
PH 2	Labial hair present
PH 3	Labial hair spreads over mons pubis
PH 4	Slight lateral spread
PH 5	Further lateral spread to form inverse triangle and reach medial thighs

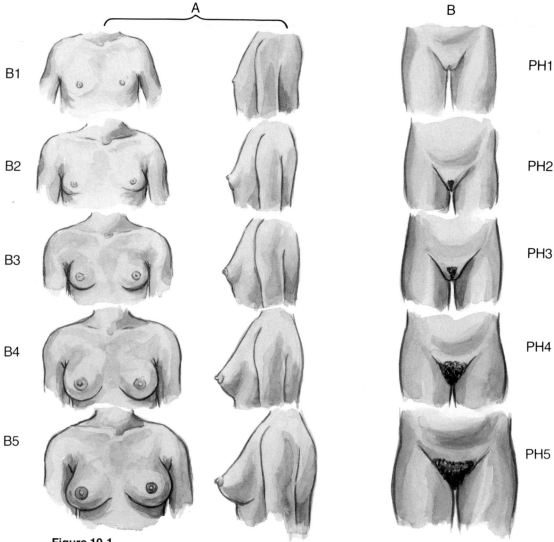

Figure 10-1
Diagrammatic representation of Tanner stages I to V of human breast maturation and development of pubic hair.

Adapted, with permission, from Marshall WA, Tanner JM: Variations in pattern of pubertal changes in girls. Arch Dis Child *44:291, 1969.*

breast maturation. The most recent data for mean age of various pubertal events in American girls are given in Table 10-5.[2]

Between 1850 and 1950, in Western nations, the mean age at first menses decreased at the rate of 3 to 4 months per decade, probably because of better nutrition. In the past 30 years, in the US, the mean age at menarche has plateaued at 12.9 years. For most girls, the earliest sign of puberty, breast budding, occurs between the ages of 8 and 13 years—approximately 2.5 years before menarche.

In 1971, Frisch and Revelle proposed a widely debated "critical-weight" theory to explain this decrease in the mean age of menarche in US and English girls.[2] They cited a body weight of about 48 kg (106 lb) as the critical weight at which menarche occurs (Table 10-5).[2] This critical body weight can be correlated with changes in body composition to achieve a minimum weight for height, representing a critical lean/fat ratio, which is thought to alter important metabolic processes. These changes are associated with a decrease in hypothalamic sensitivity to the inhibitory effects of circulating sex steroids. This, in turn, leads to release of GnRH and gonadotropins, which are necessary to initiate menarche. When urinary gonadotropin levels were correlated with changes in body composition associated with changing pubertal stages, investigators found that gonadotropin changes did not precede the onset of pubertal development.[3] Hence, these data could not confirm the Frisch and Revelle theory, because the change in lean/fat ratio and the achievement of critical body weight did not occur before gonadotropin output from the pituitary increased.[3] Thus the validity of the critical-weight theory has not been established.

The age of menarche varies greatly from one culture to another and may be influenced by several factors. Inheritance seems to be an important determinant for the onset of menstruation. Girls tend to have a late menarche if their

Table 10-3
Sequence of events in female puberty

Event	Mean (years)	SD
Breast budding (B2) (thelarche)	11.2	1.10
Onset of pubic hair (PH2) (pubarche)	11.7	1.21
Peak height velocity (PHV)	12.1	0.88
Menarche (M)	13.5	1.02

Data compiled from Marshall WA, Tanner JM: Variations in pattern of pubertal changes in girls. Arch Dis Child 44:291, 1969.

Table 10-4
Pubertal intervals

Interval	Mean (years)	SD
B2-PHV*	1.0	0.77
B2-M†	2.3	1.03
B2-PH5	3.1	1.04
B2-B5 (average duration of puberty)	4.5	2.04

*PHV, peak height velocity.   †M, menarche.

Data compiled from Marshall WA, Tanner JM: Variations in pattern of pubertal changes in girls. Arch Dis Child 44:291, 1969.

Table 10-5
Pubertal events in US girls

Event	Mean ± SD
Initiation of breast development (B2)	10.8 ± 1.10 years
Appearance of pubic hair (PH2)	11.0 ± 1.21 years
Menarche	12.9 ± 1.20 years
Height at menarche	158.5 ± 6.80 cm
Weight at menarche	47.8 ± 6.90 kg

Data compiled from Frisch RE, Revelle R: Height and weight at menarche and a hypothesis of menarche. Arch Dis Child 46:695, 1971.

mothers had their first menses relatively late, and an early onset of menses if there is a family history of early menarche. Certain diseases and adverse physical conditions alter the onset of menstruation. Blind women have an earlier onset of menses than women with normal vision. Diabetic girls are reported to have a later menarche than girls with normal carbohydrate metabolism. An increase of 20% to 30% over ideal body weight is associated with an earlier menarche than is seen in girls of normal weight. Obesity of more than 30% above ideal body weight, however, is associated with delayed menarche. Socioeconomic factors have been reported to influence the timing of the menarche; many of these are probably related to nutrition. Colder climate, rigorous exercise programs, rural living, and higher altitudes have been reported to be associated with a later onset of menstruation.

Recently, the critical-weight theory has been refined to place greater emphasis on body composition. The ratio of fat to total body weight or of fat to lean body weight is related both to the time of initiation of puberty and also to fertility. As children mature, their percentage of body fat increases and the percentage of body water decreases.[4] The body weight of the mature female is approximately 52% water and 27% fat.

During puberty, the concentrations of gonadotropins in the peripheral circulation coincidentally increase as the amount of body fat increases.[3] Malnutrition delays puberty and the adolescent growth spurt. The importance of the ratio of fat to lean body weight is supported by evidence that onset of menarche is delayed to approximately 15 years of age in ballet dancers, swimmers, and runners if they began their arduous exercise programs before menarche (Figure 10-2).[5] Thus, exercising results in taller and lighter girls at menarche. Individuals who exercise strenuously before menarche are more likely to be oligomenorrheic or amenorrheic, in contrast with those who began such activities after menarche.[6] These exercising girls, as well as those who have anorexia nervosa, have gonadotropin patterns similar to those normally found in the prepubertal years of normal girls.[7] The exact mechanism by which the critical ratio of fat to lean body weight affects puberty is not known. One mechanism, however, may be the effect of the body composition of fat on the metabolism of estrogens. Obese women have lower levels of 2-hydroxylated estrogen compounds

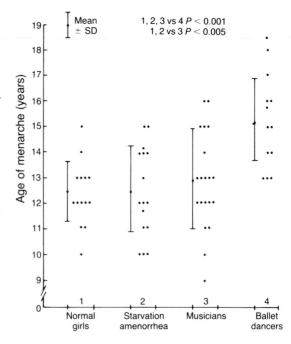

Figure 10-2
The age of menarche in ballet dancers compared with three other groups.

Reproduced, with permission, from Warren MP: The effects of exercise on pubertal progression and reproductive function in girls. J Clin Endocrinol Metab 51:1150, 1980.
© 1980 The Endocrine Society.

(catechol estrogens), whereas those with anorexia nervosa or thin athletes have an increase of these compounds.[8] These metabolites have been shown to reduce LH secretion, which in turn produces clinical hypoestrogenism.

Injury leading to forced inactivity by girls involved in these strenuous activities has frequently been associated with the initiation of spontaneous menses, regardless of changes in body weight. This suggests that stress may be a factor in delaying menarche or causing oligomenorrhea or amenorrhea.[5] However, Warren found that girls pursuing serious and stressful musical careers initiated before menarche did not have a significant delay in the age of menar-

Table 10-6
Height and weight of US adolescents

Mean age (years)	At menarche		At age 18	
	Mean height ± SD (cm)	Mean weight ± SD (kg)	Mean height ± SD (cm)	Mean weight ± SD (kg)
11.4	156.4 ± 0.97	47.9 ± 1.10	165.9 ± 1.10	59.5 ± 1.50
12.4	158.0 ± 0.73	48.7 ± 0.95	165.8 ± 0.71	58.4 ± 0.99
13.4	159.1 ± 1.00	47.2 ± 0.93	165.2 ± 0.95	55.9 ± 0.89
14.5	160.9 ± 1.40*	47.2 ± 1.20	165.8 ± 1.40	57.1 ± 0.57
All patients:				
12.9 ± 0.1	158.5 ± 0.50	47.8 ± 0.51	165.6 ± 0.48	57.1 ± 0.57

*Different from earliest group, P < 0.02.

Data compiled from Frisch RE, Revelle R: Height and weight at menarche and a hypothesis of menarche. Arch Dis Child 46:695, 1971.

Table 10-7
Clinical implications of events related to puberty

Event	Implication
No breast development by 14 years	Sexual infantilism
Complete breast development, no pubic hair	Testicular feminization
Complete pubic hair, no breast development	Androgen excess
Peak height velocity reached	Menarche imminent
Menarche	Final height predicted
Sexual maturation before 8 years	Precocious puberty
No menses by age 16.5	Primary amenorrhea
Duration of puberty > 4.5 years	Deranged pubertal development

che and the pattern of menstrual cycles was similar to controls.[5] Thus stress, per se, may not explain the incidence of delayed menarche or altered menstrual cyclicity. The high energy drain that is associated with intensive athletic activities may, in part, account for the increased incidence of oligomenorrhea or amenorrhea in these girls.[5]

Closer examination of weight and height data collected from US pubertal girls suggests that although girls with late menarche are taller than girls with early menarche at the time of the first menses, by age 18 there is no significant difference in height between girls with early and those with late menarche (Table 10-6).[2] The rea-

son for this lack of difference in ultimate height is that the final height is determined with first menses. Linear growth averages 10 cm for girls with early menarche and 6 for girls with late menarche. In contrast with the height observations, the girls with late menarche weighed less at age 18 than girls who had early menarche.

The rate of skeletal change is not uniform in all parts of the body.[9] Sex steroids are primarily responsible for the growth of the trunk, which reaches its maximum growth rate about 6 months after the peak for the legs and arms, which is growth-hormone dependent. Similarly, foot and hand growth accelerates before that of the lower leg and forearm, which, in turn, pre-

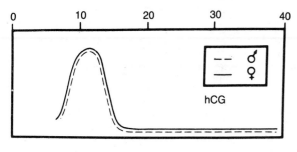

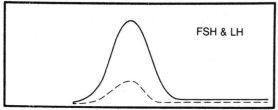

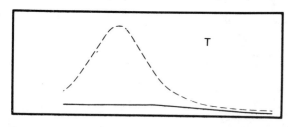

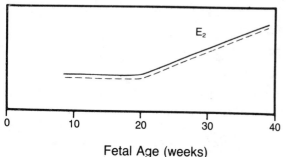

Fetal Age (weeks)

Figure 10-3

Schematic representation of hormonal patterns (mean serum levels) in both sexes during human fetal life. T, testosterone; E_2, estradiol.

From Faiman D, Winter JSD, Reyes FI: Patterns of gonadotropins and gonadal steroids throughout life. Clin Obstet Gynecol 3:467, 1976.

cedes that of the thigh and upper arm. Thus, the frequent concern about "big feet" is unjustified, because the foot approaches its adult size at an earlier age than does the leg and will stop growing earlier. Gonadotropin-deficient individuals have long legs and arms, probably because of continued growth hormone effect in the absence of the epiphyseal maturing effect of sex steroids. Conversely, individuals with growth hormone deficiency have relatively long trunks with short limbs. The clinical implications of these data are outlined in Table 10-7.

Prepubertal endocrine events

In order to gain an understanding of the current concepts of the initiation of puberty, it is necessary to review certain prepubertal endocrine events. In female rodents, there is both a tonic center and a cyclic center in the hypothalamus for the release of gonadotropins from the pituitary. Only a tonic center is found to exist in the hypothalamus of male rodents. Such a difference between the sexes is thought to exist also in humans.

Fetal period

The "imprinting" of the fetal hypothalamus to be male (possessing a tonic center) or to be female (possessing both a tonic and a cyclic center) has been ascribed to testosterone.[10,11] The steroids secreted by the fetal ovary apparently do not play an active role in this determination. Instead, as in the development of the internal genital structures, they play a passive role. There is indirect evidence that a tonic center for the secretion of gonadotropins operates during fetal life. The ovaries of anencephalic fetuses who have reduced serum levels of follicle-stimulating hormone (FSH) and luteinizing hormone (LH) show reduced weight, decreased numbers of interstitial cells, and arrested follicular develop-

Normal endocrinology

Table 10-8
Hormone levels in girls*

Age or pubertal stage	FSH (μg LER-907/dL)	LH (μg LER-907/dL)	E$_2$ (ng/dL)	Testosterone (ng/dL)	Androstenedione (ng/dL)	DHEA (ng/dL)
5–7 days	5 (3–70)	2.3 (1.3–3.5)	1.0 (0–3.2)	14 (11–28)	26 (16–57)	
8–60 days	18 (3–88)	3.3 (1.3–8.5)	1.5 (0–5.0)	11 (3–24)	25 (4–68)	
2–12 months	13 (2–160)	2.8 (0.8–7.3)	1.1 (0–7.5)	5 (3–17)	13 (2–23)	
1–4 years	9 (3–25)	1.7 (0.8–3.5)	1.1 (0–2.0)	8 (3–15)	8 (2–16)	
4–8 years	7 (4–17)	2.0 (0.8–3.3)	0.5 (0–1.7)	6 (3–14)	18 (12–27)	29 (19–42)
8–10 years	7 (4–13)	2.3 (1.2–5.0)	0.5 (0–3.1)	8 (4–20)	32 (22–47)	54 (12–187)
10–12 years	11 (6–21)	2.5 (1.0–6.3)	1.6 (0–6.3)	18 (5–47)	65 (42–100)	82 (24–289)
12–14 years	14 (7–22)	4.5 (1.1–12)	4.2 (0.5–12)	26 (11–60)	123 (80–190)	261 (50–916)
14–16 years	19 (6–51)	8.7 (2.4–45)	8.6 (1–25)	34 (16–72)	133 (177–224)	473 (93–2,000)
P1†	8.2 ± 0.6	2.1 ± 0.1	0.8 ± 0.3	7 ± 1	26 ± 2	75 (19–300)
P2†	9.4 ± 0.9	2.1 ± 0.1	1.3 ± 0.5	17 ± 3	60 ± 3	293 (45–1,600)
P3†	14.2 ± 1.1	3.7 ± 0.3	2.5 ± 0.5	30 ± 2	70 ± 5	465 (125–1,700)
P4†	19.5 ± 1.2	7.6 ± 1.0	7.6 ± 0.8	38 ± 2	130 ± 3	471 (153–1,620)

*Mean (range) or mean ± standard error.

†P1 through P4 designate developmental stages arrived at by combining B and PH stages of Marshall and Tanner.

From Faiman C, Winter JSD, Reyes FI: Patterns of gonadotropins and gonadal steroids throughout life. Clin Obstet Gynecol 3:467, 1976.

ment. Direct evidence that the fetal pituitary secretes gonadotropins has been obtained from studies on serum gonadotropin measurements in the human fetus (Figure 10-3).[12] Before 10 weeks of fetal age, serum FSH and LH levels are indistinguishable and low in both sexes. Between 10 and 20 weeks of fetal life, serum FSH and LH levels rise in both sexes but reach adult castrate levels only in females. The female has a maximal number of germ cells and experiences early follicular development at this time, in response to the elevated gonadotropin levels. The lower serum FSH and LH levels found in males are thought to be the result of the elevated serum testosterone levels found between 8 and 20 weeks of fetal life. The testosterone production is believed to reflect Leydig cell stimulation by human chorionic gonadotropin (hCG) of the fetal testes. In males, the serum testosterone then acts to suppress the hypothalamic gonadotropin-releasing hormone (GnRH) release from the arcuate nucleus of the medial basal hypothalamus. This negative feedback is believed to

result in reduced gonadotropin release from the pituitary.[13]

GnRH is present in the hypothalamus as early as 6 to 8 weeks of fetal life. It is released in pulses in fetuses of both sexes and regulates the episodic pituitary production and release of gonadotropins. In the brain, testosterone is capable of being aromatized to estradiol. This conversion is thought to effect inhibition of GnRH. Dihydrotestosterone, a testosterone metabolite that cannot be aromatized, has no such effect. Also, testosterone effects can be blocked by the administration of an estrogen antagonist, MER-25. This blockade suggests that local brain estrogen levels, and not testosterone, imprint the hypothalamus to be male (tonic center) or to be female (tonic and cyclic centers) during a critical period of neuronal organization.

Serum estradiol levels in fetuses, regardless of sex, are mainly of placental origin, indistinguishable, and low up to 20 weeks' gestation. Thereafter, estradiol levels rise at similar rates and are associated with a concomitant reduction of gonadotropins. This indicates that a negative feedback effect operates in both sexes until delivery. Circulating serum estradiol, therefore, cannot be implicated as the agent that programs the fetal brain.

It is possible (although not proven) that female fetal exposure to synthetic estrogens, androgens, or 19-nortestosterone compounds during a critical period of neuronal organization may lead to anovulatory sterility in the adult.

In summary, the hypothalamic-pituitary-gonadal axis differentiates during the fetal peri-

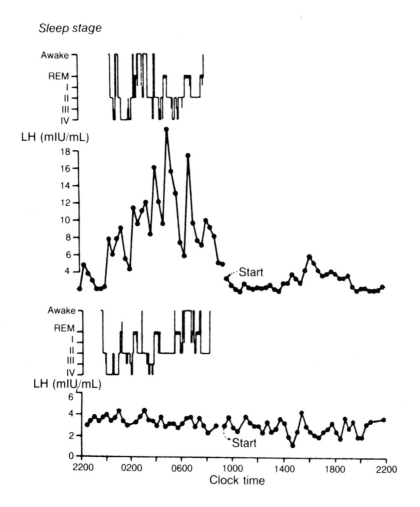

Figure 10-4
Plasma LH concentration and sleep stage in an early pubertal girl (upper panel) and in a normal prepubertal girl (lower panel).

Adapted from Boyar RM, Katz J, Finkelstein JW, et al: Anorexia nervosa: Immaturity of the 24-hour luteinizing hormone secretory pattern. N Engl J Med 291:861, 1974.

Normal endocrinology

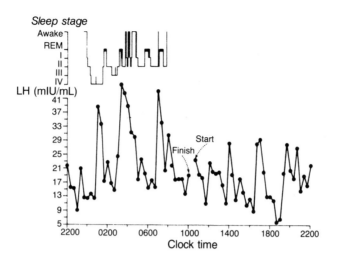

Figure 10-5

Plasma LH concentration and sleep stage in a late pubertal girl.

Adapted from Boyar RM, Katz J, Finkelstein JW, et al: Anorexia nervosa: Immaturity of the 24-hour luteinizing hormone secretory pattern. N Engl J Med 291:861, 1974.

od, is suppressed by the time of late gestation (through an operative negative feedback system of sex hormones of placental origin on the higher centers), and remains suppressed until puberty reactivates the system. Some authorities have referred to this negative feedback mechanism as a "gonadostat."[14]

Infancy (birth to 4 years)

When the placenta separates, levels of sex steroids drop abruptly (Table 10-8).[12] The negative feedback action of the sex steroids of placental origin on the hypothalamus and the pituitary is removed and gonadotropins are released from the pituitary. In the newborn girl, FSH levels peak at 18 µg LER-907/dL between 2 and 5 months, and fall to basal levels as late as 4 years. The simultaneously low circulating sex steroid and gonadotropin levels are thought to be the result of the increased sensitivity of the gonado-

stat to sex steroids that turn off gonadotropin release. Serum LH levels reach a maximum of 3.3 µg LER-907/dL at 2 to 3 months and then fall to baseline levels by 4 months, for the same reason FSH decreases.

Serum estradiol decreases to basal levels (10 pg/mL) within 5 to 7 days after birth and persists at approximately this level until puberty. Occasionally, there is increased estradiol production and release coincident with transient elevations in FSH in the first few months of life. This may result in transient breast development by the age of 6 months. Testosterone levels in girls at birth are the same as in women (45 ng/dL); however, during the second month of life they are reduced to prepubertal levels (5 ng/dL), presumably because of the removal of hCG. In girls, by approximately 4 years of age, low levels of gonadotropins coexist with low levels of gonadal steroids. This finding indicates that the gonadostat is operative and exquisitely sensitive to circulating levels of sex steroids.

Childhood (4 to 10 years)

The period between 4 and 10 years of age is characterized by low levels of gonadotropins and ovarian steroids (Table 10-8).[12] However, the ovaries are fully developed and capable of being stimulated by gonadotropin. If human menopausal gonadotropin (hMG) is given to a prepubertal girl, ovulation can be induced.

The first endocrine change associated with puberty in both sexes is the increase in the adrenal production of androgens. Plasma levels of dehydroepiandrosterone (DHEA) and its sulfate ester (DHEA-S) increase between 5 and 10 years of age, and those of androstenedione (A) rise between 8 and 10 years. This increase, which precedes the onset of clinical adrenarche, does not appear to be under the control of gonadotropin, adrenocorticotropin (ACTH), or prolactin. The mechanism for its increase is unknown.[15] Parker and associates have suggested that there are adrenal androgen-stimulating hormones, proopiomelanocortin-related peptides, that may play a role in stimulating androgen production in the peripubertal period.[16,17] Their role, however, is as yet undetermined. The steroids DHEA and DHEA-S are almost exclusively of adrenal origin, as suggested by their very low concentrations in patients with Addison's disease and their normal levels in those with hypogonadotropic hypogonadism. Furthermore, the low concentrations found when adrenarche is clinically delayed suggest that DHEA is the adrenal androgen responsible for development of axillary hair and growth of pubic hair. DHEA-S, the steroid present in the largest concentration during prepuberty and puberty, has been shown to increase sebum production and to cause vaginal cornification—two signs of secondary sexual development associated with puberty. Vaginal cornification is thought to occur after small amounts of DHEA-S are converted to estrogens. Like the pubertal changes in the reproductive axis, which begin earlier in girls than in boys, the changes in pubertal androgen function also occur at an earlier mean age in girls than in boys.

The increase in adrenal androgen production precedes the other endocrine changes associated with puberty.[18] The role of the increase in adrenal androgens in the initiation of puberty, if any, has not been agreed upon.[19] Investigators have suggested that this increased adrenal secre-

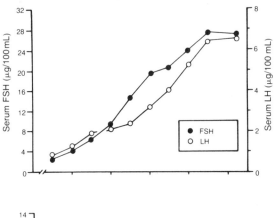

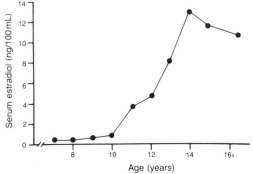

Figure 10-6

Mean serum concentrations of FSH, LH, and estradiol observed during a mixed longitudinal study of 58 adolescent girls.

Adapted, with permission, from Faiman C, Winter JSD: Gonadotropins and sex hormone patterns in puberty: Clinical data. In Grumbach MM, Grave GD, Mayer FE (eds): Control of the Onset of Puberty. New York, John Wiley & Sons, 1974, p 46.

Normal endocrinology

tion of DHEA and A may play a necessary role in reducing the sensitivity of the gonadostat.[19,20] Both DHEA and A could affect this change directly or indirectly after being converted to estrogens at the level of the hypothalamus or pituitary, in a manner analogous to that of testosterone during the fetal period. The observation by Boyar et al[21] that sleep-related episodic secretion of LH occurred at ages 6 and 9 in two children who had congenital adrenal hyperplasia suggests a temporal relationship between an increase in adrenal androgens and the hormonal events commonly associated with early puberty.[18] However, children with Addison's disease taking only glucocorticoids as replacement therapy have normal pubertal develop-

ment, and individuals with gonadal dysgenesis experience adrenarche but not gonadarche. These findings suggest that these two endocrine events associated with puberty have independent control mechanisms.[22]

In summary, before the onset of puberty, the hypothalamic-pituitary axis is intact and able to respond to GnRH stimulation with an increased release of FSH and LH. The magnitude of this release, however, is less than during the pubertal and adult periods. The sensitive negative feedback center in the hypothalamus responds to the administration of low dosages of such synthetic estrogens as ethinylestradiol or weak estrogens like clomiphene citrate by decreasing basal FSH and LH levels. The transition to an adult hypothalamic-pituitary-ovarian relationship requires a decreased sensitivity of the hypothalamus to sex steroids (decreased sensitivity of the gonadostat) and development of the positive feedback system that results in increased secretion of LH.

Endocrine events of puberty

The first gonadotropin pattern changes of puberty appear during sleep. Boyar and associates found episodic secretion of LH, and to a lesser extent FSH, in pubertal girls during sleep that did not occur when the girls were awake (Figure 10-4, upper panel). This pattern was absent in prepubertal girls (Figure 10-4, lower panel).[21,23,24] In the adult, as in the late pubertal girl, the episodic pattern of gonadotropin secretion occurs whether the individual is awake or asleep (Figure 10-5).[24] Thus the initiation of the episodic release of GnRH occurs at first mainly during sleep.

With the initiation of puberty, the hypothalamic gonadostat (the arcuate nucleus) and possibly the pituitary, which are exquisitely sensitive to the suppressive effect of sex steroids, become

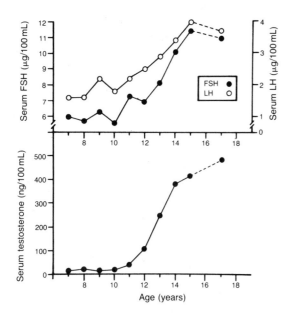

Figure 10-7
Mean serum concentrations of FSH, LH, and testosterone obtained during a mixed longitudinal study of 56 healthy adolescent boys.

Adapted, with permission, from Faiman C, Winter JSD: Gonadotropins and sex hormone patterns in puberty: Clinical data. In Grumbach MM, Grave GD, Mayer FE (eds): Control of the Onset of Puberty. New York, John Wiley & Sons, 1974, p 39.

less sensitive to the sex steroids. The mechanisms are unknown, but the result is an increased pattern of pulsatile GnRH release. This pattern is similar to the episodic release of GnRH in the fetal period, before the initiation of the negative feedback mechanism.

The occurrence of the pulsatile LH release during sleep is found in children with precocious puberty.[21] This hormonal activity is advanced for the patient's chronologic age, but is normal for the stage of puberty. Its action is not blocked by the administration of the androgen antagonist cyproterone acetate. The episodic secretion of gonadotropins synchronized with sleep is seen in patients who have primary gonadal dysgenesis.[25] This finding indicates that the initiation of the gonadotropin changes of early puberty are independent of normal ovarian function and suggests that changes in the central nervous system (CNS) control the initiation of puberty. Biologically active LH, which is undetectable during the prepubertal years and then increases markedly during the pubertal period, may be a more sensitive marker of peripubertal change than the sleep-associated rise of serum LH.[26]

From birth to puberty, inhibition of the hypothalamic release of GnRH is the only functional restraint on the endocrine changes and clinical events characteristic of puberty. The inhibition of hypothalamic GnRH secretion is due to two mechanisms: the negative feedback of gonadal sex steroids on the CNS and an intrinsic CNS inhibitory phenomenon. Individuals with streak gonads have a qualitative pattern of gonadotropin secretion similar to that of normal girls, but the peripheral concentrations of FSH and LH are quantitatively elevated when they are under 4 years of age. These elevated gonadotropins fall between the ages of 4 and 11, despite the absence of gonadal steroids. This finding suggests that the intrinsic CNS inhibition mechanism dominates in the years 4 to 11.

At puberty, the hypothalamic-pituitary-gonadal axis is reactivated after a decade of suppression. It is characterized by a reduced sensitivity of the CNS to sex steroids. The increased release of gonadotropins by the pituitary results

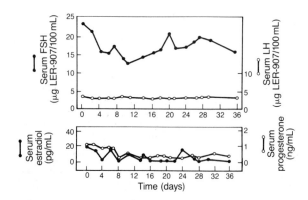

Figure 10-8
Serum FSH, LH, estradiol, and progesterone in a girl at thelarche.

From Winter JSD, Faiman C: The development of cyclic pituitary-gonadal function in adolescent females. J Clin Endocrinol Metab 37:714, 1973.

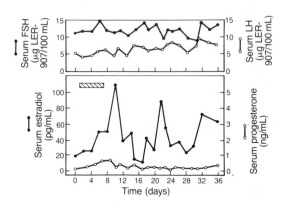

Figure 10-9
Serum FSH, LH, estradiol, and progesterone in a girl at menarche.

From Winter JSD, Faiman C: The development of cyclic pituitary-gonadal function in adolescent females. J Clin Endocrinol Metab 37:714, 1973.

Normal endocrinology

in an increased ovarian stimulation and enhancement of steroidogenesis.

Most studies have shown that basal levels of FSH are higher than those of LH, until maturity of the reproductive axis is attained. There is a progressive, but slight, increase in levels of both FSH and LH with age before puberty and a greater increase during the advancing stages of puberty (Figure 10-6).[27] Female gonadotropin patterns are correlated with pubertal stage. FSH levels plateau after midpuberty, whereas LH levels rise slowly throughout puberty. The latter's sixfold increase eventually produces levels higher than those of FSH (Table 10-8).[12] The pubertal increases of both gonadotropins occur approximately 2 years earlier in girls than in boys (Figure 10-7).[27]

Higher serum estradiol levels reflect the increased gonadotropin production that occurs with advancing pubertal stage. By midpuberty, the pituitary responsiveness to GnRH is enhanced. Administration of low levels of synthetic estrogens does not lower the basal level of gonadotropins, as is seen in the prepubertal period. However, a bolus of estradiol will not elicit an LH surge in either early or midpuberty. The positive feedback mechanism by which estradiol induces an LH surge becomes operative only at the end of puberty.

In a longitudinal study, serial determinations of gonadotropins and estrogens were performed in the same girls over a 35-day interval in four groups of subjects: (1) prepubertal, (2) pubertal and premenarcheal, (3) menarcheal, and (4) postmenarcheal.[28] Episodic fluctuations of FSH and estradiol begin in early puberty (Figure 10-8).[28] At menarche, an 11-day estradiol rhythm with peaks of 120 pg/mL occurred without progesterone elevations, indicating anovulatory bleeding cycles (Figure 10-9).[28] This anovulatory pattern, somewhat common the first year after menarche, is followed by the hormonal pattern associated with ovulatory cycles. Baseline LH values exceed those of FSH only after menarche.

Prolactin has been detected in girls as young as 2 years. Its levels progressively increase after age 8, doubling in value within the next 7 years—probably in relation to the increase in circulating estradiol (Figure 10-10).[29] Neither the onset of puberty nor the acceleration of linear skeletal growth appears to be solely growth-hormone dependent. Levels of growth hormone remain unchanged at these times.[30,31] However, growth hormone clearly does have an important role in the achievement of ultimate height. Nat-

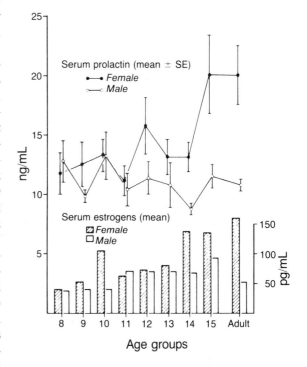

Figure 10-10

Mean ± SE of serum PRL concentrations in boys and girls and in adult men and women, analyzed according to age groups. The bar graph represents the mean total estrogen levels in corresponding age groups.

Reproduced, with permission, from Ehara Y, Yen SSC, Silver TM: Serum prolactin levels during puberty. Am J Obstet Gynecol 121:995, 1975.

ural and synthetic growth hormones have been used successfully to accelerate linear growth in individuals with growth hormone deficiency.[32]

Summary

The responsibility for imprinting the fetal hypothalamus to have a male (tonic) or a female (tonic and cyclic) center has been ascribed to testosterone, through its conversion to estrogen in the brain. At term, the human fetus has an operative negative feedback system; that is, low serum gonadotropins secondary to high placental estrogens are evident. This negative feedback system has been called a gonadostat (Figure 10-11).[14]

By about 4 years of age, low levels of gonadotropins coincide with low levels of gonadal steroids. These low levels indicate that the gonadostat is operative and exquisitely sensitive to the suppressive effect of low circulating levels of sex steroids. During childhood, the period from 4 to 10 years, adrenarche occurs. The production of adrenal androgens precedes the other endocrine events associated with puberty, but is most likely independent of the hormonal changes associated with gonadarche.

During childhood, the gonadostat responds to synthetic estrogens with a reduction of gonadotropin secretion. An infusion of GnRH will elicit a release of FSH and LH from the pituitary. This release, however, is not of the magnitude seen in the late pubertal period, nor does it display the greater response of LH than of FSH that occurs in late puberty.

A sleep-associated rise of LH is the first event heralding puberty. This episodic secretion of LH during sleep does not occur during prepuberty, and after menarche the episodic secretions occur whether the individual is asleep or

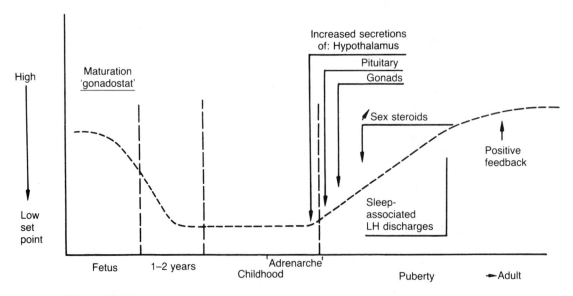

Figure 10-11
Schematic diagram illustrating the evolution of the regulatory factors governing the hypothalamic, pituitary, and gonadal maturation from fetus to adult.

From Forest MG, de Peretti E, Bertrand J: Hypothalamic-pituitary-gonadal relationships in man from birth to puberty. Clin Endocrinol 5:551, 1976.

awake. In contrast with prepubertal LH, pubertal LH is biologically active. Measurement of bioactive LH may be used as an additional marker heralding the initiation of puberty. As the critical weight is approached, the pituitary responds to increasing secretions of GnRH, from the arcuate nucleus of the hypothalamus, with an increasing release of FSH and LH, which, in turn, causes follicular maturation and increased estrogen secretion by the ovary. The last event in puberty is activation of the positive feedback response. Rising levels of estradiol stimulate the hypothalamic-pituitary axis to release a surge of LH. After a variable period of anovulatory menstruation, ovulation eventually occurs.

The earlier age of menarche experienced by Western girls has some important implications. Recent studies have shown that early menarche leads to early onset of ovulatory cycles. When age at first full-term pregnancy is delayed until after age 25, these women have been found to have a higher risk for developing breast cancer. Additionally, psychological and emotional maturity generally occurs much later than menarche. At present, it is difficult to know what useful purpose is served by early menarche.

References

1. Marshall WA, Tanner JM: Variations in pattern of pubertal changes in girls. *Arch Dis Child* 44:291, 1969

2. Frisch RE, Revelle R: Height and weight at menarche and a hypothesis of menarche. *Arch Dis Child* 46:695, 1971

3. Penny R, Goldstein IP, Frasier SD: Gonadotropin excretion and body composition. *Pediatrics* 61:294, 1978

4. Frisch RE: Pubertal adipose tissue: Is it necessary for normal sexual maturation? Evidence from the rat and human female. *Fed Proc* 39:2395, 1980

5. Warren MP: The effects of exercise on pubertal progression and reproductive function in girls. *J Clin Endocrinol Metab* 51:1150, 1980

6. Frisch RE, Gotz-Welbergen AV, McArthur JW, et al: Delayed menarche and amenorrhea of college athletes in relation to age of onset of training. *JAMA* 246:1559, 1981

7. Katz JL, Boyar RM, Weiner H, et al: *Hormones, Behavior and Psychopathology.* New York, Raven Press, 1976, p 279

8. Schneider J, Bradlow HL, Strain G, et al: Effects of obesity on estradiol metabolism: Decreased formation of non-uterotropic metabolites. *J Clin Endocrinol Metab* 56:973, 1983

9. Brook CGD: Endocrinological control of growth at puberty. *Br Med Bull* 37:281, 1981

10. Reyes FI, Winter JSD, Faiman C: Studies on human sexual development. I. Fetal gonadal and adrenal sex steroids. *J Clin Endocrinol Metab* 37:74, 1973

11. Reyes FI, Boroditsky RS, Winter JSD, et al: Studies on human sexual development. II. Fetal and maternal serum gonadotropin and sex steroid concentrations. *J Clin Endocrinol Metab* 38:612, 1974

12. Faiman C, Winter JSD, Reyes FI: Patterns of gonadotropins and gonadal steroids throughout life. *Clin Obstet Gynecol* 3:467, 1976

13. MacLusky NJ, Naftolin F: Sexual differentiation of the central nervous system. *Science* 211:1294, 1981

14. Forest MG, DePeretti E, Bertrand J: Hypothalamic-pituitary-gonadal relationships in man from birth to puberty. *Clin Endocrinol* 5:551, 1976

15. Parker LN, Sack J, Fisher DA, et al: The adrenarche: Prolactin, gonadotropins, adrenal androgens and cortisol. *J Clin Endocrinol Metab* 46:396, 1978

16. Parker LN, Odell WD: Evidence for existence of cortical androgen stimulating hormone. *Am J Physiol* 236:E616, 1979

17. Parker LN, Lifrak ET, Odell WD: A 60,000 molecular weight human pituitary glycopeptide stimulates adrenal androgen secretion. *Endocrinology* 113:2092, 1983

18. Grumbach MM, Richards GE, Conte FA, et al: Clinical disorders of adrenal androgen function and puberty: An assessment of the role of the adrenal cortex in normal and abnormal puberty in man and evidence for an ACTH-like pituitary adrenal androgen stimulation hormone. In James VHT, Serio M, Giusti G, et al (eds): *The Endocrine Function of the Human Adrenal Cortex.* London, Academic Press, 1978, p 583

19. Cutler GB Jr, Loriaux DL: Adrenarche and its relationship to the onset of puberty. *Fed Proc* 39:2384, 1980

20. Ducharme JR, Forest MG, De Peretti E, et al: Plasma adrenal and gonadal sex steroids in human pubertal development. *J Clin Endocrinol Metab* 42:468, 1976

21. Boyar RM, Finkelstein JW, David R, et al: Twenty-four hour patterns of plasma luteinizing hormone and follicle stimulating hormone in sexual precocity. *N Engl J Med* 289:282, 1973

22. Sklar CA, Kaplan SL, Grumbach MM: Evidence for dissociation between adrenarche and gonadarche: Studies in patients with idiopathic precocious puberty, gonadal dysgenesis, isolated gonadotroph deficiency, and constitutionally delayed growth and adolescence. *J Clin Endocrinol Metab* 51:548, 1980

23. Boyar R, Finkelstein J, Roffwarg H, et al: Synchronization of augmented luteinizing hormone secretion with sleep during puberty. *N Engl J Med* 287:582, 1972

24. Boyar RM, Katz J, Finkelstein JW, et al: Anorexia nervosa: Immaturity of the 24-hour luteinizing hormone secretory pattern. *N Engl J Med* 291:861, 1974

25. Weitzman ED, Boyar RM, Kapen S, et al: The relationship of sleep and sleep stages to neuroendocrine secretion and biological rhythms in man. *Recent Prog Horm Res* 31:399, 1975

26. Lucky AW, Rich BH, Rosenfield RL, et al: LH bioavailability increases more than immunoreactivity during puberty. *J Pediatr* 97:205, 1980

27. Faiman C, Winter JSD: Gonadotropins and sex hormone patterns in puberty: Clinical data. In Grumbach MM, Grave GD, Mayer FE (eds): Control of the Onset of Puberty. New York, John Wiley & Sons, 1974

28. Winter JSD, Faiman C: The development of cyclic pituitary-gonadal function in adolescent females. *J Clin Endocrinol Metab* 37:714, 1973

29. Ehara Y, Yen SSC, Silver TM: Serum prolactin levels during puberty. *Am J Obstet Gynecol* 121:995, 1975

30. Tanner JM, Whitehouse RH, Hughes PCR, et al: Relative importance of growth hormone and sex steroids for the growth at puberty of trunk length, limb length, and muscle width in growth hormone deficient children. *J Pediatr* 89:1000, 1976

31. Laron Z, Roitman A, Kauli R: Effect of human growth hormone therapy on head circumference in childhood with hypopituitarism. *Clin Endocrinol* 10:393, 1979

32. Frasier SD: Human pituitary growth hormone (hGH) therapy in growth hormone deficiency. *Endocr Rev* 4:155, 1983

Suggested reading

Chipman JJ: Pubertal control mechanisms as revealed from human studies. *Fed Proc* 39:2391, 1980

Ducharme JR, Collu R: Pubertal development: Normal, precocious, and delayed. *Clin Endocrinol* 11:57, 1982

Grumbach MM: The neuroendocrinology of puberty. *Hosp Prac* 51-60, March 1980

Kaplan SL, Grumbach MM, Aubert ML: The ontogenesis of pituitary hormones and hypothalamic factors in the human fetus: Maturation of central nervous system regulation of anterior pituitary function. *Recent Prog Horm Res* 32:161, 1976

Kawano N, Miyao M: Studies on gonadotropin secretion during sleep in patients with abnormal sexual development: The role of the CNS in the onset of puberty. *Brain Dev* 4:421, 1982

Ojeda SR, Andrews WW, Advis JP, et al: Recent advances in the endocrinology of puberty. *Endocr Rev* 1:228, 1980

Reiter EO, Grumbach MM: Neuroendocrine control mechanisms and the onset of puberty. *Ann Rev Physiol* 44:595, 1982

Roberts DF: Race, genetics and growth. *J Biosoc Sci* (suppl) 1:43, 1969

Winter JSD: Nutrition and the neuroendocrinology of puberty. *Curr Concepts Nutr* 11:3, 1982

Normal endocrinology

Chapter 11

Menopause

Daniel R. Mishell Jr., M.D.
Paul F. Brenner, M.D.

The menopause is defined as permanent cessation of menstruation due to decreased ovarian steroidogenesis with adequate gonadotropin stimulation. Climacteric is defined as the physiologic period in a woman's life during which ovarian function regresses. Ovarian function declines gradually, not suddenly, and the cessation of menses is only one facet of the process. In practice, the terms menopause and climacteric are used interchangeably. The mean age at menopause in the US is about 51 years, with a normal distribution curve and 95% confidence limits between ages 45 and 55 (Figure 11-1).[1] If a woman stops menstruating before age 40, the condition should be called premature ovarian failure instead of premature menopause, because of the severe psychological connotations of the latter term. If a woman continues to menstruate after the age of 55, the possibility increases that the endometrium will be hyperplastic or have a malignancy. Therefore, it is best to take a biopsy of her endometrium.

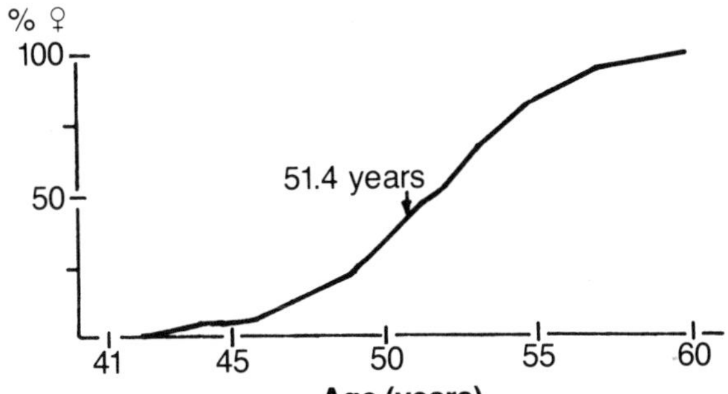

Figure 11-1
Frequency distribution of age at menopause.

From Jaszmann LJB: Epidemiology of the climacteric syndrome. In Campbell S (ed): Management of the Menopause and Post-Menopausal Years. *Lancaster, England, MTP Press Ltd, 1976, p 12.*

Age at menopause

The mean age at menopause has been increasing slightly during the past century; however, this increase is not due to better nutrition, which has accounted for an earlier age at menarche. The age at menarche is related to body mass; while the age at menopause is genetically predetermined. A century ago, the mean age at menopause was approximately 40 years; now it is about 50, because women are living longer and those who genetically would have a later menopause are living past that age (Figure 11-2).[2]

The age at menopause is not related to the number of ovulations; that is, pregnancy, lactation, use of oral contraceptives, or failure to ovulate spontaneously. It is also unrelated to race, socioeconomic conditions, education, height, weight, age at menarche, or the age at the last

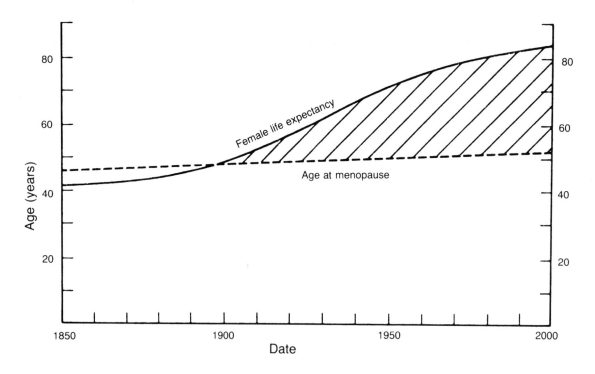

Figure 11-2
Female life expectancy.

Reproduced, with permission, from Cope E: Physical changes associated with the post-menopausal years. In Campbell S (ed): Management of the Menopause and Post-Menopausal Years. *Lancaster, England, MTP Press Ltd, 1976, p 33.*

pregnancy. The age at menopause may be affected by smoking, since it has been reported that cigarette smokers experience an earlier spontaneous menopause than nonsmokers.

In the US, where the average life expectancy for a woman is approximately 78 years, about 28 years will be lived after the menopause. More than one-third of a woman's life will be spent postmenopausally—a time when many women seek medical care. Thus, physicians (gynecologists, internists, and family practitioners) will devote a large proportion of their time to the care of postmenopausal women. In 1980, when there were 113 million women in the US, about 32 million were over 50 years of age, an increase in both numbers from the 1970 census.

Characteristics

The basic feature of the menopause is depletion of ovarian follicles, with degeneration of the granulosa and theca cells. As these cells degenerate, they fail to react to endogenous gonadotropins. As a result, less estrogen is produced, and there is a decrease in the negative feedback on the hypothalamic-pituitary axis. With less inhibition, gonadotropin production increases in an attempt to stimulate the ovary. As reported by Sherman and associates, this process begins about 5 years before the actual menopause.[3] At this time, follicle-stimulating hormone (FSH) levels increase and estradiol levels decrease,

Normal endocrinology

whereas luteinizing hormone (LH) and progesterone levels remain unchanged, indicating the cycles probably remain ovulatory (Figure 11-3).[3] As estrogen concentrations decline, there is an associated decrease in prolactin levels. The decrease in estradiol before the actual menopause accounts for the occurrence of hot flushes in some women during the 5 years or so before menses stop completely. Patients over 40 who are having regular menstrual cycles as well as hot flushes should be treated with very low doses of estrogen (0.3 mg of conjugated equine estrogen or 0.3 mg of estrone sulfate from the fifth day after menstruation begins until the onset of the next menses) to relieve these symptoms.

In contrast with the follicle cells, the stromal cells of the ovary continue to produce androgens, androstenedione and testosterone, as a result of increased LH stimulation after the menopause. The physiologic process of a decrease in the estrogen/androgen ratio is the cause of the increased facial hair growth that frequently occurs postmenopausally. Also, the rate of conversion of androstenedione to estrone, which occurs in the peripheral body fat, increases as individuals age. Postmenopausally, about 3,000 μg of androstenedione are produced daily, approximately 95% by the adrenals and 5% by the ovaries. In a slim postmenopausal woman, about 1.5% of the androstenedione is converted to estrone, producing approximately 45 μg/day. With a greater amount of fat, more estrone is produced: In an obese woman, as much as 7% of androstenedione is converted, producing about 200 μg of estrone a day. For this reason, obese women are less likely to develop symptoms of estrogen deficiency and may not require estrogen replacement therapy, but they are also more likely to develop endometrial hyperplasia and adenocarcinoma of the endometrium.

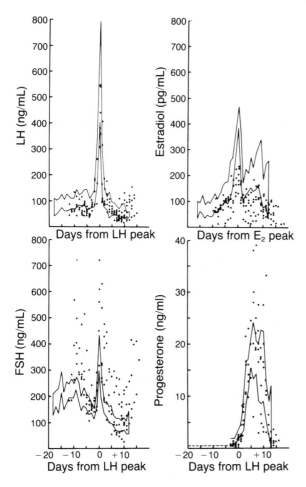

Figure 11-3
Serum concentrations of LH, FSH, estradiol, and progesterone in eight cycles from perimenopausal women. Mean levels ± 2 SE in ten normal ovulatory cycles from women under 30 years are in the enclosed area.

From Sherman BM, West JH, Korenman SG: The menopausal transition: Analysis of LH, FSH, estradiol, and progesterone concentrations during menstrual cycles of older women. J Clin Endocrinol Metab *42:629, 1976.*

Urogenital tract changes

There are a number of changes in a woman's body after the menopause. The lack of ovarian follicular function produces amenorrhea and sterility. Also, decreasing estrogen production leads to atrophy of the vagina, which can produce the very distressful symptoms of senile or atrophic vaginitis. This type of vaginitis can cause itching, burning, discomfort, dyspareunia, and also vaginal bleeding when the epithelium becomes very thin. Senile vaginitis is best treated with estrogen replacement therapy. Local therapy can be used for the first few months. However, because the vaginal administration of estrogen results in irregular systemic absorption, the patient is best treated with systemic estrogen for long-term prevention of vaginal atrophy as well as osteoporosis.

The trigone of bladder and the urethra are embryologically derived from estrogen-dependent tissue, and estrogen deficiency can result in atrophy of these urinary tissues and produce urgency incontinence, dysuria, and urinary frequency. Because there is less estrogen stimulation of the elastic tissue around the vagina postmenopausally, support of the urethra lessens and patients can develop urinary stress incontinence. All these urinary symptoms are best treated with estrogen replacement.

Hot flushes

Besides these changes in the urogenital tract, changes also occur in the rest of the body. The pathognomonic symptom of the menopause is the hot flush, which is related to a decrease in normal circulating estrogen levels. Women who have had low estrogen levels throughout their lives, such as those without gonads, will not have hot flushes. If such patients receive estrogen therapy that is eventually discontinued, they may also experience menopausal symptoms when the estrogen is stopped. The change in estrogen levels leads to alterations in the hypothalamus that are probably mediated through the central nervous system. When the change in estrogen levels is not gradual but sudden, as occurs after castration, hot flushes are more likely.

About 75% of all postmenopausal women develop hot flushes. The obese are less likely to develop flushes because they do not have as

great a decrease in estrogen levels. Erlik and co-workers have shown that postmenopausal women with hot flushes have lower circulating estrone and estradiol levels as well as less sex hormone-binding globulin (SHBG)-bound estradiol than postmenopausal women without hot flushes (Figure 11-4).[4] These investigators reported that women with hot flushes had less total body weight and more normal ideal body weight, compared with those without hot flushes. About one-third of the patients who have hot flushes have symptoms severe enough to require medical assistance. About one-half of patients with flushes have at least one a day, and about 20% have more than one a day. These flushes frequently occur at night, awaken the woman, and then make returning to sleep difficult (Figure 11-5).[5] Most women do not have hot flushes for more than 2 or 3 years, and it is uncommon for them to last more than 5 years after the menopause.

Hot flushes are not a psychological but a physiologic phenomenon. Mashchak and co-workers have shown that a sudden, explosive, systemic physiologic phenomenon takes place throughout the body.[6] The flush, which lasts about 4 minutes, is preceded by an increase in digital perfusion, followed by an increase in peripheral skin temperature and circulating epinephrine and LH, as well as an increase in heart rate (Figure 11-6).[6] With each flush, the levels of LH, adrenocorticotropic hormone (ACTH), and cortisone rise, but not those of FSH or estradiol. The LH increase is an effect of the change in the hypothalamic-pituitary axis, rather than a cause of the hot flush. Women without pituitary glands also have hot flushes.

The best treatment for the hot flush is estrogen. In a randomized, double-blind, crossover study conducted by Coope, women with hot flushes were given either a placebo or estrogen first and after 3 months crossed over to the other therapy.[7] The placebo diminished the frequency of hot flushes. However, when the pa-

Normal endocrinology

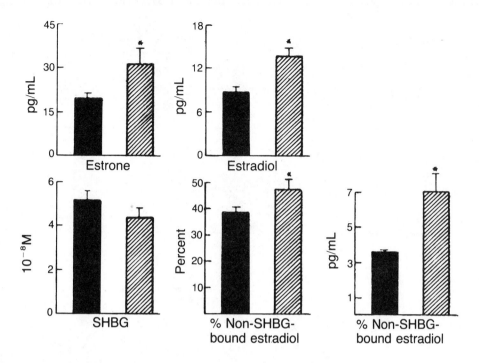

Figure 11-4

Mean levels ± SE of estrone, estradiol, sex hormone-binding globulin (SHBG), percentage of non-SHBG-bound estradiol, and non-SHBG-bound estradiol in 24 women with hot flushes (solid bars) compared with 24 asymptomatic women (striped bars).

*Significantly different from asymptomatic women.

From Erlik Y, Meldrum DR, Judd HL: Estrogen levels in postmenopausal women with hot flashes. Obstet Gynecol 59:403, 1982. Reprinted with permission from The American College of Obstetricians and Gynecologists.

tients receiving placebo were crossed over to estrogen, their hot flushes disappeared (Figure 11-7).[7] The patients who were treated with estrogen first had a marked diminution of hot flushes, significantly more than the placebo-treated controls, and when they were crossed over to placebo, the incidence of hot flushes exceeded pretreatment levels. This study demonstrates that estrogen is more effective treatment than placebo. Because most hot flushes occur at night, it is best for the patient to take the estrogen tablet before bedtime. Initially a dosage equivalent to 0.625 mg of conjugated estrogen should be tried, but frequently 1.25 mg is needed to relieve the symptoms. Occasionally a patient may need parenteral estrogen to relieve her symptoms.

Some patients, such as those with cancer of the breast or endometrium, cannot take estrogen. The next best therapy is a progestogen. Schiff and associates showed in a randomized, double-blind, crossover study that oral medroxyprogesterone acetate (MPA), 20 mg/day, relieved hot flushes significantly better than placebo (Figure 11-8).[8] Unfortunately, MPA does not prevent vaginal or urethral atrophy and is

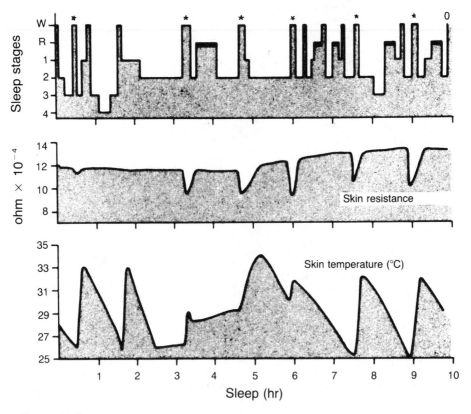

Figure 11-5
Sleepgram and recordings of skin resistance and temperature in postmenopausal woman with severe hot flushes.

*Objectively measured hot flush.

From Erlik Y, Tataryn IV, Meldrum DR, et al: Association of waking episodes with menopausal hot flushes. JAMA 245:1741, 1981. Copyright 1981, American Medical Association.

expensive. Several investigators have shown that injections of depo-MPA (DMPA), 150 mg once every 3 months, relieve hot flushes very well. When Lobo and associates compared the use of DMPA with a dosage of 0.625 mg of conjugated equine estrogens in the treatment of hot flushes, DMPA was as effective as the estrogens in relieving the symptoms.[9] Also, DMPA decreased markers of bone resorption, urinary calcium, and hydroxyproline urinary excretion to an extent similar to the changes produced by conjugated equine estrogen. Other agents that have been shown to reduce hot flushes substantially include clonidine, naloxone, and methyldopa.

A cluster of symptoms

A number of other symptoms—anxiety, depression, irritability, and fatigue—increase postmenopausally. There has been controversy over whether estrogen relieves these symptoms directly, or, because it prevents hot flushes and al-

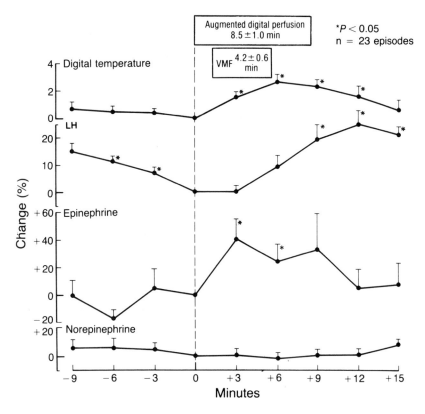

Figure 11-6
Composite graph of objective measurements obtained in five symptomatic postmenopausal women. Data are normalized to the beginning of augmented digital perfusion (zero time). VMF, vasomotor flush.

Reproduced, with permission, from Mashchak CA, Kletzky OA, Artal R, et al: The relation of physiological changes to subjective symptoms in postmenopausal women with and without hot flushes. Maturitas, in press.

lows the patient to sleep better, the other symptoms are relieved indirectly. Campbell studied 64 women who had severe menopausal symptoms.[10] The subjects were treated for 4 months in double-blind, crossover fashion with estrogen and a placebo. The frequency of symptoms was determined and psychological testing was performed. Among the women with hot flushes, estrogen treatment produced a significantly greater reduction in the following symptoms, compared with placebo: hot flushes, insomnia,

irritability, headaches, and urinary frequency. The following symptoms were significantly more improved with estrogen than with placebo in symptomatic women with and without flushes: vaginal dryness, poor memory, anxiety, and worry about self. Psychological tests indicated an increase in optimism and good spirits.

Certain symptoms were not significantly improved by estrogen compared with placebo in this study. These included arthralgias, backache, and vaginal discomfort. Estrogen also had no

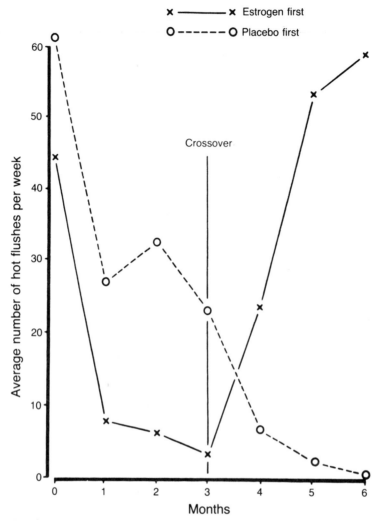

Figure 11-7
The average number of hot flushes per week in a randomized, double-blind, 6-month crossover study of estrogen and placebo therapy.

From Coope J: Double-blind crossover study of estrogen replacement therapy. In Campbell S (ed): Management of the Menopause and Post-Menopausal Years. Lancaster, England, MTP Press Ltd, 1976, p 167.

significant effect on skin condition or on coital satisfaction and frequency of orgasm. Thus, although many systemic symptoms are improved by estrogen, it is not a panacea for all the problems associated with aging.

Osteoporosis

Postmenopausal osteoporosis is an asymptomatic disorder that is difficult to diagnose early in its

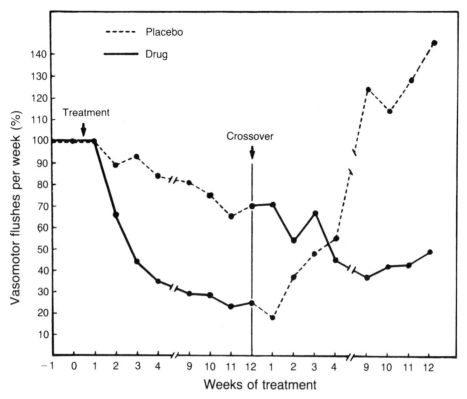

Figure 11-8

Percentage change in mean number of vasomotor flushes as a percentage change over pretreatment level (week −1 to 0) as a result of treatment with MPA. Change of treatment regimen (crossover) occurred at 12 weeks.

From Schiff I, Tulchinsky D, Cramer D, et al: Oral medroxyprogesterone in the treatment of postmenopausal symptoms. JAMA 244:1443, 1980. Copyright 1980, American Medical Association.

course. Once it has developed to the extent that it produces symptoms (fractures), it becomes difficult to treat. However, the condition can be prevented. Osteoporosis is defined as a reduction in the quantity of structural bony material in trabecular bone. Bone mass is increased in black, obese, and tall women and is decreased in small, frail, thin-skinned, sedentary women. Thus, women in the former group usually do not develop osteoporosis, whereas women in the latter may lose about 1% to 1.5% of bone mass each year after the menopause. Fractures begin to occur between ages 60 and 65 in structures

such as the vertebral spine and radius, where there is less bone mass. By age 60, 25% of white and oriental women develop spinal compression fractures.

Bone mass is greater in the femoral neck, so osteoporotic fractures of the femur do not begin to occur until about age 70 to 75 (Figure 11-9).[11] By age 90, 20% of all white women will develop hip fractures, and one-sixth of these will be fatal within 3 months. It has been estimated that each year in the US there are about 190,000 osteoporotic hip fractures, about 100,000 radius fractures, and about 400,000 other fractures, mainly

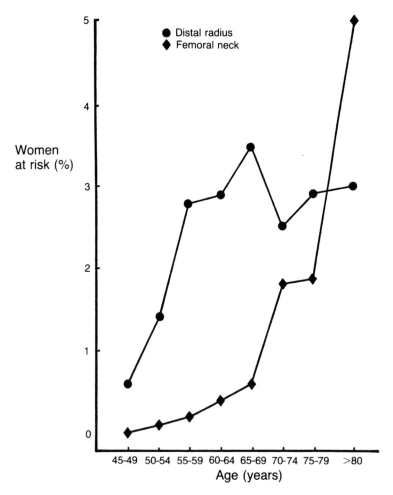

Figure 11-9
Relationship between the incidence of distal radius and femoral neck fractures and age in women.

From Aitken JM: Bone metabolism in post-menopausal women. In Beard RJ (ed): The Menopause: A Guide to Current Research and Practice. *Lancaster, England, MTP Press Ltd, 1976, p 99.*

thoracic vertebral fractures, due to osteoporosis.[12] About 15,000 women die of osteoporosis or its complications annually in the US, where total health care costs from osteoporosis are in excess of $1 billion per year. The fatal consequence of osteoporotic fractures is such that they represent the twelfth most frequent cause of death in American women. This costly, painful, possibly fatal disease can be prevented by estrogen treatment. Women whose ovaries are removed premenopausally are more likely to develop osteoporosis than are women who have a hysterectomy without oophorectomy. Young, castrated women have the highest risk for devel-

Normal endocrinology

oping osteoporosis. Therefore, if the ovaries are removed before age 45, white and oriental non-obese women should receive estrogen replacement therapy to prevent osteoporosis.

We do not know how estrogen prevents osteoporosis. Postmenopausally, serum levels of calcium and phosphorus are slightly increased and serum parathyroid hormone levels are decreased. The active form of vitamin D, 1,25-dihydroxy-D, is decreased and calcium absorption drops. Calcitonin levels are also lowered. Serum calcium levels need to be maintained within a fairly narrow range. Calcium is regulated by parathyroid hormone production. Parathyroid hormone increases serum calcium levels by three mechanisms: increasing bone resorption, increasing tubal resorption of calcium in the kidney, and producing an enzyme, 1α-hydroxylase, that changes vitamin D from its inactive form, which occurs in the diet or sunlight, to its active form, which increases calcium absorption from the gut. It has been postulated that sex steroids, including estrogen, androgens, and progestins, block the action of parathyroid hormone on bone, possibly by increasing levels of calcitonin (which inhibits bone resorption), so that less calcium is resorbed into the circulation. Therefore, parathyroid hormone levels remain high and exert their other actions (Figure 11-10).[13] After the menopause, as estrogen levels decline, the action of parathyroid hormone on bone is inhibited less, so that serum calcium levels increase, serum parathyroid hormone levels decrease, and there is less tubular reabsorption of calcium. Less 1α-hydroxylase and active vitamin D are produced, so less dietary calcium is absorbed (Figure 11-11).[13] Most of the serum calcium is then derived from bone. This drain causes the steady loss of about 1.5% of bone mass each year after the menopause.

Systemic estrogen therapy will stabilize the process or prevent it from starting. The best way to prevent loss of calcium from bone in post-menopausal or castrated women is to give estro-

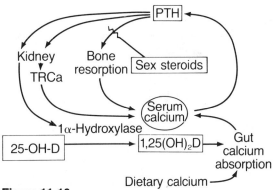

Figure 11-10
Hormonal control of calcium hemostasis in normal premenopausal women. Parathyroid hormone (PTH) increases bone resorption, increases renal tubular reabsorption of filtered calcium (TRCa), and increases the conversion of 25-hydroxyvitamin D (25-OH-D) to 1,25-dihydroxyvitamin D (1,25(OH)$_2$D).

From Riggs BL, Gallagher JC: Evidence for bihormonal deficiency state (estrogen and 1,25 dihydroxyvitamin D) in patients with postmenopausal osteoporosis. In Norman AW, et al (eds): Vitamin D. Biochemical, Chemical and Clinical Aspects Related to Calcium Metabolism. Berlin, Walter de Gruyter & Co, 1977, p 643.

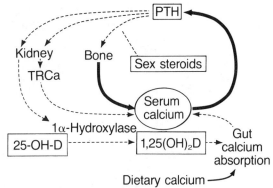

Figure 11-11
Postulated changes in hormonal control of calcium hemostasis in postmenopausal women with osteoporosis. Bone-resorbing cells have an increased sensitivity to PTH action; bone resorption increases in spite of decreased PTH. Decreased PTH results in decreased production of 1,25-dihydroxyvitamin D, leading to increased intestinal calcium absorption.

From Riggs BL, Gallagher JC: Evidence for bihormonal deficiency state (estrogen and 1,25 dihydroxyvitamin D) in patients with postmenopausal osteoporosis. In Norman AW, et al (eds): Vitamin D. Biochemical, Chemical and Clinical Aspects Related to Calcium Metabolism. Berlin, Walter de Gruyter & Co, 1977, p 643.

gens. Data in support of this mechanism were provided by Riggs and Gallagher, who took biopsies from patients with postmenopausal osteoporotic fractures and measured bone resorption and formation before and after they received estrogen therapy.[13] Patients with osteoporosis had a higher than normal rate of bone resorption (Figure 11-12).[14] With estrogen treatment, levels of bone resorption returned to normal. Bone

formation in patients with osteoporosis was normal both before and after the estrogen therapy (Figure 11-13).[14]

Prevention of bone loss

One of the first studies showing that estrogen prevented osteoporosis was performed by Albright's group. Patients treated with estrogen

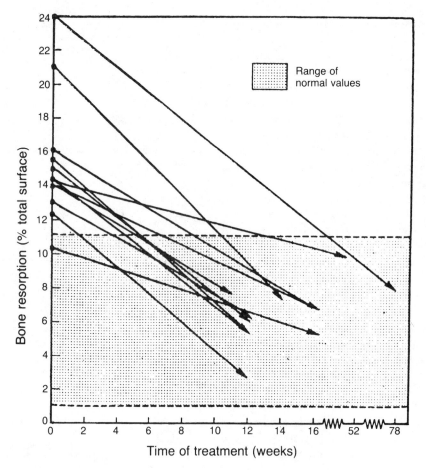

Figure 11-12
Effect of sex hormone on bone resorption.

Reproduced, with permission, from Riggs BL, Jowsey J, Kelley PJ, et al: Effect of sex hormones on bone in primary osteoporosis. J Clin Invest 48:1065, 1969. Copyright 1969, The American Society for Clinical Investigation.

Normal endocrinology

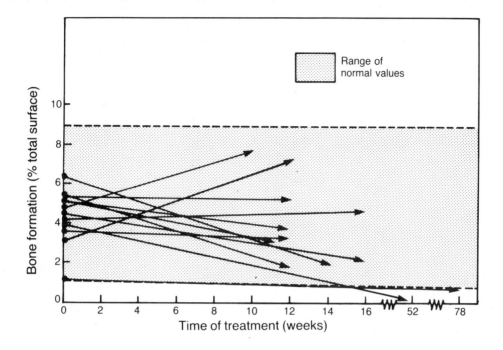

Figure 11-13
Effect of sex hormone on bone formation.

Reproduced, with permission, from Riggs BL, Jowsey J, Kelley PJ, et al: Effect of sex hormones on bone in primary osteoporosis. J Clin Invest 48:1065, 1969. Copyright 1969, The American Society for Clinical Investigation.

before the menopause did not lose height.[15] Patients with osteoporosis who had lost height when treated with estrogen usually did not lose any more height. These studies were the first to suggest that estrogen could prevent osteoporosis or stabilize the process after it had developed. Confirmation of this finding has been reported by Lindsay and his co-workers, who studied a group of young oophorectomized women in Scotland.[16,17] Half of them were treated with 20 µg of mestranol and half with placebo. Bone density was measured at yearly intervals. After 10 years, the group receiving estrogen had no decrease in bone density, whereas those who received the placebo had a steady decline in bone density (Figure 11-14).[17] Some of the placebo group developed loss of anterior vertebral

height, indicating compression fractures had occurred. One group of women received the estrogen for 4 years and then stopped taking it. Although they did not lose bone mass in the 4 years they took estrogen, once they stopped taking it they started losing bone at the same rate as the placebo group (Figure 11-15).[16] Therefore, estrogen treatment needs to be continued for long periods—to at least age 75 or 80—to prevent osteoporosis. Once estrogen therapy is stopped, bone loss begins.

Two studies in which bone density was recorded have shown the minimal dosage of estrogen needed to prevent osteoporosis to be 0.625 mg of conjugated equine estrogens.[17] Bone density studies with other estrogen formulations have not been published.

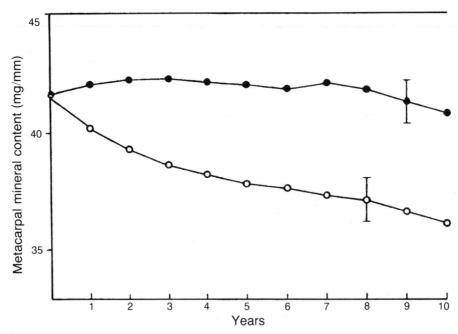

Figure 11-14
Bone mineral content (± maximum SE) in patients treated with estrogen (upper line) and placebo (lower line).

Reproduced, with permission, from Lindsay R, Hart DM, Forrest C, et al: Prevention of spinal osteoporosis in oophorectomized women. Lancet 2:1151, 1980.

Prevention of fractures

Several epidemiologic studies have shown that estrogens prevent fractures. A retrospective case-cohort study by Paganini-Hill and associates showed that a group of women who took estrogen had less than half as many fractures as a group who did not ingest estrogen.[18] Calcium also appeared to prevent fractures, but was not as effective as estrogen. Horowitz and colleagues found that patients who did not take estrogen had three times the number of fractures as a group that did take estrogen.[19] Another recent study, by Weiss and co-workers, reported that the reduction in fractures occurred mainly in those patients who had taken estrogen for more than 5 years (Table 11-1).[20] Patients who took estrogen for more than 5 years had less than half the number of fractures as the controls. Thus, at least three epidemiologic studies reported a decreased number of fractures in estrogen users when they were compared with controls who were not using estrogen.[21]

Riggs and colleagues have shown that patients with osteoporotic fractures treated with calcium had a higher incidence of recurrent fractures than those treated with calcium plus estrogen.[22] Estrogen is the best therapy to prevent osteoporosis, but 1 to 2 g of elemental calcium should also be ingested daily. Women receiving estrogen and who have an adequate diet should either drink $1\frac{1}{2}$ glasses of low-fat milk a day and take two 500-mg calcium carbonate tablets at night to supplement their dietary intake, or take three 500-mg calcium carbonate tablets each day. It is not necessary for postmenopausal women to receive vitamin D. Riggs and co-work-

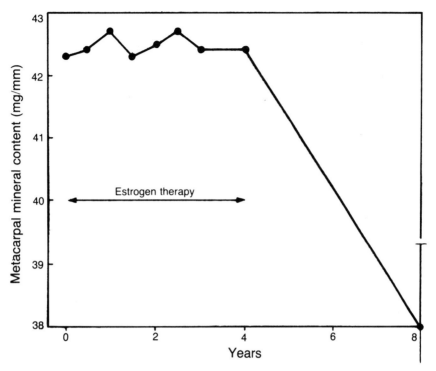

Figure 11-15
Effects of withdrawal of estrogen therapy on bone mineral content after 4 years of active treatment.

Reproduced, with permission, from Lindsay R, Hart DM, MacLean A, et al: Bone response to termination of oestrogen treatment. Lancet 1:1325, 1978.

Table 11-1
Menopausal estrogen use and osteoporotic fractures

Duration of use (yr)	Cases (%)	Controls (%)	Relative risk*	95% confidence interval†
0‡	66	48	1.0	
1–2	10	9	0.84	0.51–1.4
3–5	9	10	0.89	0.54–1.4
6–9	5	12	0.38	0.22–0.66
≥10	11	21	0.46	0.30–0.69

Standardized for age group (50 to 59, 60 to 69, and 70 to 74 years), history of hysterectomy, and current use versus past use of estrogens, by the method of Mantel and Haenszel.

†Approximate values, by the method of Miettinen.

‡Includes women using estrogens for less than 1 year.

From Weiss NS, Ure CL, Ballard JH, et al: Decreased risk of fractures of the hip and lower forearm with postmenopausal use of estrogen. N Engl J Med 303:1195, 1980.

ers showed that women with osteoporosis treated with various regimens, with and without vitamin D, had no difference in incidence of osteoporotic fractures.[22] Weight-bearing exercise, however, is important in preventing bone loss. Therefore, postmenopausal women should be encouraged to exercise.

Osteoporosis is insidious, because its presence is usually not detected until a compression fracture occurs many years after disease onset. At least 25% of the bone needs to be lost before osteoporosis is diagnosed by routine x-ray. At present, the methods available for establishing the early diagnosis of osteoporosis, specifically bone density studies and CT scans, are complicated and expensive. If they can be improved, they may be adopted for routine use. Thus, until scanning techniques or tests to measure urinary calcium excretion are refined, it will continue to be difficult to determine which patients are developing osteoporosis until a large amount of bone is lost. Perhaps a morning urinary calcium/creatinine ratio, obtained 3 hours after first voiding and then drinking 1 L of distilled water, may be used to screen patients at risk. If the urinary calcium/creatinine ratio is above 0.15, the woman is at risk for developing osteoporosis; if it is 0.10 or less, she is not.[23] Although not all nonobese white women develop osteoporosis, it may be best to treat all of them with estrogen at menopause to prevent this disorder. Factors known to increase the risk of osteoporosis are shown in Table 11-2.

In summary, estrogens increase calcium absorption, prevent bone resorption, and inhibit bone remodeling. They do not stimulate new bone growth, but will stabilize osteoporosis if it is present. Most important, estrogen treatment will prevent osteoporosis if started at menopause. Not all women need estrogen, because not all women are going to develop osteoporosis. However, for the nonobese white or oriental woman, estrogen offers the best way to prevent this debilitating and painful disease.

Table 11-2
Factors thought to place
women at increased risk for osteoporosis

Race: white or oriental
Reduced weight for height
Early spontaneous menopause
Early surgical menopause
Family history of osteoporosis
Diet: low calcium intake
     low vitamin D intake
     high caffeine intake
     high alcohol intake
     high protein intake
Cigarette smoking
Sedentary lifestyle

Need for estrogen therapy

In the past, vaginal cytology was used to determine the need for estrogen therapy. The karyopyknotic index and maturation index, the most popular methods of measuring estrogen effect on vaginal cytology, both correlate poorly with circulating estrogen levels. The problem with vaginal cytology is that because measurement is subjective, there are variations in results among laboratories for patients with the same circulating estrogen levels. Also, such local factors as the amount of thinning of the vaginal mucosa can change the karyopyknotic index, whereas circulating levels of estrogen are constant. Infection or bacteria can also change the karyopyknotic index, and the patient's vaginal mucosa can become refractory to estrogen therapy. Finally, drugs such as digitalis may alter vaginal cytology. For these reasons, we do not recommend that vaginal cytology be used to determine whether the patient needs estrogen replacement therapy.

With any drug, there is a benefit/risk ratio, but the risks of estrogen replacement therapy are minimal. Exogenous estrogen administration affects serum proteins, specifically by increasing serum globulins. One of these globulins, angiotensinogen, can be converted to angiotensin and raise blood pressure. Other globulins may produce a hypercoagulable state and even thrombosis. Exogenous estrogens may also alter lipid and glucose metabolism. However, the changes in protein, lipid, and glucose metabolism are related to the dosage and type of estrogen administered. The dose and type of estrogen given for hormone replacement therapy differ from the dose and type used in oral contraceptives (OCs). For prevention of osteoporosis, bone density studies have shown that at least the equivalent of 0.625 mg of conjugated equine estrone needs to be ingested. Patients with hot flushes sometimes need to receive the equivalent of 1.25 mg of conjugated equine estrogen or more for relief of these symptoms.

Drug regimens

Even a dosage of 2.5 mg of conjugated equine estrogen causes less of an increase in liver globulins than does 30 μg of ethinylestradiol (Figure 11-16).[24] Because of the presence of the ethynyl group at position 17, ethinylestradiol, the estrogen used in OCs, causes a much greater increase in liver globulin production than does estrone sulfate. We recently compared the potency of various doses of three types of natural oral estrogens (estrone sulfate, conjugated equine estrogen sulfate, and micronized estradiol) and two synthetic estrogens (diethylstilbestrol and ethinylestradiol).[25] Ethinylestradiol was much more potent in increasing globulin levels than any of the natural estrogens. In terms of equivalent weight, when an increase in liver globulins was used to measure estrogenic activity, we found ethinylestradiol to be about 90 times more potent than conjugated equine estrogen (Table 11-3).[25] Thus, 30 or 35 μg of ethinylestradiol, the dosage of estrogen in most of the new OC formulations, are the equivalent of about 2.5 mg of conjugated equine estrogens. The usual estro-

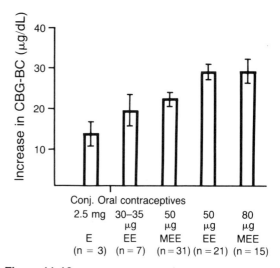

Figure 11-16

Increase in corticosteroid-binding globulin binding capacity (CBG-BC) in relation to the dose of synthetic estrogen. Conj E, conjugated equine estrogen; EE, ethinylestradiol; MEE, mestranol.

From Moore DE, Kawagoe S, Davajan V, et al: An in vivo system in man for quantitation of estrogenicity. II. Pharmacologic changes in binding capacity of serum corticosteroid-binding globulin induced by conjugated estrogens, mestranol, and ethinylestradiol. Am J Obstet Gynecol 130:482, 1978.

gen replacement dosage, 0.625 mg/day, is about one-fifth as potent as the usual dose of estrogen in OCs.

OCs raise the blood pressure of some women, but there is no evidence that the doses of natural oral estrogens used to treat menopausal women do. Pfeffer and co-workers measured systolic and diastolic blood pressure in postmenopausal women before and after taking estrogen, and compared these measurements with those of a control population during the same interval. They showed that neither group had a significant change in mean blood pressure (Table 11-4).[26] Aylward and colleagues also showed that the natural estrogens, in the dosages used for hormonal replacement, do not increase clotting factors,[27] while ethinylestradiol alone did produce a hypercoagulable state. No study has demonstrated an increased incidence of throm-

Table 11-3
Relative potency according to four specific measures of estrogenicity

Estrogen preparation	Serum FSH	Serum CBG-BC*	Serum SHBG-BC	Serum angiotensinogen
Piperazine estrone sulfate	1.0	1.0	1.0	1.0
Conjugated estrogens	1.4	2.5	3.2	3.5
Micronized estradiol	1.3	1.9	1.0	0.7
Diethylstilbestrol	3.8	7.9	2.8	13
Ethinylestradiol	(80–200)†	(1,000)†	614	232

*Corticosteroid-binding globulin binding capacity.

†Estimate in absence of parallelism.

From Mashchak CA, Lobo RA, Dozono-Takano R, et al: Comparison of pharmacodynamic properties of various estrogen formulations. Am J Obstet Gynecol 144:511, 1982.

Table 11-4
Blood pressure (BP) in matched users and nonusers of estrogen

Estrogen group	Before* (mean ± SD)	During (mean ± SD)
Users (n = 162)		
Systolic BP	144.7 ± 16.2	143.9 ± 18.3
Diastolic BP	82.1 ± 8.1	81.9 ± 9.0
Nonusers (n = 162)		
Systolic BP	147.6 ± 17.2	147.0 ± 17.9
Diastolic BP	82.9 ± 8.9	83.0 ± 8.8

*For nonusers of estrogens, time intervals are defined by use-periods for matched user.

From Pfeffer RI, Kurosaki TT, Charlton SK: Estrogen use and blood pressure in later life. Am J Epidemiol 110:469, 1979.

bophlebitis or thromboembolism in postmenopausal estrogen users compared with controls. Several studies, however, have reported no increased incidence of these disorders in postmenopausal women taking estrogen in contrast with the increased incidence found in OC users.[28] Furthermore, there is no evidence that postmenopausal women with a past history of thrombophlebitis have an increased incidence of thrombophlebitis with estrogen replacement therapy.

Atherosclerosis

Epidemiologic evidence indicates that arterial thrombosis, not atherosclerosis, is the cause of the increased incidence of myocardial infarction in OC users over 35 who smoke. The risk of myocardial infarction is not related to duration of OC use and has not been shown to be increased in former OC users. Because natural estrogen in the dosages used by postmenopausal women does not alter clotting factors as much as the dosage of ethinylestradiol in OCs, the former agents should not increase the risk of coronary arterial thrombosis. In fact, several studies have shown no increased relative risk of myocardial infarction in patients who take estrogen postmenopausally. In most of these studies, the relative risk was about 1 or less, indicating that, in contrast with older OC users, postmenopausal women taking estrogen do not have an increase in myocardial infarction. Epidemiologic studies by Pfeffer and co-workers showed that neither the relative risk of heart attack nor stroke is increased in postmenopausal patients who take estrogen compared with controls.[29,30]

Another epidemiologic study, by Ross and associates, compared the mortality rates from ischemic heart disease in postmenopausal women using estrogen with the rates in both living and deceased controls who had not used estrogen.[31] Their data showed that diabetes, hypertension, and smoking increased the chance of dying from ischemic heart disease, but that estrogens, as well as alcohol intake, decreased the

Table 11-5
Matched risk ratios for death from ischemic heart disease

| | Living controls | | Deceased controls | |
Variable	Discordant pairs (No.)	Risk ratio	Discordant pairs (No.)	Risk ratio
Stroke	31	3.43*	32	2.20‡
Hypertension	72	3.24†	80	2.33†
Angina pectoris	53	6.57†	42	2.50*
Myocardial infarction	50	7.33†	44	3.89†
Diabetes before age 65	11	2.67	14	2.50
Family history of MI	37	2.29	23	0.95
Cholesterol ≥ 300 mg/dL	25	1.27	24	3.00*
Cigarettes > 1 pack/day	13	3.33‡	20	1.00
Alcohol	33	0.38*	45	0.88
Conjugated estrogens	57	0.43*	55	0.57‡

*$P \leq 0.01$
†$P \leq 0.001$
‡$P \leq 0.05$

From Ross RK, Mack TM, Paganini-Hill A, et al: Menopausal oestrogen therapy and protection from death from ischemic heart disease. Lancet 1:858, 1981.

chance of dying from ischemic heart disease (Table 11-5).[31] This study showed a protective effect of estrogens against myocardial infarction; even women who smoked and took estrogen had a significantly decreased chance of dying from myocardial infarction compared with controls. Therefore, it appears that, in contrast with OC users, postmenopausal women who smoke and take natural estrogen replacement therapy do not have an increased risk of developing myocardial infarction.

Levels of low-density lipoprotein (LDL)-cholesterol have a positive correlation with coronary heart disease, whereas levels of high-density lipoprotein (HDL)-cholesterol have an inverse relation to coronary heart disease. Thus, individuals with naturally high LDL-cholesterol and low HDL-cholesterol are at greater risk of having coronary heart disease. However, to date there is no evidence that altering these lipid fractions in normal people reduces the chance of developing coronary heart disease.

Nevertheless, it should be reassuring to postmenopausal estrogen users that the results of a recent Lipid Research Clinics Program study revealed that, in contrast with some OC users who had increased levels of LDL-cholesterol, postmenopausal estrogen users had decreased levels of LDL-cholesterol.[32] The latter also had increased levels of HDL-cholesterol when compared with postmenopausal non-estrogen users (Table 11-6).[32] Another recent study from this same NIH program indicated that age-adjusted, all-causes mortality rates were significantly lower in estrogen users as compared with nonusers, whether or not they had a previous hysterectomy or oophorectomy (Table 11-7).[33] Although a few studies have shown a statistically increased risk of gallbladder disease in postmenopausal estrogen users, others have reported no such risk. Perhaps, like OCs, estrogens accelerate cholelithiasis in individuals destined to develop this disorder. Also, studies of the effect of estrogen on glucose tolerance have been equivocal. Several recent studies have shown no decrease in glucose tolerance in patients treated with doses of estrogen equivalent to 1.25 mg of conjugated equine estrogen.

Table 11-6
**Concentrations of lipids and lipoproteins
in users and nonusers of estrogen**

Lipid profile	Nonuser: mean ± SD (median)	Equine estrogen: mean ± SD (median)
Cholesterol	230 ± 44.3 (226)	219 ± 33.9 (218)*
Triglyceride	174 ± 66.9 (100)	141 ± 71.5 (126)*
HDL cholesterol	61 ± 15.6 (61)	69 ± 17.7 (67)*
LDL cholesterol	154 ± 43.8 (147)	133 ± 33.9 (131)*
VDL cholesterol	16 ± 13.8 (13)	18 ± 12.5 (16)

*Significantly different from nonusers at the 0.05 level.

From Wahl P, Walden C, Knopp R, et al: Effect of estrogen/progestin potency on lipid/lipoprotein cholesterol. N Engl J Med 308:862, 1983.

Cancer and estrogen replacement

Breast cancer
Much concern has been raised about the neoplastic risks associated with postmenopausal estrogen replacement therapy. Even though the preponderance of evidence from well-designed case-control studies shows no increased risk of breast cancer in postmenopausal estrogen users, the possibility exists that estrogen can stimulate a nonpalpable breast cancer.[34] Carcinoma of the breast may exist in the preclinical state for as long as 8 years before it is palpable. Thus, it is advisable to obtain a mammogram to rule out subclinical breast cancer in all patients before initiating estrogen therapy.

Endometrial cancer
Several epidemiologic studies have reported that there is a three- to sevenfold increased risk of developing endometrial cancer in postmenopausal women who are ingesting estrogen, compared with non-estrogen users. When the data for these studies were carefully evaluated, Hulka showed that this increased risk occurred mainly with high doses of estrogen given for long periods of time.[34] For an increased risk of endometrial cancer, the estrogen needed to be ingested for more than 4 years and the daily dosage needed to be at least 1.25 mg of conjugated estrogen. Furthermore, the actual increased risk that a woman would develop endometrial cancer, even if the relative risk was sevenfold, was only about 1/500. Actually, the risk is not even this great, because a substantial number of the controls in the various epidemiologic studies who were presumed not to have endometrial cancer probably did have undiagnosed endometrial cancer.

A study of three large series of routine autopsies during the past 30 years in New England indicated that about 1/300 women who died of other causes had undiagnosed and unsuspected endometrial cancer. Therefore, it appears that a certain number of women in the control groups of all epidemiologic studies linking endometrial cancer with estrogen use had undiagnosed endometrial cancer. The disease may have become manifest by uterine bleeding if the women had received exogenous estrogen, thus spuriously increasing the risk ratio. Therefore, the risk of developing endometrial cancer with estrogen therapy is substantially overestimated and is related to the dosage of estrogen and duration of use. Furthermore, the endometrial cancer that develops in estrogen users is usually well differentiated and cured by simple hysterectomy.

A report by Collins and co-workers showed that women who had endometrial cancer, and were not receiving estrogen, had a 10-year survival rate of about 50%.[35] A control population without cancer, matched for age and also not taking estrogen, had about an 80% survival rate at the end of 10 years (Figure 11-17).[35] A group of patients who had endometrial cancer, and were also taking estrogen, had a survival rate similar to the control population taking estrogen (90%). These rates indicate that the well-differentiated endometrial carcinoma occurring with estrogen treatment can be adequately treated by hysterectomy and usually is not lethal. Furthermore, this estrogen-induced carcinoma can be prevented by giving the patient progestogens.

Estrogen acts only if a specific receptor is present within the target cell. The estrogen-receptor complex is translocated into the nucleus, where it activates messenger RNA, which then changes DNA to initiate cell division and also produces new receptors. Progesterone, which normally is produced in the last half of the menstrual cycle, blocks receptor synthesis so that no new receptors are formed. Therefore, the endometrium does not proliferate in the latter half of the menstrual cycle because progesterone prevents receptor synthesis and further growth and division of the cells, despite estrogen production. To summarize, estrogen increases the synthesis of both estrogen and progesterone receptors; progesterone and synthetic progestins decrease the synthesis of both these receptors and thus have an antiproliferative action.

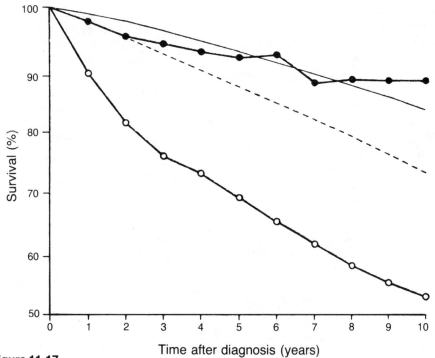

Figure 11-17
Survival of women with endometrial cancer and history of estrogen use (solid circles) compared with estrogen-user controls (age-adjusted mortality), (solid line), women with endometrial cancer who were not estrogen users (open circles), and non-estrogen-user controls (age-adjusted mortality), (dashed line).

Reproduced, with permission, from Collins J, Donner A, Allen LH, et al: Oestrogen use and survival in endometrial cancer. Lancet 2:961, 1980.

Role of progestins

Progestins have been shown to prevent endometrial hyperplasia. Sturdee and co-workers performed endometrial biopsies annually in women receiving sex steroids.[36] They found that 23% of the women receiving continuous estrogen alone developed cystic or adenomatous hyperplasia and 12% of patients taking cyclic estrogen alone developed endometrial hyperplasia. When progestins were added to the estrogen for 5 days each month, the incidence of hyperplasia decreased to 8%. When progestins were added to the regimen for more than 12 days each month for 4 years, no hyperplasia developed.

These and other investigators have found the duration of progestin therapy is more important than the dosage. Small amounts of progestin administered for more than 12 days each month will reduce the incidence of carcinoma. Hammond and colleagues showed that patients receiving a progestin along with estrogen were less likely to develop cancer than patients receiving estrogen alone.[37] All the patients in this retrospective series were treated for more than 5 years. Gambrell reported that during a 5-year period at a large referral center, eight endometrial cancers developed in patients given estrogen alone, for a rate of 4/1,000.[38] In patients receiving no steroid therapy, the rate was 2/1,000. In patients receiving an estrogen-progestin combination, only 0.5/1,000 developed endometrial carcinoma—substantially fewer women than those receiving estrogen alone.

Thus, all the evidence indicates that progestins appear to lower the chances that postmenopausal estrogen users will develop cancer of the endometrium. Therefore, to reduce the risk of endometrial cancer, a progestin should probably be given to postmenopausal women receiving estrogen. Progestin-estrogen therapy does not cause an increase of any other systemic disease, according to a 10-year study performed by Nachtigall's group.[39] In this study, as well as a double-blind placebo study performed by Christiansen et al,[40] estrogen-progestin therapy not only prevented loss of bone density but also actually caused a slight increase in bone density in postmenopausal women.

The dosage and type of progestin necessary to prevent endometrial cancer have not been determined. Whitehead and his colleagues showed that in patients receiving 0.625 mg of conjugated estrogens, as little as 1 mg of norethindrone and 150 µg of norgestrel were sufficient to decrease the receptor and DNA activity in endo-

Table 11-7
Age-adjusted, all-cause mortality rates (per 1,000/year) by hysterectomy status and estrogen use (95% confidence limits on rates)

Hysterectomy status	Estrogen use		
	Nonuser	User	Total
Intact	9.0 (6.5–12.0)	4.9 (1.8–10.7)	8.2 (6.1–10.8)
Hysterectomy	8.2 (3.3–16.8)	2.8 (0.3–10.0)	5.7 (2.6–10.8)
Oophorectomy	11.8 (5.9–21.2)	1.4 (0.0–7.6)	7.2 (3.7–12.6)
Total	9.3 (7.2–11.9)	3.4 (1.5–6.4)	

From Bush TL, Cowan LD, Barrett-Connor E, et al: Estrogen use and all-cause mortality. Preliminary results from the Lipid Research Clinics Program Follow-Up Study. JAMA 249:903, 1983.

metrial cells to a level similar to the secretory phase of the normal cycle.[41] These investigators recently reported that 350 µg of norethindrone produced the same degree of protection as 1 mg. A recent report by Gibbons indicated that in patients receiving 0.625 mg of conjugated estrone, 2.5 mg of MPA reduced nuclear and cytosol estrogen receptor levels to those found prior to estrogen administration.[42] With a daily dose of 1.25 mg of conjugated estrogen, 5 mg of MPA were necessary to decrease receptor synthesis to the same degree.

Currently, we are recommending that 0.625 mg of conjugated equine estrogen or estrone sulfate be administered for 25 days each month. Beginning on the 15th day of estrogen treatment, 2.5 to 10 mg of MPA are added daily for 10 days. Although less than 10 mg doses of MPA have not been shown to decrease the risk of cancer by decreasing receptor levels, they decrease mitotic activity and also reduce the incidence of withdrawal bleeding. Studies of lipid metabolism indicate that MPA has a weak effect on lipid metabolism and does not substantially alter levels of serum cholesterol, triglycerides, HDL-cholesterol, LDL-cholesterol, or the ratio of the two lipid fractions.[43] Thus, the addition of MPA to the management of the menopause should not significantly alter the risk of cardiovascular disease. Whitehead et al advise that patients take 0.625 mg of conjugated equine estrogen every day, along with 350 µg of norethindrone for the first 10 days of the month.[41] Other therapeutic regimens are also used.

A treatment regimen of 0.625 mg of conjugated equine estrone or estrone sulfate, together with 2.5 mg of MPA administered each week from Monday to Friday, reduces the chance of breakthrough bleeding. This method also avoids a week-off treatment, during which symptoms may appear. This regimen is especially convenient for women without a uterus, as well as for those who develop breast tenderness or have cystic breast disease. A pretreatment endometrial biopsy is advisable, but routine annual biopsies are unnecessary if adequate progestogen is given, unless abnormal bleeding (not withdrawal) occurs.

To summarize, indications for estrogen therapy after menopause include the presence of vasomotor symptoms as well as prevention of atrophic vaginitis, atrophic urethritis, osteoporosis, and possibly atherosclerosis. Until diagnostic methods are perfected to detect bone loss when it initially occurs, it would appear prudent to prescribe estrogen-progestins for all postmenopausal women who are at risk for developing osteoporosis and to continue treatment indefinitely.

References

1. Jaszmann LJB: Epidemiology of the climacteric syndrome. In Campbell S (ed): *Management of the Menopause and Post-Menopausal Years.* Lancaster, England, MTP Press Ltd, 1976, p 12

2. Cope E: Physical changes associated with the post-menopausal years. In Campbell S (ed): *Management of the Menopause and Post-Menopausal Years.* Lancaster, England, MTP Press Ltd, 1976, p 33

3. Sherman BM, West JH, Korenman SG: The menopausal transition: Analysis of LH, FSH, estradiol, and progesterone concentrations during menstrual cycles of older women. *J Clin Endocrinol Metab* 42:629, 1976

4. Erlik Y, Meldrum DR, Judd HL: Estrogen levels in postmenopausal women with hot flashes. *Obstet Gynecol* 59:403, 1982

5. Erlik Y, Tataryn IV, Meldrum DR, et al: Association of waking episodes with menopausal hot flushes. *JAMA* 245:1741, 1981

6. Mashchak CA, Kletzky OA, Artal R, et al: The relation of physiological changes to subjective symptoms in postmenopausal women with and without hot flushes. *Maturitas,* in press

7. Coope J: Double-blind crossover study of estrogen replacement therapy. In Campbell S (ed): *Management of the Menopause and Post-Menopausal Years.* Lancaster, England, MTP Press Ltd, 1976, p 167

8. Schiff I, Tulchinsky D, Cramer D, et al: Oral medroxyprogesterone in the treatment of postmenopausal symptoms. *JAMA* 244:1443, 1980

9. Lobo RA, McCormick W, Singer F, et al: Depo-medroxyprogesterone acetate compared with conjugated estrogens for the treatment of postmenopausal women. *Obstet Gynecol* 63:1, 1984

10. Campbell S: Double blind psychometric studies on the effects of natural estrogens on post-menopausal women. In Campbell S (ed): *Management of the Menopause and Post-Menopausal Years.* Lancaster, England, MTP Press Ltd, 1976, p 152

11. Aitken JM: Bone metabolism in post-menopausal women. In Beard RJ (ed): *The Menopause: A Guide to Current Research and Practice.* Lancaster, England, MTP Press Ltd, 1976, p 99

12. Marx JL: Hormones and their effects in the aging body. *Science* 206:805, 1979

13. Riggs BL, Gallagher JC: Evidence for bihormonal deficiency state (estrogen and 1,25 dihydroxyvitamin D) in patients with postmenopausal osteoporosis. In Norman AW, et al (eds): *Vitamin D. Biochemical, Chemical and Clinical Aspects Related to Calcium Metabolism.* Berlin, Walter de Gruyter & Co, 1977, p 643

14. Riggs BL, Jowsey J, Kelley PJ, et al: Effect of sex hormones on bone in primary osteoporosis. *J Clin Invest* 48:1065, 1969

15. Wallach S, Henneman PH: Prolonged estrogen therapy in postmenopausal women. *JAMA* 171:1637, 1959

16. Lindsay R, Hart DM, MacLean A, et al: Bone response to termination of oestrogen treatment. *Lancet* 1:1325, 1978

17. Lindsay R, Hart DM, Forrest C, et al: Prevention of spinal osteoporosis in oophorectomized women. *Lancet* 2:1151, 1980

18. Paganini-Hill A, Ross RK, Gerkins VR, et al: Menopausal estrogen therapy and hip fractures. *Ann Intern Med* 95:28, 1981

19. Horowitz RI, Feinstein AR: Alternative analytic methods for case-control studies of estrogens and endometrial cancer. *N Engl J Med* 299:1089, 1978

20. Weiss NS, Ure CL, Ballard JH, et al: Decreased risk of fractures of the hip and lower forearm with postmenopausal use of estrogen. *N Engl J Med* 303:1195, 1980

21. Kreiger N, Kelsey JL, Holford TR, et al: An epidemiologic study of hip fracture in postmenopausal women. *Am J Epidemiol* 116:141, 1982

22. Riggs BL, Seeman E, Hodgson SF, et al: Effect of the fluoride/calcium regimen on vertebral fracture occurrence in postmenopausal osteoporosis. *N Engl J Med* 306:446, 1982

23. Nordin BEC, Gallagher JC, Aaron JE, et al: Post-menopausal osteopenia and osteoporosis. Estrogens in the post-menopause. *Front Hormone Res* 3:131, 1975

24. Moore DE, Kawagoe S, Davajan V, et al: An in vivo system in man for quantitation of estrogenicity. II. Pharmacologic changes in binding capacity of serum corticosteroid-binding globulin induced by conjugated estrogens, mestranol, and ethinylestradiol. *Am J Obstet Gynecol* 130:482, 1978

25. Mashchak CA, Lobo RA, Dozono-Takano R, et al: Comparison of pharmacodynamic properties of various estrogen formulations. *Am J Obstet Gynecol* 144:511, 1982

26. Pfeffer RI, Kurosaki TT, Charlton SK: Estrogen use and blood pressure in later life. *Am J Epidemiol* 110:469, 1979

27. Aylward M, Maddock J, Rees PL: Natural oestrogen replacement therapy and blood clotting. *Br Med J* 1:220, 1976

28. Boston Collaborative Drug Surveillance Program: Surgically confirmed gallbladder disease, venous thromboembolism, and breast tumors in relation to postmenopausal estrogen therapy. *N Engl J Med* 304:560, 1981

29. Pfeffer RI, Whipple GH, Kurosaki TT, et al: Coronary risk and estrogen use in postmenopausal women. *Am J Epidemiol* 107:479, 1978

30. Pfeffer RI: Estrogen use, hypertension and stroke in postmenopausal women. *J Chron Dis* 31:389, 1978

31. Ross RK, Mack TM, Paganini-Hill A, et al: Menopausal oestrogen therapy and protection from death from ischaemic heart disease. *Lancet* 1:858, 1981

32. Wahl P, Walden C, Knopp R, et al: Effect of estrogen/progestin potency on lipid/lipoprotein cholesterol. *N Engl J Med* 308:862, 1983

33. Bush TL, Cowan LD, Barrett-Connor E, et al: Estrogen use and all-cause mortality. Preliminary results from the Lipid Research Clinics Program Follow-Up Study. *JAMA* 249:903, 1983

34. Hulka BS: Effect of exogenous estrogen on postmenopausal women: The epidemiologic evidence. *Obstet Gynecol Surv* 35:389, 1980

35. Collins J, Donner A, Allen LH, et al: Oestrogen use and survival in endometrial cancer. *Lancet* 2:961, 1980

36. Sturdee DW, Wade-Evans T, Paterson MEL, et al: Relations between bleeding pattern, endometrial histology, and estrogen treatment in menopausal women. *Br Med J* 1:1575, 1978

37. Hammond CB, Jelovsek FR, Lee KI, et al: Effects of long-term estrogen replacement therapy—II. Neoplasia. *Am J Obstet Gynecol* 133:537, 1979

38. Gambrell RD Jr: The menopause: benefits and risks of estrogen-progestogen replacement therapy. *Fertil Steril* 37:457, 1982

39. Nachtigall LE, Nachtigall RH, Nachtigall RD, et al: Estrogen replacement therapy I: A 10-year prospective study in the relationship to osteoporosis. *Obstet Gynecol* 53:277, 1979

40. Christiansen C, Christiansen MS, Transbol I: Bone mass in postmenopausal women after withdrawal of oestrogen/gestagen replacement therapy. *Lancet* 1:459, 1981

41. Whitehead MI, Townsend PT, Pryse-Davies J, et al: Effect of estrogens and progestins on the biochemistry and morphology of the postmenopausal endometrium. *N Engl J Med* 305:1599, 1981

42. Gibbons WE: Personal communication, 1984

43. Hirvonen E, Mälkönen M, Manninken V: Effects of different progestogens on lipoproteins during postmenopausal replacement therapy. *N Engl J Med* 304:560, 1981

Normal endocrinology

Part II
Abnormal Endocrinology

Chapter 12

Disorders of Sexual Differentiation

Daniel R. Mishell Jr., M.D.
Uwe Goebelsmann, M.D.

There are several characteristics whereby the sex of an individual can be identified. In a normal individual, all these characteristics are consistently either male or female; where a discrepancy exists, hermaphroditism or intersexuality is present. Jones and Scott have described five organic and two psychological characteristics for defining the sex of an individual.[1] The organic characteristics are (1) sex chromosomes, (2) gonadal histology, (3) morphology of the external genitalia, (4) morphology of the internal genitalia, and (5) hormonal status. The psychological characteristics are (6) sex of rearing and (7) gender role of the individual. Intersexuality exists only when the first four organic (morphogenetic) criteria are not all characteristic of the same sex. The hormonal status may be male in a woman with a virilizing ovarian tumor, for example, without the presence of intersexuality. Certain individuals without any morphologic or organic evidence of intersexuality may assume the opposite gender role solely because of a psychological disorder, such as transvestism or transsexualism.

The psychological characteristics are usually related to the morphology of the external genitalia. Therefore, when intersexuality exists in a newborn, it is important to determine and designate the infant's sex soon after birth—before the infant leaves the hospital. This will avoid a change in the gender role later in life, with its accompanying psychological trauma.

Normal sexual development

Familiarity with normal sexual development provides a basis for understanding disorders of intersexuality. There are three major stages in sexual development. In chronologic order, these are (1) gonadal development, (2) differentiation of the internal genitalia, and (3) differentiation of the external genitalia (Figure 12-1).

Gonadal development

The sex chromosomes of the zygote determine the type of gonad that will be developed. In both

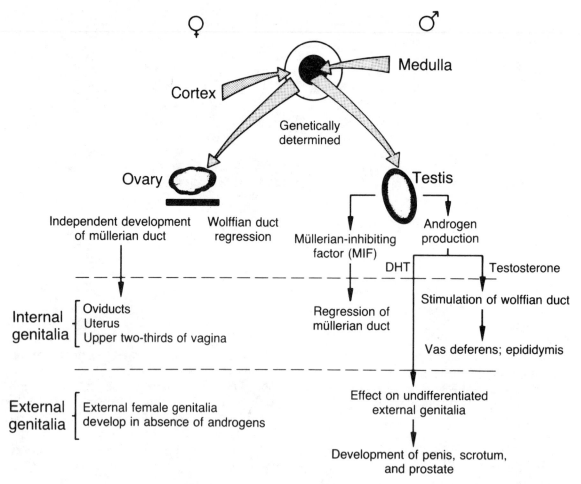

Figure 12-1
Outline of male and female sexual development.

sexes an undifferentiated gonad appears at about the fourth week of embryonic life. This gonad consists of an inner medullary portion and an outer cortex. During the fourth to sixth weeks of gestation, germ cells migrate into this gonad from the endoderm of the yolk sac. After the germ cells reach it, the gonad begins to differentiate into an ovary or testis. If no germ cells reach the gonad, gonadal agenesis results: The gonad does not develop and persists only as a streak of fibrous tissue.

For a testis to develop, a Y chromosome must be present. Jost and associates postulated that the undifferentiated gonad develops as an ovary unless a testicular organizer or inducer (not an androgen), produced by cells within the gonad, imposes testicular organogenesis on the other cells of the gonadal primordium.[2] It is thought that the genes responsible for development of the testes are located on the short arm of the Y chromosome near the centromere. More recent evidence suggests that several genes, which appear to be located on both X and Y chromosomes, are necessary for sex differentiation of the mammalian gonad. Whereas the Y chromosome is mandatory for testicular development, a gene on the X chromosome appears to regulate the testis-organizing gene on the Y chromosome. Furthermore, as reported by Wachtel et al,[3] a cell surface antigen (H-Y antigen) appears to be the organizer or inducer responsible for testicular development. The gene for this antigen is on the short arm of the Y chromosome. Another gene regulates a specific receptor for the H-Y antigen on the gonadal cells to facilitate the antigen's action in inducing testicular development. When the testis develops, the medullary portion of the undifferentiated gonad persists and differentiates, while the cortex disappears. The mechanism of gonadal differentiation has not been completely elucidated.

Initiation of testicular differentiation occurs earlier than initiation of ovarian differentiation; the former at about 7 weeks of fetal life, and the latter at about 12 weeks. In the testes, the seminiferous tubules are formed first, followed by Leydig cell differentiation beginning at about 8 weeks of gestation. Leydig cell hyperplasia and testosterone secretion occur subsequently. Fetal serum testosterone levels peak between 15 and 18 weeks' gestation, while maternal serum human chorionic gonadotropin (hCG) reaches peak levels by the end of the first trimester.

When at least two X chromosomes and no Y chromosomes are present, the gonad differentiates into an ovary. In ovarian development, the outer cortex persists and the inner medulla regresses. A complete 46,XX chromosomal complement is necessary for development of normal ovaries. Deletion of any portion of an X chromosome will result in streak gonads.

Differentiation of internal genitalia

Originally, in embryos of both sexes, müllerian and wolffian duct primordia are both present.

In the female, the müllerian ducts grow caudally and fuse to form the oviducts, uterus, and the upper portion of the vagina. The wolffian ducts regress. In the male, the wolffian ducts differentiate to form the vas deferens, seminal vesicles, and epididymis, while the müllerian ducts disappear. Müllerian duct regression is brought about by the local action of a testicular agent, müllerian-inhibiting factor (MIF). Müllerian duct regression commences at 8 weeks' gestation and is completed by 11 weeks, whereas wolffian duct development, being about 1 week behind müllerian duct regression, occurs between 9 and 12 weeks of pregnancy. It is believed that MIF, which has not as yet been completely identified, is secreted by the Sertoli cells within the seminiferous tubules of the embryonic testis and is probably a high-molecular-weight polypeptide. MIF is definitely not an androgen. Wolffian duct development, however, can be produced experimentally by high concentrations of testosterone administered locally in the form of a testosterone crystal, indicating that this hormone is important in the differentiation of the male internal genitalia. In the absence of a gonad, müllerian duct development and wolffian duct regression occur.

Differentiation of external genitalia

In the final stage of sexual development, the external genitalia of both sexes develop from a common undifferentiated anlage. Specifically, the genital tubercle becomes the clitoris in the female and the penis in the male. The genital folds form the labia minora in the female, but fuse to form the ventral medial raphe in the male. The genital swellings develop into the labia majora in the female and the scrotum in the male. Wolffian duct degeneration and development of the female external genitalia take place between 10 and 14 weeks of gestation. Dihydrotestosterone (DHT) stimulation is necessary for development of the male external genitalia, which occurs between 9 and 14 weeks' gestation, and for development of the prostate. DHT is converted from testosterone in these target tissues by the enzyme 5α-reductase. Without DHT formation, female differentiation of the external genitalia occurs, even in the presence of adequate testosterone levels.

Sexual ambiguity

Classification

There are numerous schemes for classifying the various disorders of sexual development. The Klebs classification, based on gonadal histology, provides a useful basis for definitions. When there is an inconsistency among the four morphogenetic sexual characteristics and the gonads are masculine, the individual is designated a male pseudohermaphrodite. When the histologic appearance of the gonads is feminine, the individual is designated a female pseudohermaphrodite. An individual with both male and female elements in the same or opposite gonads is classified as a true hermaphrodite.

Recent advances in cytogenetics and biochemistry have made a more definitive classification possible (Table 12-1). This system is based on Federman's monograph as modified by findings of Imperato-McGinley and Peterson and of Wilson and co-workers.[4-6] Disorders of sexual ambiguity are divided into two major categories on the basis of etiology: (1) disorders of gonadal development, in which the basic defect is usually a major chromosomal lesion, and (2) disorders of fetal endocrinology, in which the individual has normal chromosomes corresponding to his or her gonadal sex, but usually has a genetic (and often hereditary) defect.

It has been estimated that the incidence of normal males with hypospadias may range from 1/600 to 1/1,800 births. By strict definition, hypospadias should be classified as a disorder of intersexuality. By common usage, however, it is not considered to be an intersex disorder. Jones and Scott state that "in order for the individual to be classified as a hermaphrodite, a vagina has to be present in addition to hypospadias. Therefore, hypospadiac males without a vagina should not be considered as male hermaphrodites."[1]

Disorders of gonadal development

Etiology

The major chromosomal lesions causing abnormal gonadal development are due to errors in meiosis or mitosis. These lesions occur by chance and are neither hereditary nor more likely to occur in siblings. The normal female has 44 autosomes and two X sex chromosomes, while the normal male has 44 autosomes and one X and one Y sex chromosome. In the male, both the first and second meiotic divisions occur during the process of spermatogenesis, which begins at puberty. Each spermatogonium produces four spermatocytes, each having 23 chromosomes. Two of the spermatocytes have an X chromosome and two have a Y chromosome. In the female, meiosis begins in the ova during the fourth month of fetal life. The first stages of the first meiotic division occur during the next 3 months. Meiosis then ceases and does not resume until puberty, when further development of 8 to 12 ova per cycle occurs. During the process of ovulation, the first meiotic division is completed with the development of the first polar body, and the second meiotic division is initiated. Following completion of the first meiotic division, the number of chromosomes is reduced to 23, but the DNA content is still equivalent to the amount in the original germ cell. The second meiotic division is not completed until after fertilization, when the second polar body is formed and the first divides. Thus, the ovum itself, containing half of the DNA present in the original germ cell, as well as each polar body, contains 22 autosomes and one X chromosome.

Abnormal endocrinology

Table 12-1
Classification of intersexuality

I. Disorders of gonadal development
   A. Klinefelter's syndrome
   B. Gonadal dysgenesis
      1. Turner's syndrome
      2. Mosaicism
      3. Structural abnormality of the second X chromosome
      4. Normal karyotype (pure gonadal dysgenesis)
   C. True hermaphroditism
   D. Male pseudohermaphroditism
      1. Primary gonadal defect
      2. Y chromosomal defect
II. Disorders of fetal endocrinology
   A. Female pseudohermaphroditism with partial virilization
      1. Congenital adrenal hyperplasia
         a. 21-Hydroxylase deficiency without salt wasting
         b. 21-Hydroxylase deficiency with salt wasting
         c. 11-Hydroxylase deficiency (hypertensive)
         d. 3β-ol Dehydrogenase deficiency
      2. Nonadrenal female pseudohermaphroditism
         a. Maternal androgenization
            (i) Exogenous androgen
            (ii) Virilizing tumors
         b. Idiopathic
   B. Male pseudohermaphroditism with partial failure of virilization
      1. Abnormalities of müllerian-inhibiting factor synthesis or action
      2. Defects in testosterone action
         a. Complete androgen-binding protein deficiency (complete testicular feminization)
         b. Partial defects of androgen cytosol receptors (incomplete testicular feminization; familial incomplete male pseudohermaphroditism type I)
         c. 5α-Reductase deficiency (familial incomplete male pseudohermaphroditism type II)
      3. Testosterone biosynthesis defect
         a. Pregnenolone synthesis defect (lipoid adrenal hyperplasia)
         b. 3β-Hydroxysteroid dehydrogenase deficiency
         c. 17α-Hydroxylase deficiency
         d. 17,20-Desmolase deficiency
         e. 17β-Hydroxysteroid dehydrogenase deficiency

Various errors in meiotic division can cause aneuploidy, an abnormality involving an incorrect number of sex chromosomes (either extra or absent), as well as structurally abnormal sex chromosomes. The mechanisms by which these abnormalities occur include nondisjunction, anaphase lag, and translocation, breakage and rearrangement, or deletion of part of the sex chromosome. When meiotic nondisjunction oc- curs, the sex chromosomes do not separate during the second meiotic division, so the resulting gamete has either no sex chromosome or two Xs (Figure 12-2)[4] or two Ys. Absence of a sex chromosome can also result from anaphase lag, an error whereby the chromosomal material fails to be included within the nuclear membrane of the new cell. When gametes with extra or absent sex chromosomes are fertilized by normal gametes,

Disorders of sexual differentiation

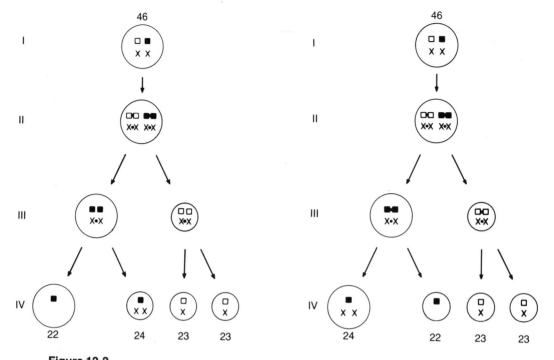

Figure 12-2
Abnormality of meiosis: nondisjunction leading to a gamete with two Xs (left) or to a hypoploid gamete when both Xs enter a polar body (right).

Reproduced, with permission, from Federman DD (ed): Abnormal Sexual Development: A Genetic and Endocrine Approach to Differential Diagnosis. Philadelphia, WB Saunders, 1967, p 18.

various forms of sexual abnormalities occur, usually gonadal dysgenesis (45,X) or Klinefelter's syndrome (47,XXY).

Nondisjunction and anaphase lag can also produce abnormalities during mitotic division. In these cases, both divided cells remain in the organism, and the resulting condition is known as mosaicism. A mosaic individual has cells of different karyotypes but of one genetic origin. Mosaicism can produce any number of chromosomal varieties, because abnormalities in chromosomal division can occur at the first or subsequent division of the zygote. Thus, more than two different cell lines may persist (Figure 12-3).[4] Since these various cell lines may appear in different tissues, mosaicism can never be excluded unless karyotypic examination is performed on every tissue in the body.

Klinefelter's syndrome

This relatively common disorder has an incidence of about 1/400 live male births. Because internal and external genitalia are completely male, there are no physical stigmata whereby the condition may be diagnosed before puberty. After puberty, the main abnormal physical findings are small testes, less than 1.5 cm long, and gynecomastia, which is present in about 80% of cases. The main histologic abnormalities found in the testes are hyalinized tubules with a lack of spermatogenesis. All patients with this syndrome have azoospermia, and infertility is a fre-

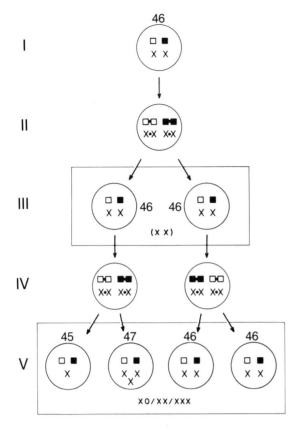

Figure 12-3
Abnormality of mitosis: nondisjunction at a step beyond the first division of the zygote resulting in mosaicism with three cell lines.

Reproduced, with permission, from Federman DD (ed): Abnormal Sexual Development: A Genetic and Endocrine Approach to Differential Diagnosis. *Philadelphia, WB Saunders, 1967, p 25.*

quent presenting complaint. It has been estimated that more than 10% of aspermic males have Klinefelter's syndrome or a variant.[4]

Serum testosterone levels in these usually taller-than-average men are generally below the range found in normal males, while gonadotropins are elevated. There is always an abnormal karyotype, most commonly 47,XXY. Various other karyotypes with more than two Xs and/or

more than one Y have been described; however, all patients with this syndrome have at least one Y and two X sex chromosomes in some or all of their cells. Mosaicism can occur; the abnormal karyotype may not be present in all cell lines. This is a disorder of intersexuality, because there is a female chromatin pattern, but the other morphologic sexual characteristics are completely male.

Gonadal dysgenesis

Gonadal dysgenesis is associated with involution of the germ cells soon after they migrate into the undifferentiated gonad during early embryonic life. Thus, the gonads fail to develop and persist only as bilateral streaks of fibrous tissue that do not produce hormones (Figure 12-4).[4] This syndrome is associated with normal female genitalia at birth and a wide range of karyotypes. It has been estimated that about half of the patients with gonadal dysgenesis have a total absence of an X chromosome, while mosaicism is present in one-third.[4]

The most common karyotype associated with gonadal dysgenesis is the 45,X originally described as a syndrome by Turner, with an incidence of about 1/7,000 newborn females. The defect is found much more commonly in abortuses. Turner's syndrome is characterized by short stature; nearly all adults with pure 45,X are less than 60 inches in height. Webbing of the neck, cardiac malformations, and lymphedema of the hands and feet are the other most common associated anomalies. Because of these malformations, the diagnosis is usually made in infancy. Both the internal and external genitalia remain immature because of estrogen deficiency. At the usual age of puberty, breast development and menarche do not occur.

Gonadal dysgenesis can also result from various types of mosaicism or a structural abnormality of the second X chromosome (e.g., deletion of a portion or an isochromosome for the long arm). Individuals with these disorders may

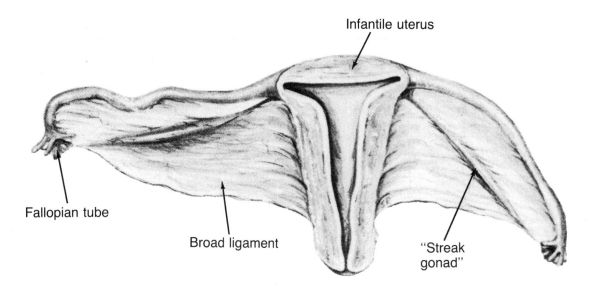

Figure 12-4
Internal genitalia of a patient with gonadal dysgenesis (Turner's syndrome), featuring a normal but infantile uterus, normal fallopian tubes, and pale, glistening streak gonads in both broad ligaments.

Reproduced, with permission, from Federman DD (ed): Abnormal Sexual Development: A Genetic and Endocrine Approach to Differential Diagnosis. *Philadelphia, WB Saunders, 1967, p 43.*

be normal in height and free of the other physical stigmata of Turner's syndrome. They may also have some breast development and a few menstrual periods. Deletion of the short arm of the X is associated with the short stature and somatic anomalies of Turner's syndrome, but long-arm deletions usually do not produce these anomalies.

Finally, another type of gonadal dysgenesis results in bilateral streak gonads in association with a normal karyotype. The term "pure gonadal dysgenesis" has been used to describe this syndrome. Affected individuals have no chromosomal abnormality, but have some genetic defect. Their only external physical abnormalities are associated with hypoestrogenism, in contrast with Turner's syndrome patients. Thus, pure gonadal dysgenesis is usually not diagnosed before puberty.

True hermaphroditism

Both male and female gonadal tissue is present in true hermaphroditism. There may be a separate ovary and testis or these elements may be combined in a single ovotestis. Histologic examination of the gonad is usually necessary to establish the diagnosis. A uterus is nearly always present, and the differentiation of the other internal genitalia corresponds very closely with the adjacent gonad. Cryptorchidism is frequent, together with some deficiency in labioscrotal fusion. The external genitalia are generally more male than female, and three-fourths of the patients are raised as males. At puberty, about three-fourths of true hermaphrodites develop gynecomastia and more than half menstruate.

More than 80% are chromatin positive, and the most frequent karyotype is 46,XX. It has been postulated that the testis-determining

Abnormal endocrinology

genes of the Y chromosome have been translocated to an X chromosome. Documentation of an H-Y antigen in these 46,XX true hermaphrodites suggests that the H-Y gene has indeed undergone such a translocation. Mosaicism occurs in a minority of cases.[7] The pathogenesis of this disorder is not completely understood, but it is thought to be a genetic abnormality, causing failure of the undifferentiated gonad to develop normally.

Male pseudohermaphroditism

This category comprises a group of disorders of testicular development or differentiation that theoretically could involve (1) abnormalities in formation of the bipotential gonad and (2) abnormalities in development of the testes from the undifferentiated gonad. Disorders of the second type involve abnormalities in the testicular-inducing genes on the short arm of the Y chromosome.

In male pseudohermaphroditism with a primary gonadal defect, absence of gonads is accompanied by a normal male 46,XY karyotype. This disorder has also been termed "gonadal agenesis" or "vanishing testes syndrome." Patients have ambiguous external genitalia with a vagina or even normal female external genitalia, but no evidence of female internal genitalia. They may first present with primary amenorrhea associated with lack of breast development (see Chapter 14).

The most common type of male pseudohermaphroditism with a Y chromosomal defect is the syndrome of asymmetric gonadal differentiation or mixed gonadal dysgenesis (Figure 12-

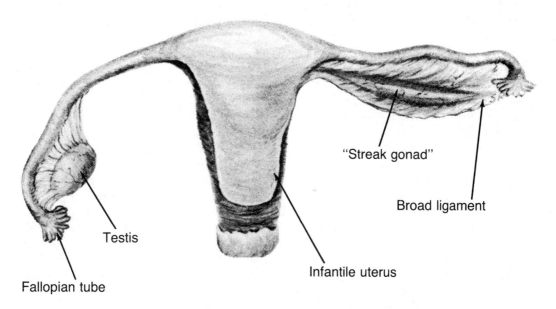

Figure 12-5
Internal genitalia in mixed gonadal dysgenesis featuring an infantile uterus, bilateral fallopian tubes, a streak gonad on one side, and a testis on the other.

Reproduced, with permission, from Federman DD (ed): Abnormal Sexual Development: A Genetic and Endocrine Approach to Differential Diagnosis. *Philadelphia, WB Saunders, 1967, p 70.*

5).[4] These patients have a testis on one side and a streak on the other. There is a high frequency of tumor formation in the testis. The internal genitalia usually have a completely normal female character. Ambiguous external genitalia are present at birth in more than half of cases. The morphology ranges from a normal male type with hypospadias to a normal female type with clitoromegaly. However, totally normal male or female external genitalia are sometimes present. Cytogenetically, X chromosomal mosaicism is almost always involved, and the most frequent sex chromosome combination is X/XY.

Disorders of fetal endocrinology

Disorders of fetal endocrinology can be subdivided into (1) female pseudohermaphroditism with some degree of virilization and (2) male pseudohermaphroditism with some degree of failure of virilization.

Female pseudohermaphroditism with partial virilization

This condition is usually due to congenital adrenal hyperplasia (CAH), although some forms have a nonadrenal etiology. CAH is the most frequent cause of ambiguous genitalia in the newborn, and it has several unique features. First, it is the only type of intersex condition with the possibility of entirely normal sexual function, including the capability of conception, as virilization involves only the external genitalia. The gonads and internal genitalia are normal female, and the external genitalia can be surgically reconstructed to those of a normal female. Second, because this is the only genetically female intersex disorder that can jeopardize survival, it is imperative to make the diagnosis at birth.

Although six different enzyme defects have thus far been reported as variants of CAH, only three—21-hydroxylase deficiency with and without salt wasting, 11-hydroxylase deficiency, and 3β-ol dehydrogenase deficiency—are associated with virilization of the external female genitalia

(Figure 12-6). Deficiency of 11-hydroxylase is associated with hypertension. Deficiency of 3β-ol dehydrogenase, the least common, is associated with the mildest virilization, but it usually is fatal because it results in severe adrenal insufficiency. In these autosomal recessive disorders, enzyme deficiency causes a lack of cortisol biosynthesis. The result is increased production of adrenocorticotropic hormone (ACTH). The excessive ACTH, in turn, causes an increased production of adrenal androgens, mainly androstenedione and dehydroepiandrosterone, and an associated increase in the excretion of their 17-ketosteroid metabolites in the urine. Only the external genitalia are affected because differentiation of the internal genitalia takes place around the 10th week of embryonic life, while the adrenal cortex does not begin to function until around the 12th week. Thus, when the external genitalia undergo differentiation, they are subjected to increased androgen stimulation.

Virilization in patients with CAH ranges from clitoromegaly with minimal labial fusion to complete scrotal fusion with the urethra opening at the tip of the phallus (Figure 12-6). With the latter morphology, the infant may resemble a completely normal male with cryptorchidism. Therefore, the obstetrician should examine every newborn boy and palpate the scrotum. If no testes are palpable, CAH should be suspected and appropriate diagnostic tests performed. It is important to establish the diagnosis soon after birth, because the 21-hydroxylase deficiency with salt wasting and the 3β-ol dehydrogenase deficiency may cause death. Once the diagnosis is suspected, it can easily be confirmed by testing for elevated levels of serum 17-hydroxyprogesterone or urinary pregnanetriol.

The nonadrenal type of female pseudohermaphroditism is usually caused by fetal exposure to excessive exogenous androgen stimulation. This exposure can come from the maternal ingestion of androgens or of 19-nortestosterone gestagens such as those found in oral contracep-

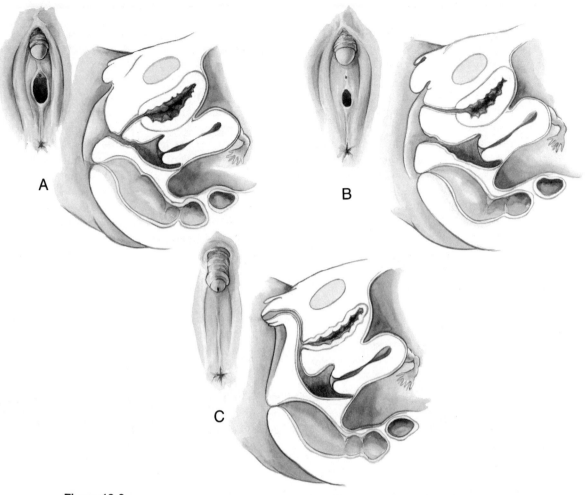

Figure 12-6
Schematic drawings of variation in degree of virilization in congenital adrenal hyperplasia. A, mildest form with minimal labial fusion; B, intermediate form; C, most severe form with urethra opening at tip of phallus.

tives (OCs). Experimental evidence indicates that small amounts of 19-nortestosterone derivatives given to mothers will virilize the external genitalia of female fetuses.[8] Maternal ingestion of OC steroids has also been reported to cause clitoral hypertrophy and labioscrotal fusion in the fetus.

Occasionally, infants with virilized external genitalia were born to mothers who have not taken exogenous androgens of any type. These infants have been classified as "idiopathic non-adrenal female pseudohermaphrodites." Rarely, a virilizing ovarian tumor or markedly increased production of ovarian testosterone by benign hyperplastic thecal luteinization (luteoma) can occur during pregnancy. Masculinization of the female fetus has been reported with both of these conditions.[9]

Because the placenta can effectively convert androstenedione and testosterone—but not 19-nortestosterone derivatives—to estrogens, virilization of a female fetus does not occur regularly in cases of maternal testosterone excess (unless the mother's serum level exceeds about 4 ng/mL). However, fetal virilization is very likely if a pregnant woman takes 19-nortestosterone between 14 and 18 weeks of gestation.

Male pseudohermaphroditism with partial failure of virilization

This disorder can be the result of abnormalities of MIF synthesis or action, defects in testosterone action, or a testosterone biosynthesis defect.

ABNORMALITIES OF MIF SYNTHESIS OR ACTION. Individuals with MIF abnormalities have bilateral testes with normal male wolffian differentiation and male external genitalia. However, because the function of MIF is lacking, they also have a uterus and oviducts. The latter frequently are present in an inguinal hernia.

DEFECTS IN TESTOSTERONE ACTION. There are three types of defective testosterone action: (1) complete androgen-binding protein deficiency, (2) partial defects of androgen cytosol receptors or familial incomplete male pseudohermaphroditism type I, and (3) 5α-reductase deficiency or familial incomplete male pseudohermaphroditism type II.

Complete androgen-binding protein deficiency. This disorder, probably the best-known form of male pseudohermaphroditism, is also called "complete testicular feminization syndrome" or "androgen insensitivity syndrome." It has been shown in tissue culture systems to be caused by absence of androgen cytosol receptors, absence of binding of androgen to the cytosol receptors

in the target tissue, or absence of binding of the androgen cytosol receptor complex to the nucleus.[10] Any of these mechanisms would prevent androgen action. These individuals, genetically males with testes, have a completely normal external female appearance and normal growth and development, including normal breast development. However, facial, body, and pubic hair is either absent or scanty. The internal genitalia are absent; the external genitalia are female in type but usually not fully developed. The vagina usually is short and ends in a blind pouch. Occasionally, the vagina may be absent.

Inguinal hernias are frequent, and the testes may be in the inguinal canal. Histologically, the testes show immature testicular tubules with a normal or increased number of Leydig cells. Testosterone levels are in the normal to upper range for men. The testes produce MIF, which accounts for the lack of female internal genitalia, but because of the end-organ androgen insensitivity, both internal and external male genitalia (other than the testes) fail to develop.

The karyotype is a normal 46,XY. The syndrome is due to absence of an X-chromosomal gene responsible for the cytoplasmic or nuclear testosterone receptor. It is either an X-linked recessive or sex-limited autosomal dominant disorder with transmission through the mother. Characteristically, the mothers of patients with testicular feminization have "sisters" with primary amenorrhea. About half the male offspring will develop the syndrome.

In most cases, the main symptom of this disorder is primary amenorrhea. Congenital absence of the uterus—a nonhereditary disorder of chromosomally and enzymatically normal females—is associated with similar morphology of the external genitalia and must be ruled out. Individuals with congenital absence of the uterus ovulate and have normal hair distribution. It has been postulated that normal breast development occurs in testicular feminization because the androgen insensitivity causes lack of suppression

Abnormal endocrinology

of the breast tissue anlage during fetal life. At puberty, with continued androgen insensitivity, the limited amounts of estradiol (only slightly above the mean for men and produced by the testes as well as by peripheral conversion of testicular androgens) suffice to achieve full breast development.

Familial incomplete male pseudohermaphroditism type I. Disorders in this subcategory result from hereditary partial defects of androgen cytosol receptors, causing varying degrees of ambiguity of the external genitalia. These range from a female appearance with partial labioscrotal fusion through a male appearance with only minimal hypospadias. Varying degrees of development of the male internal genitalia are also seen. Breast development occurs at puberty. "Incomplete testicular feminization," "Reifenstein's syndrome," and other terms have been applied to some of these disorders.

Familial incomplete male pseudohermaphroditism type II. This disorder results from 5α-reductase deficiency in the androgen target tissues of the urogenital sinus, originally described by Walsh et al.[11] The defect causes decreased conversion of testosterone to dihydrotestosterone (DHT), with resulting normal testosterone levels and a decrease in plasma DHT. It is not known whether the biochemical error involves the synthesis, structure, or metabolism of 5α-reductase.

This inherited biochemical defect is an autosomal recessive disorder found in certain families. The chromosomal complement is a normal male 46,XY. Affected individuals may be born as apparently normal phenotypic females, with or without palpable labial or labio-inguinal gonads (testes), or they may have a prominent or enlarged clitoris and other ambiguities of the external genitalia. At puberty, with greatly increased testosterone production and resultant conversion to DHT, there is marked virilization with growth of the phallus and descent of the testes into the labioscrotal folds,

which become rugated and hyperpigmented. Gynecomastia does not occur, as normal levels of testosterone are present during fetal life, and testosterone is the major androgen suppressing the breast anlage in utero.

These patients possess cytoplasmic and nuclear androgen receptors, readily recognized by their signs of hirsutism and virilization beginning at puberty. Particularly impressive is their pronounced muscle development and physical strength in comparison with their female peers. This may have a severe psychological impact. Both testosterone and DHT are necessary for complete differentiation of the male external genitalia. The fetal testes secrete testosterone, which acts directly on the wolffian ducts to cause their differentiation into the vas deferens, epididymis, and seminal vesicles. However, DHT is necessary for the differentiation of the external genitalia as well as development of the prostate (Figure 12-7). Thus, the external genitalia remain ambiguous in this disorder, with a lack of both labioscrotal fusion and phallic enlargement. After puberty, penile erection, ejaculation, and fertility occur in some.

It is important to establish the diagnosis as soon as possible, ideally at the time of delivery, and to differentiate it from familial incomplete male pseudohermaphroditism type I. Individuals with type I should usually be raised as females, while a few with type II should be raised as males.

Imperato-McGinley and Peterson reported that a large number of patients with 5α-reductase deficiency belonging to the same large family in the Dominican Republic were raised as females and, postpubertally, were found to function reasonably well in the male gender role.[5] However, in the United States and elsewhere, 5α-reductase deficiency patients who were initially raised as girls became emotionally distraught when they virilized at puberty. Had these individuals undergone gonadectomy before puberty, they would not have questioned

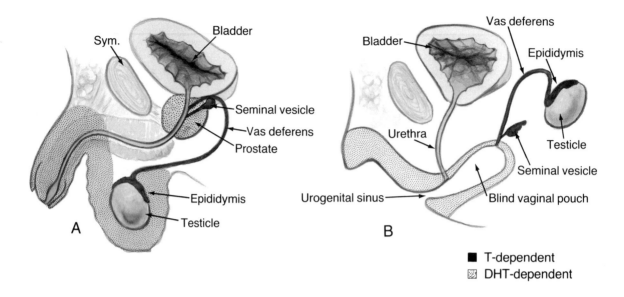

Figure 12-7
A, Development in utero of normal male internal and external genitalia. Tissues dependent upon testosterone (dark) and dihydrotestosterone (stippled) for maturation are indicated. B, Development in utero of male internal and external genitalia in individuals with 5α-reductase deficiency, indicating normal maturation of testosterone-dependent tissues and lack of maturation of dihydrotestosterone-dependent tissues.

their female gender identity. Except under unusual circumstances, newborns and children with 5α-reductase deficiency should be raised as girls. Gonadectomy and reduction clitoroplasty, if indicated, should be performed as soon as the diagnosis is made by assessing the conversion of testosterone to DHT in genital skin fibroblasts. This syndrome used to be called pseudovaginal perineoscrotal hypospadias.

DEFECTS IN BIOSYNTHESIS OF TESTOSTERONE. Patients with these defects have a 46,XY karyotype, male gonads, and ambiguous external genitalia, and they may develop breasts at puberty. The fetal testes differentiate normally and produce normal amounts of MIF, so no müllerian structures remain. But the inadequate testosterone production causes incomplete differentiation of the external genitalia; ambiguity results.

The degree of ambiguity depends on the severity of the enzymatic defect. The lowered testosterone production fails to suppress the fetal breast anlage, so at puberty those individuals with sufficient adrenal and/or testicular estrogen develop gynecomastia.

There are five basic steps in biosynthesis of testosterone from cholesterol. Deficiencies of those enzymes that are also necessary for cortisol synthesis constitute forms of the adrenogenital syndrome. The enzyme deficiencies occur in both the adrenal glands and the gonads, and inheritance is autosomal recessive. Only a few isolated patients have been reported with each of these genetic deficiencies. One of these disorders, a defect in pregnenolone synthesis, has been called lipoid adrenal hyperplasia due to defects in 20α-hydroxylase, 22β-hydroxylase, or 20,22-desmolase. Other disorders so far identi-

Abnormal endocrinology

fied include deficiencies of 3β-hydroxysteroid dehydrogenase, 17α-hydroxylase, 17,20-desmolase, and 17β-hydroxysteroid dehydrogenase. Pathways of steroid biosynthesis are depicted in Figure 12-8.

Diagnosis and management

The newborn infant with ambiguous genitalia represents a medical emergency. Regardless of the complexity of the anomaly, appropriate and rapid gender assignment at the time of delivery, or soon thereafter at referral hospitalization, will often determine the success of the final outcome for the child and the family. Gender assignment is based on the existing anatomy and a full understanding of the pathologic and endocrine reasons for the sexual ambiguity. It should be stressed that the objective is to assign a gender concordant with the child's best future anatomic and sexual functioning. The sex chromosome pattern and gonadal histology are entirely immaterial with regard to gender assignment.

It is imperative that the parents be informed immediately in a nontraumatic manner. They should be told that the baby's sex organs are incompletely developed and that this birth

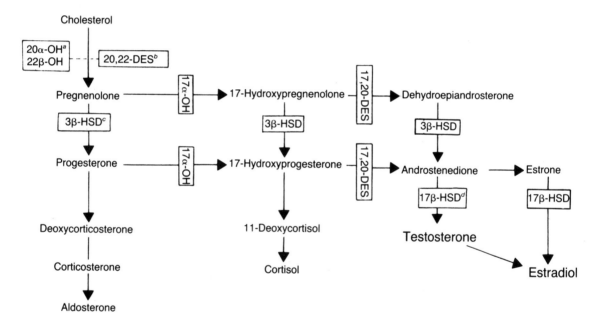

[a] OH = hydroxylase
[b] DES = desmolase
[c] 3β-HSD = 3β-hydroxysteroid dehydrogenase + Δ[5]-isomerase
[d] 17β-HSD = 17β-hydroxysteroid dehydrogenase

Figure 12-8
Pathways of steroid biosynthesis indicating various reported enzymatic defects in testosterone biosynthesis causing nonvirilizing forms of congenital adrenal hyperplasia and male pseudohermaphroditism.

defect precludes immediate gender assignment. However, diagnostic studies will commence at once to determine the gender of the baby. Until then, the sex of the child should not be announced and a birth certificate cannot be completed. Giving the baby a name that would suit a girl as well as a boy can only reinforce the idea of sexual ambiguity, which should be avoided under all circumstances. The parents should be allowed to examine the baby and its genitalia with the physician. It is important not to convey to the parents the idea of sexual ambiguity: The physician assigns the gender based on the following considerations and presents the assigned gender as the de facto diagnosis.

The diagnostic workup should begin immediately. If inspection of the external genitalia reveals a transposition of the phallus and scrotum (i.e., if the phallus originates posterior to the scrotum), the physician should at once search for additional malformations that may be life-threatening such as tracheoesophageal fistula, imperforate anus, or cardiac anomalies. In such instances, the extragenital malformations may be much more serious than the abnormal sexual development, or even incompatible with life.

In the absence of genital transposition, the physician should direct attention to the size of the phallus, the position of the urethral orifice, the degree of hypospadias if present, and the extent of labioscrotal fusion. Following inspection, the most important part of the physical examination is the palpation for gonads. Gonads palpable in the inguinal canal, in the labioinguinal area, or the labioscrotal folds are virtually always testes. Thus, the presence of one or two palpable gonads rules out virilization of an otherwise normal female, the most common form of ambiguous genitalia. Conversely, the infant born with ambiguous genitalia without palpable gonads most often represents virilization of a genetic female, usually as the result of CAH. Thus, determining the presence or absence of palpable gonads is the key in the initial evaluation.

The initial anatomic evaluation of the infant without palpable gonads is designed to establish whether a cervix and uterus are present. This is accomplished by ultrasonography and/or genitography. It should be noted that ultrasonography is best performed within 24 to 48 hours after delivery, because the estrogens of pregnancy that stimulate endometrial growth disappear rapidly in the neonatal period. Infants *with* a cervix and uterus will almost always be assigned the female gender irrespective of phallus size, because they are either virilized genetic females with full reproductive potential (CAH, exogenous androgens, maternal virilizing disorders), individuals with mixed (asymmetric) gonadal dysgenesis, or true hermaphrodites.

Infants *without* a cervix and uterus (consistent with MIF of testicular origin) present a problem. Their gender assignment will often depend on the adequacy of the phallic structure. The infant with cryptorchidism or anorchia usually has an adequate phallus and is assigned the male gender. Hormonal studies and surgical exploration can be performed later, and testosterone therapy will assure appropriate development and function as a male. Infants with an inadequate phallus and/or severe hypospadias are best assigned the female gender unless there is good potential for phallic reconstruction, as determined by a competent urologic surgeon. Errors in testosterone action tend to preclude adequate virilization, and infants born with these disorders usually should be assigned the female gender. The same holds true for most infants with 5α-reductase deficiency.

When an infant with ambiguous genitalia does have palpable gonads, the assessment should be as follows. First, one should distinguish between infants with unilaterally and those with bilaterally palpable gonads. A unilaterally palpable gonad may indicate asymmetric development of the internal genitalia and be consistent with either mixed gonadal dysgenesis or true hermaphroditism. A genitourogram

Abnormal endocrinology

may show unilateral or complete müllerian duct development. Such infants are best assigned the female gender. But infants with ambiguous genitalia and symmetric labioscrotal or inguinal gonads usually represent cases of incomplete androgen insensitivity of type I or type II or defects in testosterone biosynthesis. It is imperative to rule out deficiency of 3β-hydroxysteroid dehydrogenase, because this disorder could result in early salt loss, dehydration, and death. No infant with bilateral palpable gonads will have a cervix or uterus. Usually, infants with ambiguous genitalia resulting from type I or type II incomplete androgen insensitivity or defects in testosterone biosynthesis are assigned the female gender.

It is unnecessary to obtain a karyotype before gender can be assigned. The karyotype is helpful only when it confirms the clinical and anatomic findings.

All intra-abdominal gonads or gonadal streaks in patients with intersex disorders and a Y chromosome have a relatively high potential for becoming malignant. The two most common tumors are dysgerminoma and gonadoblastoma. Manuel and associates have reported that tumor incidence markedly increases about the time of puberty in all intersex disorders with a Y chromosome other than testicular feminization.[12] These include gonadal dysgenesis, asymmetric gonadal differentiation (mixed gonadal dysgenesis), and other types of male pseudohermaphroditism. Therefore, the gonads should be removed before puberty from individuals with these disorders and a Y chromosome. Manuel et al have reported that tumors are uncommon before the age of 25 in individuals with testicular feminization. Since the gonadal secretion of these individuals induces normal pubertal feminization, including breast development, removal of their gonads may be delayed until after age 20 with relative safety. Intersex patients without a Y chromosome rarely develop gonadal tumors, so their gonads or streaks should not be removed.

Disorders such as pure gonadal dysgenesis and testicular feminization usually do not become manifest until after the time of puberty, when affected individuals present with primary amenorrhea. The differential diagnosis of these disorders is discussed in detail in Chapter 14.

References

1. Jones HW, Scott WW (eds): *Hermaphroditism, Genital Anomalies and Related Endocrine Disorders,* ed 2. Baltimore, Williams & Wilkins, 1971

2. Jost A, Vigier B, Prépin J, et al: Studies on sex differentiation in mammals. *Rec Prog Horm Res* 29:1, 1973

3. Wachtel SS, Ohno S, Koo GC, et al: Possible role for H-Y antigen in the primary determination of sex. *Nature* 257:235, 1975

4. Federman DD (ed): *Abnormal Sexual Development: A Genetic and Endocrine Approach to Differential Diagnosis.* Philadelphia, WB Saunders, 1967

5. Imperato-McGinley J, Peterson RE: Male pseudohermaphroditism: The complexities of male phenotypic development. *Am J Med* 61:251, 1976

6. Wilson JD, Harrod MJ, Goldstein JL, et al: Familial incomplete male pseudohermaphroditism, type 1. Evidence of androgen resistance and variable clinical manifestations in a family with the Reifenstein syndrome. *N Engl J Med* 290:1097, 1974

7. Wachtel SS, Koo GC, Breg WR, et al: Serologic detection of a Y-linked gene in XX males and XX true hermaphrodites. *N Engl J Med* 295:750, 1976

8. Wilkins L: Masculinization of female fetus due to use of orally given progestins. *JAMA* 172:1028, 1960

9. Hensleigh PA, Woodruff JD: Differential maternal-fetal response to androgenizing luteoma or hyperreactio luteinalis. *Obstet Gynecol Surv* 33:262, 1978

10. Keenan BS, Meyer WJ III, Hadjian AJ, et al: Syndrome of androgen insensitivity in man: Absence of 5α-dihydrotestosterone binding protein in skin fibroblasts. *J Clin Endocrinol Metab* 38:1143, 1974

11. Walsh PC, Madden JD, Harrod MJ, et al: Familial incomplete male pseudohermaphroditism, type 2. Decreased dihydrotestosterone formation in pseudovaginal perineoscrotal hypospadias. *N Engl J Med* 291:944, 1974

12. Manuel M, Katayama KP, Jones HW: The age of occurrence of gonadal tumors in intersex patients with a Y chromosome. *Am J Obstet Gynecol* 124:293, 1976

Suggested reading

Donahoe PK, Hendren WH: Evaluation of the newborn with ambiguous genitalia. *Pediatr Clin North Am* 23:361, 1976

Lippe BM: Ambiguous genitalia and pseudohermaphroditism. *Pediatr Clin North Am* 26:91, 1979

Park IJ, Aimakhu VE, Jones HW: An etiologic and pathogenic classification of male hermaphroditism. *Am J Obstet Gynecol* 123:505, 1975

Rimoin DL, Schimke RN: *Genetic Disorders of the Endocrine Glands*. St Louis, CV Mosby Company, 1971

Chapter 13

Precocious Puberty in the Female

Paul F. Brenner, M.D.

At puberty, when the hypothalamic negative and positive feedback mechanisms mature, cyclic pituitary and gonadal function results. This, in turn, causes development of the secondary sex characteristics, the adolescent growth spurt, follicular maturation, and eventually ovulation.

In the prepubertal human, both the gonads and the pituitary gland possess the capacity for normal adult function. At this period, however, the hypothalamus is extremely sensitive to the negative inhibitory feedback of low levels of circulating sex steroids. According to a current theory explaining the onset of puberty, when a certain "critical weight" is achieved, the sensitivity of the hypothalamic negative feedback response to sex steroids decreases.[1]

The following sequence of events is usually associated with puberty: breast development, appearance of pubic hair, appearance of axillary hair, and the menarche. Breast development is a very early pubertal phenomenon, and menarche a late one. Axillary and pubic hair growth is less predictable. Menarche precedes the appearance of either axillary or pubic hair in approximately 10% of girls.

Marshall and Tanner reported that breast budding, the earliest event associated with puberty, occurs at a mean age of 11.2 with a standard deviation (SD) of 1.1 years (Figure 13-1).[2] Assuming a normal frequency distribution, precocious puberty occurs when any event in the series of pubertal changes begins more than 3 SD

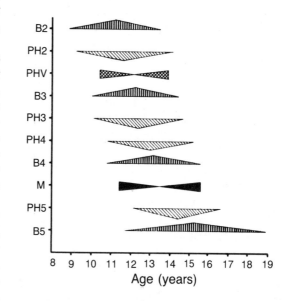

Figure 13-1
Age on reaching each stage of puberty, based on the scheme of Marshall and Tanner (see Chapter 10). B, breast development; PH, pubic hair; M, menarche; PHV, peak height velocity. The center of each symbol represents the mean, and the length of the symbol is equivalent to 2 SD on either side of the mean.

Reproduced, with permission, from Marshall WA, Tanner JM: Variations in pattern of pubertal changes in girls. Arch Dis Child 44:291, 1969.

earlier than the mean. In girls, the diagnosis of precocious puberty is made when breast budding occurs before the age of 8. Menarche occurring before age 9 is a second, but less commonly used, definition of precocious puberty.

The disorder encompasses a wide spectrum of changes, which depend on the source, quantity, duration of stimulus, and identity of the hormones involved. The classification of female precocious puberty is presented in Table 13-1.

If the secondary sex characteristics that appear early agree with the genetic and phenotypic sex, the term isosexual precocious puberty is used. If the early secondary sex characteristics disagree with the genetic and phenotypic sex, the term heterosexual precocious puberty is used. The distinction is an obvious one, based on history and physical examination. The evaluation of heterosexual precocious puberty in the female is designed to determine the source of the androgen.

Incomplete isosexual precocious puberty

Incomplete isosexual precocious puberty in the female is defined as the early appearance of a single clinical pubertal change without any other evidence of an estrogen effect. The incomplete forms are designated premature thelarche, premature adrenarche, and premature pubarche.

It is not always possible to confirm the diagnosis of an incomplete form of precocious puberty at the initial evaluation. Any one pubertal event (breast development, appearance of axillary or pubic hair) may be the first in a series of changes in precocious puberty. Patients should be reevaluated at least at 6-month intervals.

Premature thelarche
Premature thelarche is the appearance of breast development before the age of 8, without clinical

Table 13-1
Classification of female precocious puberty

I. Heterosexual precocious puberty
II. Isosexual precocious puberty
   A. Incomplete isosexual precocious puberty
      1. Premature thelarche
      2. Premature adrenarche
      3. Premature pubarche
   B. Complete isosexual precocious puberty
      1. True isosexual precocious puberty
         a. Constitutional
         b. Organic brain disease
      2. Pseudoisosexual precocious puberty
         a. Ovarian
         b. Adrenal
         c. Exogenous
         d. Hypothyroidism
         e. McCune-Albright syndrome
         f. Hemihypertrophy

evidence of other estrogen effects such as vaginal cornification or advancement of the bone age. It is most commonly found between ages 1 and 4. This is a benign condition, not associated with pubic or axillary hair growth, menarche, an early growth spurt, premature epiphyseal closure, follicular maturation, or fertility.

The etiology of premature thelarche is still unclear. Theories include: (1) that the target organ, the breast, has increased sensitivity to the small normal amounts of endogenous estrogens found in the peripheral circulation; (2) that ovarian follicles undergo cystic changes and luteinization, independent of the hypothalamic-pituitary control, and thus produce increased amounts of estrogen; and (3) that partial activation of the reproductive axis occurs, affecting follicle-stimulating hormone (FSH) but not luteinizing hormone (LH).[3]

Spontaneous regression of the breast development is the rule, and therapy is unnecessary. Several laboratory tests can help to distinguish girls with premature thelarche from those with the first changes of constitutional precocious puberty. The latter condition should be treated. Escobar and associates have measured serum estradiol levels in children with these conditions.[4] Normal low prepubertal levels (<20 pg/mL) indicate premature thelarche. Elevated levels (>25 pg/mL), especially if accompanied by prolactin elevation, indicate the more serious constitutional precocious puberty (Figure 13-2).[4]

Concentrations of serum LH measured by radioimmunoassay are higher in girls with constitutional precocious puberty than in those with premature thelarche. However, because there is an overlap of LH levels between the two groups, this assay does not conclusively separate them.[5] Lucky and co-workers reported that bioassay of LH, using the in vitro secretion of testosterone by rat interstitial cells when LH is added to the culture medium, is reliable.[6] This method can distinguish constitutional precocious puberty from premature thelarche (Figure 13-3).[6] Unfortunately, it is usually impractical to perform this test because of its limited availability.

Normal prepubertal girls show little or no increase in gonadotropins following the administration of gonadotropin-releasing hormone (GnRH). Girls with constitutional precocious puberty respond with an increase in both FSH and LH; those with premature thelarche have an increase in FSH but not LH (Figure 13-4).[3] The GnRH stimulation test has been suggested as a

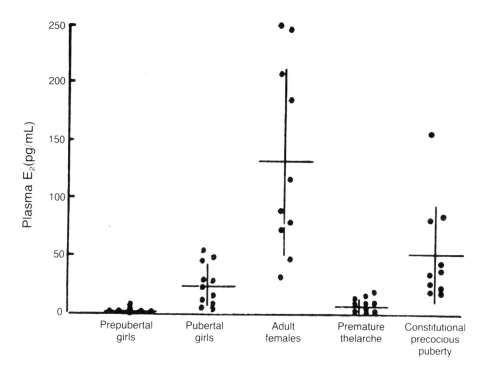

Figure 13-2
Estradiol (E$_2$) plasma values in normal females and in those with premature thelarche and constitutional precocious puberty. Mean values are indicated by horizontal lines, and standard deviations by vertical lines.

Reproduced, with permission, from Escobar ME, Rivarola MA, Bergadá C: Plasma concentration of oestradiol-17β in premature thelarche and in different types of sexual precocity. Acta Endocrinol 81:351, 1976.

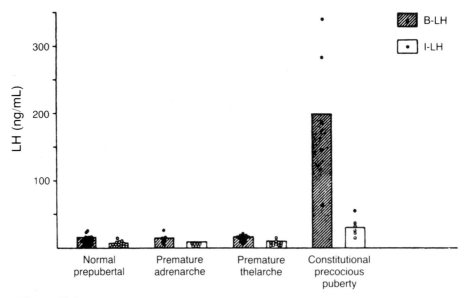

Figure 13-3
Bioactive LH (B-LH) and immunoreactive LH (I-LH) in normal prepubertal girls and in girls with disorders of puberty, including premature adrenarche, premature thelarche, and true precocious puberty.

Reproduced, with permission, from Lucky AW, Rich BH, Rosenfield RL, et al: Bioactive LH: A test to discriminate true precocious puberty from premature thelarche and adrenarche. J Pediatr 97:214, 1980.

means for distinguishing between these conditions.[3] The test is performed by giving 50 μg of synthetic GnRH as an IV bolus. Blood samples are obtained just before and at 10, 20, 30, 60, and 90 minutes after the injection to determine LH and FSH concentrations in the serum.

Premature adrenarche
Premature adrenarche is defined as the isolated appearance of axillary hair before 8 years of age. Breast development, pubic hair growth, and menstruation do not occur, and there is no estrogen effect on the bone age or vaginal mucosa. Furthermore, there is no linear growth acceleration, premature epiphyseal fusion, or fertility. This is also a benign condition that does not require treatment. Presumably, the adrenal gland increases androgen production earlier than normal for an unknown reason. The circulating levels of the adrenal androgens dehydroepiandrosterone (DHEA) and dehydroepiandrosterone sulfate (DHEA-S) are normal.

Premature pubarche
Premature pubarche is the isolated appearance of pubic hair before the age of 8. The hair growth is considered to be the consequence of a functional increase in the adrenal production of DHEA and DHEA-S. This increased androgen production results from changes in biosynthesis of adrenal androgens.

Stimulation with adrenocorticotropic hormone (ACTH), following overnight dexamethasone suppression, accentuates alterations in the biosynthetic pathways of adrenal androgens and cortisol. Rich and associates, using the ACTH stimulation test, found that patients with premature pubic hair growth had increased conversion

Abnormal endocrinology

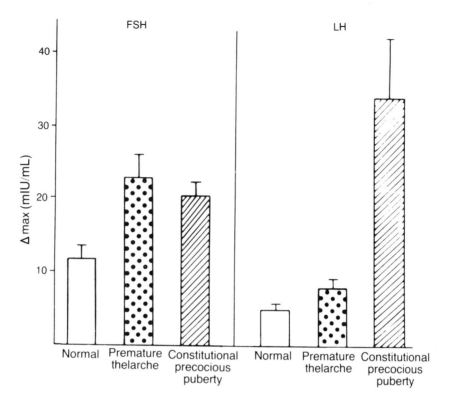

Figure 13-4
FSH and LH maximum increment following GnRH administration in normal prepubertal girls and in girls with premature thelarche and constitutional precocious puberty.

Reproduced, with permission, from Pasquino AM, Piccolo F, Scalamandre A, et al: Hypothalamic-pituitary-gonadotropic function in girls with premature thelarche. Arch Dis Child 55:941, 1980.

of 17α-hydroxypregnenolone to DHEA and decreased conversion of DHEA to androstenedione.[7] With the increased availability of DHEA from these two mechanisms, sulfokinase activity produces an increase in DHEA-S (Figure 13-5).[7] DHEA levels in normal prepubertal, premature pubarcheal, and adult females are 63 ng/dL, 243 ng/dL, and 332 ng/dL, respectively.[7] Approximately half the patients with premature pubarche have organic brain disease. The reason for this association has never been elucidated.

Complete isosexual precocious puberty

In the complete form of isosexual precocious puberty, the initial presenting pubertal change is accompanied by additional estrogen effects elsewhere in the body. Complete isosexual precocious puberty is divided into two major categories: true and pseudo. In both groups, there is an increase in circulating estrogen levels, and

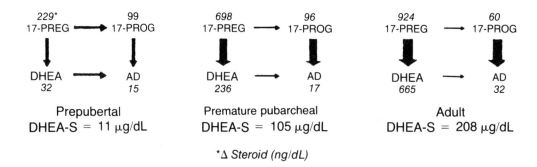

Figure 13-5
Summary of the apparent maturational shift in adrenal steroidogenic pathways. 17-PREG, 17α-hydroxypregnenolone; 17-PROG, 17α-hydroxyprogesterone; DHEA, dehydroepiandrosterone; AD, androstenedione; DHEA-S, dehydroepiandrosterone sulfate. The control DHEA-S level of each group is shown. Italicized numbers are increments (ng/dL) 30 minutes after ACTH administration. Size of arrow indicates relative activity of each pathway compared with the prepubertal state. With progressive maturation, there is an apparent decrease in 3β-ol dehydrogenase efficiency and an apparent increase in lyase efficiency.

Reproduced, with permission, from Rich BH, Rosenfield RL, Lucky AW, et al: Adrenarche: Changing adrenal response to adrenocorticotropin. J Clin Endocrinol Metab 52:1129, 1981. © 1981, The Endocrine Society.

pubertal development may progress to the stage of uterine bleeding. There may be an initial rapid acceleration of linear growth, and the distal epiphyses may close prematurely. Thus, these patients, who are usually taller than their peers when the precocious development is first manifested, will ultimately have short stature. In the true form, there is cyclic release of gonadotropins and fertility is possible; in the pseudo form, gonadotropin levels remain low and ovulation does not occur.

True isosexual precocious puberty

Of all girls with complete isosexual precocious puberty, 90% have the true form. Puberty occurs early, but the sequence of endocrine events is normal. Cyclic function of the hypothalamic-pituitary-ovarian axis and the negative and positive feedback mechanisms develop prematurely. The result is adult levels and patterns of gonadotropin and sex steroid secretion. Secondary sex characteristics appear, and follicular maturation and ovulation occur. Because the etiology always involves the central nervous system, the term cerebral isosexual precocious puberty is also used. True isosexual precocious puberty may be constitutional or result from organic brain disease.

Constitutional

Most (90%) of girls with true isosexual precocious puberty have a constitutional, or idiopathic, disorder. The underlying etiology for the premature activation of hypothalamic function is unknown. The progression of endocrine events of normal puberty occurs at an early age and leads to the clinical manifestations of pubertal development. Sleep-associated enhancement of gonadotropin secretion is followed by the augmented release of LH and FSH during the waking hours, leading to increased ovarian estrogen production (Figure 13-6).[8] Basal levels of gonadotropins are elevated for the chronologic age, but normal for the stage of puberty.[8] The gonadotropins show a positive response to GnRH stimulation. Levels of prolactin are higher than in normal prepubertal girls of the same age and normal girls at the same pubertal stage.

Abnormal endocrinology

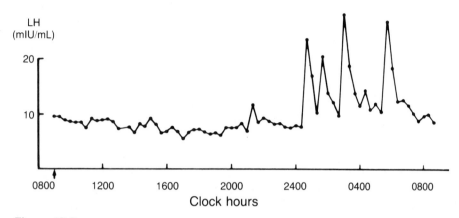

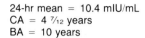
24-hr mean = 10.4 mIU/mL
CA = 4 ⁷/₁₂ years
BA = 10 years

Sleep

LH
(mIU/mL)

20

10

0800   1200   1600   2000   2400   0400   0800

Clock hours

Figure 13-6
The 24-hour LH secretory pattern in a girl with constitutional precocious puberty whose chronologic age (CA) was 4 ⁷/₁₂ years. The height age was equivalent to 7 ½ years. The bone age (BA) was equivalent to 10 years.

Reproduced, with permission, from Chipman JJ: Pubertal control mechanisms as revealed from human studies. Fed Proc 39:2391, 1980.

The early appearance of secondary sex characteristics can cause psychological difficulties for both the patient and her family. Often, great emotional trauma is inflicted on these girls by their peers. It can be difficult for girls with precocious puberty to adjust to the appearance of menstruation at an early age. At first, these girls are much taller than their peers, but ultimately they will be very short. Premature closure of the distal epiphyses results from the high levels of circulating estrogens. Growth is rapid, but of short duration. The earlier the disorder begins, the shorter will be the final height.

The growth potential of girls with precocious puberty is less than would be predicted from their advanced bone age. Methods normally used to predict adult height (Roche-Wainer-Thissen and Tanner), which are based on the rate of bone maturation in normal children, yield predictions for children with precocious puberty that are far too high (Figure 13-7).[9] The Bayley-Pinneau method, based on percentages of adult height, is acceptably accurate in predicting the adult height of children with precocious puberty, although the estimates tend to be slightly low.

The onset of pubertal symptoms may occur at any age before 8, but is extremely rare in the first year of life. The progression of symptoms may be rapid or slow, and the sequence of pubertal changes may vary considerably. Spontaneous remissions are rare. The general health of these girls is excellent, although the precocity may cause emotional problems. Approximately 50% of these patients have electroencephalogram (EEG) patterns consistent with epilepsy. A

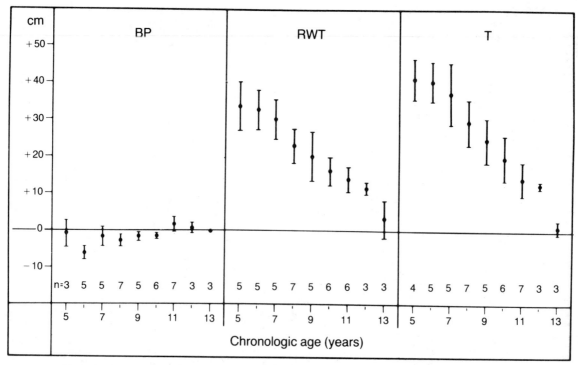

Figure 13-7

Deviation of height predictions from adult height in patients with constitutional precocious puberty.

Reproduced, with permission, from Zachmann M, Sobradillo B, Frank M, et al: Bayley-Pinneau [BP], Roche-Wainer-Thissen [RWT], and Tanner [T] height predictions in normal children and in patients with various pathologic conditions. J Pediatr 93:749, 1978.

few patients with constitutional precocious puberty have been tested in adult life and found to have normal psychic development and superior intelligence quotient scores.[10] Follicular cysts have been detected by ultrasound in patients with this disorder.[11] This finding might be expected in the presence of cyclic gonadotropin stimulation and should not be an indication for surgical exploration. The diagnosis of constitutional precocious puberty is made by exclusion, because there is no pathognomonic adjunctive laboratory test.

Organic brain disease

The remaining 10% of girls with true isosexual precocious puberty have organic brain disease.

The cause may be a tumor (craniopharyngioma, glioma, hamartoma, astrocytoma, astroblastoma, pineal tumor, or suprasellar cyst), a congenital defect, an obstructive process (hydrocephalus), neurofibromatosis, or a postinfective lesion. These lesions usually involve the hypothalamus, particularly the area of the tuber cinereum and mammillary bodies.

In the general population, the incidence of craniopharyngiomas is about 3% of all intracranial tumors and 20% of all suprasellar tumors.[12] The incidence of this tumor in children increases to 10% of all intracranial tumors and 50% of all suprasellar tumors. When hypothalamic-pituitary dysfunction occurs as the result of a craniopharyngioma, the clinical result is usually hypopituitarism. The decrease of gonadotropins in children leads to retarded or absent sexual development. There are only three reported cases of craniopharyngiomas associated with female precocious puberty.

Hamartomas located in, or adjacent to, the hypothalamus, causing precocious puberty, occur twice as often in males as in females.[13] Pineal tumors also occur far more frequently in males than in females, and in males, 25% are associated with precocious puberty.[14] Females with pineal tumors do not usually present with a clinical endocrinopathy. However, there is one reported case of a pineal tumor producing human chorionic gonadotropin (hCG) that caused precocious puberty in a 5-year-old girl.[15]

Patients with precocious puberty and organic brain disease almost always manifest neurologic symptoms and signs of their disease process before the appearance of the stigmata of precocious puberty. Inappropriate laughter in association with seizures (gelastic seizures) is an unusual neurologic presentation occurring infrequently in patients with precocious puberty and intracranial neoplasms.[16] Unfortunately, most of the intracranial lesions that cause precocious puberty cannot be successfully treated.

Pseudoisosexual precocious puberty

Patients with this type of precocious puberty do not attain cyclic function of the reproductive axis, and follicular maturation and ovulation do not occur. There are increased levels of estrogens, however, causing development of the secondary sex characteristics. The "pseudo-" prefix is used because the potential for fertility does not exist. Disorders of this type are categorized as (1) ovarian, (2) adrenal, or (3) exogenous; or they may be due to (4) hypothyroidism, (5) McCune-Albright syndrome, or (6) hemihypertrophy syndrome.

Ovarian

Estrogen-secreting tumors of the ovary (granulosa-theca cell tumors) are the most common cause of pseudoisosexual precocious puberty in girls. These tumors are almost always palpable on rectoabdominal examination, as well as detectable by ultrasonography. Fewer than 5% of granulosa-theca cell tumors occur in prepubertal girls; 95% are confined to one ovary at the time of surgical exploration. Most granulosa-theca cell tumors are benign; the usual treatment is unilateral oophorectomy.

Choriocarcinoma, originating in the ovary or as a component of an extragonadal teratoma, is a rare cause of precocious puberty. This type of tumor secretes hCG, which may act on the ovary to stimulate estrogen production. The diagnosis is made by detection of elevated hCG levels in the blood or urine.

Adrenal

Estrogen-secreting adrenal tumors are a rare cause of pseudoisosexual precocious puberty. Clinically, these tumors usually produce masculinizing signs and symptoms before the feminizing effects of excess estrogen appear.

Exogenous

Oral or topical use of estrogens (in cleansing creams, cosmetics, creams for diaper rash, or pharmaceutical preparations contaminated with estrogens) is sometimes a cause of pseudoisosexual precocious puberty. It is important to question all the people with whom the patient has close contact. Ask carefully about all medications, cosmetics, creams, and powders that the patient could possibly have used. Uncovering an exogenous source of estrogen depends on a detailed history. Sometimes even an examination of medication and cosmetic containers in the home is necessary.

Hypothyroidism

Advanced hypothyroidism is characterized by a marked reduction in thyroxine. Therefore, the negative feedback on the pituitary and the positive feedback on hypothalamic dopamine are abolished. The result is increased production of thyroid-stimulating hormone (TSH). There may be a concomitant increase in gonadotropins stimulating the ovary. If production of prolactin is also increased, galactorrhea may result.[17] A theory of hormone overlap has been proposed to provide a basis for these effects.

Hypothyroidism as a cause of pseudoisosexual precocious puberty is limited almost entirely to females.[18] It is the only cause of precocious puberty associated with retarded bone age. Ovarian cysts due to gonadotropin stimulation have been reported in juvenile hypothyroid patients.[19] If a euthyroid state is reestablished, the gonadotropin levels return to the prepubertal range, the pubertal changes regress, and the ovarian cysts decrease in size spontaneously.[20] Surgical extirpation of asymptomatic ovarian cysts is not indicated in patients with hypothyroidism and precocious puberty. Surgery might compromise ovarian function. Prolactin levels also return to normal in response to thyroid replacement therapy.

McCune-Albright syndrome

This syndrome is characterized by sexual precocity, multiple areas of fibrous or cystic dysplasia of bone, and brown or café-au-lait spots on the skin. Facial asymmetry and/or skeletal deformities are pathognomonic of polyostotic fibrous dysplasia. The skin pigmentation appears most commonly on the face, neck, shoulders, and back, and may be present at birth. Sexual precocity is usually not manifested until after 2 years of age. Sclerotic changes at the base of the skull may be responsible for cranial nerve defects. This rare syndrome is much more common in girls than in boys. Whether it is a pseudo or true form of isosexual precocious puberty is controversial. Elevated gonadotropins and ovarian cysts have been reported in some patients; undetectable gonadotropin concentrations have been reported in others.[21] Cyclic hypothalamic-pituitary function does not occur.

Hemihypertrophy

In the rare hemihypertrophy syndrome of Wilkins, unilateral sexual precocity is associated with various vascular anomalies. Only three cases have been reported.

Differential diagnosis

The specific diagnosis of precocious puberty requires a careful history, physical examination, and the sequential selection of a few laboratory tests. Heterosexual precocious puberty in the female can be distinguished from isosexual forms by a history and physical examination that show male secondary sex characteristics resulting from abnormally high androgen levels.

The incomplete forms of precocious puberty (premature thelarche, premature adrenarche, and premature pubarche) are diagnosed when serial observations, several months apart, indicate no peripheral estrogen effects (i.e., only one pubertal change and a bone age corresponding to the chronologic age). Such tests as serum estradiol and prolactin, bioassay of LH, and the GnRH stimulation test are also helpful in distinguishing incomplete forms from true precocious puberty. Incomplete forms are associated with normal prepubertal levels of serum estradiol and prolactin, low quantities of bioassayable LH, and a significant increase in the level of FSH, but not of LH, 30 to 60 minutes after rapid IV injection of 50 μg of GnRH.[3] Patients with premature thelarche have approximately twice the maximum FSH increment (22.9 ± 2.9 mIU/mL) when compared with normal prepubertal girls (11.8 ± 1.8 mIU/mL).[3]

Hemihypertrophy syndrome and McCune-Albright syndrome are associated with unique findings on physical examination that confirm the diagnosis. Exogenous sources of estrogen can be identified only by a meticulous history. Laboratory tests cannot identify all the exogenous agents that might cause precocious puberty. Hypothyroid patients have short stature and a retarded bone age as distinguishing features. The very rare choriocarcinoma is diagnosed by elevated levels of hCG in the blood or urine. The granulosa-theca cell tumor causing precocious pubertal changes is usually palpable on recto-abdominal examination or detectable by ultrasonography. Patients with underlying organic brain disease have neurologic signs and symptoms and confirmatory findings before indications of early pubertal development appear.

Most cases of isosexual precocious puberty are constitutional. This diagnosis can be made only by excluding all other possible disease entities. The diagnostic criteria used in evaluating precocious puberty are outlined in Table 13-2.

The diagnosis of any reproductive endocrinopathy can be established by logical sequential selection of adjunctive laboratory aids. Nowhere is this more apparent than in the evaluation of patients with precocious puberty. Bone age should be determined first. The hypothyroid patient will have a retarded bone age, and no further diagnostic evaluation will be required. TSH, triiodothyronine (T_3), and thyroxine (T_4) levels will be confirmatory and serve as a baseline for judging the effects of therapy.

A bone age that agrees with the chronologic age is compatible with incomplete forms of precocious puberty. The advancement of bone age above the 95th percentile for the chronologic age indicates a peripheral estrogen effect. Whether this increase in estrogen is due to elevated gonadotropins (as in the true forms) or to excess estrogen secretion without elevated gonadotropins (as in the pseudo forms) can be determined by measuring serum FSH. In the true forms, the sensitivity of the hypothalamic negative feedback response to circulating estrogens is decreased. The result is increased production of GnRH and a rise in gonadotropins to the levels that occur in the adult female. In the pseudo forms, the exquisite sensitivity of the hypothalamus to circulating estrogens from any source persists. The levels of pituitary gonadotropins

Table 13-2
Diagnosis of precocious puberty

Form	Diagnostic criteria
Isosexual precocious puberty	
Complete forms	
True	
Constitutional	Exclusion
Organic brain disease	History, neurologic exam
Pseudo	
Ovarian	
Granulosa-theca cell tumor	Rectoabdominal exam
Choriocarcinoma	Human chorionic gonadotropin excess
Adrenal	Ultrasound
Exogenous	History
Hypothyroidism	Bone age
Fibrous dysplasia (McCune-Albright syndrome)	Physical exam
Hemihypertrophy syndrome	Physical exam
Incomplete forms	Bone age
Heterosexual precocious puberty	Androgen excess

are very low—in the range found in the normal prepubertal girl.

Advanced bone age and low serum FSH indicate a pseudo cause of isosexual precocious puberty. The specific entities can be further distinguished by history and physical examination. Advanced bone age and normal levels of serum FSH indicate a true cause of isosexual precocious puberty. An abnormal neurologic exam suggests the possibility of organic brain disease. Finally, the diagnosis of constitutional precocious puberty is made by the exclusion of other possible causes.

Treatment

The treatment of precocious puberty depends on the specific underlying cause. Incomplete forms are usually self-limited and will spontaneously regress without any therapy. Thyroid hormone replacement therapy is the choice for the hypothyroid patient. Thyroid medication produces negative feedback on the hypothalamus and pituitary gland, and the concomitant release of gonadotropins ceases. If ovarian cysts are present, they will disappear without surgery. Exogenous sources are often difficult to identify, but once recognized, they are easy to eliminate. Unilateral oophorectomy is indicated for estrogen-secreting ovarian tumors.

In constitutional precocious puberty, the ideal therapy would cause regression of the secondary sex characteristics and cessation of menstruation, and would prevent fertility and the accelerated growth and premature fusion of the distal epiphyses. Depo-medroxyprogesterone acetate, danazol, and cyproterone acetate have all been used.[22,23] Danazol has been associated with virilization and is not recommended. Cyproterone acetate is only partially effective in suppressing menstruation and fails to reduce the effect of sex steroids on the long bones, but it

does inhibit ovulation. This medication, used in Europe, is currently unavailable in the US.

Depo-medroxyprogesterone acetate, a potent gonadotropin inhibitor, stops menstruation and inhibits ovulation, thereby preventing fertility. But it has little or no effect on epiphyseal closure or secondary sex characteristics. A lessening of the estrogen effect on the vaginal mucosa may be noted, but there is little regression of breast development or pubic hair growth. Doses of 100 to 200 mg are administered every 2 to 4 weeks. These high doses may slightly suppress both adrenocortical and ovarian function for 1 to 2 years after the medication is discontinued. These potential disadvantages must be weighed in each patient against the advantages of prevention of menses and ovulation. There is no universal agreement on when to discontinue therapy; but in general, stopping therapy somewhere between the ages of 10 and 12 will allow the resumption of age-concordant pubertal events.

Recently, it has been shown that the chronic administration of GnRH agonists initially enhances, but then inhibits, the pituitary release of gonadotropins. The inhibitory effect then persists for as long as the agonists are given. The paradoxical failure of the pituitary gland to respond to chronic GnRH agonist administration (pituitary "desensitization") has led to the theory that chronic GnRH agonist therapy would be effective in patients with precocious puberty.[24] Currently, GnRH agonists are available for such use in only a few medical centers in the US, but they are expected to become widely available shortly.

Carefully monitored clinical investigations are being conducted by Crowley's team in Boston.[25] At least 40 girls with constitutional precocious puberty are receiving the GnRH agonist D-Trp[6]-Pro[9]-NEt-LHRH (GnRHa), 4 μg/kg/day subcutaneously, for as long as 2 years.

All of the endocrine and clinical findings of precocious puberty are reversed by daily subcutaneous GnRH agonist therapy. Basal levels of

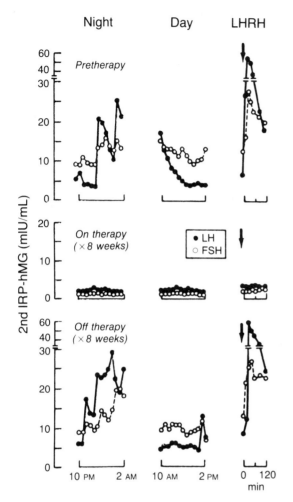

Night Day LHRH

Figure 13-8

LH and FSH levels in a 2-year-old girl with constitutional precocious puberty. Levels were determined on samples collected from 10 PM to 2 AM (night), 10 AM to 2 PM (day), and following administration of 100 μg of synthetic LHRH. Following a baseline assessment (pretherapy), the patient was treated with daily injections of 4 μg/kg of D-Trp⁶-Pro⁹-NEt-LHRH. Repeat evaluation occurred after 8 weeks of treatment (on therapy). Then injections were discontinued for 8 weeks and followed by repeat evaluation (off therapy). 2nd IRP-hMG, Second International Reference Preparation–human menopausal gonadotropin.

Reproduced, with permission, from Crowley WF Jr, Comite F, Vale W, et al: Therapeutic use of pituitary desensitization with a long-acting LHRH agonist: A potential new treatment for idiopathic precocious puberty. J Clin Endocrinol Metab 52:370, 1981. © 1981, The Endocrine Society.

gonadotropins and estradiol fall to the prepubertal range. Both the day and night pulsatile discharges of gonadotropins disappear. The response of FSH and LH to exogenous GnRH stimulation is eliminated (Figure 13-8).[25] Removal of the sex-steroid stimulation of target organs causes the following: regression of breast development and pubic hair growth; amenorrhea; the absence of superficial cells observed with vaginal cytology; and, most important, slowing of the bone age advancement to a rate that is normal for the patient's chronologic age. This is the first therapeutic modality for precocious puberty that prevents premature epiphyseal closure.[26] With the exception of a transitory rash at the site of injection in a few patients, no side effects have been reported. All of the suppressive endocrine effects of the therapy are reversed when the injections are discontinued.

Agonist and antagonist analogs of GnRH have been synthesized, but so far only the former have sufficient potency to be used clinically. Eventually, antagonist analogs of greater potency may be synthesized and used to treat constitutional precocious puberty. These agents provide the most effective treatment for this uncommon, but very distressing, endocrinopathy.

References

1. Feek CM, Sawers JSA, Brown NS, et al: Influence of thyroid status on dopaminergic inhibition of thyrotropin and prolactin secretion: Evidence for an additional feedback mechanism in the control of thyroid hormone secretion. *J Clin Endocrinol Metab* 51:585, 1980

2. Marshall WA, Tanner JM: Variations in pattern of pubertal changes in girls. *Arch Dis Child* 44:291, 1969

3. Pasquino AM, Piccolo F, Scalamandre A, et al: Hypothalamic-pituitary-gonadotropic function in girls with premature thelarche. *Arch Dis Child* 55:941, 1980

4. Escobar ME, Rivarola MA, Bergadá C: Plasma concentration of oestradiol-17β in premature thelarche and in different types of sexual precocity. *Acta Endocrinol* 81:351, 1976

5. Bidlingmaier F, Butenandt O, Knorr D: Plasma gonadotropins and estrogens in girls with idiopathic precocious puberty. *Pediatr Res* 11:91, 1977

6. Lucky AW, Rich BH, Rosenfield RL, et al: Bioactive LH: A test to discriminate true precocious puberty from premature thelarche and adrenarche. *J Pediatr* 97:214, 1980

7. Rich BH, Rosenfield RL, Lucky AW, et al: Adrenarche: Changing adrenal response to adrenocorticotropin. *J Clin Endocrinol Metab* 52:1129, 1981

8. Chipman JJ: Pubertal control mechanisms as revealed from human studies. *Fed Proc* 39:2391, 1980

9. Zachmann M, Sobradillo B, Frank M, et al: Bayley-Pinneau, Roche-Wainer-Thissen, and Tanner height predictions in normal children and in patients with various pathologic conditions. *J Pediatr* 93:749, 1978

10. Schambach H, Schneemann K, Muller E: Psychic and intellectual development in girls with precocious puberty. *Endokrinologie* 74:47, 1979

11. Lester PD, McAlister WH: Asymmetric ovarian enlargement in idiopathic precocious puberty. *South Med J* 71:738, 1978

12. Cabezudo JM, Perez C, Vaquero J, et al: Pubertas praecox in craniopharyngioma. *J Neurosurg* 55:127, 1981

13. Zuniga OF, Tanner SM, Wild WO, et al: Hamartoma of CNS associated with precocious puberty. *Am J Dis Child* 137:127, 1983

14. Giovannelli G: Pineal region tumors: Endocrinological aspects. *Childs Brain* 9:267, 1982

15. Kubo O, Yamasaki N, Kamijo Y, et al: Human chorionic gonadotropin produced by ectopic pinealoma in a girl with precocious puberty. *J Neurosurg* 47:101, 1977

16. Matustik MC, Eisenberg HM, Meyer WJ: Gelastic (laughing) seizures and precocious puberty. *Am J Dis Child* 135:837, 1981

17. Van Wyk JJ, Grumbach MM: Syndrome of precocious menstruation and galactorrhea in juvenile hypothyroidism: An example of hormonal overlap in pituitary feedback. *J Pediatr* 57:416, 1960

18. Hayles AB: Precocious sexual maturation in juvenile hypothyroidism. *Fertil Steril* 27:1220, 1976

19. Riddlesberger MM Jr, Kuhn JP, Munschauer RW: The association of juvenile hypothyroidism and cystic ovaries. *Radiology* 139:77, 1981

20. Hancock KW, Stitch SR, Chapman C: Precocious puberty associated with primary hypothyroidism in a mongol girl. *Clin Endocrinol* 11:611, 1979

21. Lester PD, McAlister WH: Fibrous dysplasia and precocious puberty (McCune-Albright syndrome). *South Med J* 72:631, 1979

22. Fonzo D, Angeli A, Sivieri R, et al: Hyperprolactinemia in girls with idiopathic precocious puberty under prolonged treatment with cyproterone acetate. *J Clin Endocrinol Metab* 45:164, 1977

23. Kaplan SH, Ling SM, Irani NG: Idiopathic isosexual precocity. Therapy with medroxyprogesterone. *Am J Dis Child* 116:591, 1968

24. Comite F, Cutler GB Jr, Rivier J, et al: Short-term treatment of idiopathic precocious puberty with a long-acting analogue of luteinizing hormone-releasing hormone. *N Engl J Med* 305:1546, 1981

25. Crowley WF Jr, Comite F, Vale W, et al: Therapeutic use of pituitary desensitization with a long-acting LHRH agonist: A potential new treatment for idiopathic precocious puberty. *J Clin Endocrinol Metab* 52:370, 1981

26. Laron Z, Kauli R, Zeev ZB, et al: D-TRP[6]-analogue of luteinising hormone releasing hormone in combination with cyproterone acetate to treat precocious puberty. *Lancet* 2:955, 1981

Chapter 14

Primary Amenorrhea

Val Davajan, M.D.
Oscar A. Kletzky, M.D.

Amenorrhea is a symptom of a number of pathophysiologic states. Because some are serious and life-endangering illnesses, it is essential to make a correct diagnosis. The normal process of sexual maturation occurs only in genetically, anatomically, and functionally normal women. A derangement of any of these factors may result in the absence of secondary sex characteristics and/or spontaneous menses. In this chapter, we present a systematic method for establishing the differential diagnosis of primary amenorrhea and instituting the correct treatment.

The diagnosis of primary amenorrhea is made when a girl has had no episode of spontaneous uterine bleeding by the age of $16\frac{1}{2}$.[1] In most patients with delayed menarche, a diagnostic workup should be performed sooner, especially in the girl who has no breast development by age 15 or who has failed to menstruate within 2 years after the onset of thelarche and adrenarche. Patients with primary amenorrhea and phenotypic female external genitalia can be placed in one of four categories depending on the presence or absence of breast development and uterus (Table 14-1).[2]

Primary amenorrhea without breast development; uterus present

In this category, the primary disorder may be due to (1) a hypothalamic failure that is caused by inadequate release of gonadotropin-releasing hormone (GnRH); (2) isolated gonadotropin insufficiency, a rare pituitary defect; or (3) failure of gonadal development and/or function due to a genetic abnormality (Table 14-2).

Hypothalamic failure secondary to inadequate GnRH release (hypothalamic hypogonadotropic hypogonadism)

Before GnRH became available for use in testing pituitary function, all hypoestrogenic patients with low serum levels of gonadotropins were considered to have primary pituitary failure (primary pituitary hypogonadotropic hypogonadism). Now it is well established that most of these patients, when stimulated with GnRH, will have a significant serum luteinizing hormone (LH) and follicle-stimulating hormone (FSH) response. This demonstrates intact pituitary gonadotropic function. Because the pituitary gland is able to secrete gonadotropins rapidly when pharmacologic doses of GnRH are administered, it is clear that some endogenous GnRH is being secreted. The defect appears to be at the hypothalamic level; either insufficient secretion of GnRH or some abnormality of the neurotransmitter(s) (norepinephrine, dopamine) necessary to induce adequate GnRH synthesis and/or release is at fault.

However, some patients with primary amenorrhea and low gonadotropins do not have a normal serum LH and FSH response when stimulated with a single bolus of GnRH. This finding does not necessarily indicate that prima-

ry pituitary hypogonadotropic hypogonadism is present. Kletzky and associates found that these patients may have a normal serum LH and FSH response if the pituitary is first primed with GnRH for as little as 4 consecutive days before the stimulation test (Figure 14-1).[3] Therefore, the diagnosis is almost invariably one of hypothalamic, not of pituitary, etiology. In rare instances, GnRH stimulation elicits no response even after proper pretreatment. Associated disorders, such as thalassemia major or retinitis pigmentosa, have been found in such cases.[4,5]

Some patients with primary amenorrhea also have anosmia and possible agenesis or altered development of the rhinencephalic brain structure (Kallmann's syndrome). Therefore, all patients with primary amenorrhea and low serum gonadotropins should have at least a qualitative test for olfaction with coffee, tobacco, orange, and cocoa. Patients with primary amenorrhea and no breast development rarely present with a pituitary tumor. However other CNS neoplasms (craniopharyngioma) may present as such, and therefore we recommend that a CT be performed in patients who fail to respond to chronic GnRH stimulation tests and who do not have thalassemia major or retinitis pigmentosa.

The logical treatment for patients with hypogonadotropic hypogonadism of hypothalamic etiology would be the chronic use of GnRH. However, this method of therapy requires an indwelling IV or subcutaneous catheter and a portable pump for prolonged periods. Because chronic GnRH administration is not yet clinically practiced, all patients with low gonadotropins require estrogen/progestin therapy for breast development, sexual development, and prevention of osteoporosis. In the short patient, no more than 0.625 mg/day of conjugated estrogens should be given, to avoid premature closure of the epiphyses. Patients of normal height can be given at least 0.625 mg/day. If a higher dose is used, it should be lowered to 0.625 mg/day after 6 months. All patients on estrogen

Table 14-1
Classification of disorders in primary amenorrhea with normal external genitalia

I. Primary amenorrhea without breast development; uterus present
  A. Hypothalamic failure secondary to inadequate GnRH release
  B. Pituitary isolated gonadotropin insufficiency
  C. Gonadal failure
    1. 45,X (Turner's syndrome)
    2. 46,X, abnormal X (e.g., short or long arm deletion)
    3. Mosaicism (e.g., X/XX, X/XX/XXX)
    4. 46,XX or 46,XY pure gonadal dysgenesis
    5. 17α-Hydroxylase deficiency with 46,XX karyotype
II. Primary amenorrhea with breast development; uterus absent
  A. Androgen insensitivity (testicular feminization)
  B. Congenital absence of uterus
III. Primary amenorrhea without breast development; uterus absent
  A. 17,20-Desmolase deficiency
  B. Agonadism
  C. 17α-Hydroxylase deficiency with 46,XY karyotype
IV. Primary amenorrhea with breast development; uterus present
  A. Hypothalamic causes
  B. Pituitary causes
  C. Ovarian causes
  D. Uterine causes

Adapted from Mashchak CA, Kletzky OA, Davajan V, et al: Clinical and laboratory evaluation of patients with primary amenorrhea. Obstet Gynecol 57:715, 1981. Used with permission from The American College of Obstetricians and Gynecologists.

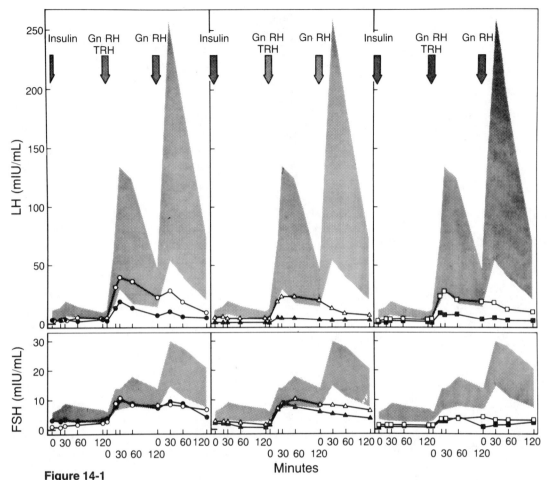

Figure 14-1

Serum LH and FSH responses to GnRH-TRH stimulation in three patients with hypothalamic hypogonadotropic hypogonadism before (solid symbols) and after (open symbols) priming with GnRH for 4 consecutive days. Shaded areas represent the 95% confidence limits of control subjects.

From Kletzky OA, Nicoloff JT, Davajan V, et al: Idiopathic hypogonadotropic hypogonadal primary amenorrhea. J Clin Endocrinol Metab *46:808, 1978.*

replacement therapy should take the estrogen on days 1 to 25 of each month. A progestin (medroxyprogesterone acetate), 10 mg/day, should be added on days 14 to 25 to prevent unopposed estrogen stimulation of the endometrium and breast. If pregnancy is desired, the treatment of choice is either human menopausal gonadotropins (hMG) or pulsatile GnRH. Clomiphene citrate is found to be ineffective in inducing ovulation in patients with hypoestrogenic amenorrhea.

Pituitary isolated gonadotropin insufficiency

A few male patients have been reported to have primary hypogonadotropic hypogonadism with

Table 14-2
Hormonal status in patients with the most common genetic defects

Disorder	FSH	LH	Estrogen
45,X (Turner's syndrome)	↑	↑	↓
46,X, abnormal X (e.g., short or long arm deletion)	↑	↑	↓
Mosaicism (e.g., X/XX, X/XX/XXX)	↑	↑	↓
46,XX or 46,XY pure gonadal dysgenesis	↑	↑	↓
17α-Hydroxylase deficiency with 46,XX	↑	↑	↓

↑ = above normal range; ↓ = below normal range.

no demonstrable pituitary tumor or deficiency of the other tropic hormones. When GnRH is administered to these patients, there is no increase in release of FSH or LH. In this situation also, the definitive diagnosis of primary pituitary isolated gonadotropin insufficiency should not be made unless the patient is first primed with daily doses of GnRH before the stimulation test. In our experience, adult isolated gonadotropin insufficiency has been found only in association with thalassemia major in both women (Figure 14-2)[4] and men. In these patients, daily priming of the pituitary with GnRH failed to elicit a normal gonadotropic pituitary response.

Gonadal failure due to genetic abnormalities and enzyme deficiency (hypergonadotropic hypogonadism)

We found that approximately 30% (17/62) of patients with primary amenorrhea had gonadal failure due to a genetic defect.[2] According to the literature, the most common disorders associated with hypergonadotropism are (1) 45,X, or Turner's syndrome; (2) structurally abnormal X chromosome; (3) mosaicism; (4) pure gonadal dysgenesis (46,XX and 46,XY with streaks); and (5) 17α-hydroxylase deficiency with a 46,XX karyotype (Table 14-2).

Individuals with any of the five disorders listed above have gonadal failure. In most instances, because these patients (except in 17α-hydroxylase deficiency) do not have primordial follicles, they cannot synthesize ovarian steroids. Therefore, they have elevated gonadotropins because they lack the negative estrogen feedback on the hypothalamic-pituitary axis (Figure 14-3).[2] Patients with 17α-hydroxylase deficiency do have primordial follicles, but cannot synthesize sex steroids. An occasional individual with mosaicism, an abnormal X, or pure gonadal dysgenesis (46,XX) may have a few follicles that develop under endogenous gonadotropin stimulation early in puberty and synthesize enough estrogen to induce breast development and a few episodes of uterine bleeding. An occasional pregnancy can occur. However, most of these patients have primary amenorrhea and show no signs of secondary sex characteristics.

45,X (Turner's syndrome)

Turner reported that the most common chromosomal abnormality causing gonadal failure is a completely absent X chromosome, the 45,X karyotype (Turner's syndrome).[6] The incidence of this disorder has been reported to be between 1/2,000 and 1/7,000 births.[7] The major features are (1) short stature (almost always less than 60 inches, or 150 cm, in height), (2) streak gonads, and (3) sexual infantilism. The patient may have numerous other somatic anomalies, such as webbing of the neck, short fourth metacarpal, cubitus valgus, and coarctation of the aorta. The birth weight of infants with Turner's syndrome is frequently at or below the third percentile.

The gonadal streaks lack the follicular apparatus and cannot synthesize ovarian steroids. Therefore, with no negative feedback on the hypothalamic-pituitary axis, the gonadotropins are elevated into the postmenopausal range. The gonadal streaks should not be surgically removed, because malignant transformation is extremely rare. The exceptions are patients with clinical evidence of excess androgen production or a Y chromosome in a karyotype of the peripheral blood leukocytes.

The diagnosis of Turner's syndrome is easily made by physical examination, an elevated serum FSH value, and a 45,X karyotype. Almost all individuals with this syndrome are sterile and need estrogen therapy. We did have one patient, with mosaic Turner's syndrome (X/XX) and gonadal streaks, who ovulated spontaneously, became pregnant, and was delivered of a normal infant. Thyroiditis and thyroid autoantibodies

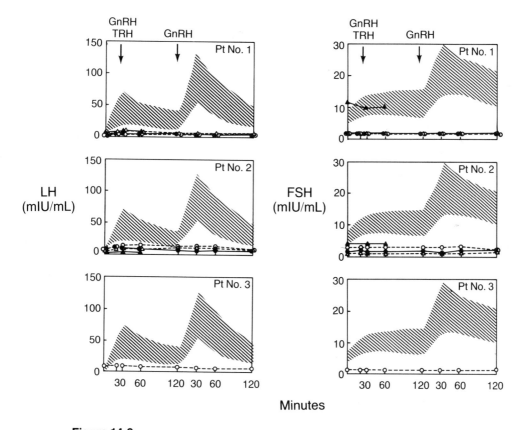

Figure 14-2
Serum LH and FSH responses in three female patients with thalassemia major to GnRH-TRH stimulation test—before any treatment (open circles; patient No. 3 was on estrogen replacement and was studied only once), after priming with GnRH for 7 days (solid circles), with E_2 for 7 days (open triangles), and after hMG treatment (solid triangles).

Reproduced, with permission, from Kletzky OA, Costin G, Marrs RP, et al: Gonadotropin insufficiency in patients with thalassemia major.J Clin Endocrinol Metab 48:901, 1979.

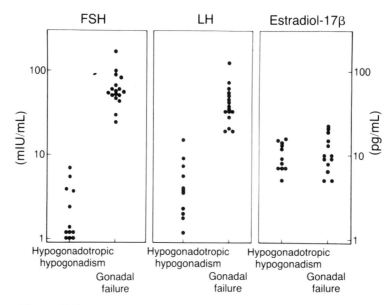

Figure 14-3
Serum levels of FSH, LH, and E₂ in patients with hypogonadotropic hypogonadism and gonadal failure.

From Mashchak CA, Kletzky OA, Davajan V, et al: Clinical and laboratory evaluation of patients with primary amenorrhea. Obstet Gynecol 57:715, 1981. Reprinted with permission from The American College of Obstetricians and Gynecologists.

have been described in patients with Turner's syndrome.[8] An increased incidence of abnormal glucose tolerance has also been reported in these patients.[9]

It has been suggested that for very short patients with Turner's syndrome, low-dose androgens be used before or with estrogen replacement therapy, in an effort to achieve maximum height. One recommended regimen is fluoxymesterone, 2.5 mg/day, to be continued until no linear growth is achieved over a 3-month interval. Then estrogen replacement therapy is instituted. To increase growth velocity, treatment with 0.1 mg/kg/day of oxandrolone, a synthetic analog of testosterone, has been recommended. According to some investigators, this therapy will ultimately result in substantially greater height.[10,11]

Structurally abnormal X chromosome

The karyotype in this disorder is 46,XX, but one of the X chromosomes is incomplete.[7] The phenotype varies, depending on the amount of material missing from the structurally abnormal X.

Patients with deletion of the long arm of the X chromosome usually, but not always, have normal stature, no somatic abnormalities, streak gonads, and sexual infantilism.[12-14] They are also sterile and need estrogen replacement therapy for breast development and prevention of osteoporosis. Some patients have delayed epiphyseal closure and are eunuchoidal in appearance. Clinically, there may be a resemblance to patients with either hypogonadotropic hypogonadism or pure gonadal dysgenesis.

Patients with short-arm deletion of the X chromosome usually have a phenotype similar to that of Turner's syndrome.[7] Patients with isochromosome of the long arm of the X, either alone or in a mosaic state, also have most of the clinical features of Turner's syndrome. A number of other chromosomal aberrations in the structurally abnormal X syndrome have been described.[15,16] These include a ring X and minute fragmentation of the X chromosome.

Mosaicism

Primary amenorrhea has been associated with a variety of mosaic states; the most common is X/XX.[15] Patients with this mosaic pattern may have positive or negative buccal smears, and they range across a broad spectrum of phenotypism. In general, the X/XX individual is taller and has fewer anomalies than someone with a pure 45,X cell line. However, it has been reported that 80% of X/XX mosaics are shorter than their peers (although taller than individuals with 45,X) and 66% have some somatic anomaly. Approximately 20% of these patients have had spontaneous menses.[15]

The clinical findings in X/XXX and X/XX/XXX mosaicism are similar to those in X/XX mosaicism. The exact status of estrogen and gonadotropin production is variable, depending on the functional capacity (presence of follicular apparatus) of the gonads.

Pure gonadal dysgenesis
(46,XX, 46,XY with gonadal streaks)

Patients with pure gonadal dysgenesis usually have primary amenorrhea, infantile secondary sex characteristics, and normal stature. However, secondary sex characteristics and a history of a few episodes of spontaneous uterine bleeding at the time of puberty have been reported in a few cases. Those patients most likely had a few primordial follicles that responded to gonadotropic stimulation, resulting in some ovarian estrogen production.

The somatic abnormalities associated with Turner's syndrome are usually absent in pure gonadal dysgenesis. It is probably a genetic disorder, because it has been reported among siblings. Because of the lack of estrogen synthesis, patients with pure gonadal dysgenesis will not have uterine bleeding after IM administration of progesterone. In addition, their serum LH and FSH levels are invariably in the postmenopausal range.

17α-Hydroxylase deficiency
with 46,XX karyotype

In 1966, a patient was described with 17α-hydroxylase deficiency and primary amenorrhea, no breast development, an intact uterus, and normal external female genitalia.[17] From 1967 to 1969, three more such patients were reported.[18,19] They were found to have a 46,XX karyotype with slightly eunuchoid habitus. The urinary gonadotropins were elevated and the sex steroids were very low. The unique feature of this disorder was the universal finding of hypertension and hypokalemia.

A reduction in cortisol production results from the diminished levels of 17α-hydroxylase characteristic of this disorder. This in turn causes an increase in adrenocorticotropic hormone (ACTH). The conversion of progesterone to deoxycorticosterone (DOC) and corticosterone does not require 17α-hydroxylation. Therefore, with the elevated ACTH, the production of mineralocorticoids becomes markedly excessive. The result is sodium retention, hypertension, and loss of potassium.

Otherwise, these patients present physically with the same findings as seen in either hypogonadotropic hypogonadism or pure gonadal dysgenesis. This deficiency disorder may be categorized with other types of gonadal failure (hypergonadotropic hypogonadism) because it is also associated with elevated gonadotropins.

The diagnosis of 17α-hydroxylase deficiency can be made by obtaining an elevated serum progesterone value (>3 ng/mL), a low 17α-hydroxyprogesterone level (<0.2 ng/mL), and

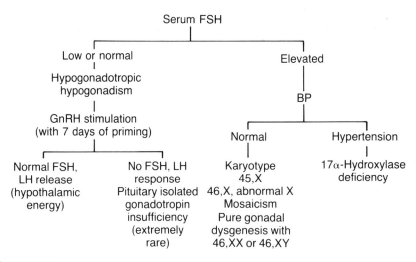

Serum FSH

Low or normal
|
Hypogonadotropic hypogonadism
|
GnRH stimulation
(with 7 days of priming)

Normal FSH, LH release (hypothalamic energy)

No FSH, LH response Pituitary isolated gonadotropin insufficiency (extremely rare)

Elevated
|
BP

Normal
|
Karyotype
45,X
46,X, abnormal X
Mosaicism
Pure gonadal dysgenesis with 46,XX or 46,XY

Hypertension
|
17α-Hydroxylase deficiency

Figure 14-4
Diagnostic workup of patients with primary amenorrhea, undeveloped breasts, and intact uterus.

an elevated serum DOC value (the normal range in adult women = 4 to 17 ng/100 mL). The diagnosis should then be confirmed by performing an ACTH stimulation test. A bolus of 0.25 mg of ACTH is administered after the baseline progesterone and 17α-hydroxyprogesterone levels are obtained. Then, 60 minutes later, a blood sample is drawn. Patients with 17α-hydroxylase deficiency have markedly increased levels of serum progesterone and essentially no change in serum 17α-hydroxyprogesterone levels.

Patients with 17α-hydroxylase deficiency have been reported to have low levels of aldosterone in the presence of elevated 11-deoxycorticosterone and corticosterone.[18] This finding can be explained by the fact that aldosterone, unlike DOC and corticosterone, is not ACTH-dependent, but is influenced by the renin-angiotensin system and by the plasma sodium concentration. Thus, the elevated DOC and corticosterone levels lead to sodium retention, which results in lowering of aldosterone levels in the serum. The hypokalemia is a result of high renal potassium excretion.[20]

The possibility of 17α-hydroxylase deficien-

cy must always be considered, because its treatment with cortisone and estrogen/progestin is markedly different from the simple estrogen/progestin replacement used in other forms of gonadal failure. 17α-Hydroxylase deficiency is a life-threatening disease, whereas the other disorders, if left untreated, place patients at risk only for developing early onset of osteoporosis.

Summary of diagnosis and treatment

The most accurate way to differentiate between CNS and gonadal failure in hypoestrogenic patients is to measure serum FSH by radioimmunoassay (RIA). Patients with hypogonadotropic hypogonadism (central failure) have low or, occasionally, normal FSH values. Patients with gonadal failure (peripheral failure) have serum FSH values elevated into the postmenopausal range (Figure 14-3).[2] Figure 14-4 is a schematic representation of the workup of patients with primary amenorrhea, undeveloped breasts, and intact uterus. The basic differences in the treatment of such patients are presented in Figure 14-5. A karyotype is necessary only if the FSH is elevated. The gonads or streaks need be removed only if a Y chromosome is present or if the patient has clinical evidence of excess androgen production (e.g., hirsutism). Laparoscopy and/or laparotomy are not necessary otherwise and should not be performed.

Essentially all patients with gonadal abnormalities are sterile, because ovulation usually cannot be induced. Exogenous estrogen/progestin replacement therapy should be given to stimulate breast development and to prevent osteoporosis. The degree of breast development does not appear to be related to the estrogen dosage. The same degree of breast development can be achieved with 0.625 mg/day of conjugated estrogens (or the equivalent) as with 2.5 mg/day. The degree of breast development is best ascertained by periodically measuring the diameter of the breast plate (between the anterior axillary line and midsternum in sitting position), rather than the distance from the tip of the nipple to the chest wall or to the surface of the examining table. Many of these patients tend to develop conical breasts during estrogen therapy; the addition of a progestin during the last 12 days of the 25-day estrogen regimen has been recommended so that the breasts will be more rounded. However, we have been unable to detect any difference in breast contour, with or without progestins. We do recommend the use of progestin therapy to prevent unopposed estrogen stimulation of the endometrium and breast tissue.

Primary amenorrhea with breast development; uterus absent

There are two disorders in this category: androgen insensitivity (testicular feminization) and congenital absence of the uterus.

Androgen insensitivity (testicular feminization, complete form)

An individual with this syndrome has a 46,XY karyotype, testes, and female phenotype.[21] In the complete form, the clinical features are total lack of axillary and pubic hair, normal breast development, and a blind vaginal pouch. This syndrome, which is either X-linked recessive or X-linked dominant, may be found in several members of a family.

The basic defect is a lack of androgen receptors, which are normally present in the cytoplasm of target cells. Ovaries, uterus, and oviducts are absent, because the testes secrete normal amounts of müllerian inhibiting factor (MIF), which does not require the presence of

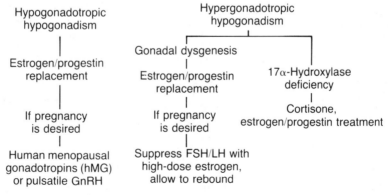

Figure 14-5
Treatment of disorders associated with primary amenorrhea, undeveloped breasts, and intact uterus.

receptors to exert its action. Because the testes also produce normal male levels of testosterone and estradiol, the serum levels of gonadotropins are normal. The presence of normal breast development, even with low levels of estradiol (<30 pg/mL), is apparently due to the lack of any androgen opposition. The small amounts of estrogen secreted by the adrenals and testes and produced by peripheral conversion of androstenedione to estrone, when unopposed by androgens, seem to be adequate for normal development of the breasts.

Serum testosterone levels (Figure 14-6) can be used to differentiate the androgen insensitivity syndrome (with normal male levels >300 ng/dL) from congenital absence of the uterus (with normal female levels of 20 to 85 ng/dL). Other distinguishing features of congenital absence of the uterus include normal pubic and axillary hair and, in most cases, normal ovulation. Thus, when patients present with primary amenorrhea, breast development, and absent uterus, the diagnosis can usually be made by physical examination, serum testosterone level, and, if testosterone is elevated, confirmation by a karyotype. Alternatively, if ovulation is documented by a biphasic basal body temperature (BBT) graph or an ovulatory level of serum progesterone (>3 ng/mL), the syndrome of androgen insensitivity can be ruled out.

As a general rule, any patient with an abnormality of sexual differentiation and a Y chromosome should have the gonads surgically removed, because of the high incidence of malignancy reported in such cases. In patients over the age of 30 with the androgen insensitivity syndrome, the incidence of malignant gonadal tumors has been reported to be 22%, with 50% having benign tumors such as adenomas and cysts.[21] The malignant gonadal tumors are usually dysgerminomas or gonadoblastomas. Because malignant tumors have not been reported in prepubertal patients with this syndrome, it is recommended that the testes not be removed

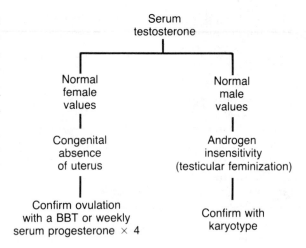

Figure 14-6
Differentiating congenital absence of the uterus from androgen insensitivity syndrome.

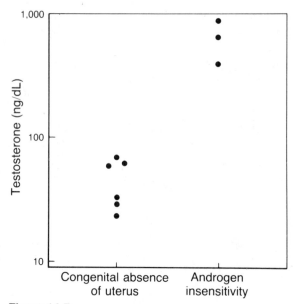

Figure 14-7
Serum testosterone levels in patients with primary amenorrhea, breast development, and no uterus.

From Mashchak CA, Kletzky OA, Davajan V, et al: Clinical and laboratory evaluation of patients with primary amenorrhea. Obstet Gynecol 57:715, 1981. Reprinted with permission from The American College of Obstetricians and Gynecologists.

Abnormal endocrinology

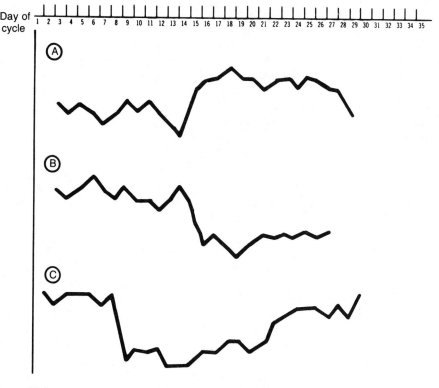

Figure 14-8
Basal body temperature (BBT) graphs illustrating various possible patterns of ovulatory cycles in patients with congenital absence of the uterus. Pattern A represents the usual biphasic curve. Pattern B is the biphasic graph of a patient starting to record her BBT in the early luteal phase. Pattern C is the biphasic graph of a patient starting her record in the middle of the luteal phase.

until the patient has undergone full sexual development, with her own endogenous testicular steroids. After sexual maturity is achieved, the testes should be removed and the patient placed on estrogen/progestin therapy to prevent osteoporosis. If necessary, progressive vaginal dilation or skin-graft vaginoplasty should be performed when the patient approaches the age of sexual function.

We recommend telling patients with androgen insensitivity syndrome that they have an abnormal sex chromosome, without specifically mentioning a Y chromosome, because most people know that an XY karyotype indicates male-

ness. In addition, because psychologically and phenotypically these individuals are females, the term gonads should be used instead of testes. However, these patients should be told that they cannot become pregnant.

Congenital absence of the uterus

In our clinic, complete uterine agenesis is a more common cause of primary amenorrhea than androgen insensitivity. Because ovaries are present, these patients have normal secondary sex characteristics and often experience cyclic breast and mood alterations compatible with ovulation. In the differential diagnosis, the incomplete form of the androgen insensitivity syndrome with normal pubic hair growth must be considered. In both conditions, the uterus is absent and the gonadotropins are normal. However, the serum testosterone levels in patients with congenital absence of the uterus are in the normal female range, whereas levels in the androgen insensitivity group are usually in the male range (Figure 14-7).[2] A 30-day record of basal body temperature will usually show a biphasic curve indicative of ovulation in the patient with congenital absence of the uterus (Figure 14-8). Weekly serum progesterone values can also be used to document ovulation. If ovulation is occurring, androgen insensitivity syndrome is obviously ruled out. Conversely, a serum testosterone level in the normal male range rules out congenital absence of the uterus.

Because patients with congenital absence of the uterus have normal ovarian function, hormone replacement is unnecessary. If the vagina is also absent (Rokitansky's syndrome), either vaginal dilation with progressively larger dilators or vaginoplasty will correct the defect. With recent in vitro fertilization advances, it may be possible, using a surrogate mother, for these patients to have their own genetic children.

Primary amenorrhea without breast development; uterus absent

Patients with primary amenorrhea who have neither breast nor uterine development are extremely rare. Such patients most often have a male karyotype, elevated gonadotropin levels, and testosterone values in or below the normal female range. They differ from patients with gonadal failure because they do not have a uterus, and from patients with androgen insensitivity syndrome because they do not have breast development or testosterone levels in the male range. At our institution, two such patients have been described, one with 17,20-desmolase deficiency, the other with agonadism. A third type of disorder has been described in association with this phenotype: 17α-hydroxylase deficiency with 46,XY karyotype (Table 14-3).

17,20-Desmolase deficiency
The patient with a deficiency of 17,20-desmolase, as reported from this institution, lacked the enzyme necessary to convert 17α-hydroxypregnenolone to dehydroepiandrosterone (Δ^5) and 17α-hydroxyprogesterone to androstenedione (Δ^4).[22] With both these pathways blocked, the patient failed to synthesize any sex steroids, but was capable of making cortisol and DOC (Figure 14-9). This patient was found to have abdominal testes, which were surgically removed.[22]

Agonadism
The other patient, also lacking both breast and uterine development, was found to have absolutely no internal sex organs (agonadism) at laparotomy. Federman distinguished this disorder, which presents with female or ambiguous external genitalia, from congenital anorchia, which is seen in patients with male external genitalia.[23] It

Table 14-3
Disorders in primary amenorrhea with neither breast nor uterine development

Disorder	FSH	T	Karyotype	Uterus	Gonads
17,20-Desmolase deficiency	↑	Low	XY	−	+
Agonadism	↑	Low	XY	−	−
17α-Hydroxylase deficiency with 46,XY	↑	Low	XY	−	+

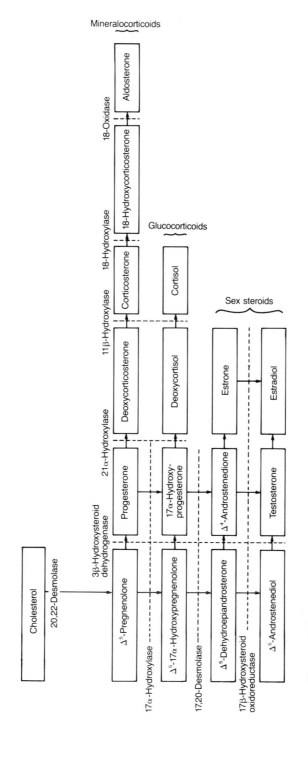

Figure 14-9

Steroid biosynthetic pathway of a patient with 17,20-desmolase deficiency.

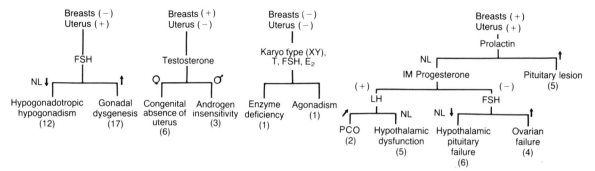

Figure 14-10

A systematic approach to diagnostic evaluation of patients with primary amenorrhea, based on presence or absence of breast development and uterus. Slanted arrow indicates moderate elevation. Positive (+) and negative (−) responses to IM progesterone refer to withdrawal uterine bleeding. Numbers in parentheses indicate distribution of diagnoses in a series of 62 patients. NL, normal.

From Mashchak CA, Kletzky OA, Davajan V, et al: Clinical and laboratory evaluation of patients with primary amenorrhea. Obstet Gynecol 57:715, 1981. Reprinted with permission from The American College of Obstetricians and Gynecologists.

is difficult to postulate why a patient with agonadism has no internal female reproductive organs. Because these patients do not have testes, they have no source of MIF; therefore, the uterus should have developed. It has been suggested that at some time in early embryonic development testicular tissue was present, and that MIF suppressed the development of the müllerian system. Then for unknown reasons, the testes disappeared after the müllerian system inhibition. Because of this theory, the syndrome of agonadism is also referred to as the vanishing testes syndrome.

17α-Hydroxylase deficiency with 46,XY karyotype

The first two cases of 17α-hydroxylase deficiency in XY patients were published in 1970.[24] These patients presented with primary amenorrhea, failure of secondary sex characteristics to develop, no uterus, and hypertension. By 1980, 12 such patients had been described.[25] The feature distinguishing these individuals from those with 46,XX and 17α-hydroxylase deficiency is the absence of a uterus. Lack of breast develop-

ment distinguishes this disorder from androgen insensitivity syndrome. The diagnosis and management of this disorder is exactly the same as for the patient with 17α-hydroxylase deficiency and 46,XX karyotype. Table 14-3 summarizes the various enzymatic deficiencies. Only the syndromes presenting with female external genitalia are discussed in this chapter.

Primary amenorrhea with breast development; uterus present

Approximately one-third (22/62) of patients with primary amenorrhea reported from this institution had both breast and uterine development.[2] Approximately 25% of these patients were found to have galactorrhea, elevated serum prolactin (PRL) levels, and abnormal tomograms of the sella turcica compatible with the presence of a pituitary adenoma. The remaining 75% to 80% of patients presenting with primary amenorrhea, normal breast development, and intact uteri had normal PRL levels. They were found to have the same categories of disorders (polycystic ovary syndrome, hypothalamic dysfunction, hypothalamic-pituitary failure, ovarian failure) as occur in patients with secondary amenorrhea. The one major difference in the workup for primary amenorrhea is the necessity to obtain a serum PRL value first. This is because it is more difficult to elicit galactorrhea from the breast of a patient who has primary amenorrhea. Therefore, to avoid missing the hyperprolactinemic patient with primary amenorrhea, we recommend a serum PRL as the initial step.

Figure 14-10 summarizes the diagnostic evaluation of the four groups of patients with primary amenorrhea categorized by presence or absence of breast development and uterus.[2] See Chapter 15 for a detailed discussion of secondary amenorrhea—which also applies to patients with primary amenorrhea and normal PRL levels in the fourth category (those with both breast development and uterus).

References

1. Frisch RE, Revelle R: Height and weight at menarche and a hypothesis of menarche. *Arch Dis Child* 46:695, 1971

2. Mashchak CA, Kletzky OA, Davajan V, et al: Clinical and laboratory evaluation of patients with primary amenorrhea. *Obstet Gynecol* 57:715, 1981

3. Kletzky OA, Nicoloff JT, Davajan V, et al: Idiopathic hypogonadotropic hypogonadal primary amenorrhea. *J Clin Endocrinol Metab* 46:808, 1978

4. Kletzky OA, Costin G, Marrs RP, et al: Gonadotropin insufficiency in patients with thalassemia major. *J Clin Endocrinol Metab* 48:901, 1979

5. Chang RJ, Davidson BJ, Carlson HE, et al: Hypogonadotropic hypogonadism associated with retinitis pigmentosa in a female sibling: Evidence for gonadotropin deficiency. *J Clin Endocrinol Metab* 53:1179, 1981

6. Turner HH: A syndrome of infantilism, congenital webbed neck and cubitus-valgus. *Endocrinology* 23:566, 1938

7. Rimoin DL, Schimke NR: *Genetic Disorders of the Endocrine Glands.* St Louis, CV Mosby, 1971, p 285

8. Hamilton CR, Moldawer M, Rosenberg HS: Hashimoto's thyroiditis and Turner's syndrome. *Arch Intern Med* 122:69, 1968

9. Forbes AP, Engel E: The high incidence of diabetes mellitus in 41 patients with gonadal dysgenesis and their close relatives. *Metab Clin Exp* 12:428, 1963

10. Urban MD, Lee PA, Dorst JP, et al: Oxandrolone therapy in patients with Turner syndrome. *J Pediatr* 94:823, 1979

11. Rudman D, Goldsmith M, Kutner M, et al: Effect of growth hormone and oxandrolone singly and together on growth rate in girls with X chromosome abnormalities. *J Clin Endocrinol Metab* 96:132, 1980

12. Hecht F, MacFarlane JC: Mosaicism in Turner's syndrome reflects the lethality of XO. *Lancet* 2:1197, 1969

13. Baughman FA, Kolk KJ, Mann JD, et al: Two cases of primary amenorrhea with deletion of the long arm of X chromosome (46,XXq−). *Am J Obstet Gynecol* 102:1065, 1968

14. Hsu LYF, Hirschhorn K: Genetic and clinical consideration of long arm deletion of the X chromosome. *Pediatrics* 45:656, 1970

15. Ferguson-Smith MA: Karyotype-phenotype correlations in gonadal dysgenesis and their bearing on the pathogenesis of malformations. *J Med Genet* 2:142, 1965

16. Ferguson-Smith MA: Phenotypic aspects of sex chromosome aberrations. *Birth Defects, Original Article Series* 5:3, 1969

17. Biglieri EG, Herron MA, Brust N: 17 hydroxylation deficiency in man. *J Clin Invest* 45:1946, 1966

18. Goldsmith O, Soloman DH, Horton R: Hypogonadism and mineralocorticoid excess. The 17 hydroxylase deficiency syndrome. *N Engl J Med* 277:673, 1967

19. Mallin SR: Congenital adrenal hyperplasia secondary to 17 hydroxylase deficiency. *Ann Intern Med* 70:69, 1969

20. Saruta T, Nagahama S, Eguchi T, et al: Renin, aldosterone and other mineralocorticoids in hyperkalemic patients with chronic renal failure showing mild azotemia. *Nephron* 29:128, 1981

21. Morris JM, Mahesh VB: Further observations on the syndrome "testicular feminization." *Am J Obstet Gynecol* 87:731, 1963

22. Goebelsmann U, Zachmann M, Davajan V, et al: Male pseudohermaphroditism consistent with 17,20 desmolase deficiency. *Gyn Invest* 7:138, 1976

23. Federman DD: *Abnormal Sexual Development: A Genetic and Endocrine Approach to Differential Diagnosis.* Philadelphia, WB Saunders, 1967

24. New MI: Male pseudohermaphroditism due to 17 alpha-hydroxylase deficiency. *J Clin Invest* 49:1930, 1970

25. Abad L, Parrilla JJ, Marcos J, et al: Male pseudohermaphroditism with 17 alpha-hydroxylase deficiency. A case report. *Br J Obstet Gynaecol* 87:1162, 1980

Chapter 15

Secondary Amenorrhea

(Without Galactorrhea or Androgen Excess)

Val Davajan, M.D.
Oscar A. Kletzky, M.D.

Secondary amenorrhea is usually defined as the absence of menses for at least 6 months in a woman who previously had been having regular menses, or the absence of menses for 12 months in a patient with a history of oligomenorrhea. Before the differential diagnosis of these patients is considered, thyroid disease, diabetes mellitus, and normal or abnormal pregnancies should be ruled out. After a careful physical examination, the patient can be placed in one of the following categories: (1) those with no evidence of galactorrhea or excess of cortisol or androgen; (2) those with galactorrhea; or (3) those with possible cortisol excess (Cushing's syndrome) and/or androgen excess. Patients in the first category are discussed in this chapter (Table 15-1); the second and third categories are discussed in the next two chapters.

Women with amenorrhea and no clinical evidence of cortisol excess, androgen excess, or galactorrhea have either a defect in the hypothalamic-pituitary-ovarian axis or uterine disease (Asherman's syndrome).[1] If a patient presents with amenorrhea following uterine curettage, particularly if the procedure was associated with pregnancy or elective pregnancy termination, the clinician should suspect the presence of intrauterine synechiae and proceed to investigate the uterine cavity by use of hysterosalpingography and/or hysterography.

CNS-hypothalamic etiology

CNS-hypothalamic dysfunction

Idiopathic

One of the most common causes of amenorrhea is idiopathic hypothalamic dysfunction, without any history of stress or drug intake. The exact mechanism has not been determined; it may involve failure of the estradiol (E_2) levels to rise high enough to trigger the luteinizing hormone (LH) surge. This dysfunction appears to be related to either a neurotransmitter alteration or a hypothalamic derangement, because in most cases ovulation can be induced with clomiphene citrate.

Some patients have been found to have a blunted prolactin (PRL) response following insulin-induced hypoglycemia.[2] Furthermore, the

Table 15-1
Differential diagnosis of amenorrhea

Causes	FSH	LH	Estrogen (E$_2$)	Uterine bleeding after progesterone
I. Hypothalamic				
A. CNS-hypothalamic dysfunction				
1. Idiopathic	N	N	N	+
2. Secondary to medications	N	N	N	+
3. Secondary to stress	N	N	N	+
B. CNS-hypothalamic dysfunction or failure due to exercise	↓ or N	↓ or N	↓ or N	±
C. CNS-hypothalamic dysfunction or failure due to weight loss				
1. Simple weight loss	↓ or N	↓ or N	↓ or N	±
2. Anorexia nervosa	↓	↓	↓	−
D. CNS-hypothalamic failure				
1. Lesions	↓	↓	↓	−
2. Idiopathic	↓	↓	↓	−
E. CNS-hypothalamic-adreno-ovarian dysfunction (polycystic ovary syndrome, PCO)	N	↗	N	+
II. Pituitary				
A. Destructive lesions (Sheehan's syndrome)	↓	↓	↓	−
B. Tumor	↓	↓	↓	−
III. Ovarian				
A. Premature ovarian failure	↑	↑	↓	−
B. Loss of ovarian function (oophorectomy, infection, cystic degeneration)	↑	↑	↓	−
IV. Uterine				
A. Uterine synechiae (Asherman's syndrome)	N	N	N	−

N = value within normal range; ↓ = value below normal range; ↑ = value above normal range. ↗ = >25 mIU/mL; <menopausal level

serum LH and follicle-stimulating-hormone (FSH) response is usually normal following gonadotropin-releasing-hormone (GnRH) stimulation (Figure 15-1).[3] This finding indicates that the hypothalamus is the site of the dysfunction. These patients usually have serum E$_2$ levels of at least 40 pg/mL and therefore usually have uterine bleeding following progesterone administration (Figure 15-2).[4] Random or daily serum FSH and LH levels are in the normal range. With measurement of gonadotropins every 15 minutes for 4 consecutive hours, maintenance of the LH fluctuations, with peaks of hormone secretion occurring every 60 to 75 minutes (Figure 15-3),[2] has been reported. More recently, with sampling every 10 minutes, a dyssynchrony of LH fluctuations was reported in women with dysfunctional amenorrhea. This would indicate a derangement in the endogenous secretion of GnRH.[5] Patients with hypothalamic dysfunction should be challenged with oral medroxyprogesterone acetate, 10 mg/day for 12 days every 60 days. If this regimen fails to induce uterine bleeding, progesterone in oil (100 mg) should be given IM. If this dose fails to cause withdrawal uterine bleeding within 2 weeks, then a 200-mg dose should be given. Even in the absence of galactorrhea, we recommend that a serum PRL be obtained to rule out hyperprolactinemia. If either failure of withdrawal uterine bleeding or hyperprolactinemia is noted, patients with hypothalamic dysfunction should have complete

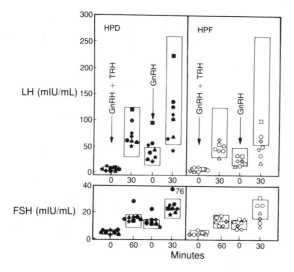

Figure 15-1

Maximum LH and FSH response following the sequential administration of GnRH in patients with hypothalamic-pituitary dysfunction (HPD) and patients with hypothalamic-pituitary failure (HPF).

Reproduced, with permission, from Kletzky OA, Mishell DR Jr, Davajan V, et al: Pituitary stimulation test in amenorrheic patients with normal or low estradiol. Acta Endocrinol 87:456, 1978.

workups of the pituitary as outlined under step 3, Table 15-2.

Dysfunction secondary to medications

Drugs most commonly associated with amenorrhea are the phenothiazine derivatives and the contraceptive steroids. The mechanism appears to be either depletion of catecholamines or a blocking effect on the neurotransmitter at the receptors. The phenothiazine-induced amenorrhea is usually associated with hyperprolactinemia and galactorrhea. The discussion and management of this condition is in Chapter 16.

From work done at this institution, it was found that contraceptive steroids also have a suppressive effect on the pituitary; and sometimes this effect persists after oral contraceptives (OCs) are discontinued, resulting in the condition referred to as postpill amenorrhea.[6-8]

Women taking OCs not only have diminished basal levels of LH and FSH, but also have a blunted gonadotropin response to GnRH (Figure 15-4).[6] OC users secrete PRL in larger quantities after both insulin-induced hypoglycemia and thyrotropin-releasing-hormone (TRH) stimulation (Figure 15-5).[8]

Most patients with postpill amenorrhea have normal baseline serum FSH and LH levels; the E_2 level is usually greater than 40 pg/mL. Therefore, uterine bleeding will usually occur following progesterone administration; we have shown that patients with E_2 levels of less than 40 pg/mL do not have uterine bleeding following administration of IM progesterone. Patients with postpill amenorrhea do not need to undergo a workup for at least 6 months, unless galactorrhea is present, the patient is especially anx-

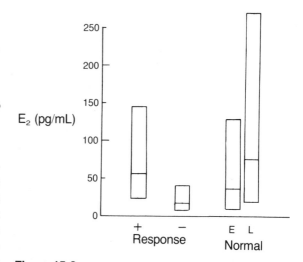

Figure 15-2

Mean and 95% confidence limits of estradiol levels in patients with secondary amenorrhea with positive and negative uterine bleeding response to IM injection of progesterone in oil, in comparison with the levels in the early (E) and late (L) follicular phase of normal ovulatory cycles.

Reproduced, with permission, from Kletzky OA, Davajan V, Nakamura RM, et al: Clinical categorization of patients with secondary amenorrhea using progesterone-induced uterine bleeding and measurement of serum gonadotropin levels. Am J Obstet Gynecol 121:695, 1975.

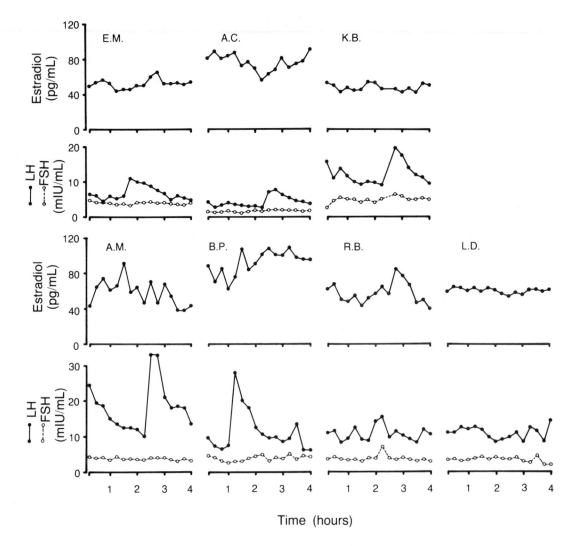

Figure 15-3
Serum LH, FSH, and estradiol (E$_2$) concentrations in samples obtained at 15-minute intervals from seven patients with hypothalamic-pituitary dysfunction.

Reproduced, with permission, from Kletzky OA, Davajan V, Nakamura, RM, et al: Classification of secondary amenorrhea based on distinct hormonal patterns. J Clin Endocrinol Metab 41:660, 1975.

ious, or conception is desired. In most women, menses resume spontaneously within 6 months after discontinuation of OCs. IM progesterone (100 or 200 mg) should be administered to determine the patient's estrogen status.

If withdrawal uterine bleeding occurs and the serum PRL level remains normal, further workup is unnecessary. If the patient wishes to conceive, clomiphene citrate should be administered. If the patient fails to have withdrawal

Abnormal endocrinology

Table 15-2
Responses to progesterone

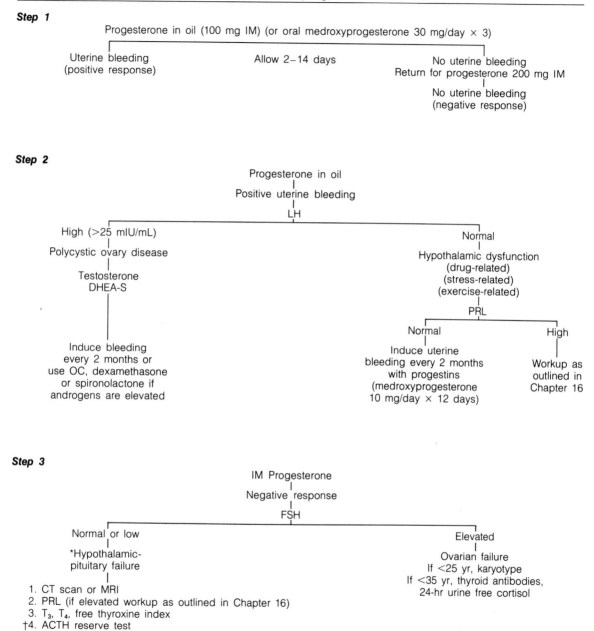

Step 1

Progesterone in oil (100 mg IM) (or oral medroxyprogesterone 30 mg/day × 3)

Uterine bleeding   Allow 2–14 days   No uterine bleeding
(positive response)   Return for progesterone 200 mg IM

No uterine bleeding
(negative response)

Step 2

Progesterone in oil

Positive uterine bleeding

LH

High (>25 mIU/mL)   Normal

Polycystic ovary disease   Hypothalamic dysfunction
                         (drug-related)
Testosterone   (stress-related)
DHEA-S   (exercise-related)

                        PRL

              Normal   High

Induce bleeding   Induce uterine
every 2 months or   bleeding every 2 months   Workup as
use OC, dexamethasone with progestins   outlined in
or spironolactone if   (medroxyprogesterone Chapter 16
androgens are elevated 10 mg/day × 12 days)

Step 3

IM Progesterone

Negative response

FSH

Normal or low   Elevated

*Hypothalamic-   Ovarian failure
pituitary failure   If <25 yr, karyotype
                          If <35 yr, thyroid antibodies,
1. CT scan or MRI   24-hr urine free cortisol
2. PRL (if elevated workup as outlined in Chapter 16)
3. T₃, T₄, free thyroxine index
†4. ACTH reserve test

Patients with simple weight loss, history of drug intake, stress or exercise, who do not have hyperprolactinemia do not need a CT scan.
†*Only in patients with history of postpartum hemorrhage*

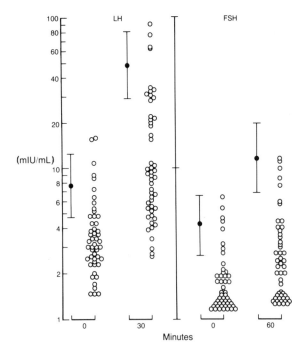

Figure 15-4
Serum LH and FSH levels in 50 subjects taking oral contraceptives at 0 (baseline), 30, and 60 minutes after stimulation with GnRH. Bars represent mean and 95% confidence limits of control subjects.

Reproduced, with permission, from Scott JZ, Brenner PF, Kletzky OA, et al: Factors affecting pituitary gonadotropin function in users of oral contraceptive steroids. Am J Obstet Gynecol 130:817, 1978.

bleeding after a progesterone challenge, her serum FSH level should be measured to rule out ovarian failure. If the FSH level is low or normal, the serum PRL level should be measured. If PRL is elevated, the patient should undergo a workup as outlined in Chapter 16.

Dysfunction secondary to stress

Some patients become amenorrheic when they encounter a stressful situation such as going away to school, divorce, or death in the family.[9] Changes in environment have been reported to cause abnormality in the reproductive processes of animals. With disruption of social structure, female monkeys have been reported to lose their LH surge.[10] In most patients with stress amenorrhea, serum levels of FSH and LH are normal, and E_2 levels are greater than 40 pg/mL. Therefore, these patients will usually have uterine bleeding following progesterone administration. If the serum PRL level is normal, no further diagnostic workup is necessary. There is usually a spontaneous recovery. An oral progestin (10 mg of medroxyprogesterone acetate) should be given for at least 12 days once every 60 days to induce uterine bleeding. A 2-month interval is chosen to allow time for the patient to have spontaneous menses. If withdrawal bleeding fails to occur in response to oral progestins and IM progesterone, the patient should undergo further investigation (step 3, Table 15-2).

Dysfunction or failure resulting from exercise

Published data have shown that the incidence of amenorrhea among a group of women engaged in collegiate cross-country running increased as the weekly training mileage increased (Figure 15-6).[11] This increase did not appear to be related to weight loss, but the frequency of amenorrhea did show a positive correlation with the number of months of intensive training per year. When these women stopped running, their normal menstrual cycles usually resumed. This is strong evidence that exercise-induced amenorrhea has its origin in the neurotransmitter-hypothalamic center. Therefore, an extensive pituitary evaluation is usually unnecessary.

It has been reported that strenuous exercise increases the level of catechol estrogens that in turn may reduce the rate of catecholamine degradation. This causes an increase in the availability of catecholamines to exert an effect in the hypothalamus.

The competition between catecholamine and catechol estrogens for catechol-O-methyl-

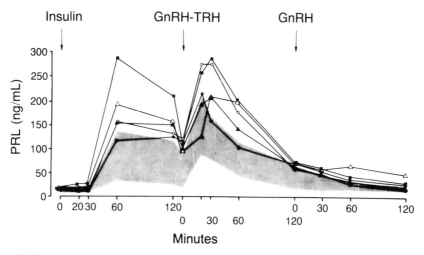

Figure 15-5
PRL levels during sequential stimulation testing on five subjects with long-term steroid ingestion. Shaded area indicates 95% confidence limits of control subjects.

From Mishell DR Jr, Kletzky OA, Brenner PF, et al: The effect of contraceptive steroids on hypothalamic-pituitary function. Am J Obstet Gynecol 128:60, 1977.

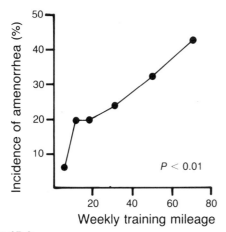

Figure 15-6
Correlation between training mileage and amenorrhea. Each point represents an average of 21 respondents. The statistical significance of the relationship was obtained by point-biserial correlation. (One mile = 1.6 km.)

From Feicht CB, Johnson TS, Martin BJ, et al: Secondary amenorrhea in athletes. Lancet 2:1145, 1978.

transferase results in increased levels of dopamine, which suppresses the release of GnRH and, thus, LH and PRL.[12] The decrease in serum PRL levels occurs in exercising amenorrheic women and not in eumenorrheic athletes.[13] In the latter, serum PRL levels increased soon after starting exercise, compared with resting levels. This acute increase in PRL may be the result of nipple stimulation by a garment and/or by movement of the breast during running.

It has also been reported that the natural opiates (endorphins) are elevated during strenuous exercise and may contribute to the development of amenorrhea.[14] The mechanism by which they do so has been said to be both a direct negative effect on GnRH secretion and a positive effect on dopamine secretion, which in turn suppresses GnRH release. This decrease in GnRH results in decrease in gonadotropin release and amenorrhea.[15]

Until recently, whether all patients with exercise-induced amenorrhea and low serum E_2 levels should be given estrogen replacement was controversial. There is no doubt that exercise-related amenorrhea is caused by reversible hypothalamic dysfunction or failure. Normal menses usually resume when the exercise is no longer a disturbing factor, and there is no danger of osteoporosis developing during a short period of amenorrhea. However, if the patient, regardless of her age, continues to exercise and remains amenorrheic with low levels of E_2, estrogen/progestin replacement therapy should be prescribed to prevent the reported decrease in bone density associated with low circulating estrogen levels.[16] These bone changes occurred in the vertebrae of amenorrheic athletes in their mid-20s.

Amenorrhea secondary to weight loss

It is probable that some patients with amenorrhea associated with acute weight loss also have a major stress factor. In many instances, it is impossible to isolate stress from weight loss as the sole cause of amenorrhea. Therefore, it should be kept in mind that there is most likely an overlap in etiology.

Simple weight loss

The CNS-hypothalamic-pituitary system appears to be extremely sensitive to environmental alterations, especially acute weight loss. Changes in reproductive capacity because of malnutrition are well documented in animal studies. Underfeeding has been reported to be directly related to reduced egg laying in hens, disturbed estrus cycles in rats, and ovarian atrophy in cats.[17] In the male, a decrease in both fertility and spermatogenesis has been reported to result from undernutrition.[18]

Age of menarche has been related to attainment of a critical body weight of 106 lb (48.2 kg).[17] More recently, this statement has been disputed with the contention that the critical level of body fat is probably different for each woman and probably changes during the various phases of life.[18] There is, nevertheless, evidence suggesting that the attainment and maintenance of normal cyclic reproductive function depend on a minimal weight per height.[19] In girls engaged in vigorous physical training, such as ballet dancing, a dichotomy in development has been noted. There is a normal pubarche but a marked delay in thelarche and menarche. This finding supports the hypothesis that the increase in adrenal androgen production occurring at the beginning of puberty is not affected by strenuous exercise and loss of body fat. In contrast, both breast development and menarche are estrogen-dependent and suppressed by loss of body fat.[19] In fact, higher-than-normal testosterone levels have been reported in thin female runners.[20] The source of increased testosterone may be decreased aromatization of androstenedione to E_2 due to the decrease in adipose tissue. Thus more androstenedione is converted to testosterone.

Weight loss related to amenorrhea may be either simple weight loss or true anorexia nervosa. The patients with simple weight loss have been divided into two groups: (1) the underweight, or those whose weight loss is below 15% to 25% of ideal body weight; and (2) the severely underweight, or those whose weight loss is greater than 25% of ideal body weight.[19] The serum E_2 levels of patients with simple weight loss can vary from low to normal. Therefore, such patients may or may not respond with uterine bleeding after the administration of progesterone. In contrast, it has been reported[21,22] that individuals with anorexia nervosa have serum E_2 levels below 10 pg/mL and therefore, based on published data from this institution,[4] will have no uterine bleeding following progesterone challenge.

In amenorrhea associated with weight loss, the administration of GnRH has been used in an effort to differentiate between hypothalamic and pituitary derangement. Patients who are severely underweight (including those with anorexia nervosa) have a blunted LH response and a lower-than-normal increase in FSH with GnRH stimulation, in comparison with the response seen in controls and amenorrheic patients who are only underweight (between 15% and 25% below ideal body weight). As these individuals regain their body weight, the FSH response to GnRH administration returns to normal in linear fashion, while the LH response returns to normal exponentially. When the response of patients with simple weight loss was compared with that of controls, it was found that only the peak LH response, not the FSH response, was delayed in the patients with simple weight loss.

Anorexia nervosa

Individuals with anorexia nervosa, besides being severely underweight, almost always have severe constipation, hypotension, bradycardia, and hypothermia. Invariably, they have an abnormal body image and aversion to food intake. The amenorrhea may occur before, during, or after the initiation of weight loss. Usually, it can be dated to the time the patient began her food restriction.[19,23] In rare cases, food aversion begins before onset of menarche, and the patient presents with primary amenorrhea.

To differentiate anorexia nervosa, a serious psychiatric disorder, from acute simple weight loss, measurement of serum triiodothyronine (T_3) by radioimmunoassay (RIA) can be used. Almost invariably, patients with anorexia nervosa have low serum T_3 in comparison with the normal T_3 levels observed in patients with simple weight loss. Thyroxine (T_4) levels in patients with anorexia nervosa may also be low but not as consistently as are the T_3 levels.

Kinetic studies of anorexia nervosa patients have shown that the time of peak LH, FSH, thyroid-stimulating hormone (TSH), and PRL response to GnRH and TRH administration is delayed compared with that of control subjects and patients with simple weight loss. All these abnormalities in endocrine functions have supported the conclusion that amenorrhea associated with weight loss is due primarily to a derangement of the hypothalamus. The defect appears to be more severe in anorexia nervosa than in simple weight loss.

The treatment in all cases appears to be primarily related to the regaining of body weight. When a patient regains her lost body weight, her endocrine abnormality corrects itself (Figure 15-7).[24] Although anorexia nervosa patients do have a hypothalamic derangement that causes amenorrhea, their primary disorder demands immediate psychiatric attention. These patients do not respond to lectures on the importance of good nutrition. It should be noted that in some patients with weight loss and amenorrhea, and in almost all patients with anorexia nervosa and hypothalamic or pituitary lesions, the levels of a single and randomly obtained serum FSH and LH may be normal despite the almost universally low circulating levels of serum E_2. With low serum E_2, the gonadotropin levels would be expected to be either below the normal range (hypogonadotropic hypogonadism) or above the normal range (hypergonadotropic hypogonadism). In a published report of hypoestrogenic amenorrheic patients, although a single value of LH could be in the normal range, when serum LH was measured every 15 minutes for 4 hours in the same patient, the LH pattern was flat, lacking the normal and prominent LH fluctuations (Figure 15-8).[2] When the area under the curve was calculated and compared with values seen in normal and menstruating women, it was found that patients with hypoestrogenic amenorrhea (negative withdrawal to progesterone challenge) were secreting approximately half as much LH as the normal subjects in the 4-hour period. Therefore, a single gonadotropin value within the normal range obtained in any patient with hypoestrogenic amenorrhea should be considered a "pseudonormal" value.

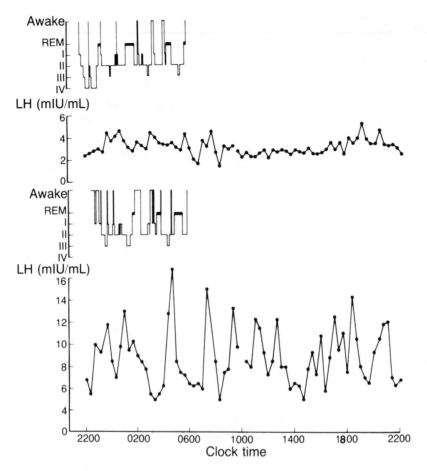

Figure 15-7
Plasma LH concentration every 20 minutes for 24 hours during acute exacerbation of anorexia nervosa (upper) and after clinical remission with a return of body weight to normal (lower). The latter panel shows a normal adult pattern.

From Boyer RM, Katz J, Finkelstein JW, et al: Anorexia nervosa: Immaturity of 24-hour luteinizing hormone secretory pattern. N Engl J Med 291:861, 1974.

CNS-hypothalamic failure

Lesions of the hypothalamus

These disorders are rare and may manifest as either primary or secondary amenorrhea. Hypothalamic lesions that have been associated with amenorrhea include craniopharyngioma, tuber-culous granuloma, and the sequelae of meningoencephalitis.

The cause of amenorrhea is most likely a lack of GnRH. These patients have low E_2 levels and will not have uterine bleeding following progesterone administration. The random serum FSH and LH levels are either low or "normal." Because the pituitary has not been primed by endogenous GnRH, many of these patients will not have a normal LH and FSH response following exogenous GnRH administration. After pretreatment, or priming, with exogenous GnRH, the pituitary will demonstrate a normal LH and FSH response. The diagnosis of a hypothalamic lesion may be made with computerized tomography (CT) scans or magnetic resonance imaging (MRI), also called nuclear magnetic resonance (NMR). The treatment is invariably directed toward the neurologic disorder and, if necessary, hormone replacement.

Idiopathic

In this type of disorder, the clinical presentation is hypogonadotropic hypogonadism with low levels of circulating E_2. There is no withdrawal uterine bleeding following administration of IM progesterone. The pituitary response to GnRH stimulation, after priming of the pituitary with GnRH, is normal. The CT scan is normal; there-

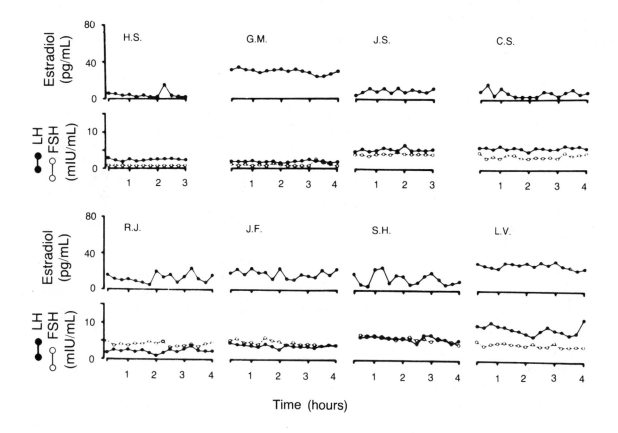

Figure 15-8
Serum LH, FSH, and estradiol (E_2) concentrations in samples obtained at 15-minute intervals from eight patients with failure of the hypothalamic-pituitary axis.

Reproduced, with permission, from Kletzky OA, Davajan V, Nakamura RM, et al: Classification of secondary amenorrhea based on distinct hormonal patterns. J Clin Endocrinol Metab 41:660, 1975.

fore, the diagnosis of idiopathic GnRH insufficiency is made by exclusion. These patients should be given estrogen/progestin replacement, because their serum E_2 levels are almost always below the physiologic levels necessary to maintain normal bone integrity.

CNS-hypothalamic-adreno-ovarian dysfunction (polycystic ovary syndrome)

It is now commonly, but not universally, accepted that patients with polycystic ovary syndrome (PCO) have a CNS-hypothalamic disorder that results in the histologic (polycystic) changes seen in the ovary. Because of this, PCO is now listed under hypothalamic causes of amenorrhea. (For a detailed discussion of PCO, see chapter 18.)

Most PCO patients present with oligomenorrhea, but some may have secondary amenorrhea or even primary amenorrhea. These patients usually have E_2 levels above 40 pg/mL. Therefore, they have uterine bleeding following IM administration of progesterone. Approximately 60% to 80% of patients with PCO have elevated serum LH values (about 25 mIU/mL) and low-normal levels of serum FSH (Figure 15-9).[25] The elevated LH value has been used to differentiate this disorder from hypothalamic dysfunction, in which serum levels of LH are normal. Although LH does have marked daily fluctuations, in patients with PCO a single measurement of LH is sufficient to make the diagnosis.[2] In our institution, the LH fluctuations were always found to be elevated within the 95% confidence limits for these patients. We found the early follicular phase LH values in normal ovulating women to be almost always (± 3 SD) under 25 mIU/mL (Figure 15-9).

Although the patients discussed in this chapter are amenorrheic without clinical evidence of androgen excess, the androgen levels in PCO patients with elevated serum LH may be high even in the absence of hirsutism. Therefore, we recommend baseline measurements of

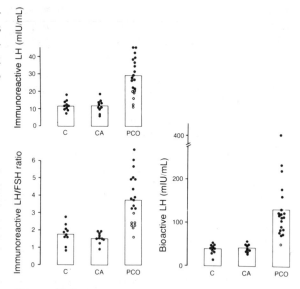

Figure 15-9
Serum measurements of immunoreactive LH, LH/FSH ratios, and bioactive LH in control subjects (C), women with chronic anovulation (CA) and women with PCO. Solid circles for women with PCO indicate values exceeding 3 SD of mean control levels.

Reproduced, with permission, from Lobo RA, Kletzky OA, Campeau JD, et al: Elevated bioactive luteinizing hormone in women with polycystic ovary syndrome. Fertil Steril 39:674, 1983.

serum testosterone and DHEA-S for these patients. If androgens are elevated, drugs that suppress androgen hypersecretion should be given.

If the patient desires pregnancy, clomiphene citrate is the therapy of choice. If the patient does not desire pregnancy, she should be given either therapy for suppression of androgen excess (dexamethasone, OCs, spironolactone) or be treated with cyclic progestin therapy. OCs are recommended only for patients in whom the major complaint is hirsutism. Cyclic progestin therapy is used to induce uterine bleeding and prevent unopposed estrogen effect on the endometrium, which may lead to either benign or atypical hyperplasia. A recommended mode of progestin therapy is 12 days of oral medroxyprogesterone acetate, 10 mg/day, each month.

Abnormal endocrinology

Pituitary etiology

Patients with amenorrhea of pituitary etiology may have nonneoplastic lesions or pituitary tumors. The most common pituitary lesion resulting in secondary amenorrhea is a PRL-secreting adenoma (Chapter 16). This chapter discusses several other pituitary adenomas.

Nonneoplastic lesions of the pituitary

Nonneoplastic pituitary lesions include those seen in Sheehan's syndrome (pregnancy-related) and Simmonds' syndrome (non-pregnancy related). The pituitary cells are damaged by anoxia, thrombosis, or hemorrhage. Because of low serum levels of LH, FSH, and E_2, withdrawal uterine bleeding will not occur following IM administration of progesterone.[4] Depending on the extent of pituitary destruction, many of these patients also have secondary hypothyroidism and adrenal insufficiency. When the pituitary is stimulated by insulin-induced hypoglycemia, levels of growth hormone (GH), PRL, and ACTH (as measured indirectly by the response of serum cortisol) may not show a normal rise (Figure 15-10).[26] Although we consider lack of cortisol response to hypoglycemia adequate for diagnosing ACTH insufficiency, it has been suggested that a metyrapone test (Chapter 21) be used before this diagnosis is made with certainty. Direct pituitary stimulation with GnRH/TRH will fail to evoke a normal response to LH, FSH, TSH, and PRL unless the pituitary is only partially destroyed (Figures 15-10 and 15-11).[26]

If the patient has a low free thyroxine index (FTI) and/or lacks a normal cortisol response, appropriate replacement therapy should be instituted. Thyroxine should be given starting at a dose of 0.05 mg/day for 2 weeks. It is then increased every 2 to 3 weeks by an increment of 0.05 mg until the patient is clinically and chemically euthyroid. The usual dose of hydrocortisone prescribed for replacement in cortisol insufficiency is 20 mg in the morning and 10 mg in

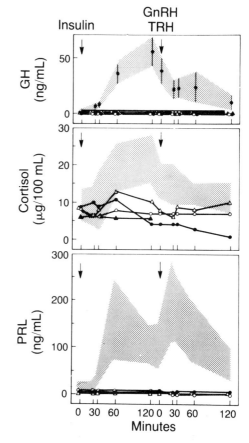

Figure 15-10
Pituitary stimulation in diagnosing Sheehan's syndrome.

Reproduced, with permission, from diZerega G, Kletzky OA, Mishell DR Jr: Diagnosis of Sheehan's syndrome using a sequential pituitary stimulation test. Am J Obstet Gynecol 132:348, 1978.

the late afternoon. All patients receiving cortisone therapy must be followed up very carefully to avoid overtreatment and the development of Cushing's syndrome. They should also be advised to carry appropriate identification, preferably permanently worn, to note their chronic cortisone therapy, and to inform all treating medical personnel.

Patients with hypogonadotropic hypogonadism need estrogen/progestin replacement therapy to prevent vaginal atrophy and osteopo-

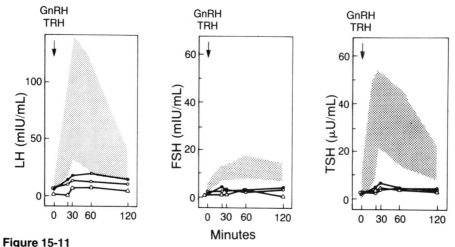

Figure 15-11
LH, FSH, and TSH response to GnRH-TRH administration in control subjects (shaded areas) and in three patients with Sheehan's syndrome.

Reproduced, with permission, from diZerega G, Kletzky OA, Mishell DR Jr: Diagnosis of Sheehan's syndrome using a sequential pituitary stimulation test. Am J Obstet Gynecol 132:348, 1978.

rosis. If the patient desires pregnancy, human menopausal gonadotropin (hMG) is the therapy of choice to induce ovulation. Clomiphene citrate is ineffective for inducing ovulation when circulating levels of E_2 are low, as in most patients with pituitary insufficiency.

Pituitary tumors

Amenorrhea may be the first symptom of a pituitary tumor. Chromophobe adenomas are the most common pituitary tumors reported in amenorrhea without galactorrhea. These tumors most often do not secrete hormones and therefore differ from the PRL-secreting adenomas associated with galactorrhea. Other types of pituitary tumors that secrete hormones are the basophilic and acidophilic adenomas. Patients with basophilic-cell tumors may have amenorrhea and clinical changes associated with excess cortisol production (Cushing's disease). The acidophilic adenomas usually produce the symptoms of gigantism or acromegaly.

Patients with amenorrhea resulting from pituitary tumors usually have very low E_2 levels (<40 pg/mL) and, therefore, do not have uterine bleeding after IM administration of progesterone. A random serum level of FSH and LH may be either low or normal. It was hoped that administration of GnRH would allow differentiation between amenorrheic patients with and without pituitary tumors. Unfortunately, this test has not been useful in determining whether a tumor is present. Many patients with proven tumors have normal gonadotropin responses; many without tumors have abnormal responses (Figure 15-12).[27] Therefore, the diagnosis of pituitary tumor has to be made by polytomography, CT scan, or MRI.

The treatment of choice in patients with nonsecreting pituitary adenomas is surgical resection, preferably transsphenoidal. The need for hormone-replacement therapy depends on the lack of specific hormones secreted by the pituitary after surgery.

In conclusion, there are four hypothalamic and two pituitary causes of amenorrhea. The patients with hypothalamic dysfunction, with or without a history of drug use or stress, and those with PCO most often have uterine bleeding after IM progesterone and, therefore, have a serum E_2 level of at least 40 pg/mL (Figure 15-2). Patients with hypothalamic or pituitary failure have serum E_2 levels below 40 pg/mL and will not have uterine bleeding after IM progesterone. Therefore, IM progesterone can be used as a bioassay for estrogenicity, instead of measuring serum E_2.

Random or even daily blood levels of LH and FSH will not differentiate between hypotha-

lamic dysfunction and hypothalamic or pituitary failure. But when blood samples are obtained at 15-minute intervals, there is a significant difference in both LH levels and the LH/FSH ratio between these two groups (Figure 15-3). Patients with dysfunction usually have LH intermittent peaks similar to those seen in normal controls, whereas patients with failure lack these intermittent peaks and, therefore, secrete less LH. This decreased amount of LH results in inadequate ovarian stimulation, decreased secretion of E_2, and inadequate proliferation of the endometrium. Therefore, patients with failure do not have uterine bleeding following progesterone administration, even though a single value of LH or

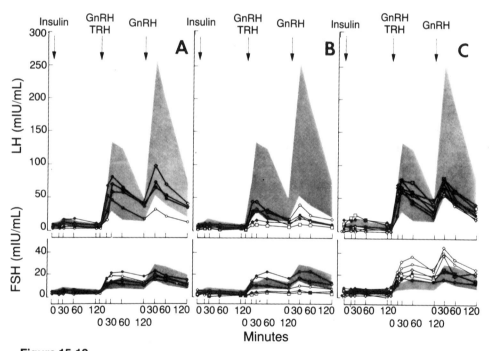

Figure 15-12
LH and FSH in control subjects (shaded areas), six patients with postpill amenorrhea-galactorrhea (C), and nine other patients with amenorrhea-galactorrhea and pituitary tumors (A and B).

Reproduced, with permission, from Kletzky OA, Davajan V, Mishell DR Jr, et al: A sequential pituitary stimulation test in normal subjects and in patients with amenorrhea-galactorrhea with pituitary tumors. J Clin Endocrinol Metab 45:631, 1977.

FSH may be within the normal range. The low serum E_2 levels that result from the absence of LH peaks are the basis for the use of the description: hypothalamic or pituitary "failure." In contrast, the term "dysfunction" refers to cases with normal serum E_2 levels and persistence of the periodic LH peaks. The functional behavior of this disorder is determined by the absence of a sustained rapid rise in E_2 that is needed to trigger the midcycle LH surge necessary to induce ovulation.

Ovarian etiology

Two different ovarian causes of amenorrhea are discussed in this section: (1) premature ovarian failure; and (2) loss of ovarian function secondary to castration, infection, hemorrhage, or compromised blood supply.

Premature ovarian failure

Premature ovarian failure (POF) has been arbitrarily defined as failure of ovarian estrogen production occurring in a hypergonadotropic state at any age between onset of menarche and 35. Some authors use 40 as the cutoff age for making the diagnosis. Biopsies obtained from the ovaries of these patients have two different histologic patterns: Some have marked generalized sclerosis similar to normal postmenopausal ovaries; others lack follicular development to the antrum stage, although primordial follicles can be seen (hypofolliculogenesis). The latter finding differs from that seen in patients with gonadal streaks, who have a total lack of follicles.

It would appear that there is a gradient between the number of follicles present. Some patients, such as those with gonadal streaks, have no follicles and present with primary amenorrhea. Others with POF are found to have either less than the normal complement of follicles or a normal number. Patients with hypofolliculogenesis can have either primary amenorrhea (with breast development) or secondary amenorrhea after only a few months or years of menstrual bleeding. Because autoantibodies against ovarian cytoplasm, as well as against other tissues such as thyroid and adrenal cortex, have been reported, a generalized autoimmune diathesis has been postulated as a potential cause of some cases of POF.[28] Ovarian enzymatic defects, such as 17-hydroxylase, desmolase, 3β-ol dehydrogenase, and 17-ketoreductase insufficiencies, have also been associated with ovarian failure.

Because the ovaries of patients with ovarian failure do not secrete sufficient amounts of E_2 to maintain the negative feedback on the hypothalamus, the gonadotropins are elevated into the postmenopausal range. Although gonadotropin levels do fluctuate, they are consistently elevated. A single serum FSH determination above 30 mIU/mL is usually adequate to make the diagnosis (Figure 15-13).[2] These patients will not have uterine bleeding following IM progesterone. Patients with secondary amenorrhea due to POF who are under age 25 should have a karyotype performed. To date, all such patients at this institution have had a 46,XX karyotype, but mosaicism has been reported by other investigators. We do not perform a karyotype on patients with secondary amenorrhea and POF after age 25 as it is rare for them to have a karyotype defect.

Because of the possibility that patients with POF may also have thyroid and/or adrenal insufficiency secondary to autoimmune disease, we screen all patients with this disorder under age 35 for thyroid antibodies. We obtain antithyroglobulin and antimicrosomal antibodies. The adrenal status is evaluated with a 24-hour urinary free cortisol level. We have not been testing these patients for the presence of ovarian antibodies, nor have we recommended that they undergo either laparoscopic or open ovarian biopsy to identify the exact nature of their follicular status.

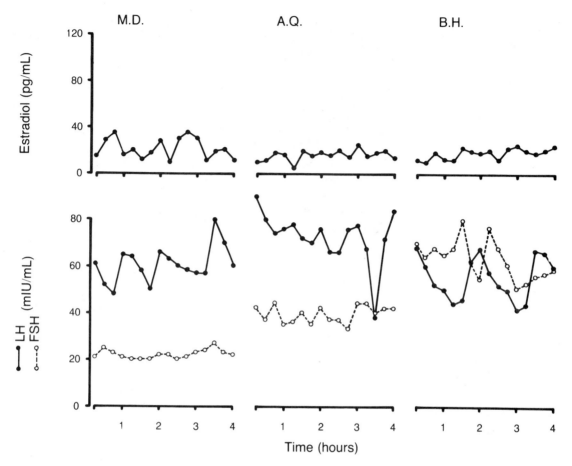

Figure 15-13
Serum LH, FSH, and estradiol (E₂) concentrations in samples obtained at 15-minute intervals from three patients with premature ovarian failure.

Reproduced, with permission, from Kletzky OA, Davajan V, Nakamura RM, et al: Classification of secondary amenorrhea based on distinct hormonal patterns. J Clin Endocrinol Metab 41:660, 1975. © 1975, The Endocrine Society.

With rare exceptions, ovulation cannot be induced with drugs in these patients. Therefore, they should be considered sterile and receive estrogen/progestin replacement therapy. It has been reported that in rare instances patients with elevated gonadotropins do have follicular development to the antrum stage. These patients have been described as having "insensitive ovaries" (Savage syndrome). There are sporadic reports of presumptive evidence of ovulation in some patients treated with extremely large doses of hMG. There is a report of a successful pregnancy in a patient with "insensitive ovaries" while having conjugated estrogen/progestin therapy.[29,30]

At our institution, patients with hypergonadotropic amenorrhea who desire a pregnancy are suppressed with high doses of conjugated estrogen (usually 5 mg/day). This is high enough to lower the serum FSH and LH values into the normal range. It usually takes at least 25 days to produce this effect. In the last 10 days (days 16 to 25), 10 mg of medroxyprogesterone acetate are added to the estrogen therapy. If the serum FSH on day 20 is found to be suppressed to a level below 15 mIU/mL, both drugs are stopped on the 25th day of therapy. If the FSH value is not in the normal range, we increase the estrogen dosage to 2.5 mg four times a day and stop the progestin. The FSH is rechecked in another 2 weeks. If the FSH is normal, we continue the estrogen and add 10 days of progestin therapy. After the drugs are stopped, the patient is instructed either to take her basal body temperature (BBT) for 30 days or to come to the office for weekly testing of serum progesterone values to see if ovulation has occurred. Using this "rebound" technique, it is hoped that these patients will ovulate when their gonadotropins begin to rise following discontinuation of estrogen/progestin therapy.

Loss of ovarian function secondary to castration, infection, or interference with blood supply

At our institution, two patients who had undergone bilateral cystectomies for dermoid cysts subsequently developed POF during their early 20s. On occasion, patients with severe bilateral tubo-ovarian abscesses respond well to antibiotic therapy and do not require surgical treatment. In rare instances, the infection completely destroys the ovarian tissue. In some patients, following hysterectomy, the ovarian blood supply is so compromised that the result is "cystic degeneration." Usually this process is unilateral and does not cause ovarian failure. However, it may occur bilaterally or in the only remaining ovary and halt ovarian function.

Because of the lack of ovarian steroids, the negative feedback to the hypothalamus is lost, and serum gonadotropin levels are elevated into the menopausal range. The loss of ovarian estrogen production leads to an atrophic endometrium. Thus, these patients do not have uterine bleeding following IM progesterone administration. They are sterile and need estrogen/progestin replacement therapy.

Uterine etiology

Before all the diagnoses of secondary amenorrhea can be considered and the appropriate laboratory tests ordered, uterine etiology must be considered and ruled out. The formation of uterine synechiae, described by Asherman, has usually been associated with dilatation and curettage (performed either in pregnancy or postpartum) and with endometritis. This condition has also been seen following myomectomy and metroplasty. In addition, three cases of total uterine cavity obliteration following cesarean sections have been seen, in which the anterior uterine wall was sutured to the posterior wall during closure of the uterine incision. The patients' postoperative fevers responded to antibiotic therapy and no probing of the cervix or endometrial cavity was attempted. The infection caused the endometrial cavity obliteration.

In some patients with partial intrauterine synechiae, uterine bleeding can be induced with estrogen/progestin therapy. Therefore, the use of estrogen/progestin as a challenge test is not always definitive in establishing the diagnosis of end-organ failure. When Asherman's syndrome is suggested by history, the patient should have an evaluation of the uterine cavity by either hysterosalpingography or hysteroscopy. Only after the uterine factor is ruled out is the endocrine workup indicated. Patients with uterine causes of amenorrhea have normal endocrine function and thus will have evidence of ovulation, e.g.: biphasic BBT graphs and/or elevated levels of serum progesterone.

Establishing the etiology of secondary amenorrhea

For a simplified and systematic approach to the workup of patients with secondary amenorrhea, the uterine factor (including pregnancy) must first be considered and ruled out. If the patient is not pregnant and does not have a history compatible with Asherman's syndrome, the workup should be started with a careful history. Special attention should be paid to possible drug ingestion or stress. A complete blood count, urinalysis, TSH determination, and at least one fasting blood sugar should be obtained. If the patient has any signs or symptoms of hyperthyroidism, T_4 and T_3 determinations by RIA and an FTI should be obtained.

Following these tests, a progesterone challenge should be performed to determine estrogen status (Table 15-2). This test has made it possible to divide patients with amenorrhea into two major categories. The progesterone challenge test is step 1 in the differential diagnosis.

The positive or negative response of the endometrium to 100 or 200 mg of IM progesterone in oil correlates well with the levels of serum E_2. In place of IM progesterone, an oral progestin (medroxyprogesterone acetate) can be used (30 mg/day for 3 days or 10 mg/day for 5 to 7 days). If withdrawal uterine bleeding occurs, the IM progesterone challenge is unnecessary. However, if bleeding does not occur following oral progestin, IM progesterone should be used before assigning the patient to the negative-response category. If there is no withdrawal bleeding within 2 weeks after 100 mg of IM progesterone, 200 mg of IM progesterone should be tried. In patients with withdrawal uterine bleeding (positive response), the E_2 value is usually greater than 40 pg/mL (Figure 15-2). In patients who fail to respond to the progesterone challenge, the E_2 value is usually below 40 pg/mL.

For the progesterone challenge test to be considered positive, uterine bleeding must occur. The amount of bleeding does not appear to be a factor, because it has been reported that even in women with normal estrogen levels only minimal spotting may occur.

At this institution, it was found that approximately two-thirds of patients with amenorrhea have uterine bleeding following IM progesterone; the rest have a negative response.[4] In patients who had uterine bleeding, we measured serum LH and FSH and analyzed the results by linear transform (probit analysis). LH values were found to be composed of two populations, one high and one normal; whereas the FSH levels revealed only one population. Because of this finding, we recommend a single LH determination in patients who have uterine bleeding after progesterone challenge. The results of the LH test further divide the patient population into two subgroups (step 2, Table 15-2).

A serum LH value over 25 mIU/mL is highly suggestive of PCO. Serum testosterone and DHEA-S should be measured in these patients. If the testosterone is elevated, its secretion can be suppressed with OCs. Preparations with 30 to 35 µg of ethinylestradiol are adequate. If the patient has an elevated DHEA-S, she should receive dexamethasone, 0.5 mg/day at bedtime, for 30 days. Then the dose should be lowered to 0.25 mg/day at bedtime.

In most instances, patients with normal LH values have hypothalamic dysfunction. In these patients, serum PRL levels should be obtained even in the absence of galactorrhea. If PRL is found to be elevated, the patient should have a total pituitary workup as outlined in Chapter 16 If the PRL level is normal, uterine withdrawal bleeding should be induced with oral medroxyprogesterone acetate (10 mg/day for 12 days every 30 to 60 days) or progesterone in oil (100 or 200 mg IM every 1 to 2 months) if the patient does not desire pregnancy.

The uterine withdrawal bleeding is recommended to prevent uninterrupted stimulation of the endometrium by E_2 produced by the ovary. In addition, some patients with hypothalamic dysfunction, if followed for a long enough time, may stop having withdrawal bleeding and present as patients in the failure group (step 3). Therefore, all women in the CNS-hypothalamic dysfunction group should have a progesterone (or oral progestin) challenge every 60 days. If withdrawal bleeding does not occur, a complete pituitary workup is indicated. As long as patients remain in the dysfunctional group and have normal serum PRL levels, it is unnecessary to perform x-ray studies or CT scans of the sella turcica, unless galactorrhea is present. If pregnancy is desired, patients with either PCO or hypothalamic dysfunction should be treated with clomiphene citrate (see Chapter 23).

We have reported that a single serum FSH level (but not LH level) in patients who do not have uterine bleeding following IM progesterone can identify two distinct populations. One group will have a low or pseudonormal serum FSH level, and the other an elevated FSH value. Those with low serum FSH levels have hypothalamic-pituitary failure; those with an elevated value have ovarian failure (step 3 of Table 15-2).

The term "hypothalamic pituitary failure" describes patients who have low E_2 secretion and therefore have no uterine bleeding following progesterone challenge. All patients with hypothalamic-pituitary failure (except those with failure secondary to drug ingestion, severe weight loss, stress, or exercise who have normal serum PRL levels) should have complete pituitary workups to determine whether a pituitary tumor is present. The evaluation should include a CT scan or MRI of the sella turcica and a serum PRL. If the CT scan reveals an adenoma with suprasellar extension, a visual-field examination should be obtained to ascertain if there is any optic nerve compression. If no tumor is found and failure of withdrawal bleeding persists, serum PRL levels should be measured every 6 to 12 months, because a radiographically undetectable microadenoma may be present.

The workup of women who develop amenorrhea related to simple weight loss, stress, drug ingestion, or exercise is directed primarily to establishing the degree of hypoestrogenicity that may exist and whether there is an undetected pathologic state unrelated to the listed contributing factors. If the patient has a serum PRL level of less than 20 ng/mL, the status of the sella turcica is not evaluated. If the patient is found to be hyperprolactinemic, then she should have a complete pituitary workup. In the euprolactinemic patient, the estrogen status should be determined since, as stated earlier, hypoestrogen status can be associated with decreased regional bone mass and early onset of osteoporosis.[16] If the patient has any amount of uterine bleeding following progesterone or progestin challenge, it can be assumed that her serum E_2 level is above 40 pg/mL and no estrogen replacement should be given. However, if the patient does not have withdrawal uterine bleeding following progesterone challenge, then a serum E_2 level should be obtained; and if the level is below 20 or 30 pg/mL, then estrogen/progestin replacement should be initiated. We recommend conjugated estrogen replacement of 0.625 mg/day given from day 1 to 25 of the month. On days 14 to 25, medroxyprogesterone acetate (Provera) 10 mg/mL should be given to avoid an unopposed estrogen effect on the endometrium and breast tissue. We have arbitrarily decided to start all hypoestrogenic amenorrheic women on estrogen/progestin therapy at age 17, since by this age most hormonally normal women have gone through menarche. This is a rather rigorous and aggressive management of these young amenorrheic women, somewhat different from our approach in the past because of the most recent published information.

All patients with x-ray, CT scan, or MRI abnormalities or a history compatible with Sheehan's syndrome should have an insulin-induced hypoglycemia test for determining pituitary GH, PRL, and ACTH reserve. The ACTH re-

Abnormal endocrinology

serve is determined indirectly by measuring the response of serum cortisol to hypoglycemia. It is the hypoglycemia, and not the insulin, that stimulates the hypothalamus and thereby mediates the pituitary hormone response.

The standard IV dose of insulin is 0.15 U/kg of body weight. A decrease in blood glucose levels of at least 50% of baseline value must be achieved to avoid false-negative results. If the blood glucose levels do not fall at least 50%, a larger dose of insulin should be given. A physician must always be present when this test is being performed, and the patient must be fed after completion of the test and before leaving the hospital. Blood samples are obtained at 0, 30, 60, and 120 minutes after administration of insulin. For results from this test to be considered normal, an increase in serum levels of GH of at least 18 ng/mL and of cortisol of 6 μg/100 mL should be obtained. The maximum response for both these hormones usually occurs between 60 and 120 minutes.

Metyrapone testing has been recommended before the diagnosis of ACTH insufficiency is made in patients with an abnormal cortisol response to hypoglycemia. Metyrapone is a synthetic drug that has the unique property of selectively inhibiting 11β-hydroxylation, an essential step in the biosynthesis of the three main corticosteroids—cortisol, corticosterone, and aldosterone. With the block in the production of cortisol, the inhibiting effect of cortisol on ACTH is removed. Therefore, the circulating levels of ACTH increase. This increase stimulates the adrenal cortex to produce more of the precursors to cortisol, corticosterone, and aldosterone, namely, 11-deoxycorticosterone and 11-deoxycortisol.

Metyrapone normally will produce a two- to fourfold increase in urinary 17-hydroxycorticosteroids above baseline value (see Chapter 21) on the day of administration (day 2) or the day after (day 3). This increase does not occur in patients with limited ACTH reserve. We do not think that this test adds any further information to that obtained from insulin-induced hypoglycemia and do not advocate its use.

Patients with pituitary failure who do not have demonstrable pituitary tumors and wish to conceive should be treated with ovulation-inducing drugs. Because these patients have very low levels of estrogen, they rarely respond to clomiphene citrate alone. It is recommended that induction of ovulation be first attempted with 250 mg/day of clomiphene given for 5 days, followed in 1 week with human chorionic gonadotropin (hCG), 5,000 U IM. If the patient fails to ovulate following this regimen, therapy with hMG should be initiated (see Chapter 23).

Patients with ovarian failure are easily diagnosed, because they invariably fail to respond to progesterone challenge and have high serum FSH values. On rare instances, they may have an abnormal karyotype, usually a mosaic of X/XX variety. Because of this, we recommend that all of these patients under age 25 have a karyotype. In addition, as stated earlier, because of the rare possibility that patients with premature ovarian failure may also have thyroid and/or adrenal insufficiency secondary to autoimmune disease, we recommend that all patients under age 35 with ovarian failure have thyroid antibodies measured and their adrenal status evaluated with a 24-hour urinary free cortisol. Until more information becomes available, we are not recommending laparoscopic or open ovarian biopsy to evaluate the patient's follicular status.

Patients with premature ovarian failure most often will not respond to any form of ovulation-inducing drug therapy, are therefore sterile, and should be given estrogen/progestin replacement therapy to prevent osteoporosis. The recommended regimen of estrogen replacement is 0.625 mg of conjugated estrogen for the first 25 days of each month with a 5- to 6-day drug-free interval. A progestin should be added during the last 12 days of estrogen intake (days 16 to 25). If the patient insists on trying to conceive, then gonadotropin suppression is attempted with high doses of estrogen, as described earlier.

In summary, a logical and categoric differential diagnosis of secondary amenorrhea has been presented (excluding patients who may have androgen or cortisol excess or galactorrhea). The least possible number of laboratory tests have been utilized in making the correct diagnosis.

References

1. Asherman JG: Traumatic intrauterine adhesions and their effects on fertility. *Int J Fertil* 2:49, 1957

2. Kletzky OA, Davajan V, Nakamura RM, et al: Classification of secondary amenorrhea based on distinct hormonal patterns. *J Clin Endocrinol Metab* 41:660, 1975

3. Kletzky OA, Mishell DR Jr, Davajan V, et al: Pituitary stimulation test in amenorrheic patients with normal or low estradiol. *Acta Endocrinol* 87:456, 1978

4. Kletzky OA, Davajan V, Nakamura RM, et al: Clinical categorization of patients with secondary amenorrhea using progesterone-induced uterine bleeding and measurement of serum gonadotropin levels. *Am J Obstet Gynecol* 121:695, 1975

5. Crowley WF, Filicori M, Spratt DI, et al: The physiology of gonadotropin-releasing hormone (GnRH) secretion in men and women. In *Recent Progress in Hormone Research*. Academic Press, 1985, p 473

6. Scott JZ, Brenner PF, Kletzky OA, et al: Factors affecting pituitary gonadotropin function in users of oral contraceptive steroids. *Am J Obstet Gynecol* 130:817, 1978

7. Scott JZ, Kletzky OA, Brenner PF, et al: Comparison of the effects of contraceptive steroid formulations containing two doses of estrogen on pituitary function. *Fertil Steril* 30:141, 1978

8. Mishell DR Jr, Kletzky OA, Brenner PF, et al: The effect of contraceptive steroids on hypothalamic-pituitary function. *Am J Obstet Gynecol* 128:60, 1977

9. Fries H, Nillus SJ, Pettersson F: Epidemiology of secondary amenorrhea: A retrospective evaluation of etiology with special regard to psychogenic factors and weight loss. *Am J Obstet Gynecol* 118:473, 1974

10. Bowman LA, Dilly SR, Keverne EB: Suppression of oestrogen-induced LH surge by social subordination in Talapoin monkeys. *Nature* 275:56, 1978

11. Feicht CB, Johnson TS, Martin BJ, et al: Secondary amenorrhea in athletes. *Lancet* 2:1145, 1978

12. Russell JB, Mitchell DE, Musey PI, et al: The role of β-endorphins and catechol estrogens on the hypothalamic-pituitary axis in female athletes. *Fertil Steril* 42:690, 1984

13. Loucks AB, Horvath SM: Exercise-induced stress responses of amenorrheic and eumenorrheic runners. *J Clin Endocrinol Metab* 59:1109, 1984

14. Gold MS, Redmond DE, Donabedian RK: Effects of opiate agonist and antagonist on serum prolactin in primates. Possible role of endorphins in prolactin regulation. *Endocrinology* 105:284, 1979

15. Reid RL, Hoff JD, Yen SSC, et al: Effects of exogenous β-endorphin on pituitary hormone secretion and its disappearance rate in normal human subjects. *J Clin Endocrinol Metab* 52:1179, 1981

16. Drinkwater BL, Nilson K, Chesnut CH, et al: Bone mineral content of amenorrheic and eumenorrheic athletes. *N Engl J Med* 311:277, 1984

17. Frisch RE: Nutrition, fatness and fertility. The effect of food intake on reproductive ability. In Mosley WH (ed), *Nutrition and Human Reproduction*. New York, Plenum Press, 1978, p 106

18. Moustgaard J: Nutritive influence upon reproduction. *J Reprod Med* 7:275, 1971

19. Warren MP, Vande Wiele RL: Clinical and metabolic features of anorexia nervosa. *Am J Obstet Gynecol* 117:435, 1973

20. Dale E, Gerlach DH, White AL: Menstrual dysfunction in distance runners. *Obstet Gynecol* 54:47, 1979

21. Vigersky RA, Loriaux DL, Anderson AE, et al: Delayed pituitary hormone response to LRF and TRF in patients with anorexia nervosa and simple weight loss. *J Clin Endocrinol Metab* 43:893, 1976

22. Vigersky RA, Anderson AE, Thompson RH, et al: Hypothalamic dysfunction in secondary amenorrhea associated with simple weight loss. *N Engl J Med* 297:1141, 1977

23. Crisp AH: Clinical and therapeutic aspects of anorexia nervosa—A study of 30 cases. *J Psychosom Res* 9:67, 1965

24. Boyer RM, Katz J, Finkelstein JW, et al: Anorexia nervosa: Immaturity of 24-hour luteinizing hormone secretory pattern. *N Engl J Med* 291:861, 1974

25. Lobo RA, Kletzky OA, Campeau JD, et al: Elevated bioactive luteinizing hormone in women with polycystic ovary syndrome. *Fertil Steril* 39:674, 1983

26. diZerega G, Kletzky OA, Mishell DR Jr: Diagnosis of Sheehan's syndrome using a sequential pituitary stimulation test. *Am J Obstet Gynecol* 132:348, 1978

27. Kletzky OA, Davajan V, Mishell DR Jr, et al: A sequential pituitary stimulation test in normal subjects and in patients with amenorrhea-galactorrhea with pituitary tumors. *J Clin Endocrinol Metab* 45:631, 1977

28. Alper MM, Garner PR: Premature ovarian failure: Its relationship to autoimmune disease. *Obstet Gynecol* 66:27, 1985

29. Shangold MM, Turksoy RN, Bashford RA, et al: Pregnancy following the "insensitive ovary syndrome." *Fertil Steril* 28:1179, 1977

30. Aiman J, Smentek C: Premature ovarian failure. *Obstet Gynecol* 66:9, 1985

Chapter 16

Hyperprolactinemia

Diagnosis and Treatment

Oscar A. Kletzky, M.D.
Val Davajan, M.D.

In the past decade, growth hormone (GH) and prolactin (PRL) were identified as separate hormones.[1] Following the isolation and purification of human PRL, a sensitive and specific radioimmunoassay (RIA) was developed.[2,3] Although GH, PRL, and human placental lactogen (hPL) are homologous hormones (belonging to the somatomammotropin family) and are considered to have lactogenic properties, only PRL is specifically related to milk production in humans.

PRL is a polypeptide hormone with 198 amino acids and a molecular weight of 22,000 daltons. It is secreted in different molecular sizes. The monomeric ("small") form is the active hormone and represents about 80% of the secreted forms. The biologic effect of the polymeric ("big" and "big-big") forms needs to be elucidated. These forms may simply represent an aggregation of monomeric molecules. PRL circulates unbound in serum and has a 20-minute half-life. It is cleared by the liver and the kidney. PRL is secreted by the lactotrophs in the anterior pituitary. They are clearly distinguished by differential staining from the somatotrophs, which secrete GH.[4] Furthermore, only the number of lactotrophs show marked increase during pregnancy and the puerperium in women and rhesus monkeys. Ultrastructural studies have shown that during pregnancy, rat lactotrophs accumulate secretory granules and deplete their granules following suckling.[5]

PRL is synthesized in the ribosomes and rough endoplasmic reticulum of the lactotrophs, concentrated in the Golgi apparatus, and stored in the form of granules in the cytoplasm, ready to be released. During the secretory process, these granules are released from the cells, either singly or in small groups, by exocytosis. During the process of exocytosis, the individual cell membrane fuses with the membrane surrounding the hormone granules.[6] Such fusion allows the granular content to dissolve into the extracellular space.

Secretion of PRL from the pituitary is controlled mainly by the inhibitory action of dopamine.[7] Dopamine was initially considered to be a prolactin-inhibiting factor (PIF). In vitro studies, using synaptosomal preparations of rat median eminence, suggest that dopamine regulates its own secretion by exerting intraneuronal negative feedback on the conversion of tyrosine to dopamine.[8] Also, dopamine turnover in the median eminence is increased in conditions associated with elevated PRL levels. Thus, the regulatory mechanism for PRL secretion may be controlled only by dopamine and PRL itself.

Alternatively, there may be a separate direct or indirect stimulatory pathway for PRL release

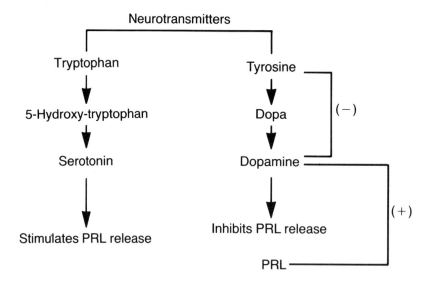

Figure 16-1
Most important pathways controlling the secretion of PRL.

modulated by the secretion of serotonin. It is now clear that activation of the CNS-serotonergic pathway results in an increase in PRL release. This stimulatory effect of serotonin on PRL release occurs even in the presence of very high levels of IV dopamine.[9] Thus, a balance may exist between dopamine and serotonin activity in regulating the secretion of PRL (Figure 16-1). Dopamine is the dominant regulatory factor, whereas serotonin may be necessary for maintaining baseline levels of circulating PRL. If the suppressive effect of dopamine is unopposed by the stimulatory effect of serotonin, we would expect total inhibition of PRL, resulting in undetectable serum levels. In normal humans, PRL is always detectable. Thyrotropin-releasing hormone (TRH), thought in the past to be a PRL-releasing factor, is effective in inducing the release of PRL when infused. However, it appears to control the secretion of PRL only minimally in normal individuals.[10,11]

Physiologic factors affecting the secretion of prolactin

PRL is secreted in a circadian rhythm in both men and women.[12] The circadian rhythm of PRL is sleep-related.[13] It increases shortly after the onset of sleep in both men and women, with a maximum release between 3 and 5 AM (Figure 16-2). The mean PRL values measured in the same person in the afternoon hours are significantly higher ($P < 0.05$) than those measured in the morning. Because of this periodicity, it is recommended that when hyperprolactinemia is suspected, the serum sample for measuring PRL be obtained between 8 AM and 12 noon, to allow the PRL concentration to decline after the nocturnal rise. Serum PRL concentration reaches its highest value during the reproductive life of a woman. Although baseline serum PRL increases from the follicular (up to 20 ng/mL) to the luteal

Abnormal endocrinology

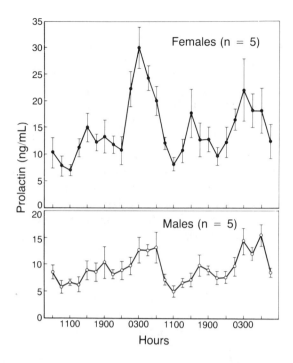

Figure 16-2
Hour-to-hour variation of serum PRL concentration in normal women and men studied throughout 48 consecutive hours.

phase (up to 30 ng/mL), this difference is not statistically significant.

Prolactin has both a mammogenic and a lactogenic action on the mammary gland. Although in some animal species, adrenal steroids, estrogens, growth hormone, and thyroxine are necessary for milk production, in the human only PRL and estrogens have a significant effect. It has been suggested that the significant increase of serum PRL observed during pregnancy is the result of increased levels of estrogens.[14] Furthermore, we reported that serum estradiol (E_2) increases from a mean of about 2.0 ng/mL in the first trimester to a mean value of about 40 ng/mL during the third trimester.[15] These high concentrations of E_2 induce hyperplasia and hy-

pertrophy of the lactotrophs, which in turn produce a significant increase of PRL, from <20 ng/mL in the nonpregnant state to a mean value of about 200 ng/mL during the third trimester (Figure 16-3).[15] The functional capacity of the lactotrophs has been shown to be preserved during pregnancy and the puerperium. During pregnancy, it is possible to stimulate the release of PRL with TRH from an already elevated PRL baseline (Figure 16-4).[15]

PRL concentrations are affected by various environmental factors. Therefore, PRL should be considered a stress hormone. One of the most dramatic environmental stimuli for inducing PRL release is major surgery with general anesthesia.[16] The intimate mechanism involved in the release of PRL during stress, exercise, or any other environmental factor has not yet been clarified. The presence of a peripheral neuroendocrine reflex responsible for the increase of PRL has been shown in experiments where tac-

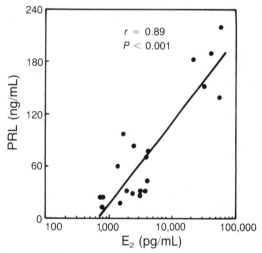

Figure 16-3
Correlation between plasma PRL and E_2 values during first, second, and third trimesters of pregnancy.

Reproduced, with permission, from Kletzky OA, Marrs RP, Howard WF, et al: Prolactin synthesis and release during pregnancy and puerperium. Am J Obstet Gynecol 136:545, 1980.

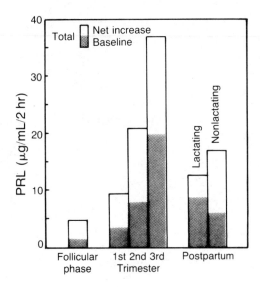

Figure 16-4
Area under the curve for plasma PRL response to TRH administration in pregnant women.

Reproduced, with permission, from Kletzky OA, Marrs RP, Howard WF, et al: Prolactin synthesis and release during pregnancy and puerperium. Am J Obstet Gynecol 136:545, 1980.

mation of Δ^5-steroids.[21] Infusion of dopamine in normal men significantly inhibited serum PRL. This was followed 16 hours later by a significant decrement of DHEA-S, but not of cortisol. This effect was maintained for the 48 hours during which dopamine was given. After the infusion was discontinued, PRL rebounded to levels higher than baseline, and DHEA-S returned to baseline values 16 hours later.

The chronic administration of bromocriptine to women with hyperprolactinemia results in the lowering of not only PRL but also DHEA-S after 3 weeks of treatment. Because it is known that there are PRL receptor sites in the adrenal gland, the above results indicate a direct effect of PRL on the adrenal secretion of DHEA-S. Furthermore, women with hyperprolactinemia were found to have elevated levels of androstenedione, but significantly lower total serum testosterone, androstenediol, dehydrotestosterone (DHT), and sex hormone-binding globulin (SHBG)-binding capacity.[22] However, unbound testosterone and unbound androstenediol levels

tile stimulation of the breast and nipple induced a significant increase of PRL (Figure 16-5).[17,18] This mechanism explains the significant increase in serum PRL 20 to 30 minutes following the initiation of breast-feeding.[19] Although sexual intercourse increases PRL secretion in some women, its intimate mechanism is unknown. It has also been found that an acute release of serum PRL and cortisol occurs following a high-protein meal at lunch, but not at breakfast.[20] It was further reported that high-fat meals, but not carbohydrates, caused release of serum PRL. It has been postulated that a link may exist between gastrointestinal hormones and the hypothalamic-pituitary system.

It has been reported that PRL has a modulatory effect on dehydroepiandrosterone sulfate (DHEA-S), perhaps by stimulating the 3-β-ol dehydrogenase enzyme and thus favoring the for-

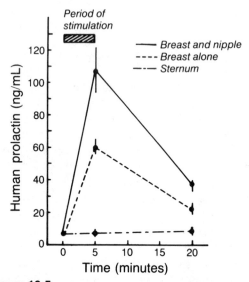

Figure 16-5
Serum prolactin response to tactile breast stimulation in normal women.

were elevated. The ratios of total and unbound testosterone to DHT were also found to be elevated. These results suggest that there is reduced 5α-reductase activity in hyperprolactinemia. This activity is normalized along with the rest of hormonal changes after hyperprolactinemia is corrected.

Symptoms and signs related to hyperprolactinemia

Galactorrhea is the most frequently observed abnormality associated with hyperprolactinemia. Galactorrhea is defined as a nonpuerperal watery or milky breast secretion that contains neither pus nor blood. The secretion may be manifested spontaneously or obtained only by breast examination. It usually is bilateral, but can be present in only one breast. Galactorrhea has the same pathophysiologic significance, whether it is reported by the patient, found during examination, or present in only one breast. The important factor is the presence or absence of milk, not the amount of secretion. Both breasts should be gently examined by expressing the gland from the periphery to the nipple. To ascertain the quality of the secretion and to determine the presence of true galactorrhea (milk), a smear is prepared and examined microscopically. If multiple fat droplets are present, the secretion contains milk (Figure 16-6).

Besides galactorrhea, hyperprolactinemia frequently, but not always, causes oligomenorrhea or amenorrhea. The mechanism(s) of menstrual irregularities varies with the etiology of hyperprolactinemia. Drugs affecting the normal pathway of dopamine secretion can produce amenorrhea by altering the secretion of norepinephrine, which is produced by the hydroxylation of dopamine. Because norepinephrine seems to be the most important neurotransmitter controlling the synthesis and secretion of GnRH, and thereby LH and FSH, any derange-

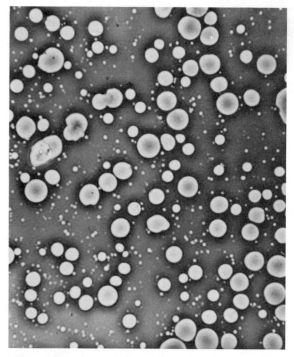

Figure 16-6
Fat droplets seen under the microscope from a patient with galactorrhea.

ment in its synthesis or secretion can result in menstrual abnormalities.

It has been suggested that hyperprolactinemia, either idiopathic or induced by a PRL-secreting pituitary adenoma, can result in primary or secondary amenorrhea by affecting the secretion of GnRH. If this is the case, the synthesis and secretion of LH and FSH should be inhibited. However, when patients with such disorders are stimulated with exogenous GnRH, levels of LH and FSH rise above normal. This rise suggests that rates of gonadotropin synthesis are preserved, but that abnormally low amounts are released and exceptionally high levels are stored, compared with baseline conditions. Therefore, it is possible that hyperprolactinemia inhibits only the release of LH and FSH by an ultrashort, intrapituitary-loop, negative feedback. This negative feedback can be overcome with exogenous GnRH, which will result in greater than normal release of gonadotropins.

It has also been reported that hyperprolactinemia can interfere with ovulation and normal corpus luteum formation by acting directly on the ovary. However, ovulation has been induced in pregnant monkeys with physiologic hyperprolactinemia. Also, we have reported that women with hyperprolactinemia due to a pituitary adenoma can secrete significantly higher than baseline levels of serum estradiol after GnRH administration.[23] When treated with bromocriptine, they can ovulate and become pregnant even in the presence of up to 50 ng/mL of serum PRL.

Hyperprolactinemia in men has been reported to diminish libido and induce impotence, but very rarely cause galactorrhea. It is usually produced by a long-standing pituitary adenoma. Because those symptoms occur late in the disease process, a macroadenoma is already present when the diagnosis is made.

Pharmacologic agents affecting the secretion of prolactin

Several pharmacologic agents can increase PRL concentration and induce galactorrhea (Table 16-1). Drug-induced hyperprolactinemia appears to be the most common etiology of nonphysiologic galactorrhea and/or hyperprolactinemia (Figure 16-7). Drugs that have been shown to produce hyperprolactinemia include tranquilizers, antihypertensive agents, narcotics, and oral contraceptive steroids. The major tranquilizers most commonly associated with hyperprolactinemia are the phenothiazines.[24] Other tranquilizers, such as chlordiazepoxide HCl and diazepam, may also cause hyperprolactinemia if taken for long periods. Tranquilizers induce hyperprolactinemia by depleting the hypothala-

Table 16-1
Pharmacologic agents affecting prolactin concentrations

Stimulators	Inhibitors
Anesthetics	L-Dopa
Psychotropics:	Dopamine
Phenothiazines	Bromocriptine
Tricyclic antidepressants	
Opiates	
Hormones:	
Estrogen	
Oral steroid contraceptives	
Thyrotropin-releasing hormone	
Antihypertensives:	
α-Methyldopa	
Reserpine	
Antiemetics:	
Sulpiride	
Metoclopramide	

mus of catecholamines or by blocking binding sites for catecholamines. This lowers the levels of dopamine or interferes with its action, which in turn deprives the pituitary of its natural inhibitor and results in the increase of PRL (Figure 16-7). Other drugs associated with causing hyperprolactinemia include tricyclic antidepressants, which block catecholamine reuptake, and propranolol, phentolamine, haloperidol, and cyproheptadine, which block hypothalamic catecholamine receptors.

Antihypertensive drugs known to cause hyperprolactinemia include reserpine and methyldopa. Reserpine depletes the catecholamines and methyldopa acts as a false neurotransmitter, thus blocking the conversion of tyrosine to dihydroxyphenylalanine (dopa). A patient with galactorrhea who is using a tranquilizer, an amphetamine, or oral contraceptive (OC) should be encouraged to discontinue the medication for at least one month. She should then be reevaluated. If galactorrhea persists, serum PRL should be measured. If the patient is taking a major

Abnormal endocrinology

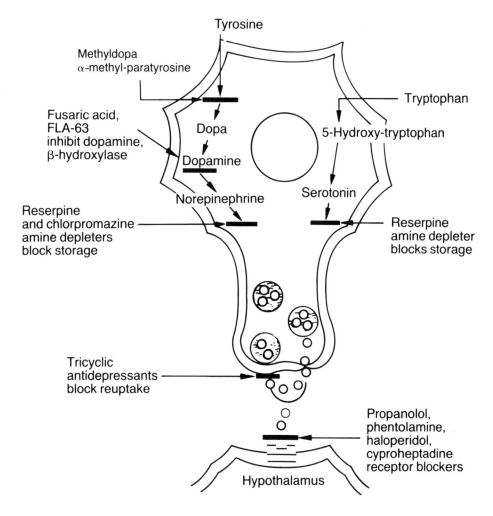

Figure 16-7
Schematic representation of inhibitory effects of drugs on synthesis and release of neurotransmitters.

tranquilizer or antihypertensive drug and cannot interrupt the medication, serum PRL should be measured and, if necessary, additional tests performed as described below to establish the cause of the galactorrhea.

About 50% of patients using OCs containing at least 50 μg of estrogen and 40% of those ingesting OCs with a lower dose of estrogen (35 μg) have elevated basal serum PRL levels of 20 to 40 ng/mL.[25] Approximately 50% of women taking the higher dose of estrogen, but only 25% taking the low-dose estrogen pill, had a PRL response greater than controls following TRH administration. A significant PRL increase, above that seen in controls, is also seen following insulin-induced hypoglycemia in women using OCs.[26] Although the exaggerated PRL response to hypoglycemia could be due to a hypothalamic effect, the greater than normal response to TRH stimulation, acting directly on the pituitary, suggests that OCs have a direct stimulatory effect upon the pituitary.

Despite the elevated serum PRL levels, most women taking OCs do not have galactorrhea, because estrogens block the binding of PRL at the receptor sites in the breast. However, some women do develop galactorrhea. If this occurs, the OCs should be discontinued and serum PRL measured one month later if galactorrhea persists. In most women, when OCs are discontinued, PRL levels fall promptly, normal ovulatory menstrual cycles resume, and galactorrhea does not occur.[27] In some, however, recovery of the hypothalamic-pituitary axis may take longer. A few patients may remain amenorrheic and note the onset of galactorrhea. Galactorrhea develops at this time because the inhibitory effect of estrogens on the breast is removed. This allows the already elevated PRL levels to stimulate the glands and induce galactorrhea. Because many patients with postpill amenorrhea and galactorrhea have been found to have radiographic changes of the sella turcica compatible with a microadenoma of the pituitary, studies have been undertaken to determine whether a causal relationship exists between OC use and the development of these tumors. Several studies have shown that women using OCs do not have a higher incidence of PRL-secreting pituitary adenomas than controls who have not used the pill.[28-31]

PRL secretion can be inhibited pharmacologically by the administration of levodopa, dopamine, or ergot alkaloids such as bromocriptine. Levodopa is decarboxylated to dopamine after crossing the blood-brain barrier. Dopamine produces the inhibitory effect by acting on the median eminence, which is outside the blood-brain barrier, and/or directly on the pituitary. Bromocriptine is a semisynthetic ergot alkaloid with potent dopamine agonist effects. It inhibits PRL secretion by acting directly on the pituitary.

Pathologic factors affecting prolactin secretion

Table 16-2 lists common pathologic factors affecting the secretion of PRL.

Hypothyroidism

In about 3% to 5% of all patients with galactorrhea and hyperprolactinemia, the underlying etiology is primary hypothyroidism. These patients have a low level of thyroxine (T_4) and therefore lack negative feedback on the hypothalamic-pituitary axis. This may result in increased secretion of TRH, which in turn overstimulates the thyrotrophs and lactotrophs, causing an increase in both thyroid-stimulating hormone (TSH) and PRL. However, because most of the negative feedback of T_4 and triiodothyronine (T_3) is exerted on the pituitary rather

Table 16-2
Pathologic factors affecting prolactin concentrations

I. Brain and pituitary disorders:
  A. Hypothalamic
    1. Destructive (tumor, encephalitis)
    2. Idiopathic (functional or biochemical)
    3. Infiltrative (histiocytosis, sarcoid)
  B. Pituitary
    1. Adenoma (micro, macro)
    2. Hyperplasia
    3. Empty sella syndrome
    4. Acromegaly
    5. Pituitary stalk section
    6. Sheehan's syndrome
II. Hypothyroidism
III. Malignant tumors with ectopic production of prolactin
IV. Renal failure

Abnormal endocrinology

than on the hypothalamus, TRH may be elevated only minimally, if at all. Also, decreased levels of T_4 and T_3 may induce changes in the sensitivity of the pituitary cell, causing an exaggerated response to normal or slightly elevated levels of TRH. Concomitant with the lack of this negative feedback, it has been postulated that patients with primary hypothyroidism also have an alteration in the positive feedback between T_4 and dopamine.[32] Thus, diminished dopamine secretion will result in elevated levels of serum TSH and PRL (Figure 16-8).

The administration of TRH to hypothyroid patients results in an exaggerated response of both serum TSH and PRL release. Similarly, serum LH, but not FSH, also shows an exaggerated response to GnRH from an elevated baseline. The concentration of free E_2 is elevated and SHBG is decreased in patients with primary hypothyroidism. Measurement of both serum PRL and TSH, as the initial tests in women with galactorrhea, identifies those who may have primary hypothyroidism as its cause (Figure 16-9). This finding is important because of the ease in

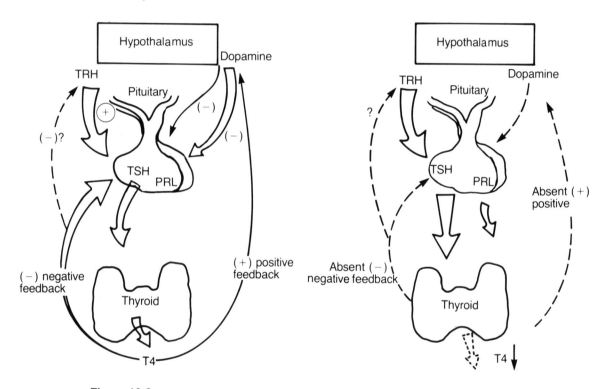

Figure 16-8
Schematic representation of mechanism(s) of normal thyroid function (left) and during primary hypothyroidism (right).

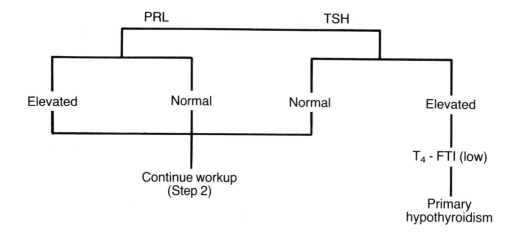

Figure 16-9
First step in the workup of patients with hyperprolactinemia: evaluation of all those with galactorrhea.

From Kletzky OA: Diagnostic approaches to hyperprolactinemic states. Seminars in Reproductive Endocrinology 2:23, 1984.

making the diagnosis and instituting the appropriate medical treatment. If serum TSH is elevated, the diagnosis is primary hypothyroidism (usually Hashimoto's thyroiditis). Although an elevated serum TSH may be seen in a patient with a TSH-secreting pituitary adenoma, such a patient actually has hyperthyroidism, not galactorrhea. Patients with primary hypothyroidism have low serum T_4 and low free thyroid index, whereas patients with a TSH-secreting adenoma have elevated T_3 levels by RIA.

If the diagnosis of primary hypothyroidism is made, no further evaluation of the hyperprolactinemia is necessary. The patient should be given thyroxine replacement therapy, starting at 0.05 mg daily for 2 weeks, and then increasing the dose by 0.05 mg every 2 weeks to a maintenance dose of 0.15 or 0.2 mg/day. This dose will effectively lower the elevated serum TSH and PRL levels into the normal range. An occasional patient may continue to have elevated serum PRL levels several weeks after the TSH has been normalized by the maintenance dose of thyrox-

ine. Such a patient should be suspected of having a combination of primary hypothyroidism and a PRL-secreting adenoma and thus should be appropriately evaluated. X-ray studies of the sella turcica are not necessary before instituting thyroxine therapy, because abnormal tomograms have been found in patients with primary hypothyroidism without a tumor.[33] The abnormal tomographic changes of primary hypothyroidism may or may not reverse after treatment.

Hypothalamic causes

Craniopharyngioma is the nonpituitary tumor most commonly associated with hyperprolactinemia. These tumors arise from epithelial remnants of Rathke's pouch, distributed along the pituitary stalk from the pars distalis to the floor of the third ventricle. These tumors are cystic in about 55%, solid in 15%, and both components are present in about 30% of cases. It has been estimated that approximately 250 cases of craniopharyngioma are diagnosed in the US annually. A craniopharyngioma is most frequently diagnosed during the second and third decades of life. Classically, plain skull x-rays or CT scans of patients with these tumors reveal calcifications during childhood, which diminish during the third decade of life.

A craniopharyngioma either damages the hypothalamus or extends into the sella turcica, where it interferes with the transport of hypothalamic hormones and neurotransmitters, resulting in pituitary dysfunction. Although some degree of impairment of pituitary function is almost universally found, the extent of impairment depends on whether the hypothalamus or the pituitary stalk is more involved. Gonadotropin deficiency is always present, resulting in amenorrhea. Galactorrhea is present in those patients with hyperprolactinemia. Diminished levels of GH, TSH, adrenocorticotropic hormone (ACTH), and antidiuretic hormone are also present.

As a craniopharyngioma expands, it produces local compression, especially of the optic chiasm. Therefore, surgical decompression is necessary. Because of the location, craniotomy may be the preferred approach, but complete resection is technically difficult. Up to 80% survival has been reported after surgical resection followed by radiotherapy. Cystic lesions require aspiration. Many patients also require hormone replacement therapy.

Pituitary causes

In recent years, there appears to be an increase in the incidence of patients with PRL-secreting pituitary adenomas (Figure 16-10). Although a tenfold increase in the incidence of all types of pituitary adenomas since 1970 has been reported, the exact incidence of PRL-secreting pituitary adenomas is still unknown.[34] In an unselected autopsy series, Burrow and co-workers found 32 (27%) microadenomas of the 120 pituitaries examined.[35] Of these, 41% stained for prolactin.

Most patients with pituitary adenomas have galactorrhea, and nearly all have hyperprolactinemia.[36] About 50% of patients with nonphysiologic hyperprolactinemia will have radiographic changes of the sella turcica compatible with an adenoma. In another 10% of patients with galactorrhea and x-ray evidence of a pituitary tumor, the serum PRL level will be in the normal range. Nearly all of these patients have empty sella syndrome.

Most patients with PRL-secreting pituitary adenomas have normal baseline levels of FSH and LH. We have shown that these patients have a normal, or even greater than normal LH or FSH response following the administration of GnRH.[37] Furthermore, the administration of two doses of GnRH every 2 hours to patients with hyperprolactinemia due to a pituitary adenoma has been reported to induce a significant increase in serum estradiol.[23] Thus, increasing levels of PRL may not interfere with ovarian estradiol secretion. Although the etiology of these adenomas is unknown, it appears likely that the underlying cause is an alteration in the hypothalamic secretion of dopamine or a dopamine receptor defect at the pituitary level.

Hyperplasia

Patients with hyperplasia of the lactotrophs cannot be distinguished from those having a microadenoma by any clinical, laboratory, or radiologic method. It is a diagnosis that can be made only at the time of surgical exploration of the pituitary gland.

Empty sella syndrome

Empty sella is characterized by herniation of the subarachnoid membrane into the sella turcica through a defective or incompetent sella diaphragm. It may be classified as primary or secondary. Primary empty sella may be due to a congenitally deficient diaphragm, coexist with PRL-, GH-, or ACTH-secreting pituitary adenomas, or result from alterations in the circulatory dynamics of the cerebrospinal fluid (CSF). Sec-

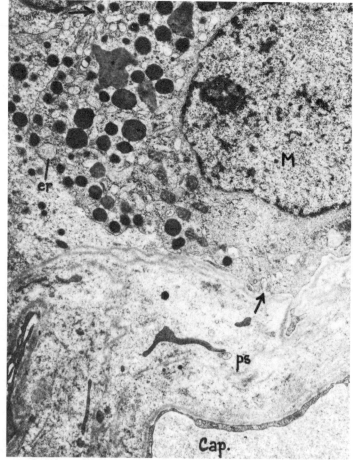

Figure 16-10
Electron microscopy of a PRL-secreting pituitary adenoma. Arrows, PRL exocytosis; PS, perivascular space; cap, capillary; er, endoplasmic reticulum; M, mitochondria.

ondary empty sella is seen after radiation therapy or surgical intervention in the sellar region. The sellar diaphragm defect allows the subarachnoid membrane, filled with CSF, to protrude into the sella turcica every time there is an increase in intracranial pressure. This results in compression of the pituitary gland and remodeling of the sella contour (Figure 16-11). Radiographically, the sella is symmetrically enlarged, with or without erosion. A definitive diagnosis can be made by CT scan with metrizamide in-

jected into the CSF through a lumbar puncture. This contrast medium fills up the intrasellar defect, thus establishing the diagnosis. It is important to make the diagnosis, because patients with an empty sella have, in general, a more benign prognosis than patients with pituitary adenomas. They require a less stringent follow-up. Although most patients with empty sella have no endocrine abnormalities, some may have pituitary dysfunction and even panhypopituitarism. However, a pituitary adenoma can coexist with

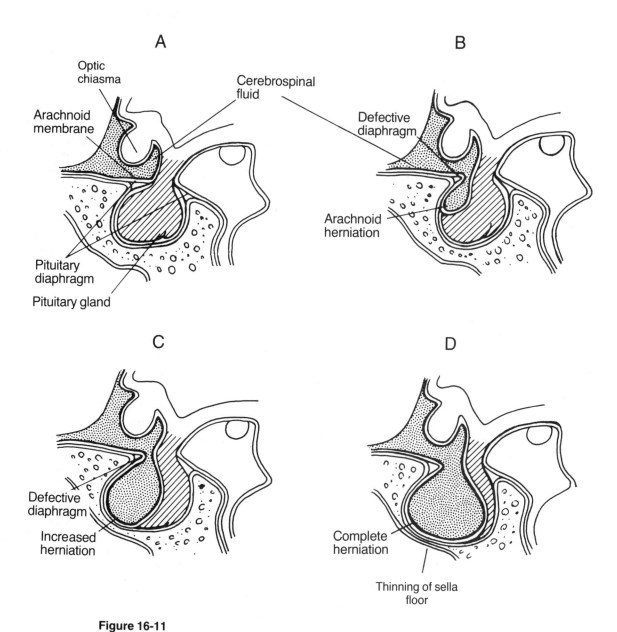

Figure 16-11
Diagrammatic representation of empty sella. A. Normal anatomic relationship. B, C, and D. Progression in the development of empty sella. Note the thinning of the floor and symmetrical enlargement of the sella turcica.

partial empty sella.[38]

Patients with an empty sella can have galactorrhea with normal or moderately elevated levels of serum PRL. It is thought that the elevation of PRL can occur because of the arachnoid herniation and compression on the pituitary stalk, interfering with the transport of dopamine. It is not known why many of these patients have galactorrhea with normal serum PRL levels. The administration of TRH to these patients results in a normal PRL increase (three times the baseline). Frequent measurements of serum PRL (every 15 minutes for 3 hours), as well as every 2 hours for 24 hours, demonstrated that the secretion levels of PRL in patients with empty sella are similar to the levels and pattern of PRL secretion observed in normal women.

Acromegaly

Patients with acromegaly can have galactorrhea and elevated serum PRL. In vitro studies with growth hormone-secreting pituitary adenomas showed that these tumors secrete PRL in addition to growth hormone. Similarly, use of the immunoperoxidase technique demonstrated the presence of both hormones within the tumor. Therefore, galactorrhea in patients with acromegaly is most likely due to the secretion of PRL rather than to the lactogenic properties of growth hormone.

Sheehan's syndrome

Sheehan's syndrome is the only known entity with lower than normal levels of serum PRL (<5 ng/mL) that is of clinical significance. These patients fail to lactate postpartum. Patients with Sheehan's syndrome lack a response of serum GH, cortisol, and PRL to insulin-induced hypoglycemia (see Figure 15-10). If the insult to the pituitary resulted in complete damage to the anterior pituitary, these women will also have a blunted LH, FSH, PRL, and TSH response following the administration of GnRH and TRH (see Figure 15-11).[39]

Other causes of hyperprolactinemia
Renal disease

Patients with acute or chronic renal failure have hyperprolactinemia because of delayed clearance of the hormone. Also, there seems to be a pituitary dysfunction, because there is a blunted PRL response to TRH stimulation. In any event, very rarely do these patients require treatment other than for the acute or chronic renal failure.

Chest surgery

Patients with previous chest surgery, including breast implants, may have galactorrhea with normal serum PRL levels. This is probably due to peripheral nerve stimulation. Further investigations must be performed to establish the mechanism by which galactorrhea, and sometimes hyperprolactinemia, is produced in these patients.

Diagnostic evaluation

The use of drugs or medications with PRL-stimulatory properties can be ruled out by the history. If possible, such agents should be discontinued and serum PRL measured 1 month later. If the PRL is still elevated, the physician should proceed with the evaluation. If the medication (tranquilizer or antihypertensive) cannot be discontinued, a complete workup to rule out a pituitary adenoma should be initiated. Primary hypothyroidism should then be ruled out as described above.

We have found that the most consistently abnormal hormone response in patients with pituitary tumors is the failure of TRH to induce a rise in serum PRL.[37] Because PRL can be inhibited in these patients by levodopa, dopamine, and bromocriptine, it appears that the stimulatory receptors are affected but the inhibitory receptors do respond normally. The administration of TRH, chlorpromazine, or arginine or induction of hypoglycemia with insulin in normal individuals results in a significant release of serum PRL.[37,40] Since this stimulatory capacity is lost, these agents have been used to distinguish patients with hyperprolactinemia who have a pituitary tumor from those who do not.

The major effort in the workup of patients with hyperprolactinemia is directed toward diagnosing pituitary adenoma, because of its serious endocrinologic and ophthalmologic implications. The measurement of serum PRL before and 20 minutes following the IV administration of 500 μg of TRH as a bolus is a valuable test, if a normal response occurs, for ruling out the presence of a pituitary adenoma in patients with galactorrhea and hyperprolactinemia.[41] Nausea and urinary urgency are the only side effects produced by IV TRH administration. These side effects are short-lived (seconds) and need no special treatment.

In normal women, pregnant women, and patients without pituitary adenomas, PRL levels are increased 200% (tripled) over baseline levels in 20 minutes (Figure 16-12).[42] If the increase is blunted or does not triple over baseline, it is compatible with the presence of a pituitary adenoma, although the tumor may not be demonstrable by CT scan. This provocative test is not universally accepted as being accurate in assessing the status of the pituitary.[43,44] However, we have recently shown that the TRH test is clinically useful in a group of patients with hyperprolactinemia of 20 to 60 ng/mL (Figure 16-13, upper).[42] Patients with a baseline serum PRL greater than 60 ng/mL were always found to have a blunted response independent of the CT scan results (Figure 16-13, lower). Thus, the discriminatory value of the test seems to have clinical applicability only for patients with mild hyperprolactinemia of no more than 60 ng/mL. Our cur-

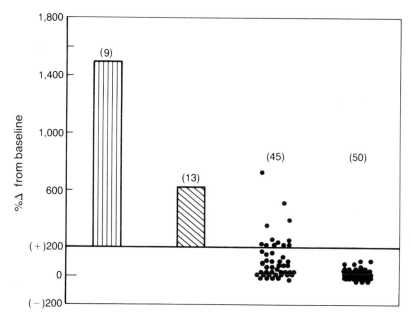

Figure 16-12

PRL increase (95% confidence limits) following TRH stimulation in normal women (vertical lines); during pregnancy (oblique lines); in 45 patients with baseline serum PRL between 20 and 60 ng/mL; and in 50 patients with serum PRL >60 ng/mL.

From Shangold GA, Kletzky OA, Marrs RP, et al: Use of TRH test to avoid sellar tomography in selected patients with hyperprolactinemia. Obstet Gynecol 63:771, 1984. Reproduced with permission from The American College of Obstetricians and Gynecologists.

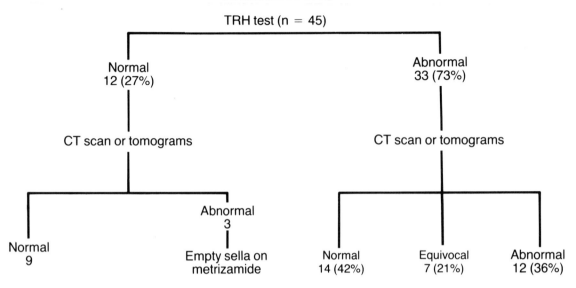

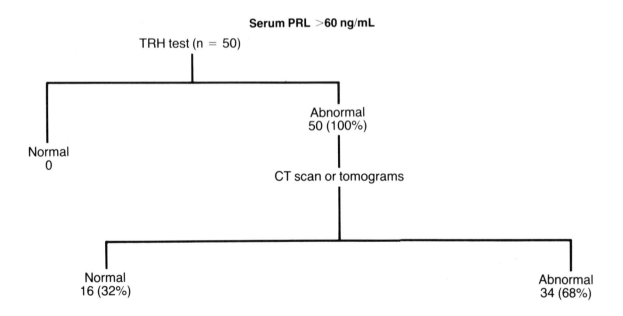

Figure 16-13
TRH test in patients with moderate (upper) and severe (lower) hyperprolactinemia.

Abnormal endocrinology

rent approach is to perform the TRH test only in patients with hyperprolactinemia of less than 60 ng/mL. Only those with an abnormal serum PRL response to TRH as well as those with a serum PRL baseline above 60 ng/mL need to have a CT scan of the sella turcica.

Hyperprolactinemia, pituitary adenomas, and the menstrual cycle

We have reported the relationships among menstrual history, serum PRL, and the presence or absence of a PRL-secreting pituitary adenoma in a large group of women with galactorrhea.[36] All patients with galactorrhea, regular menses, and normal serum PRL values (<20 ng/mL) had normal tomograms, indicating that these women represent a low-risk group for having a PRL-secreting pituitary adenoma (Figure 16-14).[36] Therefore, we recommend that patients with galactorrhea, normal menses, and normal serum PRL be followed up once a year with measurement of serum PRL. As long as serum PRL remains within the normal range, there is no need for an x-ray study of the sella. However, if serum PRL is elevated, further workup is necessary, even in the presence of normal menses, since it was reported that 6 of 20 women with regular menses, galactorrhea, and hyperprolactinemia had abnormal tomograms compatible with an adenoma. Thus, in the presence of an elevated serum PRL, a pituitary adenoma should be ruled out independent of the patient's menstrual history (Figure 16-15).

If the serum PRL is between 20 and 60 ng/mL, a TRH test is indicated. The TRH test is fully described in Chapter 21. If the test is normal, the patient should be followed up yearly with a TRH test; a CT scan is not necessary. If the test becomes abnormal (less than three times the baseline), then a CT scan with 1.5-mm cuts is

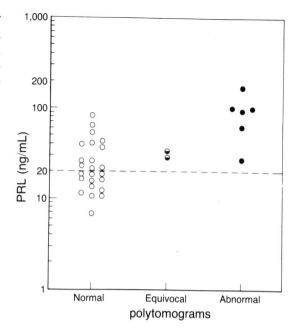

Figure 16-14
Correlation of serum PRL and polytomograms in 32 galactorrheic patients with normal menses. Broken line represents upper limits of normal for PRL.

Reproduced, with permission, from Davajan V, Kletzky OA, March CM, et al: The significance of galactorrhea in patients with normal menses, oligomenorrhea, and secondary amenorrhea. Am J Obstet Gynecol 130:894, 1978.

indicated. If the initial serum PRL is greater than 60 ng/mL, we recommend a CT scan be performed without doing a TRH test. In contrast to patients with normal menses, some patients with irregular menses, galactorrhea, and normal serum PRL levels have been shown to have an abnormal x-ray of the sella turcica. On further evaluation, these patients were found to have a normal TRH test, and CT scan demonstrated a completely empty sella. Therefore, in patients with galactorrhea, normal prolactin levels, and oligomenorrhea or amenorrhea, AP and lateral cone view x-rays of the sella turcica are indicated. If these are normal, the patient is

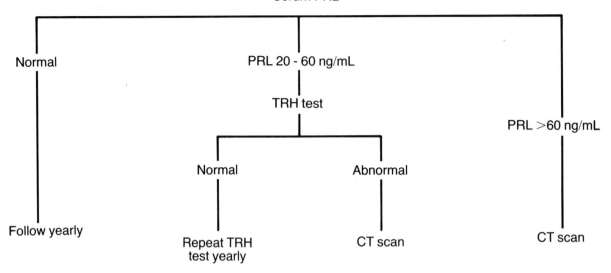

Figure 16-15
Second step in the workup of hyperprolactinemic patients with normal menses and galactorrhea.

followed up with a yearly serum PRL, as patients with the empty sella syndrome frequently have an abnormal AP and lateral cone view of the sella turcica. If the cone view is abnormal, in the presence of normal PRL, an empty sella should be ruled out with a CT scan with metrizamide given through a lumbar puncture. As stated before, in patients with a serum PRL between 20 and 60 ng/mL, a TRH test is indicated. Patients with a normal test should have a cone view and, if abnormal, an empty sella should be ruled out. Those with normal cone views should be followed up yearly with a TRH test. In those women with an abnormal TRH test, as well as in those with an initial serum PRL greater than 60 ng/mL, a CT scan is indicated (Figure 16-16). Patients with secondary amenorrhea and low levels of estrogen (<40 pg/mL) have a significantly greater proportion of abnormal tomograms and therefore they represent the group at

highest risk for having a pituitary adenoma (Figure 16-17).[36]

The new generation of CT scanners is capable of viewing the pituitary at 1.5-mm intervals.[45] It is the preferred radiologic method to confirm or rule out the presence of a pituitary adenoma. It provides information on the bony structure of the sella turcica, as well as the shape, size, and degree of extrasellar extension of the soft tissue.

A relatively new imaging modality, nuclear magnetic resonance imaging (MRI), is based on the fact that hydrogen *nuclei* in a *magnetic* field *resonate* when exposed to radio waves of specific frequency. This method uses a combination of static magnetic fields, radio waves, and atomic nuclei instead of the ionizing radiation used in CT scans. MRI tomographic slices depict tissue hydrogen density. They are more descriptive (because of better contrast resolution), potentially more useful, and may in fact replace CT scans. Further studies are required to completely evaluate MRI's usefulness in neuroendocrine disorders.

If CT scanners are not available, the sella turcica should be evaluated by hypocycloid tomography. However, it has been shown that many patients with galactorrhea and hyperprolactinemia can benefit from cone views of the sella turcica. It was reported that if the cone view and serum PRL level are normal, no further radiographic tests are necessary, because all these patients were found to have normal tomograms.[46] If serum PRL is elevated and the cone view is normal, the patient should then have a polytomogram (or CT scan if available), because about 10% were found to have abnormalities. If the initial cone view x-ray is abnormal (independent of serum PRL), a tomogram is not indicated, since the presence of an abnormal sella tur-

cica has already been demonstrated. However, these patients need a CT scan to determine the size and extension of the pituitary lesion.

Patients in whom a pituitary macroadenoma (>1 cm in diameter) has been demonstrated should have an insulin tolerance test (ITT) to determine the adequacy of ACTH reserve.[47] A dose of 0.15 U/kg of insulin is administered after an overnight fast, and blood samples are obtained before and 30, 60, and 120 minutes afterward. Serum or plasma glucose, PRL, cortisol, and GH are measured in each sample. The dose of insulin should be sufficient to decrease plasma glucose levels to at least 50% of baseline. If this is achieved, the minimal normal increase from baseline for plasma cortisol is 6 μg/100 mL; for GH, 18 ng/mL; and for PRL, 270%. In patients with an abnormal cortisol response who undergo pituitary surgery, the ITT should be repeated 8 to 10 weeks after the procedure.

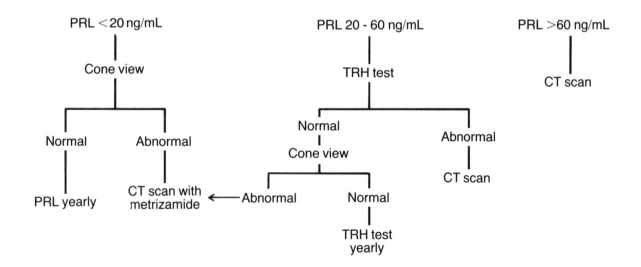

Figure 16-16
Third step in the workup of patients with hyperprolactinemia causing oligomenorrhea or amenorrhea and galactorrhea.

From Kletzky OA: Diagnostic approaches to hyperprolactinemic states. Seminars in Reproductive Endocrinology 2:23, 1984.

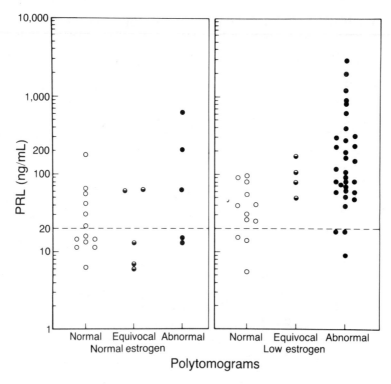

Figure 16-17
Correlation of serum PRL and polytomograms in patients with galactorrhea. There were 23 who had secondary amenorrhea with normal estrogen status, and 48 had secondary amenorrhea with low estrogen status. Broken line represents upper limits of normal for PRL.

Reproduced, with permission, from Davajan V, Kletzky OA, March CM, et al: The significance of galactorrhea in patients with normal menses, oligomenorrhea, and secondary amenorrhea. Am J Obstet Gynecol 130:894, 1978.

Alternatively, the ITT can be done only after surgery to rule out an ACTH deficiency, because all of these patients receive hydrocortisone supplementation for the surgical procedure independent of the results of a preoperative ITT.

Treatment of galactorrhea and/or hyperprolactinemia

The objectives of therapy in patients with galactorrhea and/or hyperprolactinemia include (1) elimination of lactation, (2) establishment of normal estrogen secretion, (3) induction of ovulation, and (4) treatment of prolactin-secreting pituitary adenomas. The recommended forms of management are periodic observation, drug therapy, radiation, and surgery.

Periodic observation
This form of management is indicated in menstruating women with galactorrhea who have normal or idiopathic elevated serum PRL levels. As long as the galactorrhea is not socially embarrassing and the patient has regular or irregular menses, there is no need to institute any treatment. Patients with oligomenorrhea can be treated with a gestagen to induce regular uterine

bleeding. Long-term treatment with bromocriptine is unnecessary, since no risk is known to occur because of idiopathic hyperprolactinemia in patients with normal serum levels of estrogen. Observation can even be extended to women with radiologic evidence of a microadenoma. Because the growth rate of microadenoma appears to be slow, follow-up with yearly measurement of serum PRL and CT scan every 2 years appears to be appropriate. Long-term studies have shown that only a small percentage of women with a microadenoma who do not receive any treatment have an increase in size of the tumor.[48,49]

A study by Koppelman and co-workers followed progression of the disease in 25 women with a PRL-secreting microadenoma for a mean time of 11.3 years. Hyperprolactinemia remained unchanged over the years (mean of 225 ng/mL vs. 155 ng/mL); 7 of 22 women with amenorrhea resumed spontaneous menses; while galactorrhea resolved in 6 of 19 patients presenting with the symptom. One patient showed progression, 2 showed improvement, and the remaining had no change in their sella abnormality.[48] Similarly, March and colleagues reported a longitudinal evaluation of 43 untreated women with radiographic evidence of a PRL-secreting microadenoma. A 3 to 20 years' follow-up revealed no change in mean baseline serum PRL (177 ng/mL vs. 218 ng/mL). Two patients had tumor enlargement and underwent successful adenomectomy. No change was observed in the remaining 41 patients. Three of these patients have resumed regular menses, with normalization of serum PRL (<20 ng/mL), and cessation of galactorrhea.[49] A study by Martin and co-workers followed the natural history of 41 patients with idiopathic hyperprolactinemia and amenorrhea-galactorrhea for 2 to 11 years. During this time, 9 patients conceived spontaneously, and 16 have resumed spontaneous menses with cessation of galactorrhea. Only one patient developed a microadenoma.[50]

Thus hyperprolactinemia with or without a microadenoma apparently follows a benign clinical course in most women. A period of observation or conservative management is therefore indicated for this disorder.

Drug therapy

Patients with primary hypothyroidism should be treated with thyroxine as described earlier. In patients with hyperprolactinemia and low estrogen status, determined by a serum E_2 level of less than 40 pg/mL or absent uterine bleeding response to an IM injection of progesterone in oil, it is necessary to institute therapy because these women have been shown to be at a higher risk for developing osteoporosis.[51] There is some evidence that all hyperprolactinemic women, independent of estrogen status, have a reduced bone mineral content and therefore may be at increased risk for osteoporosis.[52] If this finding is confirmed, it will indicate the need to treat all women with hyperprolactinemia, regardless of their estrogen status. Although estrogen replacement could be attempted in women without any evidence of a pituitary adenoma, the administration of bromocriptine induces more physiologic estrogen secretion.

In women with evidence of a pituitary adenoma and low estrogen, only bromocriptine should be used. Of women without an adenoma, 95% require 5 mg/day and 53% of those with an adenoma require higher doses to resume regular menses (Figure 16-18),[53] which occurs at about 6 weeks of treatment in those women without an adenoma and in about 9 weeks in those with an adenoma.[53] Galactorrhea will resolve in about 6 weeks of treatment in women without evidence of an adenoma and in about 11 weeks ($P < 0.001$) of treatment in those with an adenoma (Table 16-3). Bromocriptine is usually well tolerated as long as the dose is slowly increased at a rate of 2.5 mg/week and is taken after a meal. The discontinuation of therapy usually results in the return of hyperprolactinemia,

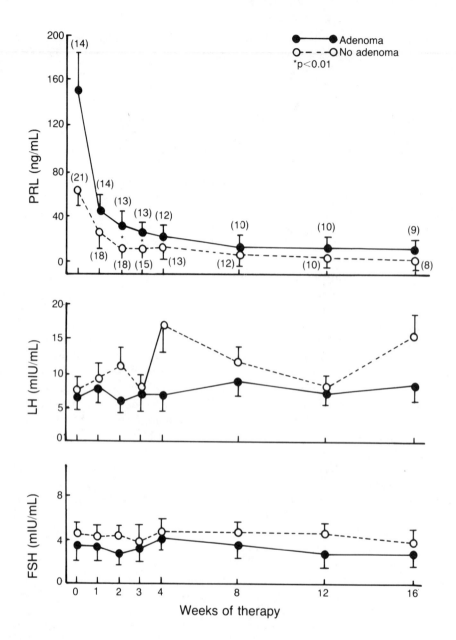

Figure 16-18
Serum PRL, LH, and FSH levels in 14 women with hyperprolactinemia with pituitary adenoma (solid circles) and in 21 without adenoma (open circles) during the initial 16 weeks of treatment with bromocriptine.

Reproduced, with permission, from Kletzky OA, Marrs RP, Davajan V: Management of patients with hyperprolactinemia and normal or abnormal tomograms. Am J Obstet Gynecol 147:528, 1983.

Abnormal endocrinology

Table 16-3
Length of bromocriptine treatment to correct symptoms

Symptom	Duration of therapy (weeks)	
	Adenoma	No adenoma
Galactorrhea	11.3 ± 2.1 (n = 17)*	5.6 ± 1.1 (n = 19)
Amenorrhea	8.7 ± 1.2 (n = 17)†	5.7 ± 0.6 (n = 15)
Infertility	16.2 ± 2.1 (n = 17)‡	9.8 ± 1.5 (n = 12)

*$P < 0.001$.
†$P < 0.01$.
‡$P < 0.02$.

From Kletzky OA, Marrs RP, Davajan V: Management of patients with hyperprolactinemia and normal or abnormal tomograms. Am J Obstet Gynecol 147:528, 1983.

leading to galactorrhea and amenorrhea; therefore, therapy should be continued indefinitely. It is recommended that these patients be followed up with measurement of serum PRL every 6 months.

Patients with a pituitary macroadenoma should have a repeat CT scan after 6 months of reaching the full dose of bromocriptine. As long as a shrinking effect on the adenoma is demonstrated, bromocriptine is continued with CT scans performed at yearly intervals. Those patients with a microadenoma should have a CT scan repeated every 2 to 3 years.

The induction of ovulation in almost all patients with hyperprolactinemia due to a pituitary adenoma can be accomplished with bromocriptine. Approximately 50% of these women will require only 5 mg/day, and the remaining patients will need larger doses of bromocriptine. The length of treatment necessary to induce ovulation in women with a pituitary adenoma (16 weeks) is significantly greater ($P < 0.02$) than in those without a tumor (10 weeks) (Table 16-3). Also, restoration of normal menstrual cycles and pregnancy may occur without complete normalization of serum PRL (Figure 16-19).[53] Bromocriptine is discontinued as soon as the diagnosis of pregnancy is confirmed.

Several studies have shown that nearly all patients with adenomas who become pregnant do not have a significant enlargement of the adenoma during their pregnancy.[37,54,55] However, the patient's visual fields should be examined at 20, 28, and 38 weeks of pregnancy. If an enlargement is suspected on the basis of visual fields, a limited CT scan is indicated. If suprasellar extension is demonstrated, bromocriptine treatment should be instituted for the rest of the pregnancy to prevent possible loss of vision.

Fetal outcomes have been reported among a relatively small group of women treated with bromocriptine during pregnancy; however, there seems to be no increased risk of fetal malformations. Bromocriptine is discontinued after the completion of pregnancy to allow unrestricted breast-feeding. Because changes occurring during pregnancy can regress, it is recommended to reevaluate the tumor status 10 to 12 weeks postpartum by CT scan. If enlargement of the tumor during pregnancy does not respond to medical treatment, surgical extirpation can be performed.[56-58] No increase in surgical morbidity has been reported when surgery was performed during pregnancy.

Women with no evidence of a pituitary adenoma who have a normal estrogen status can be induced to ovulate with clomiphene citrate. If this agent fails, bromocriptine should be given. Patients with amenorrhea who have a low estrogen status will always require bromocriptine. It may be concluded that bromocriptine is the drug of choice for inducing ovulation in women with hyperprolactinemia, even if there is evidence of a microadenoma.

Radiation therapy

The use of 4,500 rads of cobalt may arrest the progressive growth of a pituitary tumor. However, following this treatment, regular menses usually do not return. It takes several months for the galactorrhea to be corrected. Because the adenoma tissue may be more resistant than the surrounding organs, secondary hypothalamic or pituitary damage can occur. Alternatively, proton beam or heavy-particle irradiation can be used. With this method, visual field defects or oculomotor palsies have been reported to be more common than with the conventional cobalt irradiation. We do not advise either form of therapy. Medical treatment with bromocriptine achieves faster results, is easier to administer, and has no major side effects.

Surgery

The introduction of the transsphenoidal route for the microsurgical exploration of the sella turcica permits removal of the pituitary adenoma while preserving the functional capacity of the remaining gland. Critical factors in determining the results of surgery include the expertise of the neurosurgeon and the size and extension of the adenoma. Using resumption of menses, euprolactinemia, and cessation of galactorrhea as the endpoints of curability, cure rates between 50% and 80% have been reported in patients with microadenomas.

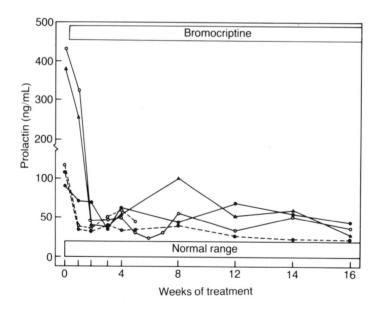

Figure 16-19

Mean serum prolactin response to bromocriptine therapy in five patients with radiographic evidence of pituitary adenoma and resistant hyperprolactinemia. Although prolactin levels remained above the normal range, four of these patients conceived.

Reproduced, with permission, from Kletzky OA, Marrs RP, Davajan V: Management of patients with hyperprolactinemia and normal or abnormal tomograms. Am J Obstet Gynecol 147:528, 1983.

Abnormal endocrinology

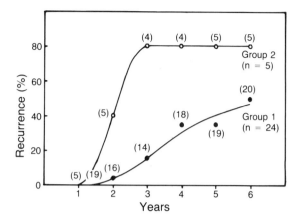

Figure 16-20
Cumulative recurrence rate in patients with microprolactinoma (group 1) or macroprolactinoma (group 2) after initially successful surgery. Figures in parentheses indicate the numbers of patients who were seen at each yearly interval.

Reproduced, with permission, from Serri O, Rasio E, Beauregard H, et al: Recurrence of hyperprolactinemia after selective transsphenoidal adenomectomy in women with prolactinoma. N Engl J Med 309:280, 1983.

Because the reported cure rate of patients with macroadenomas varies between 10% and 30%, it has been suggested that therapy be instituted before the adenoma reaches a diameter greater than 1 cm. However, morbidity should be considered before recommending this modality of therapy. Various degrees of complications, such as transient or definitive diabetes insipidus, hemorrhage, meningitis, cerebrospinal fluid leak, panhypopituitarism, and the finding of normal glands at the time of surgery have been reported. Long-term follow-up (5 to 10 years) after successful adenomectomies has recently been reported (Figure 16-20).[59] Although there was no radiologic evidence of tumor recurrence, serum PRL levels increased to a mean of about 60 ng/mL in 12 of the 24 patients successfully operated for a microadenoma and in 4 out of 5 patients with macroadenomas. Following the increase of baseline serum PRL, these pa-

tients were found to have a blunted PRL response to TRH stimulation, similar to that seen before surgery.

These results seem to strengthen the hypothesis of a dopamine receptor defect or a hypothalamic derangement of dopamine secretion as the cause of PRL-secreting adenomas. Considering the good results obtained with medical therapy (bromocriptine), the low rate of side effects, and the possibility of reducing the adenoma size, we recommend surgery only for patients having a pituitary macroadenoma.

Patients with macroadenomas or with extrasellar extension of the tumor should be treated first with bromocriptine and have surgery only after maximum reduction of the tumor size has been obtained.[60,61] Surgery should be performed without discontinuing bromocriptine, because a rapid regrowth of the adenoma has been reported.[62] These patients with suprasellar extension should be treated surgically, because the adenoma has already shown signs of aggressiveness, and bromocriptine alone is insufficient for complete resolution of the adenoma. This is especially important if the patient desires fertility, because bromocriptine is usually discontinued during pregnancy. Also, patients who must receive bromocriptine for long periods of time (years) demonstrate poor compliance, which may result in further growth of the adenoma.

References

1. Friesen H, Guyda H, Hardy J: Biosynthesis of human growth hormone and prolactin. *J Clin Endocrinol Metab* 31:611, 1970

2. Lewis UJ, Singh RNP, Seavey BK: Human prolactin: Isolation and some properties. *Biochem Biophys Res Commun* 44:1169, 1971

3. Hwang P, Guyda H, Friesen H: Purification of human prolactin. *J Biol Chem* 247:1955, 1972

4. Pasteels JL, Gausset P, Danguy A, et al: Morphology of the lactotropes and somatotropes of man and rhesus monkeys. *J Clin Endocrinol Metab* 34:959, 1972

5. Shiino M, Williams MG, Rennels EG: Ultrastructural observations of pituitary release of prolactin in the rat by suckling stimulus. *Endocrinology* 90:176, 1972

6. Vila-Porcile E, Olivier L, Racadot O: Functional polarization of the prolactin cell: An electron microscopic study in the female rat during lactation and after weaning. In Pasteels JL, Robyn C (eds): *Human Prolactin.* New York, American Elsevier, 1973, pp 56-59

7. Gibbs DM, Neill JD: Dopamine levels in hypophysial stalk blood in the rat are sufficient to inhibit PRL secretion in vivo. *Endocrinology* 102:1895, 1978

8. Annunciato L, Cerrito F, Balsamo S: Dopamine biosynthesis regulation in the terminals of tuberoinfundibular neurons. In Tolis G, Stefanis C, Mountokalakis T, et al (eds): *Prolactin and Prolactinomas.* New York, Raven Press, 1983, pp 57-69

9. Pilotte NS, Porter JC: Dopamine in hypophysial portal plasma and PRL in systemic plasma in rats treated with 5-hydroxytryptamine. *Endocrinology* 108:2137, 1981

10. Szabo M, Frohman LA: Dissociation of PRL-releasing activity from TRH in porcine stalk median eminence. *Endocrinology* 98:1451, 1976

11. Boyd AE, Spencer E, Jackson IMD, et al: Prolactin releasing factor (PRF) in porcine hypothalamic extract distinct from TRH. *Endocrinology* 99:861, 1976

12. Robyn C, Delboye P, Nokin J, et al: Prolactin in human reproduction. In Pasteels JL, Robyn C (eds): *Human Prolactin.* New York, American Elsevier, 1973, pp 167-188

13. Sassin JF, Frantz AG, Weitzman ED, et al: Human prolactin: 24 hr pattern with increased release during sleep. *Science* 177:1205, 1972

14. Rigg LA, Yen SSC, Lein A: The pattern of increase in circulating PRL levels during human gestation. *Am J Obstet Gynecol* 129:454,1977

15. Kletzky OA, Marrs RP, Howard WF, et al: Prolactin synthesis and release during pregnancy and puerperium. *Am J Obstet Gynecol* 136:545, 1980

16. Noel GL, Suh HK, Stone JG, et al: Human PRL and GH release during surgery and other conditions of stress. *J Clin Endocrinol Metab* 35:840, 1972

17. Kolodny RC, Jacobs LS, Daughaday WH: Mammary stimulation causes PRL secretion in non-lactating women. *Nature* 238:284, 1972

18. Frantz AG, Kleinberg DL, Noel GL: Studies on prolactin in man. *Recent Prog Horm Res* 28:527, 1972

19. Noel GL, Suh HK, Frantz AG: Prolactin release during nursing and breast stimulation in postpartum and nonpostpartum subjects. *J Clin Endocrinol Metab* 38:413, 1974

20. Ishizuka B, Quigley ME, Yen SSC: Pituitary hormone release in reponse to food ingestion: Evidence for neuroendocrine signals from gut to brain. *J Clin Endocrinol Metab* 57:1111, 1983

21. Lobo RA, Kletzky OA, Kaptein EM, et al: Prolactin modulation of DHEA-S secretion. *Am J Obstet Gynecol* 138:632, 1980

22. Lobo RA, Kletzky OA: Normalization of androgen and SHBG-levels after treatment of hyperprolactinemia. *J Clin Endocrinol Metab* 56:562, 1983

23. Kletzky OA, Davajan V, Mishell DR Jr: The effect of gonadotropin-releasing hormone on ovarian estradiol secretion. *Am J Obstet Gynecol* 142:427, 1982

24. Anden NE, Dahlstrom A, Fuxe K, et al: The effect of haloperidol and chlorpromazine on the amine levels of central monoamine neurons. *Acta Physiol Scand* 68:419, 1966

25. Scott JZ, Kletzky OA, Brenner PF, et al: Comparison of the effects of contraceptive steroid formulations containing two doses of estrogen on pituitary function. *Fertil Steril* 30:141, 1978

26. Mishell DR Jr, Kletzky OA, Brenner PF, et al: The effect of contraceptive steroids on hypothalamic-pituitary function. *Am J Obstet Gynecol* 128:60, 1977

27. Klein TA, Mishell DR Jr: Gonadotropin, PRL and steroid hormones after discontinuation of oral contraceptives. *Am J Obstet Gynecol* 127:585, 1977

28. March CM, Mishell DR Jr, Kletzky OA, et al: Galactorrhea and pituitary tumors in postpill and non-postpill amenorrhea. *Am J Obstet Gynecol* 134:45, 1979

29. Maheaux R, Jenicek M, Cleroux R, et al: Oral contraceptives and prolactinomas: A case-control study. *Am J Obstet Gynecol* 143:134, 1982

30. Coulam CB, Annegers JF, Abboud CF, et al: Pituitary adenoma and oral contraceptives: A case control study. *Fertil Steril* 31:25, 1979

31. NIH Pituitary Adenoma Study Group: Pituitary adenomas and oral contraceptives: A multicenter case-control study. *Fertil Steril* 39:753, 1983

32. Feek CM, Sawers JSA, Brown NS, et al: Influence of thyroid status on dopaminergic inhibition of TSH and PRL secretions: Evidence for an additional feedback mechanism in the control of thyroid hormone secretion. *J Clin Endocrinol Metab* 51:585, 1980

33. Tolis G, Hoyte K, McKenzie JM, et al: Clinical, biochemical and radiographic reversibility of hyperprolactinemic galactorrhea-amenorrhea and abnormal sella by thyroxine in a patient with primary hypothyroidism. *Am J Obstet Gynecol* 131:850, 1978

34. Annegers JF, Coulam CB, Abboud CF, et al: Pituitary adenoma in Olmstead County, Minnesota 1935-1977. A report of an increasing incidence of diagnosis in women of childbearing age. *Mayo Clin Proc* 53:641, 1978

35. Burrow GN, Wortzman G, Rewcastle NB, et al: Microadenomas of the pituitary and abnormal sellar tomograms in an unselected autopsy series. *N Engl J Med* 304:156, 1981

36. Davajan V, Kletzky OA, March CM, et al: The significance of galactorrhea in patients with normal menses, oligomenorrhea, and secondary amenorrhea. *Am J Obstet Gynecol* 130:894, 1978

37. Kletzky OA, Davajan V, Mishell DR Jr, et al: A sequential pituitary stimulation test in normal subjects and in patients with amenorrhea-galactorrhea with pituitary tumors. *J Clin Endocrinol Metab* 45:631, 1977

38. Domingue JN, Wing SD, Wilson CB: Coexisting pituitary adenomas and partially empty sellas. *J Neurosurg* 48:23, 1978

39. diZerega G, Kletzky OA, Mishell DR Jr: Diagnosis of Sheehan's Syndrome using a sequential pituitary stimulation test. *Am J Obstet Gynecol* 132:348, 1978

40. Rakoff JS, Siler TM, Sinha YN, et al: PRL and GH release in response to sequential stimulation by arginine and synthetic TRF. *J Clin Endocrinol Metab* 37:641, 1973

41. Marrs RP, Bertolli SJ, Kletzky OA: The use of TRH in distinguishing PRL-secreting pituitary adenoma. *Am J Obstet Gynecol* 138:620, 1980

42. Shangold GA, Kletzky OA, Marrs RP, et al: Use of TRH test to avoid sellar tomography in selected patients with hyperprolactinemia. *Obstet Gynecol* 63:771, 1984

43. Lamberts SW, Birkenhager JC, Kwa HG: Basal and TRH stimulated PRL in patients with pituitary tumors. *Clin Endocrinol* 5:709, 1976

44. Samaan NA, Leavens ME, Jesse JH Jr: Serum PRL in patients with functionless chromophobe adenoma before and after therapy. *Acta Endocrinol* 84:449, 1977

45. Gyldensted C, Karle A: Computed tomography of intra and juxtasellar lesions. *Neuroradiology* 14:5, 1977

46. Marrs RP, Kletzky OA, Teal J, et al: Comparison of serum PRL, plain radiography and hypocycloidal tomography of the sella turcica in patients with galactorrhea. *Am J Obstet Gynecol* 135:467, 1979

47. Morente C, Kletzky OA, Davajan V: Pituitary response to insulin-induced hypoglycemia in patients with amenorrhea of different etiologies. *Am J Obstet Gynecol* 148:375, 1984

48. Koppelman MCS, Jaffe MJ, Rieth KG, et al: Hyperprolactinemia, amenorrhea, and galactorrhea. *Ann Intern Med* 100:115, 1984

49. March CM, Kletzky OA, Davajan V: Longitudinal evaluation of patients with untreated prolactin-secreting pituitary adenomas. *Am J Obstet Gynecol* 139:835, 1981

50. Martin TL, Kim M, Malarkey WB: The natural history of idiopathic hyperprolactinemia. *J Clin Endocrinol Metab* 60:855, 1985

51. Klibanski A, Neer RM, Beitins IZ, et al: Decreased bone density in hyperprolactinemic women. *N Engl J Med* 303:1511, 1980

52. Schlechte J, Sherman B, Martin R: Decreased bone mineral and prolactin tumors. Is hyperprolactinemia a risk factor for osteoporosis? Endocrine Society Meeting, San Francisco, abstr 563, 1982

53. Kletzky OA, Marrs RP, Davajan V: Management of patients with hyperprolactinemia and normal or abnormal tomograms. *Am J Obstet Gynecol* 147:528, 1983

54. Jewelewicz R, Vande Wiele RL: Clinical course and outcome of pregnancy in 25 patients with pituitary microadenomas. *Am J Obstet Gynecol* 136:339, 1980

55. Archer DF, Lattanzi DR, Moore EE, et al: Bromocriptine treatment of women with suspected pituitary PRL-secreting microadenomas. *Am J Obstet Gynecol* 143:620, 1982

56. Bergh T, Nillius SJ, Wide L: Clinical course and outcome of pregnancies in amenorrheic women with hyperprolactinemia and pituitary tumors. *Br Med J* 1:875, 1978

57. Falconer MA, Stafford-Bell MA: Visual failure from pituitary and parasellar tumors occurring with favorable outcome in pregnant women. *J Neurol Neurosurg* 38:919, 1975

58. Nelson PB, Archer DF, Moroon JC: Symptomatic pituitary tumor enlargement after induced pregnancy. *J Neurosurg* 49:283, 1978

59. Serri O, Rasio E, Beauregard H, et al: Recurrence of hyperprolactinemia after selective transsphenoidal adenomectomy in women with prolactinoma. *N Engl J Med* 309:280, 1983

60. McGregor AM, Scanlon MF, Hall K, et al: Reduction in size of a pituitary tumor by bromocriptine. *N Engl J Med* 300:291, 1979

61. Nillius SJ, Bergh T, Lundberg PO, et al: Regression of a PRL-secreting pituitary tumor during long-term treatment with bromocriptine. *Fertil Steril* 30:710, 1978

62. Thorner MO, Perryman RL, Rogol AD, et al: Rapid changes of prolactinoma volume after withdrawal and reinstitution of bromocriptine. *J Clin Endocrinol Metab* 53:480, 1981

Chapter 17

Androgen Excess

Uwe Goebelsmann, M.D.
Rogerio A. Lobo, M.D.

Hirsutism and virilization are the clinical signs of androgen excess. It is important to distinguish between them, because hirsutism can occur in women with normal or mildly to moderately elevated serum or plasma testosterone (T) levels (usually <1.5 ng/mL). In contrast, virilization is associated with serum or plasma T levels in excess of 2 ng/mL. Such markedly elevated levels are commonly associated with more serious underlying disorders, frequently ovarian or adrenal tumors. Hence, virilization is a much more alarming sign than hirsutism alone.

Hirsutism is defined as the presence of hair in locations where hair is not commonly found in women. It refers particularly to "midline" hair (see Table 17-1); that is, facial hair on the cheeks (sideburns), above the upper lip (mustache), and on the chin (beard); chest and/or intermammary hair; a male escutcheon; hair on the inner aspects of the thighs; and midline lower back hair entering the intergluteal area. A moderate amount of hair on the forearms and lower legs by itself may not be abnormal, although it may be viewed by the patient as undesirable and may be mistaken for hirsutism.

Virilization results from excessive amounts of T, with its defeminizing (antiestrogenic) and masculinizing actions. Any or all of the following signs constitute virilization: temporal balding, deepening of voice, decreased breast size, increased muscle mass, loss of female body contours, clitoral enlargement, and amenorrhea.

Origin of androgens in women

The three principal androgens produced in women are: dehydroepiandrosterone (DHEA), androstenedione (A), and testosterone (T). As outlined in Chapter 3, these steroids, with 19 carbon atoms, are "androgens" by chemical definition and not by androgenic action. Only T has androgenic potency; DHEA and A are merely biologically inactive precursors of T. In women, these C_{19} steroids originate exclusively in the

Table 17-1
Signs of androgen excess

Hirsutism: "midline" hair

Hair on upper lip (mustache)
Hair on chin (beard)
Hair on cheeks (sideburns)
Intermammary hair
Male escutcheon
Hair on inner aspects of thighs
Hair on mid-lower back/intergluteal region

Virilization

Temporal balding
Deepening of voice
Decreased breast size
Increased muscle mass
Loss of female body contours
Clitoral enlargement
Amenorrhea

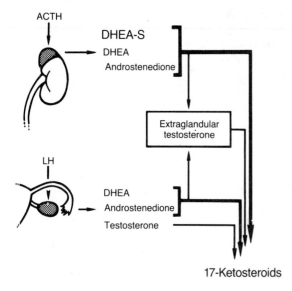

Figure 17-1
Origin of androgens in women.

Reproduced, with permission, from Goebelsmann U: Polycystic ovary syndrome. In Endocrinology and Metabolism, Continuing Education and Quality Control Program, *American Association for Clinical Chemistry, 1983, p 1.*

ovaries and adrenals. Hence, androgen excess can be the result of only adrenal or ovarian androgen overproduction. This limits the number of possible underlying disorders in women who have increased androgen levels.

The adrenals secrete dehydroepiandrosterone sulfate (DHEA-S), DHEA, and A, but little or no T; whereas the ovaries secrete DHEA, A, and T (Figure 17-1).[1] DHEA-S is secreted exclusively by the adrenals in amounts of 6 to 24 mg/24 hr and is quantitatively the most important androgen. DHEA and A originate in both the adrenals and ovaries. In addition to its ovarian secretion, T originates from peripheral (extraglandular) conversion of DHEA and A. This conversion proceeds at a low rate: Only 5% of circulating A and much smaller quantities of DHEA are converted to circulating T.

When the amounts of DHEA-S, DHEA, A, and T secreted daily by adrenals and ovaries are compared (Table 17-2), it becomes obvious that the adrenals contribute the bulk of androgens by their DHEA-S production of 6 to 24 mg/day. Thus, DHEA-S is an excellent measure of adrenal androgen production. It is present in high concentrations in the blood, has a long half-life, and is not subject to diurnal or episodic variation. Its measurement is ideal for diagnostic purposes, particularly because it can be measured easily and conveniently in the serum or plasma.

DHEA, DHEA-S, A, and T are metabolized into and excreted as urinary 17-ketosteroids (17-KS), which are comprised of DHEA, androsterone, and etiocholanolone as well as some corticosteroid metabolites. Because adrenal DHEA-S is quantitatively their most important androgenic precursor, urinary 17-KS can serve as an indicator of adrenal androgen production. Serum DHEA-S levels and urinary 17-KS levels correlate well (Figure 17-2).[2] However, serum DHEA-S is much more convenient to measure. Urinary 17-KS measurement requires simultaneous creatinine determination. In addition, urinary 17-KS normally vary with body weight. Serum (or plasma) DHEA-S levels in normal women average 1.7 ± 0.1 μg/mL (mean $\pm$ SE), and 95% confidence limits range from 0.5 to 2.8 μg/mL. Levels greater than 2.8 μg/mL are abnormally elevated.

Table 17-2
Comparison of adrenal and ovarian C_{19} steroid ("androgen") secretion in women

Steroid	Secretion rate (mg/24 hr)	
	Adrenals	Ovaries
DHEA-S	6–24	
DHEA	<1	<1
A	1–2	1–2
T		0.1

Abnormal endocrinology

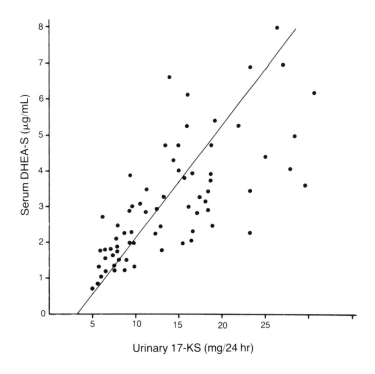

Figure 17-2
Correlation between serum dehydroepiandrosterone sulfate (DHEA-S) and urinary 17-ketosteroids (17-KS) in 71 patients ($r = 0.7$, $P < 0.0005$).

From Lobo RA, Paul WL, Goebelsmann U: Dehydroepiandrosterone sulfate as an indicator of adrenal androgen function. Obstet Gynecol 57:69, 1981. Reprinted with permission from The American College of Obstetricians and Gynecologists.

Testosterone and its metabolites 5α-dihydrotestosterone (DHT) and 5α-androstane-3α,17β-diol (Adiol) are biologically active androgens. DHEA and A, as such, are not androgenic, but they are converted peripherally to T (Figure 17-1). Serum or plasma T levels are a measurement of a biologically active androgen derived from both ovarian secretion and peripheral conversion of DHEA and, particularly, A. These T precursors originate in approximately equal amounts from the adrenals and ovaries (Table 17-3). About 60% to 67% of all the T produced

by a woman originates directly or indirectly in the ovaries; thus, T levels primarily reflect ovarian androgen production, which is controlled by luteinizing hormone (LH).

Table 17-3
Origin of testosterone in women

Ovarian secretion	0.1 mg/day
Peripheral conversion	
A → T	0.2 mg/day
DHEA → T	0.05 mg/day
Total T production	0.35 mg/day

The normal adrenals secrete little, if any, T. Adrenal tumors, however, may secrete T directly and may also secrete large amounts of DHEA-S, DHEA, or A. When extraordinarily large quantities of these T precursors are produced, peripheral conversion of A and DHEA to T increases, although the process is less efficient than gonadal A to T conversion. If the daily production of T reaches or exceeds 2 mg in a woman, virilization may result. The production of T in normal men and women averages 6 mg/24 hr and 0.35 mg/24 hr, respectively.

In conclusion, if T is secreted directly (more commonly by an ovarian than an adrenal tumor), serum (or plasma) T levels increase and serum (plasma) DHEA-S and urinary 17-KS are just within the normal range. However, if DHEA-S, DHEA, and/or A are secreted in large quantities, DHEA-S and 17-KS levels are markedly elevated; whereas T levels may be just above the normal range or moderately or severely elevated. Both serum T and either serum DHEA-S or urinary 17-KS must be measured in patients with hirsutism or virilization.

Most circulating testosterone (approximately 85%) is bound to sex hormone-binding globulin (SHBG).[3] This bound fraction is considered biologically inactive. Thus, an increased concentration of total serum T is not the only cause of androgen excess; an increase in the proportion of unbound serum T must also be considered a causal factor. A woman with a normal total serum T may have a significant elevation of unbound serum T—one explanation of hirsutism in a woman with normal serum T levels.

The fraction of serum T not bound to SHBG consists mainly of albumin-associated (10% to 15%) and entirely unbound or "free" (1% to 2%) T. These are the biologically active moieties. Non-SHBG-bound T, considered the androgenic fraction of circulating T, is elevated in approximately 60% to 70% of hirsute women, and levels found in normal and hirsute women have shown considerable overlap (Figure 17-

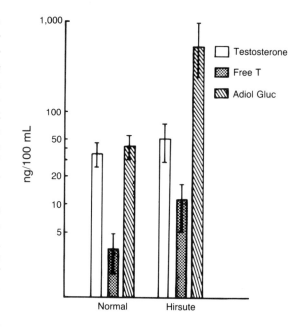

Figure 17-3
Plasma total testosterone, unbound testosterone (free T) and 5α-androstane-3α, 17β-diol-glucuronide (Adiol Gluc) in normal and hirsute women. Note the insignificant elevation with overlap for T and free T and the highly significant increase in Adiol Gluc without overlap between the two groups of women.

Reproduced from Horton R, Hawks D, Lobo RA: 3α,17β-androstanediol glucuronide in plasma. A marker of androgen action in idiopathic hirsutism. J Clin Invest 69:1203, 1982, by copyright permission of The American Society for Clinical Investigation.

3).[4-6] An explanation for this discrepancy may come from a better understanding of the mechanism of androgen action. For T to exert its biological effect, it must be converted to its active metabolite, DHT, in target tissues such as skin. The enzyme 5α-reductase is required in the conversion process. Therefore, the identification of a marker of peripheral (target tissue) androgen metabolism would be extremely useful in understanding the source of abnormality in hirsutism. To this end, serum DHT has been measured, but it does not appear to be reflective of the degree of target tissue androgen metabolism.

Abnormal endocrinology

Most recently, a metabolite of T, 5α-andro-stane-3α,17β-diol-glucuronide (Adiol Gluc), believed to originate peripherally, and possibly within the pilosebaceous apparatus (hair follicle), has been measured in hirsute women.[6,7] It was found that this 5α-reduced T metabolite was elevated in 98% of hirsute patients but normal in all nonhirsute controls in our original study (Figure 17-3).[6] With recent refinements in the assay, it appears that there may be a 25% overlap in values between hirsute and nonhirsute patients. Nevertheless, Adiol Gluc appears to be a most accurate indicator of peripheral androgen metabolism in women. Although it was hoped that this marker would be useful in evaluating a patient's response to antiandrogen therapy for the control of hirsutism, recent data have cast doubt on the usefulness of measuring Adiol Gluc to determine the efficacy of treatment.

Causes of androgen excess

Only a limited number of disorders can cause hirsutism or virilization (Table 17-4). If one eliminates (1) iatrogenic or drug-induced androgen excess, (2) abnormal gonadal or sexual development (i.e., androgen excess in conjunction with primary amenorrhea), and (3) conditions unique to pregnancy (luteoma of pregnancy and hyperreactio luteinalis), there remain only seven causes of androgen excess:

- "Idiopathic" androgen excess
- Polycystic ovary syndrome
- Stromal hyperthecosis
- Androgen-producing ovarian tumors
- Cushing's syndrome/disease
- Adult manifestation of congenital adrenal hyperplasia
- Androgen-producing adrenal tumors

When androgen excess is associated with primary amenorrhea, abnormal gonadal or sexual development should be strongly suspected. Furthermore, before embarking on a major workup for hirsutism or virilization, the physician is well advised to rule out exogenous androgens. It is best to ask the patient to list all medications that she takes on her own or by prescription, including injections. This is usually more rewarding than simply asking the patient whether she takes any androgens.

Medications that can cause hirsutism if given in moderate doses, and virilization if given in large doses, contain or are related to testosterone. These include anabolic steroids; 19-nor-steroids, or synthetic progestins (e.g., norethindrone, norgestrel); and similar compounds (e.g., danazol, which is an isoxazole derivative of 17α-ethinyltestosterone).

A description of disorders associated with androgen excess and a simplified approach to the differential diagnosis of hirsutism and virilization follow. An outline of appropriate therapy for the various disorders concludes the chapter.

"Idiopathic" androgen excess

Hirsutism labeled "idiopathic" (also referred to as constitutional or familial hirsutism) occurs more frequently in certain ethnic populations, particularly in women of Mediterranean ancestry. This is the most common disorder associated with androgen excess. It is defined as hirsutism in conjunction with regular menstrual cycles and normal levels of serum T, serum DHEA-S, and

Table 17-4
Differential diagnosis of androgen excess

"Idiopathic" hirsutism
Polycystic ovary syndrome
Stromal hyperthecosis
Androgen-producing ovarian tumors
Cushing's syndrome/disease
Adult manifestation of congenital adrenal hyperplasia
Androgen-producing adrenal tumors
Androgen excess in pregnancy: luteoma
  or hyperreactio luteinalis
Exogenous/iatrogenic androgen excess
Abnormal gonadal or sexual development

urinary 17-KS. Idiopathic hirsutism is never associated with any sign of virilization. Its cause remained enigmatic for a long time. A relative increase in unbound or non-SHBG-bound plasma or serum T has been thought to be responsible. However, as noted above, unbound T is not elevated in all women with clinical signs of the disorder, and levels in normal and hirsute women overlap (Figure 17-3).[6]

A plausible hypothesis for the cause of idiopathic hirsutism is altered T action at the pilosebaceous apparatus due to increased affinity of T to androgen receptors or increased cellular T metabolism to DHT and Adiol (increased 5α-reductase activity). As noted above, Adiol Gluc has been found to be elevated in almost all hirsute patients (Figure 17-3).[6] Recent work in our laboratory has also confirmed that there is increased 5α-reductase activity in the skin of patients with idiopathic hirsutism.[8] This suggests (1) that "idiopathic" hirsutism is a misnomer, and is, in fact, a disorder of the peripheral androgen metabolism that is possibly genetically determined and (2) that antiandrogen therapy (cyproterone acetate, spironolactone, and cimetidine), which interferes with T action and 5α-reduction at the hair follicle, should be specific therapy for this type of hirsutism.

Polycystic ovary syndrome (PCO)

PCO, the second most common disorder associated with hirsutism, is described in detail in Chapter 18. Hence, only the most important features of PCO will be mentioned here to highlight the history, physical, and laboratory findings that distinguish PCO from other disorders of androgen excess.

In brief, PCO is a combination of androgen excess and anovulation, usually manifested as hirsutism with oligomenorrhea, amenorrhea, or dysfunctional uterine bleeding. This disorder begins with menarche: Both hirsutism and menstrual irregularities are typically of perimenarcheal onset. Serum or plasma T levels are normal or mildly to moderately elevated, usually below 1.5 ng/mL; levels of DHEA-S and 17-KS may be normal or elevated, indicating an adrenal component of the disorder. Serum LH and the LH:FSH ratio are typically elevated.

Hirsutism is present in most (about 70%)—but not all—PCO patients. Virilization, which requires serum or plasma T levels of at least 2 ng/mL, is never encountered in PCO. The presence of virilization should raise the physician's suspicion of a more serious disorder than PCO.

Stromal hyperthecosis

An occasional patient may give a history consistent with PCO and present with slowly but persistently progressing signs of virilization, such as temporal balding, decreased breast size, and clitoral enlargement. Usually such patients gain weight and muscle strength through the anabolic effect of their markedly increased ovarian T production. Their urinary levels of 17-KS may be slightly elevated, but are usually commensurate with their increase in body weight. Serum or plasma T levels, however, are markedly elevated above those seen in PCO.

By the time this disorder, known as stromal hyperthecosis, has progressed to virilization, serum (plasma) T levels will exceed 2 ng/mL and may be as high as in patients with androgen-producing tumors (Sertoli-Leydig-cell tumor, hilus-cell tumor, and testosterone-producing adrenal adenomas). However, stromal hyperthecosis is associated with a long history of anovulation and/or amenorrhea, and of slowly but relentlessly progressing androgen excess; whereas androgen-producing tumors characteristically cause rapidly progressing signs of androgen excess.[9]

If retrograde ovarian vein catheterization is carried out and testosterone measured in the ovarian venous effluent, it will be found that both ovaries produce large quantities of T. Ovarian biopsy will reveal nests of luteinized theca cells within the stroma of bilaterally enlarged ovaries, which will have thickened capsules but lack the subcapsular cysts characteristic of PCO.[10] The theca cells are thought to be the source of the excessive T production.

Androgen-producing ovarian tumors[11]

This category includes: (1) Sertoli-Leydig-cell tumors (formerly known as arrhenoblastomas), (2) hilus-cell tumors, (3) lipoid-cell (adrenal rest) tumors, and (4) infrequently, granulosa-theca tumors and (5) androgen-producing ovarian stroma in association with pseudomucinous cystadenomas, cystadenocarcinomas, Brenner tumors, or Krukenberg tumors. Sertoli-Leydig-cell tumors, which account for less than 1% of all solid ovarian tumors, tend to occur during the second to fourth decades of life; whereas hilus-cell tumors occur more frequently in postmenopausal women.

By the time the signs and symptoms of androgen excess cause the patient to seek medical assistance, Sertoli-Leydig-cell tumors are usually (in more than 85% of cases) so large that they are readily palpable on pelvic exam, while hilus-cell tumors are still small. In women with either type of tumor, serum T is much more elevated than serum DHEA-S or urinary 17-KS. Granulosa-theca tumors primarily produce estradiol (E_2). They produce T less frequently.

Rapidly progressing symptoms of androgen excess should always suggest the presence of an androgen-producing tumor. This rapid progression, typical of both ovarian and adrenal androgen-producing tumors, is also known as a "short history of androgen excess." Hirsutism is usually the first sign, because it requires less T than virilization. As the tumor continues to grow, more and more T is produced, resulting in rapidly worsening hirsutism and progressive virilization. With all ovarian tumors except the lipoid-cell tumors, serum T is characteristically elevated in conjunction with normal or mildly elevated serum DHEA-S or urinary 17-KS levels. The lack of significant increase in DHEA-S or 17-KS, which originate in the adrenals, distin-

guishes ovarian from adrenal androgen-producing tumors.

Cushing's syndrome

Cushing's syndrome is caused by excessive production of glucocorticoid hormones due to (1) increased hypothalamic-pituitary ACTH secretion, resulting in bilateral adrenal hyperstimulation (Cushing's disease); (2) adrenal adenoma or carcinoma; or (3) ectopic ACTH elaborated by neoplasms such as bronchogenic carcinoma. The well-known clinical findings of Cushing's syndrome are centripetal obesity; abdominal striae; supraclavicular and dorsal neck fat pads; muscle wasting and weakness; thin skin with easy bruising; fine hair (lanugo hair) on face, back, and extremities; hypertension, potassium loss, and alkalosis; overt or latent diabetes mellitus; osteoporosis; amenorrhea; and psychosis. Serum cortisol levels are increased and lack the typical diurnal cyclicity.

If, on the basis of the clinical findings, Cushing's syndrome cannot be ruled out, an overnight dexamethasone suppression test is indicated (Figure 17-4). Dexamethasone, 1.0 mg, is given orally at 11 PM, and plasma cortisol is measured at 8 AM (next morning). If plasma cortisol is suppressed to less than 5 μg/100 mL, Cushing's syndrome is ruled out. Otherwise, the

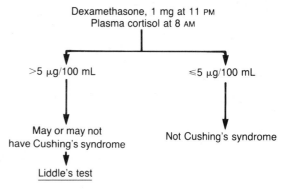

Figure 17-4
Outline of overnight dexamethasone suppression test.

patient may or may not have Cushing's syndrome and a full-scale dexamethasone suppression test (Liddle's test) must be done. Usually, it is performed by the medical rather than the gynecologic endocrinologist.

The catabolic effects of glucocorticoid excess are obvious and easily distinguished from the anabolic effects of T excess. If virilization is evident, an adrenal adenoma or carcinoma that secretes both androgens and glucocorticoids should be suspected. Its hallmark will be a marked increase in DHEA-S and 17-KS.

Adult manifestation of congenital adrenal hyperplasia (CAH)

Defects in cortisol biosynthesis causing CAH in the female are usually detected at birth, because they are manifest as genital ambiguity of the genetically female newborn. Incomplete or mild defects, however, may go unnoticed throughout the neonatal period, childhood, and puberty. They may become clinically evident in the late teens or early 20s as a combination of menstrual abnormalities and signs of androgen excess; and this entity probably accounts for about 5% of hirsute women. A history of initially (at ages 6 to 8) accelerated and subsequently (at the time of puberty) decreased linear growth should arouse suspicion of CAH.

The adult manifestation of CAH due to incomplete 21-hydroxylase or 11β-hydroxylase deficiency may mimic PCO. As a result of inadequate cortisol production, the secretion of ACTH is increased, stimulating adrenal steroid production that leads to adrenal hyperplasia and increased biosynthesis of steroids proximal to the enzymatic defect. In both 21-hydroxylase deficiency and 11β-hydroxylase deficiency, the levels of serum 17-hydroxyprogesterone and urinary pregnanetriol are markedly elevated. Conversions of 17-hydroxypregnenolone and 17-hydroxyprogesterone to DHEA and A, respectively, are the only open pathways in these disorders. Hence, C_{19} steroid ("androgen") production is elevated in CAH. Peripheral conversion of these prehormones results in increased serum or plasma T concentrations and androgen excess. Increases in levels of circulating A usually exceed those of serum T.

Simultaneously, the normal hypothalamic-pituitary-ovarian hormonal feedback system is interrupted and anovulation occurs, resulting in oligomenorrhea or amenorrhea. As hypothesized by Lobo and Goebelsmann,[12] increased adrenal androgen production causes decreased SHBG binding capacity and raises the levels of both total and non-SHBG-bound T and E_2. The increase in E_2 may lead to increased LH secretion, stimulation of ovarian androgen production, and inhibition of follicle maturation, resulting in anovulation.[12]

Suppression of excess ACTH by exogenous corticosteroids reduces adrenal C_{21} and C_{19} steroid output. Because hypothalamic-pituitary and ovarian functions are intact, ovulatory cycles are promptly reestablished. As CAH is readily treated by exogenous corticosteroids, it is advisable to obtain 17-hydroxyprogesterone levels in all young PCO-like patients with markedly elevated serum DHEA-S and/or urinary 17-KS levels.[13] Measurement of serum or plasma 17-hydroxyprogesterone is preferable to that of urinary pregnanetriol, because the former assay is more precise and urine collection is not a problem. Unfortunately, there is no absolute criterion for when to order the test in cases of PCO symptoms that may reflect an adult manifestation of CAH. When in doubt, it is highly advisable to obtain a serum 17-hydroxyprogesterone level. If a random level exceeds 8 ng/mL, the diagnosis of CAH is established.

To confirm the diagnosis of CAH in cases of borderline 17-hydroxyprogesterone levels (between 3 and 8 ng/mL), an ACTH stimulation test should be done. The patient takes 1.0 mg of oral dexamethasone at 11 PM the night before the test and returns to the clinic the following morning at 8 or 9 AM for a baseline serum 17-

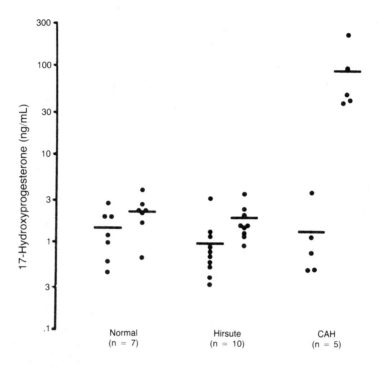

Figure 17-5
Serum 17-hydroxyprogesterone before and 60 minutes after a single IV
bolus of 0.25 mg ACTH in normal women, hirsute patients, and patients with
adult manifestation of congenital adrenal hyperplasia (CAH) after 1 mg of
dexamethasone at 11 PM. Note the markedly increased response (log scale)
only in patients with adult manifestation of CAH.

*Reproduced, with permission, from Lobo RA, Goebelsmann U: Adult manifestation of
congenital adrenal hyperplasia due to incomplete 21-hydroxylase deficiency mimicking
polycystic ovarian disease. Am J Obstet Gynecol 138:720, 1980.*

hydroxyprogesterone level and to receive 0.25
mg of cosyntropin (25 IU synthetic ACTH) IV
as a single bolus. One hour after the ACTH injection, another blood sample is drawn for 17-
hydroxyprogesterone. CAH is characterized by
a marked increase in serum 17-hydroxyproges-
terone in response to ACTH (Figure 17-5).[13] In
all patients with CAH, the level will exceed 20
ng/mL. It has been demonstrated that a rare hirsute patient may have hidden or "cryptic" CAH,
i.e., normal baseline levels of 17-hydroxyproges-
terone but a marked increase after ACTH administration. Because CAH is readily treated
with glucocorticoids, reestablishing ovulatory cycles and eliminating androgen excess, it appears
wise to do an unnecessary 17-hydroxyprogester-
one test rather than miss the diagnosis of adult
manifestation of CAH.

Androgen-producing adrenal tumors

These can be classified as: (1) adenomas and carcinomas (non-T-producing) and (2) T-producing adenomas. T-producing adrenal adenomas are extremely rare. Their cells resemble the ovarian hilus cells that are analogous to Leydig cells. These tumor cells are most efficient T producers and are stimulated by LH and hCG. Thus, T secretion decreases following LH suppression and increases upon hCG stimulation in patients with T-producing adrenal adenomas.

Most commonly, androgen-producing adrenal adenomas and carcinomas secrete large quantities of DHEA-S, DHEA, and A; T is produced by extraglandular conversion of these prehormones and may also be secreted directly by the tumor. Levels of serum DHEA-S and urinary 17-KS are very highly elevated. Often, by the time the signs of androgen excess are apparent, the tumors are already large enough to be easily diagnosed on an IV pyelogram (IVP) or renal scan. When DHEA-S levels exceed 8 μg/mL, a CAT scan is the preferred test for ruling out an adrenal tumor.

Adrenal adenomas and carcinomas may produce various corticosteroids and sex hormones in various combinations. It is, therefore, impossible to establish a definite hormonal pattern that is pathognomonic of all tumors of this type. Yet, by and large, highly elevated levels of serum (plasma) DHEA-S (>8 μg/mL) or urinary 17-KS suggest adrenal adenoma or carcinoma. If virilization has occurred, the serum or plasma T levels will be markedly elevated (>2 ng/mL). Women with androgen-producing adrenal tumors present with the same "short history of androgen excess" as do women with androgen-producing ovarian tumors. However, marked elevations in DHEA-S or 17-KS are characteristic of only the adrenal tumors, and can serve to distinguish them from ovarian tumors. Because of the highly malignant potential and metastatic tendency of adrenal carcinomas, surgical intervention is most urgent.

Androgen excess during pregnancy

Due to increased production of SHBG during pregnancy, serum T levels normally increase two- to threefold, and more T is SHBG-bound than before. When virilization occurs during pregnancy, it is usually due to a luteoma or to hyperreactio luteinalis.

Luteomas of pregnancy are unilateral or bilateral solid ovarian tumors that usually are not palpable. These benign neoplasms regress spontaneously after pregnancy with no adverse effects on the mother's health or fertility. Not all luteomas cause maternal virilization. But if the mother is virilized, some female fetuses will be virilized and others will not be affected at all.

Hyperreactio luteinalis always affects both ovaries and, in contrast to luteomas, is often associated with increased hCG levels. The ovaries are grossly enlarged in this disorder, with multiple clear or hemorrhagic fluid-filled cysts. The ovarian enlargement regresses within weeks following termination of pregnancy. As with luteomas of pregnancy, hyperreactio luteinalis may cause maternal virilization; however, there is never any virilization of the female offspring.[14] The features of luteomas and hyperreactio luteinalis are summarized in Table 17-5.[14] Today's high-resolution ultrasonography instruments should allow differentiation between luteomas and hyperreactio luteinalis.

The phenomenon of maternal virilization without fetal virilization in hyperreactio luteinalis and some cases of luteoma can be explained by the fact that the placenta protects the fetus against maternal androgens through extensive metabolism, or aromatization, of androgens into estrogens. If the maternal T levels rise beyond the placental aromatizing capacity, the danger of virilization of female offspring arises. To effect sexual ambiguity in a female fetus, androgen excess must be present before 12 to 16 weeks' gestation. The minimum maternal serum T level that places a female fetus in danger of virilization has not yet been determined.

Abnormal endocrinology

Table 17-5
Differences between luteoma of pregnancy and hyperreactio luteinalis

Luteoma	Hyperreactio luteinalis
Solid, uni- or bilateral	Multiple cysts, bilateral
Not associated with excessive hCG	Often associated with increased hCG
More common in multigravidas	More common in primigravidas
About 50% of female fetuses are virilized if mother is virilized	No reported case of virilization of a female fetus even in a virilized mother

Adapted from Hensleigh PA, Woodruff JD: Differential maternal-fetal response to androgenizing luteoma or hyperreactio luteinalis. Obstet Gynecol Surv 33:262, 1978.

Differential diagnosis of androgen excess

Based on a thorough understanding of the various causes of androgen excess, a tentative diagnosis can often be made following a detailed history and a careful physical examination. A "long history" of androgen excess is inconsistent with either ovarian or adrenal androgen-producing tumors. Rapidly progressing hirsutism and, particularly, virilization, associated with highly elevated serum T concentrations (>2 ng/mL) suggest ovarian or adrenal tumors, until proven otherwise. Markedly elevated levels of serum DHEA-S and/or urinary 17-KS indicate adrenal adenoma or carcinoma.

A CAT scan often allows a definitive diagnosis of adrenal adenoma or carcinoma. The majority of adrenal tumors produce large quantities of DHEA-S, but only a small fraction is converted by extraglandular metabolism to A, and even less is converted to T. Only T levels can affect the development of hirsutism or virilization; thus, these tumors must grow quite large before enough A and, finally, T is produced peripherally to cause noticeable signs of androgen excess. By then, the tumors are usually large enough for easy recognition by IVP or CAT scan. Only the very rare gonadotropin-dependent adrenal adenoma secretes T. This type of tumor is still small when its daily production of T reaches several milligrams. These tumors also secrete DHEA-S. Therefore, in the absence of an ovarian tumor, if T levels exceed 1.5 ng/mL and DHEA-S levels are markedly (>8 ng/mL) elevated, the rare T-producing adrenal adenoma should be considered.

It is sometimes impossible to distinguish between ovarian and adrenal androgen-producing tumors, and the use of differential suppression and stimulation tests (dexamethasone, ACTH, oral contraceptive steroids, and hCG) are usually not helpful. In this setting, retrograde catheterization of adrenal and ovarian veins and assay of the blood obtained may be helpful at times. However, ultrasonography and computerized tomography are the most diagnostically useful modalities. Surgery will always provide a definitive diagnosis.

The following practical scheme has been developed for the evaluation of patients with androgen excess:

A careful history will usually be sufficient to rule out pregnancy-related disorders, exogenous and iatrogenic causes, and abnormal gonadal/sexual development. It will also provide clues to help distinguish more serious (neoplastic) causes from benign causes of androgen excess. By physical examination, abnormal sexual development, abdominal/pelvic masses (ovarian or adrenal tumors), and signs of Cushing's syndrome can be detected.

Following the history and physical, if Cushing's syndrome or CAH is suspected, additional workup as outlined above is necessary. Severe hirsutism at a young age, abnormally short stature, a strong family history of androgen excess, extremely high androgen levels, and coexisting hypertension are characteristic of CAH.

T, DHEA-S, and, if possible, Adiol Gluc levels should be measured in all patients. This functional approach identifies the source of androgen excess, but does not necessarily differentiate between PCO, stromal hyperthecosis, and "idiopathic" androgen excess. While the history and laboratory findings help distinguish between hyperthecosis and PCO, a specific distinction between PCO and idiopathic androgen excess is unnecessary for treatment.

Therapy

Therapy for androgen excess should be directed toward its various causes.

Ovarian and adrenal tumors

For ovarian and adrenal androgen-producing tumors, surgery is indicated immediately. More than 95% of all Sertoli-Leydig-cell tumors are unilateral. These are commonly seen in young women; stage IA cases may be treated by unilateral salpingo-oophorectomy if the patient wishes to maintain reproductive potential. The less frequent, poorly differentiated Sertoli-Leydig-cell tumors that have grown beyond surgical control will require additional therapeutic measures. Hilus-cell tumors occur most often in postmenopausal women; the preferred therapy is total abdominal hysterectomy with bilateral salpingo-oophorectomy.

Adrenal androgen-producing tumors may be adenomas or carcinomas. These tumors are usually large at the time of diagnosis; signs of androgen excess are usually not apparent when the tumors are small. Surgery should be performed as early as possible to reduce the chance of (primarily hepatic) metastases. Once hepatic metastases have developed, the prognosis is poor despite chemotherapy, which includes mitotane (o,p'-DDD) and 5-fluorouracil. The very rare T-producing adrenal adenomas are benign and require simple surgical removal.

Once an androgen-producing tumor has been removed, serum levels of androgens, particularly T, will fall to normal. Subsequent measurement of hormone levels can be used to check for recurrence. The successfully treated patient will experience disappearance of acne and oily skin, resumption of regular menses (unless bilateral oophorectomy was performed), normalization of breast size, and some decrease in clitoral enlargement. The hair that developed during androgen excess will not disappear, but it will grow less rapidly and become finer (with smaller hair-shaft diameter). It is suggested that such patients, after successful removal of the source of androgen excess, undergo electrolysis for facial hair. Hair on extremities can be removed by shaving or waxing, or can be made less visible by bleaching.

Stromal hyperthecosis

Stromal hyperthecosis is best treated by bilateral oophorectomy in conjunction with total abdominal hysterectomy. These ovaries, as a rule, do not respond to ovulation induction with clomiphene citrate, and suppression with oral contraceptives (OCs) and/or glucocorticoids appears ineffective. Following surgery, estrogen and progesterone replacement, unless contraindicated, is advisable.

Polycystic ovary syndrome (PCO)

Treatment of PCO patients complaining of androgen excess has been outlined in Chapter 18. In brief, these patients are best treated with OCs. If serum (plasma) DHEA-S is significantly elevated, indicating substantial adrenal "androgen" overproduction, 0.5 mg of oral dexamethasone should be administered each evening in lieu of or in conjunction with OCs. The oligomenorrheic or amenorrheic PCO patient needs a 10-day course of oral progestins (e.g., medroxyprogesterone acetate, 10 mg/day, or norethindrone acetate, 5 mg/day) at least every other month. This regimen converts the proliferated endometrium and causes regular uterine withdrawal bleeding. Neither dexamethasone nor cyclic progestins prevent pregnancy, but spontaneously occurring pregnancy without the use of ovulation stimulatory drugs is uncommon in PCO patients. As noted above, chemical normalization of circulating androgens will not eliminate existing excess body hair. It will only decrease the rate of hair growth and the diameter of the hair shaft.

Ovarian wedge resection is followed by an immediate decrease in serum levels of T and A.[15] However, the drop in serum A is only temporary, and no conclusive evidence predicts how long decreased T levels will persist. Clinical experience shows that wedge resection is not an effective therapy for hirsutism. For women over 35 who do not want further childbearing, and who are severely affected by androgen excess of primary ovarian origin (i.e., suppressible by OCs), bilateral oophorectomy (and hysterectomy) is a useful procedure.

Adult manifestation of congenital adrenal hyperplasia (CAH)

To correct anovulation and androgen excess, patients with CAH are best treated with oral glucocorticoids: 20 to 25 mg of hydrocortisone; 5 to 7.5 mg of prednisone; or 0.5 to 0.75 mg of dexamethasone daily in divided doses. Frequently, lower doses may be therapeutic. (Glucocorticoids must be given parenterally when nausea and vomiting are present.) These doses suppress the production of ACTH, and the adrenals will decrease in size. The patient must wear a Medic Alert bracelet that identifies her disorder and medication, as well as the need to increase gluco-

corticoid dosage in case of surgery, stress, etc. Glucocorticoid therapy restores hypothalamic-pituitary-ovarian feedback so promptly that ovulation resumes within a few weeks. Pregnancy may occur, and the patient should be so advised. An appropriate contraceptive method, if desired, should be supplied. A barrier technique is preferred.

"Idiopathic" androgen excess

The treatment of "idiopathic" hirsutism has been one of the more disappointing therapeutic ventures. Although a benign and essentially cosmetic disorder, hirsutism is frequently of great concern to the patient. Besides mechanical means of removing hair (shaving, clipping, waxing) or making it less visible (bleaching), three therapeutic modalities are currently available: (1) OCs, (2) dexamethasone, and (3) antiandrogens (spironolactone, cimetidine). At present, some degree of success is achieved in approximately 70% of patients treated for hirsutism with these agents. Cyproterone acetate, a potent antiandrogen that has been used for years in European and other countries, is not available for use in the US.

OCs primarily decrease LH levels, thereby lowering ovarian androgen production and increasing levels of SHBG.[16] In addition, certain OC formulations reduce adrenal androgen secretion by about 30%.[17,18] Low-dose OCs (with 35 μg of ethinylestradiol) are as effective as higher-dose OCs. Norgestrel-containing OCs (Ovral, Lo/Ovral) should never be used for treatment of hirsutism; norgestrel is a very androgenic progestin.

Corticosteroid therapy should be used only in cases of adrenal androgen excess (DHEA-S > 4 μg/mL). Dexamethasone principally, but not exclusively, reduces the adrenal production of androgens. We prescribe 0.25 to 0.50 mg of dexamethasone to be taken at bedtime. An 8:30 AM cortisol level between 2 and 5 μg/dL measured once androgen levels have been sup-

Table 17-6
Treatment of hirsutism according to source of androgen excess

Androgen	Treatment
↑ T	Oral contraceptives
↑ DHEA-S (<4 µg/mL)	Oral contraceptives
↑ DHEA-S (>4 µg/mL), normal T	Dexamethasone
↑ T, ↑ DHEA-S (>4 µg/mL)	Oral contraceptives + dexamethasone
Normal T, normal DHEA-S, ↑ Adiol Gluc	Spironolactone*

Spironolactone may also be substituted for any of the above regimens if no improvement is noted after 3 months of treatment.

pressed (about 2 months) demonstrates that a patient on dexamethasone therapy is not at increased risk from excessive pituitary suppression of ACTH.[19] In some patients with high levels of both ovarian (T > 1.0 ng/mL) and adrenal (DHEA-S > 4 µg/mL) androgens, we have used combined therapy with both OCs and dexamethasone, as advocated by Casey.[20]

Spironolactone and cimetidine belong to a class of compounds called antiandrogens. Their mode of action is more complex; they reduce androgen production and also appear to exert interference at the site of androgenic action (the pilosebaceous apparatus).[21-23] This effect appears to be shared by C_{21} steroids with progestational activity or related steric configuration.

Therapeutic success with spironolactone has occurred in both idiopathic hirsutism and PCO. Oral dosages have ranged from 100 to 200 mg/day. Regression of hirsutism, as measured by hair-shaft diameter, density, and rate of facial hair growth, was reported in 19 of 20 women treated for 2 months.[21] Another study also reported regression of hirsutism as well as restoration of regular but anovulatory menstrual cycles and decreased levels of circulating androgens in 34 PCO patients after 3 months of spironolactone.[24] These findings have been confirmed by a study that also found 200 mg/day more effective than 100 mg/day.[22] The higher-dose regimen was apparently nontoxic; tests of liver function and plasma electrolytes remained normal.

Cimetidine has also been used with reason-able success, but results have been reported on only a small number of women.[23] More studies are needed to assess cimetidine's efficacy, safety, and mode of action for this indication.

Medication for hirsutism should be chosen according to the source of androgen excess. Table 17-6 provides a general outline for making the initial choice. In this context, elevated T signifies ovarian androgen excess; elevated DHEA-S indicates adrenal androgen excess. Ideal therapeutic agents would exert exclusively local (hair follicle) antiandrogenic action without affecting ovarian or adrenal steroidogenesis. It is likely that such compounds will eventually be developed for systemic or, possibly, local use. They would be welcomed by all who share the present dilemma of treating "idiopathic" hirsutism.

References

1. Goebelsmann U: Polycystic ovary syndrome. In *Endocrinology and Metabolism, Continuing Education and Quality Control Program.* American Association for Clinical Chemistry, 1983

2. Lobo RA, Paul WL, Goebelsmann U: Dehydroepiandrosterone sulfate as an indicator of adrenal androgen function. *Obstet Gynecol* 57:69, 1981

3. Anderson DC: Sex hormone-binding globulin. *Clin Endocrinol* 3:69, 1974

4. Lobo RA, Paul WL, Goebelsmann U: Serum levels of DHEA-S in gynecologic endocrinopathy and infertility. *Obstet Gynecol* 57:607, 1981

5. Lobo RA, Goebelsmann U, Horton R: 5α-androstane-3α,17β-diol-glucuronide (3αAG): An index of increased peripheral androgen action in hirsutism. *Proc Soc Gynecol Invest* (Abstract #367), Dallas, March 1982

6. Horton R, Hawks D, Lobo RA: 3α,17β-androstanediol glucuronide in plasma. A marker of androgen action in idiopathic hirsutism. *J Clin Invest* 69:1203, 1982

7. Lobo RA, Goebelsmann U, Horton R: Evidence for the importance of peripheral tissue events in the development of hirsutism in polycystic ovary syndrome. *J Clin Endocrinol Metab* 57:393, 1983

8. Serafini P, Aflan R, Lobo RA: 5α reductase activity in the genital skin of hirsute women. *J Clin Endocrinol Metab* 60:349, 1985

9. Judd HL, Scully RE, Herbst AL, et al: Familial hyperthecosis: Comparison of endocrinologic and histologic findings with polycystic ovarian disease. *Am J Obstet Gynecol* 117:976, 1973

10. Behrman SJ, Scully RE: Case records of the Massachusetts General Hospital: Infertility and irregular menses in a 27-year-old woman. *N Engl J Med* 287:1192, 1972

11. Ireland K, Woodruff JD: Masculinizing ovarian tumors. *Obstet Gynecol Surv* 31:83, 1976

12. Lobo RA, Goebelsmann U: Effect of androgen excess on inappropriate gonadotropin secretion as found in polycystic ovary syndrome. *Am J Obstet Gynecol* 142:394, 1982

13. Lobo RA, Goebelsmann U: Adult manifestation of congenital adrenal hyperplasia due to incomplete 21-hydroxylase deficiency mimicking polycystic ovarian disease. *Am J Obstet Gynecol* 138:720, 1980

14. Hensleigh PA, Woodruff JD: Differential maternal-fetal response to androgenizing luteoma or hyperreactio luteinalis. *Obstet Gynecol Surv* 33:262, 1978

15. Judd HL, Rigg LA, Anderson DC, et al: The effects of ovarian wedge resection on circulating gonadotropin and ovarian steroid levels in patients with polycystic ovary syndrome. *J Clin Endocrinol Metab* 43:347, 1976

16. Givens JR, Andersen RN, Wiser WL, et al: The effectiveness of two oral contraceptives in suppressing plasma androstanedione, testosterone, LH and FSH, and stimulating plasma testosterone-binding capacity in hirsute women. *Am J Obstet Gynecol* 124:333, 1976

17. Wild RA, Umstot ES, Andersen RN, et al: Adrenal function in hirsutism. II. Effect of an oral contraceptive. *J Clin Endocrinol Metab* 54:676, 1981

18. Klove KL, Roy S, Lobo RA: The effect of different contraceptive treatments on the serum concentration of dehydroepiandrosterone sulfate. *Contraception* 29:319, 1984

19. Boyers P, Buster JE, Marshall JR: Hypothalamic-pituitary-adrenocortical function during long-term low-dose dexamethasone therapy in hyperandrogenized women. *Am J Obstet Gynecol* 142:330, 1982

20. Casey J: Chronic treatment regimens for hirsutism in women: Effect on blood production rates of testosterone and on hair growth. *Clin Endocrinol* 4:313, 1975

21. Cummings D, Yang JC, Rebar RW, et al: Treatment of hirsutism with spironolactone. *JAMA* 247:1295, 1982

22. Lobo RA, Shoupe D, Serafini P, et al: The effect of two doses of spironolactone on serum androgens and anagen hair in hirsute women. *Fertil Steril* 43:200, 1985

23. Vigersky RA, Mehlman I, Glass AR, et al: Treatment of hirsute women with cimetidine. *N Engl J Med* 303:1042, 1980

24. Silber D, Kirschner MA: Therapeutic effects of spironolactone in polycystic ovary syndrome. *Obstet Gynecol* 61:429, 1983

Chapter 18

Polycystic Ovary Syndrome

Rogerio A. Lobo, M.D.

In 1935, Stein and Leventhal described a syndrome in which amenorrhea, hirsutism, and obesity were associated with enlarged polycystic ovaries.[1] Since that time, the morphologic finding of polycystic or sclerocystic ovaries has been important clinically. Although this morphologic finding was associated with a variety of clinical symptoms and signs, the diagnosis of polycystic ovary (PCO) disease was previously made on the anatomic findings alone. The spectrum of symptoms and signs of PCO was compiled in 1963 by Goldzieher and Axelrod from 1,079 cases reported in the scientific literature (Table 18-1).[2] Although the incidence of PCO has not been ac-

Table 18-1
Incidence of symptoms associated
with polycystic ovary syndrome*

| Symptom | Incidence (%) | | No. of usable cases |
	Mean	Range	
Infertility	74	35–95	596
Hirsutism	69	17–83	819
Amenorrhea	51	15–77	640
Obesity	41	16–49	600
Functional bleeding	29	6–65	547
Dysmenorrhea	23		75
Corpus luteum at surgery	22	0–71	391
Virilization	21	0–28	431
Biphasic body temperature	15	12–40	288
Cyclic menses	12	7–28	395

*Tabulated from 187 references with a total of 1,079 cases. The number of usable cases indicates how many of the 1,079 total cases could be evaluated for the presence or absence of a particular symptom.

Adapted from Goldzieher JW, Axelrod LR: Clinical and biochemical features of polycystic ovarian disease. Fertil Steril 14:631, 1963. Used with permission of the publisher, The American Fertility Society.

curately determined, it is believed that cystic ovarian changes occur in up to 7.2% of women.

Although early studies of PCO have focused on ovarian morphology, there is evidence that this emphasis is misplaced. Enlarged polycystic ovaries may occur in Cushing's syndrome, congenital adrenal hyperplasia, in association with some ovarian or adrenal tumors, and, occasionally, in normal young children.[3-7] Furthermore, women with otherwise classic aspects of this syndrome may have ovaries of normal size. Therefore, in recent years, the research into this heterogeneous syndrome has shifted away from ovarian morphology and toward hormonal characteristics.

In this syndrome, there is nothing inherently abnormal in the ovary itself. Furthermore, the finding of adrenal hyperfunction is not uncommon. These findings suggest that this clinical disorder is a syndrome rather than a disease. In fact, it is not purely an ovarian syndrome. Therefore, although for the sake of convention this disorder will be referred to as polycystic ovary syndrome or PCO, it might well be renamed as a syndrome of hyperandrogenism with chronic anovulation (HCA).

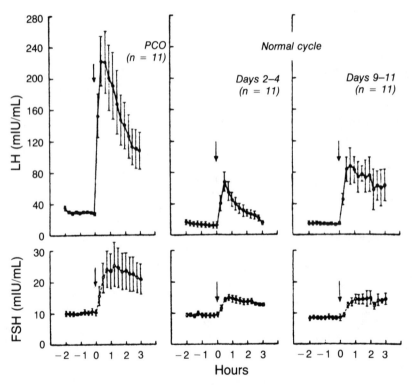

Figure 18-1
Comparison of quantitative LH and FSH release in response to a single bolus of 150 μg of GnRH in PCO patients and in normal women during low estrogen (early follicular) and high estrogen (late follicular) phases of their cycles.

Hormonal characteristics

The most characteristic biochemical abnormality in PCO is inappropriate gonadotropin secretion (IGS). IGS is primarily manifest by an elevated serum level of luteinizing hormone (LH) (>21 mIU/mL) and a normal or low serum level of follicle-stimulating hormone (FSH). Further, it has been well documented that there is an exaggerated response of serum LH, but not FSH, to gonadotropin-releasing hormone (GnRH), compared to that which occurs in various phases of the normal menstrual cycle (Figure 18-1).[8] Because serum FSH may be low and LH may not always be elevated, it has been suggested that the use of the LH:FSH ratio would be most discriminatory for hormonal diagnosis. In our experience, an LH:FSH ratio over 3, provided the serum LH level is not below 8 mIU/mL, is virtually diagnostic of PCO.

Recently, we have assessed the measurement of bioactive LH in serum, using a sensitive in vitro assay described by Van Damme, and have compared this measurement with serum LH and the LH:FSH ratio.[9,10] Serum immunoreactive LH values and LH:FSH ratios in patients with characteristic features of PCO both exceeded the upper 98th percentile of the control population approximately 70% of the time and had a similar accuracy when used diagnostically. However, serum bioactive LH was elevated above the 98th percentile in all but one patient with PCO (Figure 18-2).[9] Further, the ratio of bioactive to immunoreactive LH is also elevated in PCO. Therefore, it appears that the finding of an elevated bioactive LH level may be the best way to establish the diagnosis of PCO and the best marker of IGS. Although IGS, as indicated by an elevated LH:FSH ratio, is the biochemical hallmark for the diagnosis of PCO, patients must also have the other clinical features as listed below. The unusual woman who is clinically normal, but may be found on occasion to have an elevated LH:FSH ratio, does not have PCO.

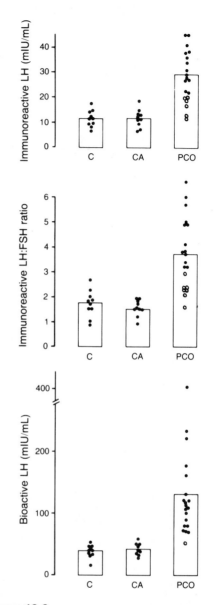

Figure 18-2
Serum measurements of immunoreactive LH, immunoreactive LH:FSH ratios, and bioactive LH in control subjects (C), women with chronic anovulation (CA), and women with PCO. Solid circles for women with PCO indicate values exceeding 3 SD of mean control levels.

From Lobo RA, Kletzky OA, Campeau JD, et al: Elevated bioactive luteinizing hormone in women with the polycystic ovary syndrome. Fertil Steril 39:674, 1983. Reproduced with permission of the publisher, The American Fertility Society.

Hirsutism

Although hirsutism was originally described as a characteristic feature of PCO, it was soon realized that hirsutism need not be present in this disorder. It has been estimated that approximately 30% of women with this syndrome do not have any hirsutism.[2] However, it has been known for several years that nearly all patients with PCO have elevated blood androgen levels.[11] Recently, we measured androgen levels of hirsute as well as nonhirsute patients with PCO.[12] It was found that levels of androgens produced by both the adrenals and ovaries were elevated in patients with PCO, regardless of the presence of hirsutism. Only by the measurement of androgens derived from peripheral tissues, such as serum 3α-androstanediol glucuronide (3α-diol G) and unconjugated 3α-androstanediol, was it possible to distinguish hirsute from nonhirsute patients with PCO (Figure 18-3).[12]

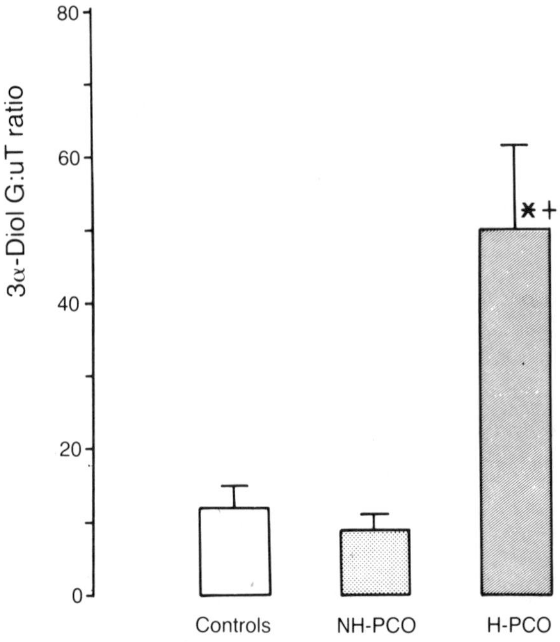

Therefore, it can be concluded that serum androgen levels are usually elevated in PCO, regardless of the presence of hirsutism. Further, the presence or absence of hirsutism depends on the peripheral production of more potent 5α-reduced androgens such as dihydrotestosterone and 3α-diol G, as reflected, most specifically, by measurements of serum 3α-diol G.

Figure 18-3
Ratios of serum 3α-diol G to unbound testosterone (uT) in controls, nonhirsute PCO patients (NH-PCO), and hirsute PCO patients (H-PCO).

*Significantly higher level compared with controls.
†Significantly higher level in hirsute PCO patients compared with nonhirsute ones.

Reproduced, with permission, from Lobo RA, Goebelsmann U, Horton R: Evidence for the importance of peripheral tissue events in the development of hirsutism in polycystic ovary syndrome. J Clin Endocrinol Metab 57:393, 1983. © 1983, The Endocrine Society.

Role of the adrenal

Serum DHEA-S serves as an important marker of adrenal androgen production and is virtually an exclusive product of the zona reticularis.[13] Therefore, by noting changes in serum DHEA-S, it has been possible to determine the extent of adrenal hyperfunction in PCO. In so doing, we have noted that about 50% of PCO patients have elevated levels of DHEA-S (Figure 18-4).[14,15]

When patients with PCO who have elevated levels of DHEA-S have been given ACTH intravenously, approximately one-third of them have exaggerated responses of DHEA-S. This suggests that while plasma ACTH levels are normal in these women, the adrenals of some patients with PCO are extremely sensitive to stimuli.[16,17] These findings suggest further that the adrenal may play an important role in PCO and, possibly, may be involved in its pathogenesis.

While there is suggestive evidence for a specific adrenal cortical androgen-stimulating hormone of approximately 60,000 daltons (CASH), its existence is still controversial. Nevertheless, whether CASH,[18] ACTH, or other factors explain the increased adrenal androgen in PCO, it

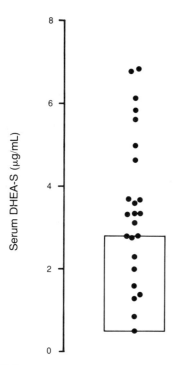

Figure 18-4
Serum DHEA-S in 24 patients with PCO (solid circles) compared with the 95% confidence limits of a control population.

Reproduced, with permission, from Lobo RA: The role of the adrenal in polycystic ovary syndrome. Semin Reprod Endocrinol 2:251, 1984.

is clear that increased adrenal androgen secretion occurs in about 50% of PCO patients.

Modulating sex hormone-binding globulin

Sex hormone-binding globulin (SHBG) is modulated by many factors. Of greatest relevance is the fact that SHBG levels are decreased by increased androgen levels and obesity and increased by hyperestrogenism.[19] Because of the hyperandrogenism and increased body weight found in PCO, it is not surprising that SHBG is significantly decreased in patients with PCO

(Figure 18-5).[20] This lower binding capacity results in an increase in biologically active (non-SHBG-bound) androgens and enhances the clinical features of hyperandrogenism.

SHBG binds estradiol (E_2) as well as testosterone. Our recent finding that non-SHBG-bound E_2 is elevated in PCO, whereas total E_2 is normal and estrone is elevated (Figure 18-6),[21] adds important information to our understanding that patients with PCO are inherently hyperestrogenic. Further, these findings provide insight into the development of IGS in PCO. The elevated levels of non-SHBG-bound E_2 were found to correlate positively with both levels of LH and the LH:FSH ratio (Figure 18-7).[21] Although this correlation was statistically significant, it is not perfect. Therefore, hyperestrogen-

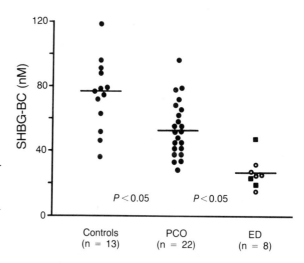

Figure 18-5
Sex hormone-binding globulin binding capacity (SHBG-BC) in control subjects, women with documented PCO, and those with subtle steroid biosynthetic enzyme deficiencies (ED). The mean SHBG-BC of the PCO patients is significantly lower ($P < 0.05$) than that of the control subjects.

Reproduced, with permission, from Lobo RA, Goebelsmann U: Effect of androgen excess on inappropriate gonadotropin secretion as found in the polycystic ovary syndrome. Am J Obstet Gynecol 142:394, 1982.

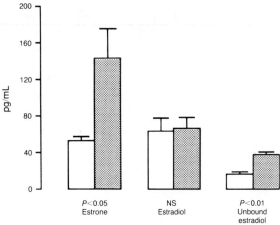

Figure 18-6
Serum estrogen concentrations in 13 normal women and 22 PCO patients (shaded areas).

Reproduced, with permission, from Lobo RA, Granger L, Goebelsmann U, et al: Elevation in unbound serum estradiol as a possible mechanism for inappropriate gonadotropin secretion in women with PCO. J Clin Endocrinol Metab 52:156, 1981. © 1981, The Endocrine Society.

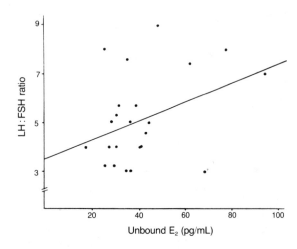

Figure 18-7
Correlation between unbound E_2 and the corresponding LH:FSH ratios of 23 women with PCO. $r = 0.39$; $P < 0.05$.

Reproduced, with permission, from Lobo RA, Granger L, Goebelsmann U, et al: Elevation in unbound serum estradiol as a possible mechanism for inappropriate gonadotropin secretion in women with PCO. J Clin Endocrinol Metab 52:156, 1981. © 1981, The Endocrine Society.

ism in PCO cannot solely explain IGS, and there must be other factors involved.

However, the central importance of SHBG binding in the development or propagation of this syndrome is illustrated in Figure 18-8.[20] Androgen excess from either the ovary or adrenal may decrease SHBG binding. The resultant increase in the free or unbound fraction of E_2 may result in IGS and chronic anovulation. The increased androgen and lowered SHBG lead to a heightened manifestation of androgen excess. Although obesity may also lower SHBG and has been considered to be a major factor in the pathogenesis of PCO,[22] it is unlikely that obesity can be responsible for the multifaceted evolution of this syndrome.

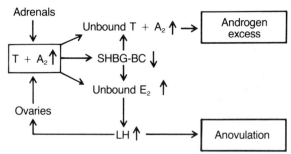

Figure 18-8
Scheme depicting the possible role of adrenal-derived androgens (T, testosterone; A_2, androstenediol) in initiating androgen excess and anovulation.

Reproduced, with permission, from Lobo RA, Goebelsmann U: Effect of androgen excess on inappropriate gonadotropin secretion as found in the polycystic ovary syndrome. Am J Obstet Gynecol 142:394, 1982.

Diagnosis of PCO

Because PCO is a heterogeneous syndrome, we have developed strict criteria for its diagnosis (Table 18-2). Historically, all patients have perimenarcheal onset of the symptom complex. Not all patients are characteristically obese, but using an obesity criterion called the ponderal index

Table 18-2
Criteria for diagnosing PCO

Perimenarcheal onset of menstrual irregularity
(oligomenorrhea and/or amenorrhea)
Increased body weight
Hormonal evidence of androgen excess
Chronic anovulation
Inappropriate gonadotropin secretion (IGS)—(LH:FSH > 3)
Euprolactinemia

(height in inches divided by the cube root of weight in pounds), all patients with PCO have a value below 12. Androgen excess is usually manifest by hirsutism and, rarely, by clitoromegaly. However, in the absence of these findings, elevated blood androgen levels are necessary for the diagnosis of PCO. Usually testosterone is in the range of 70 to 120 ng/dL, signifying that the ovary is producing excessive amounts of androgen. However, when testosterone levels approach 150 to 200 ng/dL, hyperthecosis or an ovarian tumor should be suspected. Serum androstenedione is usually elevated (3 to 5 ng/mL), but may signify either ovarian or adrenal production. For this reason, androstenedione measurements are not useful clinically. As previously stated, serum DHEA-S may be elevated in at least half of PCO patients, suggesting adrenal hyperfunction. All patients exhibit menstrual irregularity, usually oligomenorrhea and amenorrhea, and have chronic anovulation. IGS is practically defined by an LH:FSH ratio above 3.

We have also insisted that patients be euprolactinemic for strict diagnosis of PCO to apply. While this latter point is a matter of controversy, and although it has been stated that up to 25% of PCO patients have hyperprolactinemia,[23,24] we consider hyperprolactinemic patients with features of PCO to be a separate subgroup of the disorder. We refer to these patients as being PCO-like as Yen has advocated.[5] It is emphasized again that while ovarian enlargement by pelvic examination or ultrasound is useful information clinically, this finding is not a criterion for the diagnosis of PCO.

These strict criteria are appropriate for the study of patients with PCO and apply to those patients who may be considered to be "classic." However, some patients may be considered to have PCO who do not meet all these criteria. Relaxation of the criterion of obesity is acceptable if the patient has all other clinical features of the syndrome. In addition, if only immunoreactive LH and LH:FSH ratios are used, up to 30% of patients with PCO may be wrongly excluded from this diagnosis.

There is also a group of overlapping disorders that do not fit our criteria for the diagnosis of PCO. These syndromes may be referred to as PCO-like or PCO-related syndromes (Table 18-3). In a practical sense, with rare exceptions, patients with PCO and PCO-related syndromes are treated similarly. Therefore, it is mainly for theoretical and research purposes that we divide patients into these two categories.

Table 18-3
PCO-related syndromes

With IGS	Without IGS
Adult manifestations of deficiencies of 21-hydroxylase, 11β-hydroxylase, or 3β-ol dehydrogenase-isomerase	Adrenal androgen hyperfunction without IGS
Hyperthyroidism	Hyperprolactinemia
Hypothyroidism	Hyperthecosis
PRL and LH hypersecretion	Ovarian neoplasm
	Simple obesity
	Cushing's syndrome

Patients with adult manifestation of enzymatic deficiencies (congenital adrenal hyperplasia) may clinically mimic PCO and exhibit IGS.[25] Many, if not all, of the features of PCO are present. We have theorized that the reason for IGS in these women is the elevated levels of androgens.[20] The elevated androgen pool leads to lowered SHBG binding and elevated free androgen and E_2 levels as schematically depicted in Figure 18-8.

Despite the lack of phenotypic similarity, hyperthyroid patients may exhibit IGS because of elevated LH levels. This increase in LH occurs, in part, because of increased peripheral production of estrogens, particularly estrone, which produces a positive feedback on LH release. Because SHBG is significantly elevated in hyperthyroidism, high levels of total testosterone result. There is also an increased conversion of estrogen to the 2-hydroxy metabolites.

Hypothyroidism may also be clinically confused with PCO. Anovulation, increased body weight, and IGS are all characteristic findings of both entities. Elevated LH levels result, in part, from an increase in non-SHBG-bound estradiol. We have shown that non-SHBG-bound estradiol is elevated in hypothyroidism as a result of the lowered SHBG. It has also been hypothesized that hypothyroid patients may have an abnormality in dopamine turnover.

It has been reported that some patients who have prolactin-secreting pituitary microadenomas have elevations in serum LH as well. This is a different subgroup of patients from the majority of hyperprolactinemic women, who have normal or low gonadotropin levels. It is attractive to hypothesize that this group of patients may have a significant central dopamine deficiency, because it would then explain the elevations of both PRL and LH.

Some patients will have one of several different syndromes that also clinically resemble PCO. However, these patients will not exhibit IGS. Patients with Cushing's syndrome fall into this category. The obesity, menstrual irregularity, and the sometimes-present androgenic manifestations of hirsutism and acne often suggest a diagnosis of PCO. However, careful evaluation of the patient will rule out PCO. If any suspicion of Cushing's syndrome exists, an overnight dexamethasone suppression test should be carried out.

Patients may present with oligomenorrhea, obesity, and hirsutism and have high levels of serum DHEA-S, indicating adrenal hyperfunction. If serum LH and PRL are normal and Cushing's syndrome is ruled out, these patients may be characterized as having adrenal androgen hyperfunction that is different from CAH. In practical terms, these patients have similar symptoms and hormonal levels as patients with PCO, although they do not exhibit IGS. Therefore, these patients are treated similarly to those with PCO.

Hyperprolactinemic patients normally do not have elevated LH, but they often have oligoamenorrhea and may exhibit manifestations of androgen excess. Although a minority of patients with hyperprolactinemia have elevated testosterone, we have found that adrenal androgen excess is very common in hyperprolactinemic women.[26,27] Also, because SHBG is decreased as well, there may be an increase in non-SHBG-bound testosterone. We and others have shown that the hyperandrogenism in hyperprolactinemia may be normalized with bromocriptine and thus is related to the PRL elevation.[26,28] Therefore, we do not consider hyperprolactinemic patients to have PCO, because they appear to be distinctly different, pathophysiologically. Thus, although mild PRL elevations (20-30 ng/mL) have been reported to occur in 25% to 30% of PCO patients, significant hyperprolactinemia constitutes a different disease entity.

The mildly elevated levels of PRL in PCO may be related to PRL release during the hyperdynamic state of LH secretion. Indeed, we have found that PRL may be released in response to GnRH in some patients with PCO.[29] These findings suggest that hyperprolactinemia in PCO may be of primary significance, or may be secondary. Since we cannot be certain of the clinical significance of the hyperprolactinemia, we have excluded hyperprolactinemic patients from our research investigation of patients with PCO.

Hyperthecosis may be considered to be a variant of PCO, and the two syndromes may overlap to some degree. Although hyperthecosis may be a severe form of PCO that has existed for many years, these patients often have characteristic histologic changes in the ovary. For this reason, hyperthecosis is considered a separate diagnostic entity. Gonadotropin levels are usually normal. Much higher levels of circulating ovarian androgens are present than in PCO, and adrenal androgens are almost never elevated. Indeed, the testosterone levels may be in the low male range, which often causes concern about the possible presence of an ovarian neoplasm. Histologically, the bilaterally enlarged ovaries found in hyperthecosis are distinctly different from "PCO ovaries" and contain nests of luteinized theca cells (Figure 18-9).[30]

Ovarian neoplasms may mimic PCO because of the presence of androgen excess and anovulation. However, gonadotropins are normal and testosterone levels are well above the PCO range (>150 ng/dL). These patients usually have virilization, which rarely, if ever, occurs in PCO. The history is one of rapid change, clearly different from the gradual perimenarcheal onset of true PCO.

Obesity itself may simulate PCO, at least phenotypically. The oligo-amenorrhea, chronic anovulation, and long-standing obesity suggest the diagnosis of PCO. However, androgen levels and gonadotropin levels are normal. For these and other reasons, we do not feel that obesity has a central role in the pathogenesis of PCO.

The ovary in PCO

There is nothing histologically pathognomonic about the ovary in PCO. This has been confirmed in many studies, as was recently reviewed by Goldzieher.[4]

It has been shown that the ovaries of patients with PCO produce excessive amounts of androgens, particularly androstenedione. It has been hypothesized that these high levels of androgens and particularly their 5α-reduced metabolites may lead to premature follicular atresia. The increased mass of follicles undergoing atresia leads further to the androgen production. In addition, it has been shown that these PCO ovaries are aromatase deficient, resulting in an inefficient conversion of androgen to estrogen.[31] The hyperestrogenism in PCO results from increased peripheral conversion of androstenedione to estrone. It is magnified by the lowered SHBG, which results in increased non-SHBG-bound E_2. The polycystic ovary does not secrete increased amounts of E_2 or E_1.

Although it has been shown that aromatase function is deficient in PCO ovaries, it does not mean that the ovaries in PCO are inherently abnormal. Aromatase function depends on FSH, and as FSH is inappropriately low in PCO (at least relative to LH), aromatase function would be expected to be decreased. Indeed, supplying FSH to the culture medium normalizes aromatase function to PCO ovaries cultured in vitro.

Inhibin has been reported to be elevated in the ovaries of some patients with PCO.[32] While it may be attractive to conclude that ovarian inhibin is responsible for the sometimes decreased FSH levels in PCO, these data cannot confirm this. Neither can they suggest that the ovary is itself abnormal in PCO. Inhibin is linked to ovarian androgen production. Therefore, the possible increased follicular fluid inhibin concentrations are probably a secondary phenomenon.

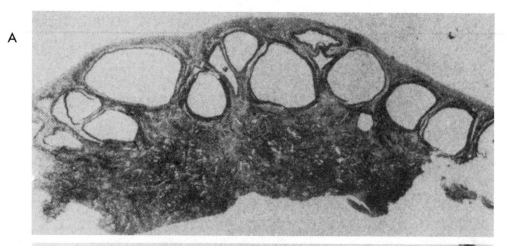

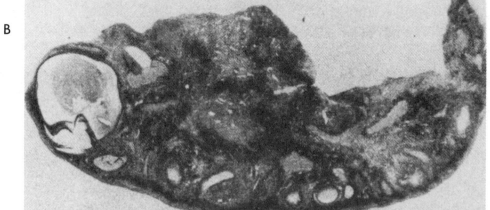

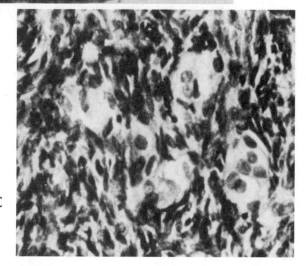

Figure 18-9

A. Sagittal section of a typical Stein-Leventhal type of polycystic ovary, illustrating the large number of follicular cysts. B. Sagittal section of a typical hyperthecotic ovary, illustrating the small number of follicular cysts and the massive amount of stromal hyperplasia. C. Islands of luteinized theca-like cells deep in the stroma of the ovary in hyperthecosis.

Reproduced, with permission, from Wilroy RS, et al: Genetic Forms of Hypogonadism, Birth Defects, vol XI, No. 4. White Plains, NY, The National Foundation, 1975.

It has been found from in vitro studies that both ovarian and adrenal tissue from at least one patient with the diagnosis of PCO were deficient in 3β-ol dehydrogenase-isomerase activity.[2] These findings agree with our data of 3β-ol hydroxysteroid dehydrogenase deficiency occurring in some patients mimicking PCO.[33] However, we have considered these patients to have a PCO-related syndrome, rather than true PCO.

Pathophysiology

Possible etiologies for the pathogenesis of PCO include heredity, central catecholamine abnormalities, psychological stress, and obesity. Other endocrine abnormalities in PCO are related to the vicious cycle of events that ensues, but are probably not related to pathogenesis. These include abnormalities in central opioid regulation and hyperestrogenism.

Heredity

There is evidence that there may be a genetic basis for the development of PCO. However, much of the older literature has reported pedigrees of patients with enlarged cystic ovaries to whom we probably would not apply the diagnosis of PCO today. Some of these patients have had karyotypic abnormalities. Givens and others have stressed that patients with PCO may have an X-linked dominant inheritance.[34] It has also been suggested that the male counterpart to PCO may present with premature baldness. HLA typing studies have been negative in families of patients with PCO.[35] Taken together, while there may be a genetic component to the pathogenesis of PCO, the data are neither clear nor convincing. An attractive hypothesis, however, is that maternal factors in utero, specifically androgens, may imprint on various fetal enzyme systems as well as hepatic SHBG production and result in progeny at risk for the development of PCO.

Central catecholamine abnormality

Yen has hypothesized that patients with PCO may have a central deficiency of dopamine resulting in increased LH secretion.[5] Supporting this hypothesis are observations of an exaggerated short-term decrement in serum LH after dopamine infusion compared with normal women in the early follicular phase.[36] There are three problems with using such data to support this hypothesis. These dopamine infusions are supraphysiologic, the decrement in LH is short-lived, and, finally, the decrement in LH may vary with the time of the menstrual cycle. Comparing this decrement of LH in PCO patients with the decrement during the late follicular phase of women with normal ovulatory cycles, there is no statistical difference. Recent data from our lab do not indicate an exaggerated decline in LH with lower doses of dopamine. Providing further support for a relative dopamine deficiency in PCO, however, are data showing that the PRL response is blunted after the administration of the dopamine receptor antagonist metoclopramide.

Other data also substantiate these findings. Dopamine metabolites, which may reflect up to 50% of central dopamine turnover, are decreased in PCO (Figure 18-10).[37] Levodopa administration increases both central and peripheral dopamine, whereas L-dopa with carbidopa will increase dopamine only within the brain. Administration of L-dopa for 1 week followed 1 month later by a week of L-dopa with carbidopa did not affect basal levels of LH or FSH. However, the exaggerated LH response to GnRH was normalized in PCO after L-dopa, but not after L-dopa with carbidopa. These data suggest that dopaminergic tone may be abnormal at the level of the hypothalamic-pituitary axis in PCO. These data do not primarily implicate a pituitary or a hypothalamic abnormality. Clearly, hyperestrogenism amplifies the system by further increasing pituitary sensitivity to GnRH. Recent data suggest increased GnRH secretion may be

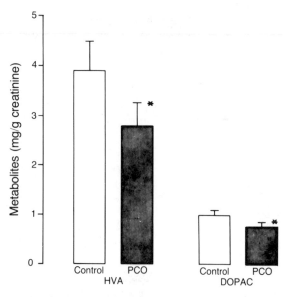

Figure 18-10
Mean (± SE) urinary homovanillic acid (HVA) and dihydroxyphenyl acetic acid (DOPAC) in controls and patients with PCO. *Significant difference from controls; $P < 0.05$.

Reproduced, with permission, from Shoupe D, Lobo RA: Evidence for altered catecholamine metabolism in polycystic ovary syndrome. Am J Obstet Gynecol 150:566, 1984.

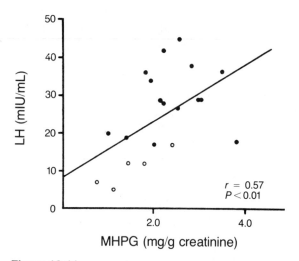

MHPG (mg/g creatinine)

Figure 18-11
The correlation between urinary levels of MHPG (3-methoxy-4-hydroxyphenyl glycol) and serum levels of LH in women with polycystic ovary syndrome (solid circles) and hypothalamic-pituitary dysfunction (open circles).

Reproduced, with permission, from Lobo RA, Granger LR, Paul WL, et al: Psychological stress and increases in urinary norepinephrine metabolites, platelet serotonin and adrenal androgens in women with polycystic ovary syndrome. Am J Obstet Gynecol 145:496, 1983.

the result of several neuromodulating factors.[37]

While dopamine decreases LH, there is evidence that norepinephrine may be important for a positive effect on LH. 3-Methoxy-4-hydroxyphenyl glycol (MHPG), a substantial central metabolite of norepinephrine, is elevated in PCO and correlates with LH levels (Figure 18-11).[17] Thus, the balance of norepinephrine (in relative excess) and dopamine (in relative deficiency) may result in abnormal LH secretion. The ratio of MHPG to homovanillic acid (HVA), a major dopamine metabolite, correlates significantly with LH (Figure 18-12).[37] Therefore, while there is no conclusive evidence, it may be suggested that abnormal central catecholamine metabolism may play a role in the pathogenesis of IGS in PCO.

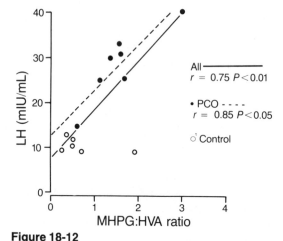

MHPG:HVA ratio

Figure 18-12
The positive correlation between the urinary MHPG:HVA ratio and serum LH in PCO patients and in all patients (PCO patients plus controls).

Reproduced, with permission, from Shoupe D, Lobo RA: Evidence for altered catecholamine metabolism in polycystic ovary syndrome. Am J Obstet Gynecol 150:566, 1984.

Abnormal endocrinology

Psychological stress

It has been hypothesized that one of the ways in which the syndrome may begin is by psychological stress inducing various hormonal changes such as altered catecholamine metabolism. We have observed that women with PCO have a higher level of psychological stress compared with other women with chronic anovulation.[17] However, this relatively crude assessment of the prevalence of stress in the adult patient with PCO, determined retrospectively, cannot be equated with peripubertal stress and the pathogenesis of the syndrome. Similarly, the stress itself may result from the syndrome rather than be its cause. Nevertheless, these observations lend promise to future investigations of psychological stress and the pathogenesis of PCO. What is clear, however, is that the stressed state of PCO is associated with certain hormonal changes that may help propagate the disorder (Figures 18-13 and 18-14[17]).

Obesity

Plymate[22] and others have hypothesized that obesity early in life may be important pathogenetically, because of the obesity-related decrease in SHBG. While this contention is noteworthy, particularly in reference to secondary changes in free estrogen and androgen, as depicted in Figure 18-8, it is unlikely that obesity is of central importance in the etiology of PCO. Against this theory are lifelong obese patients who do not have PCO, and thin patients who otherwise have characteristic features of the syndrome. Rather, it is more plausible that obesity is an important contributor to the propagation and/or enhancement of the syndrome, because of the decrease in SHBG associated with obesity.

Whatever the initiating cause(s) may be, and it may well be a combination of factors, a vicious cycle of events ensues, as pointed out by Yen and colleagues.[38] Chronic anovulation and IGS result in increased ovarian androgen production. The increased adrenal androgens may be pro-

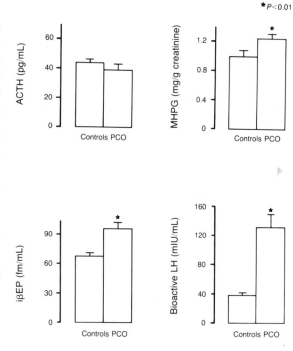

$*P < 0.01$

Figure 18-13
Hormonal changes associated with PCO. iβEP, immunoreactive β-endorphin.

duced by elevated levels of bioactive LH, but may be the result of concomitant CASH secretion or due to other factors. The increased androgen pool may lead to early follicular atresia, and, in turn, this population of atretic follicles may contribute to the ovarian stromal production of androstenedione and testosterone. Peripheral conversion of androstenedione results in tonic hyperestrogenism, which increases the pituitary sensitivity to GnRH. The result is increased LH release, yet normal or decreased FSH secretion. Thus, chronic stimulation of the ovaries results.

While it is clear that the pathogenesis of PCO remains unknown, many of the interconnecting bridges of this complex puzzle have

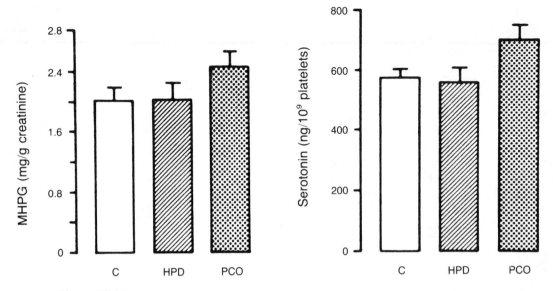

Figure 18-14
Urinary MHPG and platelet serotonin levels in control subjects (C), women with hypothalamic-pituitary dysfunction (HPD), and women with polycystic ovary syndrome (PCO).

Reproduced, with permission, from Lobo RA, Granger LR, Paul WL, et al: Psychological stress and increases in urinary norepinephrine metabolites, platelet serotonin and adrenal androgens in women with polycystic ovary syndrome. Am J Obstet Gynecol 145:496, 1983.

been identified. In Figure 18-15, we have attempted to illustrate a working hypothesis for this complex picture.

Insulin resistance

It has been recognized for years that patients with PCO-variant syndromes, such as hyperthecosis, may have acanthosis nigricans and insulin resistance. Only recently has it been determined that PCO itself may be a syndrome associated with hyperinsulinemia and insulin resistance. This hyperinsulinism is unrelated to body weight, but is highly correlated with the elevated androgen levels, particularly testosterone (Figure 18-16).[39] While patients with PCO exhibit hyperinsulinemia in response to glucose, thus typifying their insulin resistance, no receptor-mediated insulin defect has been demonstrated. This insulin resistance is mild and patients with

PCO are not overtly diabetic, but these findings are important. Insulin resistance may be an example of one of several abnormal tissue responses in this syndrome. Further, there is the theoretical possibility that patients with PCO are at risk for developing type II diabetes mellitus.

Treatment

The treatment of PCO is directed according to the particular complaints of the patient. These generally fall into three categories. Patients may request restoration of normal menses if they have oligo-amenorrhea or dysfunctional uterine bleeding (DUB) due to anovulation. Alternatively, the major concern may be hirsutism. Not infrequently, either or both of these symptoms may coexist with a problem of infertility, and the patient will require the induction of ovulation.

Either DUB or oligo-amenorrhea is due to

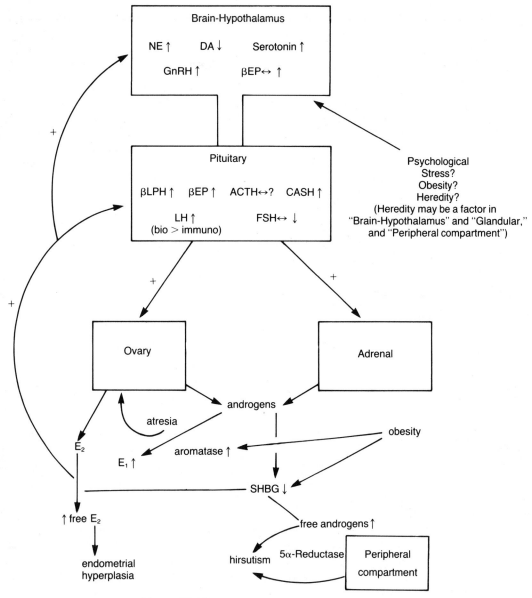

Figure 18-15
The pathophysiology of polycystic ovary syndrome.

anovulation, once pregnancy has been ruled out. Since there is an increased incidence of endometrial pathology (hyperplasia or even carcinoma) in young patients with PCO, it is important to perform an endometrial biopsy before treatment in the patient who has excessive bleed-

ing. It is important to realize that PCO patients are inherently hyperestrogenic and, over time, at risk for endometrial hyperplasia. For this reason, progestin therapy is necessary to oppose the estrogen effects. A method of treatment is to give medroxyprogesterone acetate (MPA) 10 mg

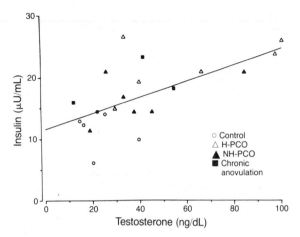

Figure 18-16
Correlation between serum testosterone and fasting serum insulin levels in control subjects, hirsute (H-PCO) and nonhirsute (NH-PCO) patients with PCO, and women with chronic anovulation.

Reproduced, with permission, from Shoupe D, Kumar DD, Lobo RA: Insulin resistance in polycystic ovary syndrome. Am J Obstet Gynecol 147:588, 1983.

orally for 10 days each month. While there are several acceptable alternatives, this regimen has been extremely effective in normalizing menstrual function. If hirsutism is present and/or contraception is desired, low-dose combination oral contraceptives (OCs) administered in the usual cyclic fashion are also appropriate.

In hirsute patients, either corticosteroids, OCs,[40,41] their combination,[42] and/or spironolactone[43,44] are used. Other patients with androgen excess are treated according to the source of the hyperandrogenism.

Wedge resection of the ovaries has been advocated for the treatment of hirsutism, as well as for the induction of ovulation. While the overall success of this procedure for hirsutism (50% to 60% response rate) and the pregnancy rate (50% to 60%) are generally satisfactory, the results are short-lived. Endocrinologically, after wedge resection, ovarian androgen secretion decreases transiently, but eventually returns to pretreatment levels.[45] Gonadotropin secretion is also transiently normalized. We strongly recommend not performing wedge resections for any reason, because (1) the success rate is comparable with medical therapy, (2) the success is short-lived, (3) infertility due to a pelvic factor often ensues because of tubo-ovarian adhesions, and (4) PCO is not an ovarian disease.

For patients requesting the induction of ovulation, clomiphene citrate is extremely successful. Ovulatory cycles are induced in close to 90% of patients, with a pregnancy rate of approximately 50%.[46] For patients who fail initially to ovulate with clomiphene, alternative regimens such as clomiphene with dexamethasone[47] or using menotropins (Pergonal) alone are possible. In recent years, pure FSH preparations have been used for ovulation induction in PCO. The overall success rate is comparable to that of menotropins, although FSH may be better suited for the PCO patient who has high levels of LH with normal or low FSH. Dexamethasone with menotropins has also achieved success.[48]

Since dopamine deficiency may be involved in PCO, the use of a dopamine agonist, bromocriptine, has been tried in order to normalize LH levels and to induce ovulation.[28] To date, our results have been disappointing. Although some success has been achieved, we have found bromocriptine to have no effect when used to treat euprolactinemic patients with PCO.

In the older patient with the long-standing diagnosis of PCO or one of its variants, hirsutism may be a persistent and worsening problem. In these patients, hyperthecosis may exist, particularly if testosterone exceeds 150 ng/dL and the patient has normal adrenal androgen levels. In such a patient, consideration may be given to performing bilateral oophorectomy (with hysterectomy) to remove the source of the androgen excess.

References

1. Stein IF, Leventhal ML: Amenorrhea associated with bilateral polycystic ovaries. *Am J Obstet Gynecol* 29:181, 1935

2. Goldzieher JW, Axelrod LR: Clinical and biochemical features of polycystic ovarian disease. *Fertil Steril* 14:631, 1963

3. Vara P, Niemineva K: Small cystic degeneration of ovaries as incidental finding in gynecological laparotomies. *Acta Obstet Gynecol Scand* 31:94, 1951

4. Goldzieher JW: Polycystic ovarian syndrome. *Fertil Steril* 35:371, 1981

5. Yen SSC: The polycystic ovary syndrome. *Clin Endocrinol* 12:177, 1980

6. Raj SG, Thompson IE, Berger MJ, et al: Clinical aspects of the polycystic ovary syndrome. *Obstet Gynecol* 49:552, 1977

7. Givens JR, Anderson RN, Wiser WL, et al: A gonadotropin responsive adrenocortical adenoma. *J Clin Endocrinol Metab* 38:126, 1974

8. Rebar R, Judd HL, Yen SSC, et al: Characterization of the inappropriate gonadotropin secretion in polycystic ovary syndrome. *J Clin Invest* 57:1320, 1976

9. Lobo RA, Kletzky OA, Campeau JD, et al: Elevated bioactive luteinizing hormone in women with the polycystic ovary syndrome. *Fertil Steril* 39:674, 1983

10. Van Damme MP, Robertson DM, Diczfalusy E: An improved *in vitro* bioassay method for measuring luteinizing hormone (LH) activity using mouse Leydig cell preparations. *Acta Endocrinol* 77:655, 1974

11. DeVane GW, Czekala NM, Judd HL, et al: Circulating gonadotropins, estrogens, and androgens in polycystic ovarian disease. *Am J Obstet Gynecol* 121:496, 1975

12. Lobo RA, Goebelsmann U, Horton R: Evidence for the importance of peripheral tissue events in the development of hirsutism in polycystic ovary syndrome. *J Clin Endocrinol Metab* 57:393, 1983

13. Lobo RA, Paul WL, Goebelsmann U: Dehydroepiandrosterone sulfate as an indicator of adrenal androgen function. *Obstet Gynecol* 57:69, 1981

14. Hoffman D, Lobo RA: The prevalence and significance of elevated DHEA-S levels in anovulatory women. *Fertil Steril* 39:404, 1983

15. Lobo RA: The role of the adrenal in polycystic ovary syndrome. *Semin Reprod Endocrinol* 2:251, 1984

16. Chang RJ, Mandel FP, Wolfsen AR, et al: Circulating levels of plasma adrenocorticotropin in polycystic ovary disease. *J Clin Endocrinol Metab* 54:1265, 1982

17. Lobo RA, Granger LR, Paul WL, et al: Psychological stress and increases in urinary norepinephrine metabolites, platelet serotonin and adrenal androgens in women with polycystic ovary syndrome. *Am J Obstet Gynecol* 145:496, 1983

18. Parker LN, Odell WD: Control of adrenal androgen secretion. *Endocr Rev* 1:392, 1980

19. Anderson DC: Sex hormone binding globulin. *Clin Endocrinol* 3:69, 1974

20. Lobo RA, Goebelsmann U: Effect of androgen excess on inappropriate gonadotropin secretion as found in the polycystic ovary syndrome. *Am J Obstet Gynecol* 142:394, 1982

21. Lobo RA, Granger L, Goebelsmann U, et al: Elevation in unbound serum estradiol as a possible mechanism for inappropriate gonadotropin secretion in women with PCO. *J Clin Endocrinol Metab* 52:156, 1981

22. Plymate SR, Fariss BL, Bassett ML, et al: Obesity and its role in polycystic ovary disease. *J Clin Endocrinol Metab* 52:1246, 1981

23. Seppala M, Hirvonen E: Raised serum prolactin levels associated with hirsutism and amenorrhea. *Br Med J* 4:144, 1975

24. Luciano AA, Chapler FK, Sherman BM: Hyperprolactinemia in polycystic ovary syndrome. *Fertil Steril* 41:719, 1984

25. Lobo RA, Goebelsmann U: Adult manifestation of congenital adrenal hyperplasia due to incomplete 21-hydroxylase deficiency mimicking polycystic ovarian disease. *Am J Obstet Gynecol* 138:720, 1980

26. Lobo RA, Kletzky OA: Normalization of androgen and sex hormone-binding globulin levels after treatment of hyperprolactinemia. *J Clin Endocrinol Metab* 56:562, 1983

27. Lobo RA, Kletzky OA, Kaptein EM, et al: Prolactin modulation of dehydroepiandrosterone sulfate secretion. *Am J Obstet Gynecol* 138:632, 1980

28. Spruce BA, Kendall-Taylor P, Dunlop W, et al: The effect of bromocriptine in the polycystic ovary syndrome. *Clin Endocrinol* 20:481, 1984

29. Shoupe D, Lobo RA: Prolactin responses after gonadotropin releasing hormone in polycystic ovary syndrome. *Fertil Steril* 43:549, 1985

30. Wilroy RS, et al: *Genetic Forms of Hypogonadism, Birth Defects*, vol XI, No. 4. White Plains, NY, The National Foundation, 1975

31. Erickson GF, Hsueh AJ, Quigley ME, et al: Functional studies of aromatase activity in human granulosa cells from normal and polycystic ovaries. *J Clin Endocrinol Metab* 49:514, 1979

32. Tanabe K, Gagliano P, Channing CP, et al: Levels of inhibin-F activity and steroids in human follicular fluid from normal women and women with polycystic ovarian disease. *J Clin Endocrinol Metab* 57:24, 1983

33. Lobo RA, Goebelsmann U: Evidence for reduced 3β-ol-hydroxysteroid dehydrogenase activity in some hirsute women thought to have polycystic ovary syndrome. *J Clin Endocrinol Metab* 53:394, 1981

34. Givens JR: Polycystic ovaries—a sign, not a diagnosis. *Semin Reprod Endocrinol* 2:271, 1984

35. Mandel FP, Chang RJ, Dupont B, et al: HLA genotyping in family members and patients with familial polycystic ovarian disease. *J Clin Endocrinol Metab* 56:862, 1983

36. Quigley ME, Rakoff JS, Yen SSC: Increased luteinizing hormone sensitivity to dopamine inhibition in polycystic ovary syndrome. *J Clin Endocrinol Metab* 52:231, 1981

37. Shoupe D, Lobo RA: Evidence for altered catecholamine metabolism in polycystic ovary syndrome. *Am J Obstet Gynecol* 150:566, 1984

38. Yen SSC, Chaney C, Judd HL: Functional aberrations of the hypothalamic-pituitary system in polycystic ovary syndrome: A consideration of the pathogenesis. In James VHT, Serio M, Ginusti G (eds): *The Endocrine Function of the Human Ovary*, 1976, pp 373-385

39. Shoupe D, Kumar DD, Lobo RA: Insulin resistance in polycystic ovary syndrome. *Am J Obstet Gynecol* 147:588, 1983

40. Givens JR, Andersen RN, Wiser WL, et al: The effectiveness of two oral contraceptives in suppressing plasma androstenedione, testosterone, LH and FSH and in stimulating plasma testosterone-binding capacity in hirsute women. *Am J Obstet Gynecol* 124:333, 1976

41. Wild RA, Umstot ES, Andersen RN, et al: Adrenal function in hirsutism. II. Effect of an oral contraceptive. *J Clin Endocrinol Metab* 54:676, 1982

42. Casey JH: Chronic treatment regimens for hirsutism in women: Effect on blood production rates of testosterone and on hair growth. *Clin Endocrinol* 4:313, 1975

43. Cumming DC, Yang JC, Rebar RW, et al: Treatment of hirsutism with spironolactone. *JAMA* 247:1295, 1982

44. Lobo RA, Shoupe D, Serafini P, et al: The effects of two doses of spironolactone on serum androgens and anagen hair in hirsute women. *Fertil Steril* 43:200, 1985

45. Judd HL, Rigg LA, Anderson DC, et al: The effect of ovarian wedge resection on circulating gonadotropin and ovarian steroid levels in patients with polycystic ovary syndrome. *J Clin Endocrinol Metab* 43:347, 1976

46. Gysler M, March CM, Mishell DR Jr, et al: A decade's experience with an individualized clomiphene treatment regimen including its effect on the postcoital test. *Fertil Steril* 37:161, 1982

47. Lobo RA, Paul W, March CM, et al: Clomiphene and dexamethasone in women unresponsive to clomiphene alone. *Obstet Gynecol* 60:497, 1982

48. Evron S, Navot D, Laufer N, et al: Induction of ovulation with combined human gonadotropins and dexamethasone in women with polycystic ovarian disease. *Fertil Steril* 40:183, 1983

Chapter 19

Dysfunctional Uterine Bleeding

Charles M. March, M.D.
David I. Hoffman, M.D.
Rogerio A. Lobo, M.D.

Dysfunctional uterine bleeding (DUB) is a very common disorder that most often occurs shortly after menarche and at the end of the reproductive years. It is defined as abnormal uterine bleeding with no demonstrable organic cause (genital or extragenital). Therefore, it is a diagnosis of exclusion, made only after complications of pregnancy, pelvic pathology, coagulation defects, systemic illnesses, or the use of medications that can influence hormonal action or clotting mechanisms have been ruled out. It has been suggested that approximately half of the patients are 40 to 50 years old; another 20% are adolescents. Anovulation is most common at such ages. Episodes of DUB are usually acyclic and painless, and they vary greatly in the amount and duration of flow. Patients with recurrent DUB are often infertile because of chronic anovulation. Numerous surgical and medical methods for treating this disorder have been described. Both the causes and treatment of DUB will be discussed in this chapter.

A thorough evaluation of abnormal bleeding usually establishes an etiology that permits specific therapy. The following eight terms are commonly used to describe abnormal uterine bleeding:

1. Dysfunctional uterine bleeding
2. Menorrhagia—prolonged and/or excessive uterine bleeding occurring at regular intervals (hypermenorrhea)
3. Metrorrhagia—uterine bleeding occurring at completely irregular but frequent intervals, the amount being variable
4. Menometrorrhagia—uterine bleeding that is prolonged and occurs at completely irregular intervals
5. Polymenorrhea—uterine bleeding occurring at regular intervals of less than 21 days
6. Intermenstrual bleeding—bleeding of variable amounts occurring between regular menstrual periods
7. Premenstrual spotting—scanty bleeding that occurs a few days to a week before menses
8. Postmenopausal bleeding—bleeding occurring more than 1 year after the last menses in a woman with ovarian failure.

Normal menstruation

The ebb and flow of estrogens and progesterone, in concert with many other factors, are responsible for normal menstruation. The broad guidelines for normal uterine bleeding are cycle length: 28 ± 7 days; duration of flow: 4 ± 2 days; and blood loss: 40 ± 20 mL.

Estrogen causes an increased flow of blood to the endometrium. This effect may be mediated by acetylcholine and histamine, and it probably is influenced by other mediators such as the prostaglandins. Theories concerning the etiology of menstruation include estrogen and/or progesterone withdrawal, inadequate lymphatic drainage and enzymatic changes leading to endometrial sloughing, and depolymerization of the acid mucopolysaccharide ground substance that supports the developing stroma and glands.

To stop the menstrual flow, the first mechanism to initiate hemostasis is the formation of platelet plugs. However, this mechanism is only partly responsible for clotting. Subsequent hemostasis is due primarily to a prostaglandin-dependent vasoconstriction. Platelets play a central role and serve three primary functions in the hemostatic pathway. First, they occlude the site of injury by adhesion and aggregation. Then, they initiate the release of potent pro-aggregatory compounds that accelerate platelet aggregation and initiate coagulation. Finally, they release substances that cause vasoconstriction. Subsequent clot retraction and thrombolysis are also mediated by platelets.

The interaction between platelets and vascular endothelium is an important one, because platelets will adhere only to damaged vascular endothelium. It is thought that collagen is the most important factor in triggering this interaction. The platelet is able to convert arachidonic acid by two pathways: The first is catalyzed by lipoxygenases and leads to the formation of 12-hydroxyeicosatetraenoic acid; the second involves the direct synthesis of prostaglandin endoperoxides via the cyclo-oxygenase pathway. These prostaglandin endoperoxides are potent inducers of platelet aggregation. The platelet can further metabolize these endoperoxides to thromboxane A_2, a very potent vasoconstrictor and inducer of platelet aggregation.[1]

The number of sanitary pads or tampons used is not a reliable indicator of menstrual blood loss (MBL). Great variability of absorption has been found among different sanitary products as well as among products within the same package.[2] Furthermore, since women differ markedly in their fastidiousness in changing sanitary products, queries about the passage of blood clots or the degree of inconvenience caused by the bleeding are more helpful in determining MBL than is recording the number of pads used, unless emphasis is placed upon the degree of departure from the norm.

Because of the unreliability of subjective assessment, objective methods have been developed to quantify MBL. The most widely used technique involves photometric measurement to quantify hematin collected on sanitary napkins.[3] Although this method is very accurate, its reliability depends on complete collection of the sanitary napkins used by the patient. This technique and others have demonstrated that the mean MBL in normal women is 35 mL and that 95% of normal women lose less than 60 mL of blood during each menses. Individuals who lose more than 80 mL of blood have significantly lower mean hemoglobin, hematocrit, and serum Fe levels.[3] Therefore, MBL greater than 80 mL should be regarded as hypermenorrhea.

Etiology

The major cause of DUB is anovulation resulting from altered neuroendocrine and/or ovarian hormonal events. The premenarcheal girl has random, episodic fluctuations in her levels of follicle-stimulating hormone (FSH), luteinizing hormone (LH), and estradiol (E_2) that are not interrelated. The FSH levels in these young girls are higher than the LH levels, and the hormonal patterns are anovulatory (Figure 19-1).[4] The administration of gonadotropin-releasing hormone (GnRH) to the postmenarcheal adolescent who has not yet developed an ovulatory pattern leads to release of greater amounts of FSH than of LH. This indicates persistence of the premenarcheal FSH dominance.

In some patients, the pathophysiology of DUB may represent exaggerated FSH release in response to normal endogenous levels of GnRH, leading to asynchronous follicular maturation. The latter condition causes the production of E_2 in amounts sufficient to stimulate the endometrium.[5] However, it has been shown that these young women do not have an LH surge following an acute rise of E_2. Thus, the basic defect is an absence of the positive feedback mechanism (Figure 19-2).[4] The negative feedback mechanism remains intact, as demonstrated by the normal gonadotropin response to the administration of estrogen.

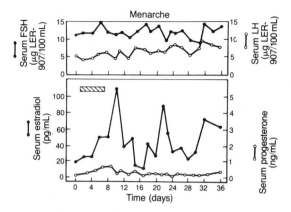

Figure 19-2
Serum FSH, LH, estradiol, and progesterone in a perimenarcheal girl at menarche.

Adapted from Winter JSD, Faiman C: The development of cyclic pituitary-gonadal function in adolescent females. J Clin Endocrinol Metab 37:714, 1973. Used with permission. © 1973, The Endocrine Society.

Following menarche, there is a change toward a normal adult pattern of LH and FSH levels, with a midcycle LH and FSH surge preceded by an E_2 peak (Figure 19-3).[4] Maturation defects persist in some perimenarcheal patients who may have anovulatory cycles or cycles characterized by a prolonged follicular phase and/or by corpus luteum defects for variable periods before a normal ovulatory pattern is established.

Because the hypothalamic-pituitary axis in the adolescent usually continues to mature, and because most bleeding episodes are not severe, most adolescent patients with DUB may be followed without active intervention. Little or no testing is needed, provided marked anemia does not develop. However, if the bleeding is very prolonged or heavy, screening should be done for coagulation disorders. Such disorders are found in about 20% of girls requiring hospitalization for abnormal uterine bleeding.[6] Coagulation defects are present in about one-fourth of

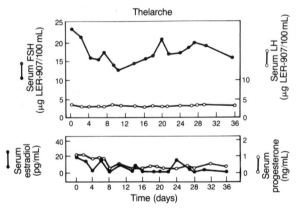

Figure 19-1
Serum FSH, LH, estradiol, and progesterone in a perimenarcheal girl at thelarche.

Adapted from Winter JSD, Faiman C: The development of cyclic pituitary-gonadal function in adolescent females. J Clin Endocrinol Metab 37:714, 1973. Used with permission. © 1973, The Endocrine Society.

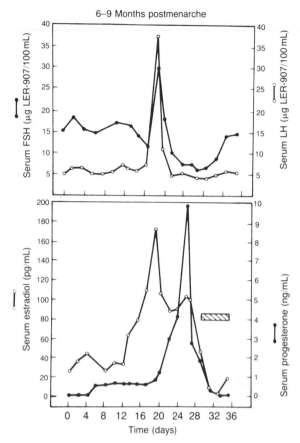

Figure 19-3
Serum FSH, LH, estradiol, and progesterone in a perimenarcheal girl 6 to 9 months after menarche.

Adapted from Winter JSD, Faiman C: The development of cyclic pituitary-gonadal function in adolescent females. J Clin Endocrinol Metab 37:714, 1973. Used with permission. © 1973, The Endocrine Society.

those whose hemoglobin falls below 10 g/100 mL and in about one-third of those who require one or more transfusions.

Women nearing the end of their reproductive years have increased variability of the intermenstrual interval. The mean length of the menstrual cycle is significantly shorter in older women than in younger women. One of several

defects causing shortening of cycle length is a shortened proliferative phase.[7] Some studies have also shown a diminished capacity of follicles in older women to secrete E_2. Initially, this diminished secretion of E_2 is accompanied by a normal production of progesterone and a luteal phase of normal length. However, as menopause approaches, progesterone secretion and the duration of the luteal phase both decrease, and DUB can result.

Other disorders that commonly cause DUB involve alterations in the life span of the corpus luteum. Prolonged life of the corpus luteum has been reported as a cause of abnormal bleeding (Halban's syndrome). This disorder is associated with a normal-appearing secretory endometrium. Its etiology is uncertain, and treatment is usually expectant. It must be differentiated from early pregnancy loss with a very sensitive serum pregnancy test. In addition, the phenomenon of irregular shedding with DUB sometimes occurs in ovulatory cycles and results from variable function or premature senescence of the corpus luteum. However, repetitive episodes are rare. Luteal phase insufficiency by itself can also present as apparent DUB.

Most patients with DUB are not ovulatory. There is continuous E_2 production without corpus luteum formation and progesterone secretion. The production of E_2, its conversion to estrone (E_1), and its metabolic clearance rate have all been reported to be normal in patients with DUB. However, the concentrations of E_2 and E_1 in follicular fluid are elevated when compared with those obtained from ovulatory women. This finding suggests inappropriate pituitary-ovarian interaction in DUB patients.

The steady state of estrogen stimulation leads to a continuously proliferating endometrium that may outgrow its blood supply or lose nutrients. Asynchronous development of stroma, glands, and blood vessels, as well as an overdeveloped Golgi-lysosomal complex capable of releasing excessive amounts of hydrolytic enzymes, may also follow unopposed estrogen stimulation. Any of these conditions could lead to the irregular endometrial shedding characteristic of DUB. Similarly, an overactive fibrinolytic system may initiate or perpetuate abnormal bleeding; however, the relationship between persistent estrogenic states and intrauterine fibrinolysis is not known. The frequency of bleeding and the degree of endometrial shedding are variable. This bleeding may be controlled by short-term increases in estrogenic stimulation. However, if the high level of exogenous endometrial stimulation is maintained continuously, estrogen breakthrough bleeding will recur.

Differential diagnosis

Pathology of pregnancy
Complications of pregnancy must be ruled out before other possible causes of bleeding are considered. Both intrauterine and ectopic pregnancies should be considered. The complications of an intrauterine pregnancy that may cause apparent DUB are: (1) threatened, incomplete, or missed abortion; (2) subinvolution of the placental site; (3) placental polyp; and (4) trophoblastic disease.

Malignancy
Cervical cancer is the most common malignancy in women during the reproductive years. Occasionally, malignancy of the vagina (especially in diethylstilbestrol-exposed patients), corpus, vulva, or fallopian tube may be the cause of abnormal uterine bleeding.

Chronic endometritis
Episodic intermenstrual spotting of varying amount and duration is the most common symptom in women with chronic endometritis. Some patients have hypermenorrhea, and those with tuberculous endometritis may present with hypomenorrhea or amenorrhea.

Intrauterine defects
Submucous myomas usually cause menorrhagia. If myomas are pedunculated, intermenstrual bleeding of variable amounts may occur. Intermenstrual spotting is the most common symptom of endometrial polyps.

Pathology of the cervix, vagina, and ovaries
Cervical erosions, polyps, and cervicitis may cause irregular bleeding that can simulate DUB. Traumatic vaginal lesions, severe vaginal infections, and foreign bodies have also been associated with abnormal bleeding. Three types of ovarian dysfunction may cause abnormal bleeding: (1) short, insufficient, or prolonged progesterone production by the corpus luteum; (2) estrogen-secreting granulosa-theca-cell and other benign or malignant tumors that do not secrete hormones but can induce abnormal steroidogenesis in the adjacent ovarian stroma; and (3) severe ovarian infections. In normal women, the physiologic midcycle fall in serum levels of E_2 may be associated with scanty uterine bleeding. Hemoglobin has been detected in midcycle vaginal secretions in over 90% of regularly menstruating women.

Systemic diseases
The mechanisms by which some systemic diseases cause abnormal bleeding are not clear, although a number of illnesses are commonly associated with DUB:

Coagulation defects
Coagulation defects, such as von Willebrand's disease and prothrombin deficiency, may become manifest initially by increased uterine bleeding. Additionally, disorders that lead to platelet deficiency or dysfunction, such as leukemias, severe sepsis, idiopathic thrombocytopenic

purpura, hypersplenism, and others, may be confused with DUB. In the absence of a history of one of these conditions, coagulation defects are most commonly found in adolescents with excessive bleeding.

Hypothyroidism
Hypothyroidism is frequently associated with menometrorrhagia. Although hyperthyroidism is usually not associated with menstrual abnormalities, hypomenorrhea, oligomenorrhea, and amenorrhea have been reported.

Adrenal pathology
Adrenal insufficiency and hyperfunction usually cause oligomenorrhea or amenorrhea. Only rarely does excessive bleeding occur.

Cirrhosis
Cirrhosis is associated with excessive bleeding because of the reduced capacity of the liver to metabolize estrogens. If the patient has hypoprothrombinemia, the tendency toward abnormal bleeding will be increased.

Iatrogenic causes
Oral or injectable steroid contraceptives and hormones used for estrogen replacement in the perimenopause (or for the management of dysmenorrhea, hirsutism, acne, or endometriosis) may lead to abnormal uterine bleeding. Tranquilizers may interfere with the neurotransmitters responsible for releasing and inhibiting hypothalamic hormones, thus causing anovulation and abnormal bleeding. An intrauterine contraceptive device may cause marked irregular and/or heavy bleeding.

Evaluation

History and physical
The initial steps are directed toward establishing the site of the bleeding with certainty and differentiating cyclic from acyclic bleeding. The history should include the earlier menstrual pattern and the dates of at least the last three bleeding episodes. The presence or absence of pain associated with the bleeding should be ascertained. The severity of the bleeding may be estimated by a history of passing clots, as well as by a significant increase in the number of pads and/or tampons used each day and the degree of saturation. A history of prior episodes of abnormal bleeding, the therapy, and the results of the therapy should be elicited. Attention should be given to any symptoms of pregnancy or of premenstrual molimina. The dates of all past pregnancies and a history of contraceptive methods, medications, trauma, extragenital sources of bleeding, easy bruising or bleeding, and clotting problems should be recorded. A complete physical examination is necessary to search for systemic disorders.

Laboratory assessment
The severity and the frequency of the abnormal uterine bleeding dictate the extent of the laboratory investigation. The following studies are used to evaluate the patient with abnormal uterine bleeding: (1) cervical cytology, (2) assay for hCG, (3) complete blood count, and (4) endometrial biopsy.

A single, high-fundal endometrial biopsy sample is usually sufficient to determine if the patient has ovulated. A more extensive "four quadrant" biopsy or vacuum aspiration should be obtained in women over 35 or with persistent anovulation, since they are at greater risk for endometrial cancer. Evaluation of the endometrial histology is extremely important in determining the etiology of DUB. Proliferative, secretory, atrophic, hyperplastic, or malignant endometria, as well as endometritis, decidual reaction, and disorders of maturation, may all be associated with abnormal bleeding.

Other laboratory studies may include tests

Abnormal endocrinology

of liver function and coagulation factors and determination of serum iron. Thyroid-stimulating hormone (TSH), triiodothyronine (T_3), and thyroxine (T_4) levels may be useful in evaluating certain patients. The clinical signs and symptoms will dictate which studies are indicated.

Hysterosalpingography and hysteroscopy

Patients with recurrent bleeding and those who do not respond to medical treatment, particularly those who have secretory endometria, may have submucous myomas or endometrial polyps. These defects are often missed even by thorough curettage, but may be detected by a hysterosalpingogram (HSG). The slow instillation of water-soluble dye under fluoroscopic control will permit their visualization. The HSG should not be performed while the patient is bleeding.

Direct inspection of the endometrial cavity is possible by hysteroscopy under local anesthesia on an outpatient basis. If high-molecular-weight dextran is used as a uterine distending medium, hysteroscopy may be performed even if the patient is bleeding actively. Polyps, submucous myomas, or hyperplastic endometria may be visualized, and biopsies may be taken under direct vision. In our institution, one-fourth of patients with presumed DUB have been found to have organic lesions by means of the HSG or hysteroscopy.

Therapy

The objectives and principles of managing patients with DUB are to control bleeding, prevent recurrences, preserve fertility, correct associated conditions, and induce ovulation in patients who wish to conceive. It must be realized that no single modality is always effective. The adequacy of therapy is best judged by a carefully kept menstrual calendar. The patient's age, the amount of bleeding, and the past history will dictate the mode of therapy selected. Guidelines are given in Table 19-1.

Medical management

Oral contraceptives (OCs), estrogens, progestins, androgens, ovulation-inducing drugs, nonsteroidal anti-inflammatory drugs (NSAIDs), and inhibitors of plasminogen activators have all been used with varying degrees of success. An endometrial biopsy should always be obtained before beginning therapy, except perhaps in the very young girl. The biopsy serves to exclude malignancy and may explain treatment failures. If the biopsy reveals atypical hyperplasia, a dilatation and curettage (D&C) should be per-

Table 19-1
Guidelines for DUB therapy

Findings	Therapy
First episode, hematocrit stable	Observation
Multiple episodes, hematocrit stable	Hormonal therapy
Multiple episodes, anemia	Hormonal and iron therapy
Hypovolemia	D&C, transfusion
>35 years old	D&C
Profuse bleeding	D&C
Failed hormonal therapy	D&C, hysteroscopy

formed to exclude malignancy. Most bleeding can be stopped quickly by appropriate hormonal therapy.

Estrogens

Estrogens have been a standard in the treatment of DUB. Estrogen causes rapid endometrial growth, proliferation of endometrial ground substance, and stabilization of lysosomal membranes. There is no evidence to suggest a direct effect upon hemostasis. Almost all acute episodes of bleeding can be stopped with estrogen. Because most episodes of DUB are associated with anovulation, the endometrium will show an unopposed estrogen effect and irregular breakdown. Although there are proponents of IV estrogen administration (25 mg every 4 hours up to three doses until bleeding stops), no study has indicated that parenteral administration stops the bleeding more quickly or effectively than oral therapy. Several hours are required to induce mitotic activity; in a placebo-controlled study, several IV injections given at 4-hour intervals were necessary to decrease bleeding.[8] Compared with oral estrogen, IV therapy produces more rapid metabolic clearance, and it is also more expensive.

We prefer giving oral conjugated estrogens, 10 mg daily in divided doses. Almost all patients who respond stop bleeding within 2 days. If the bleeding persists, a few patients will respond if the estrogen dose is doubled. However, most nonresponders require curettage. If the bleeding stops, the same dose of estrogen is continued for 21 days and medroxyprogesterone acetate (MPA), 10 mg/day, is added on days 17 to 21 of the estrogen therapy to prevent further endometrial growth. On day 22, both steroids are stopped to allow withdrawal bleeding.

It is important to understand that estrogen therapy controls the acute bleeding problem but does not alter the underlying cause. Therefore, a diagnosis should be made on the basis of the endometrial biopsy. Appropriate treatment can be instituted after the sequential estrogen/progestin regimen has controlled the acute episode and withdrawal bleeding has occurred.

Progestins

Most women experience occasional anovulatory bleeding, although it is usually not profuse or prolonged. After these patients have been evaluated and uterine pathology has been ruled out, they can be treated with progestin. MPA, 10 mg daily for 10 days, is satisfactory. Progestins are beneficial because they are antiestrogens in pharmacologic doses. They diminish the effect of estrogen on target cells by inhibiting estrogen receptor replenishment and inducing the activation of 17-hydroxysteroid dehydrogenase in endometrial cells. This converts E_2 to the less active E_1. These findings account for the antimitotic, antigrowth effect of progestins, and support the rationale for their use in the treatment of endometrial hyperplasia. If the episode involves very heavy bleeding, it is best to use estrogen therapy first. This will induce endometrial growth, stimulate production of progesterone receptors, and permit the progestin to act.

In anovulatory adolescents who exhibit immaturity of the hypothalamic-pituitary axis, progestin therapy for 10 days every month or every other month is reasonable until maturity of the axis is achieved. This therapy will not interfere with the normal resumption of spontaneous menses. OCs should be avoided in these adolescents because they may perpetuate hypothalamic-pituitary inhibition and delay the onset of normal function. Cyclic progestin therapy is also mandatory for older women with chronic anovulation and DUB to prevent recurrences or the development of endometrial hyperplasia.

Combined therapy

In young (aged 18 to 35) patients with acute DUB, combined estrogen/progestin therapy has been advocated in the form of OCs. In one regimen, one tablet is taken four times a day for 5 to

7 days. After the acute bleeding episode ceases, no OCs are given for 1 week; then three 21-day standard pill cycles follow. Any OC may be used. If the bleeding fails to stop after the initial high-dose therapy, a D&C should be performed.

Although the OC regimens are more convenient, they are usually not as effective as the high-dose estrogen treatment. Possibly, the combined use of estrogen and progestin does not stimulate endometrial growth as rapidly as estrogen alone, because the progestin decreases the estrogen receptors and increases estradiol dehydrogenase in the endometrial cell.[9] This action may inhibit the growth-promoting action of estrogen.

An unpublished study of 90 patients with DUB was performed in our clinic. The patients were between 18 and 35 years of age, none had a systemic illness, and all had normal pelvic exams. All were actively bleeding at the time of referral. The patients were randomly assigned to one of three treatment groups. Patients in the first group received norethynodrel, 5 mg, and mestranol, 75 μg (Enovid), twice a day for 20 days; the second group received norethindrone acetate (Norlutate), 5 mg, twice a day for 20 days; the third received conjugated estrogens (Premarin), 2.5 mg, four times a day for 20 days, plus MPA (Provera), 10 mg, on days 17 to 21.

The patients were reevaluated within a week and were scheduled to return to the clinic 1 month and again 4 months after starting treatment. Medication was prescribed for only one cycle. Treatment was considered successful if the bleeding stopped within 5 days.

Both of the estrogen-containing formulations were found to be significantly more effective than norethindrone acetate in stopping the bleeding (Table 19-2). In women who stopped bleeding, the mean number of days until bleeding ceased was 2.3. Irrespective of the treatment regimen, approximately half of the patients had side effects. Nausea, breast engorgement, abdominal bloating, and headache were the most common.

Of the 90 patients, 43 returned for a 4-month follow-up visit (Table 19-3). Only one of 17 patients treated by the sequential estrogen/progestin regimen had recurrent DUB. This was a significantly lower proportion than with the other methods of therapy. Therefore, sequential estrogen/progestin therapy is the regimen of choice for treating the acute episode of DUB. Therapy should begin with conjugated estrogens, 2.5 mg four times a day. If the bleeding stops, the estrogen should be continued for 21 days, and MPA, 10 mg daily, should be added during the last 5 days of estrogen administration. If the bleeding persists beyond 2 days, the dose of estrogen should be doubled, and then continued as above. If the bleeding still persists, a D&C and hysteroscopy should be performed.

This method of therapy should be used for the acute episode only. In subsequent months, patients with anovulatory bleeding should receive MPA, 10 mg daily, for the first 10 days of every month, to produce a secretory endometrium. This therapy will prevent recurrences of heavy bleeding by preventing unopposed estrogenic stimulation of the endometrium. Patients with cyclic bleeding who desire contraception may continue to use OCs at the usual dosage; however, OCs are not recommended for anovulatory patients following control of acute bleeding episodes. These women have an underlying hypothalamic-pituitary defect that cannot be monitored during OC use.

Table 19-2
Results of therapy for DUB

Drug	Success (%)
Conjugated estrogens	85*
Norethynodrel and mestranol	82*
Norethindrone acetate	54
Mean	75

*Significantly more effective (P < 0.05) than norethindrone acetate.

Table 19-3
Subsequent menstrual pattern following one course of medical therapy for DUB

Drug	No. of patients	Patients with normal cycle	Patients with recurrent DUB
Conjugated estrogens	17	16	1*
Norethynodrel and mestranol	12	6	6
Norethindrone acetate	14	9	5
Total	43	31	12

Significantly lower rate of recurrence (P < 0.05).

Patients with anovulatory bleeding who wish to become pregnant should be treated with clomiphene citrate to induce ovulation after the acute bleeding episode has been resolved. The induction of ovulation should be used only in women who wish to conceive, and not for the control of bleeding problems. Cyclic progestin treatment is less expensive and less complicated than treatment with clomiphene citrate.

Some case reports have indicated that long-term suppression of hypermenorrhea can also be achieved by the use of progesterone-releasing IUDs, which deliver progesterone directly to the endometrial cavity.[10] This mode of therapy is not suitable for all patients but can be considered an alternative for patients who have contraindications to OCs.

Androgens

Although androgens are usually effective in mild-to-moderate bleeding, they have no advantage over other agents and may cause masculinization. However, danazol has been used for the treatment of menorrhagia (blood loss greater than 80 mL in one menses).[11-14] Dosages of 200 mg and 400 mg daily have been effective when given over a 12-week period. These studies demonstrated both a reduction in blood loss from a mean of 200 mL to 25 mL and an increased interval between bleeding episodes (Figure 19-4).[14] The most common side effects of danazol were weight gain and acne. Other anabolic effects include a slight increase in clotting efficiency and stimulation of erythropoiesis. Reduction of dosage from 400 to 200 mg daily decreased the side effects but did not change the efficacy (Figure 19-5).[14] Smaller doses of danazol are ineffective. Danazol appears to be most effective for menorrhagia associated with ovulation, rather than for anovulatory DUB or acute bleeding. Its expense and side effects also limit its use.

Nonsteroidal anti-inflammatory drugs (NSAIDs)

NSAIDs, inhibitors of platelet aggregation and the platelet release reaction, also block fatty acid cyclo-oxygenase, which catalyzes the conversion

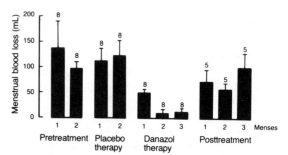

Figure 19-4
Mean menstrual blood loss (± SE) in eight patients with menorrhagia, before treatment, on placebo therapy, on danazol (200 mg daily), and after treatment. The number of patients studied is shown above each histogram.

Reproduced, with permission, from Chimbria TH, Anderson ABM, Nash C, et al: Reduction of menstrual blood loss by danazol in unexplained menorrhagia: Lack of effect of placebo. Br J Obstet Gynaecol 87:1152, 1980.

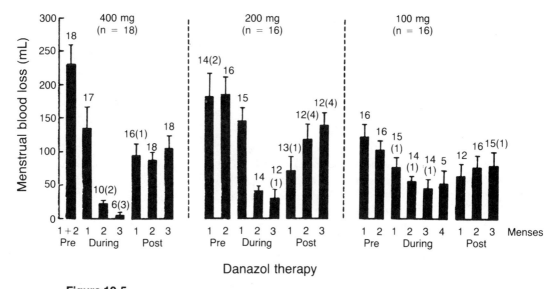

Figure 19-5
Mean menstrual blood loss (±SE) in three groups of patients with menorrhagia treated with 400 mg, 200 mg, or 100 mg of danazol daily for 12 weeks. Menstrual blood loss measurements are shown for each group before, during, and after danazol therapy. The number of patients menstruating is shown above each histogram, with the number of missing menstrual loss collections in parentheses.

Adapted from Chimbria TH, Anderson ABM, Nash C, et al: Reduction of menstrual blood loss by danazol in unexplained menorrhagia: Lack of effect of placebo. Br J Obstet Gynaecol 87:1152, 1980. Used with permission.

of arachidonic acid to prostaglandins. Among the most important is PGG_2 (thromboxane), a potent prostaglandin endoperoxide that stimulates platelet aggregation. The NSAIDs also block the formation of prostacyclin (PGI_2), an antagonist of thromboxane that relaxes vessel walls and reverses platelet aggregation. Thus, the key to reducing endometrial bleeding is to selectively block PGI_2 synthesis.[15,16] Unfortunately, there is no NSAID that works exclusively at this one site. All NSAIDs block the prohemostatic functions of thromboxane simultaneously and more extensively than the prostacyclin pathway. However, prostaglandin inhibitors have been used successfully for treatment of menorrhagia associated with ovulation. Some women with this condition have been found to have increased levels of PGI_2 in the endometrium and myometrium in vitro.

However, NSAIDs are not useful for women with anovulatory DUB. Levels of PGE_2 and $PGF_{2\alpha}$ are normally increased in endometrial tissue during the luteal phase and reach very high levels during menstruation. In some women with anovulatory DUB, the ratio of endometrial $PGF_{2\alpha}$ to PGE_2 is significantly lower than in controls.[17] All NSAIDs exhibit a nonspecific inhibition of PGE_2, $PGF_{2\alpha}$, thromboxane, and other prostaglandin endoperoxides. This generalized effect cannot correct a specific defect in prostaglandin physiology.

The benefits of the NSAIDs in reducing excessive bleeding are difficult to explain solely by the effects on the biosynthesis of prostaglandins, thromboxane, or prostacyclin. Few studies have measured $PGF_{2\alpha}$ and thromboxane simultaneously and the vasoconstriction that is the result of the thromboxane formation of these compounds; nor have they determined the degree of inhibition of the synthesis of PGI_2, PGE_2, or leukotrienes. One important effect may be on leukotriene synthesis; however, the control of leukotriene synthesis remains poorly understood at this time.

In a study of patients with unexplained menorrhagia, mefenamic acid, a potent NSAID, reduced MBL by 30%.[18] The patients were given 500 mg of mefenamic acid three times a day for 3 days. Another study also found mefenamic acid effective in reducing MBL (Figure 19-6 and Table 19-4).[19] Naproxen has been shown to be effective in reducing MBL in women with unexplained menorrhagia and in those with increased MBL following the insertion of an IUD (Table 19-4).[20] A regimen of 750 mg/day in divided doses for 3 days was found to be effective.

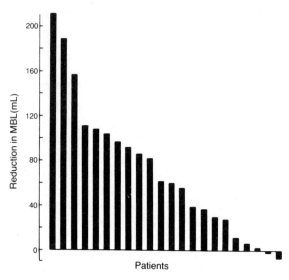

Figure 19-6
Mean reduction in menstrual blood loss during two menses in 22 patients taking mefenamic acid during menstruation, compared with blood loss during two pretreatment menses. Each histogram represents mean reduction in loss in one patient.

Reproduced, with permission, from Haynes PJ, Flint APF, Hodgson H, et al: Studies in menorrhagia: (a) mefenamic acid, (b) endometrial prostaglandin concentrations. Int J Gynaecol Obstet 17:567, 1980.

Table 19-4
Menstrual blood loss (mL)
before and during treatment
with mefenamic acid and naproxen

Treatment	Mean blood loss (mL)	
	Pretreatment	Treatment
Mefenamic acid[19]	137	76
Naproxen[20]	141	107

To date, very few studies have compared NSAIDs with other treatments. The effectiveness of NSAIDs in reducing MBL in ovulatory women is probably similar to that of antifibrinolytic agents and combination OCs.

Antifibrinolytic agents

Because *p*-aminomethylbenzoic acid (PAMBA), ε-aminocaproic acid (EACA), and tranexamic acid (AMCA) are all potent inhibitors of fibrinolysis, they have been used for the treatment of various hemorrhagic conditions.[21] All of these amino acids are potent inhibitors of the activation of plasminogen to plasmin. Endometrial tissue contains a high concentration of plasminogen activators, and the concentration is highest at the onset of menses.

Investigators compared the effect on MBL of EACA, AMCA, and combination OCs with the effect of curettage and methylergonovine maleate in 215 women with menorrhagia (Table 19-5).[22] EACA was given in a dosage of 18 g/day for 3 days and then 12, 9, 6, and 3 g daily on successive days. The total dose was always at least 48 g. AMCA was administered in a dosage of 6 g/day for 3 days followed by 4, 3, 2, and 1 g daily on successive days. The total dose of AMCA was at least 22 g. Combination OCs were administered on the usual 21-day schedule. Curettage was performed in the usual fashion, and the uterine-contracting agent methylergonovine maleate was given in a dosage of 0.75 mg daily for the first 4 days of menses. Blood loss was measured according to the method of Hallberg and Nilsson.[3] There was a significant reduction

Abnormal endocrinology

Table 19-5
Mean menstrual blood loss and percentage reduction before and during various treatments

Treatment	Mean blood loss (mL)		
	Pretreatment	Treatment	Decrease
EACA	164	87	47
AMCA	182	84	54
Oral contraceptives	158	75	52
Methylergonovine maleate	164	164	0

Adapted from Nilsson L, Rybo G: Treatment of menorrhagia. Am J Obstet Gynecol 110:713, 1971.

in MBL by EACA, AMCA, and OCs of approximately 50%. Methylergonovine maleate caused no significant reduction in MBL. Curettage decreased MBL only in the first cycle following the procedure; thereafter, there was no reduction.

The reduction in blood loss by antifibrinolytic agents was greatest among women with the greatest MBL before treatment. No significant differences in efficacy were found in a comparative study using either antifibrinolytic agents or OCs to treat women with menorrhagia.[23] Side effects occur commonly with antifibrinolytic agents, and are more frequent with EACA than with AMCA. They include nausea, dizziness, diarrhea, headaches, abdominal pain, and allergic manifestations. Other investigators have compared AMCA with placebo in double-blind investigations and found no significant differences in the occurrence of side effects. This might make AMCA the drug of choice. Antifibrinolytic agents are contraindicated in renal failure.

Ergot derivatives

These agents are not recommended for therapy because they are rarely effective and have a high incidence of side effects (nausea, vertigo, abdominal cramps). No reduction in MBL was found among 82 women with menorrhagia who were treated with methylergonovine maleate (Table 19-5).[22]

Surgical management

D&C and hysterectomy are commonly used to control abnormal bleeding. D&C is usually required when the patient is over 35 (to exclude malignancy) and in cases of very profuse bleeding, hypovolemia, and failure of medical management. Although curettage may be used to stop acute bleeding, it has no place in the long-term management of DUB. Recurrences of abnormal bleeding occur in more than 60% of patients with DUB treated with curettage alone. Therefore, following curettage, patients with histologic evidence of anovulatory bleeding should receive MPA each month as described above. For those with ovulatory menorrhagia, MBL is unchanged more than 1 month after D&C.[22] Hysteroscopic examination of the endometrial cavity at the time of D&C will help rule out the presence of a polyp or submucosal myoma. Hysterectomy, the last resort for the treatment of abnormal bleeding, is indicated when all other modalities fail or when there is associated pelvic pathology.

Laser photovaporization of the endometrium has been investigated for treatment of menorrhagia.[24] A neodymium-YAG laser was used under hysteroscopic visualization. Before the procedure, all patients were given danazol, 800 mg/day for 2 to 3 weeks. An additional 2 weeks of danazol treatment followed the laser procedure. This regimen cured 203 of 210 patients, including many with organic lesions such as submucosal myomas. Photovaporization causes varying degrees of uterine contraction, scarring, and adhesion formation, as follow-up HSGs and hysteroscopy showed. It is an alternative to hysterectomy when other modalities have failed, are contraindicated, or are undesirable. The investigators contend that there is little postoperative morbidity, discomfort, or disability.

Short- and long-term treatment

The prognosis for DUB depends on the etiology of the bleeding, the existence of other gynecologic or systemic disorders, and the desire for fertility. We advocate an initial approach aimed at determining whether or not the patient is ovulatory. Then we divide patients into those requiring acute management and those with a more chronic problem. Acute bleeding is best controlled with estrogen, unless a D&C is warranted on the basis of age, evidence of hypovolemia, and/or severe anemia. After the diagnosis of anovulation is confirmed in the majority of cases, long-term therapy should be directed by the needs of the patient.

When the patient is an adolescent, 10 mg of MPA should be given for 10 days each month and continued for at least 3 months, and the patient should be followed up carefully thereafter. Diagnostic studies to detect possible defects in the coagulation process should be performed in these young patients, particularly if bleeding is severe. In the woman of reproductive age, long-term therapy depends on whether the patient requires contraception, induction of ovulation, or treatment of DUB alone. In the last circumstance, MPA is administered for 10 days each month, continuing for at least 6 months. OCs and clomiphene citrate are used for the other indications. In the perimenopausal patient, who characteristically has lower levels of circulating estrogen, the use of cyclic MPA alone is frequently ineffective. These patients may require cyclic use of conjugated estrogens, 0.625 to 1.25 mg for 25 days, with 10 mg of MPA added from days 16 to 25, after absence of abnormal endometrial histology has been demonstrated.

The chronic ovulatory patient with menorrhagia is the most difficult type of DUB patient to treat. After cavity defects have been ruled out, long-term treatment is directed at a reduction in MBL. For these patients, NSAIDs, antifibrinolytic agents, prolonged progestin use, OCs, and danazol are part of the therapeutic armamentarium. A combination of two or more of these agents is often required to prevent the need for a hysterectomy.

References

1. Granstrom E, Swahn ML, Lundstrom V: The possible roles of prostaglandins and related compounds in endometrial bleeding. *Acta Obstet Gynecol Scand Suppl* 113:91, 1983

2. Grimes DA: Estimating vaginal blood loss. *J Reprod Med* 22:190, 1979

3. Hallberg L, Nilsson L: Determination of menstrual blood loss. *Scand J Clin Lab Invest* 16:244, 1964

4. Winter JSD, Faiman C: The development of cyclic pituitary-gonadal function in adolescent females. *J Clin Endocrinol Metab* 37:714, 1973

5. Fraser IS, Michie EA, Wide L, et al: Pituitary gonadotropins and ovarian function in adolescent dysfunctional bleeding. *J Clin Endocrinol Metab* 37:407, 1973

6. Claessens EA, Cowell CL: Acute adolescent menorrhagia. *Am J Obstet Gynecol* 139:277, 1981

7. Sherman BM, West JH, Korenman SG: The menopausal transition: Analysis of LH, FSH, estradiol, and progesterone concentrations during menstrual cycles of older woman. *J Clin Endocrinol Metab* 42:629, 1976

8. DeVore GR, Owens O, Kase N: Use of intravenous Premarin in the treatment of dysfunctional uterine bleeding—a double-blind randomized control study. *Obstet Gynecol* 59:285, 1982

9. Whitehead MI, Townsend PT, Pryse-Davies J, et al: The effects of estrogens and progestins on the biochemistry and morphology of the postmenopausal endometrium. *N Engl J Med* 305:1599, 1981

10. Parmer J: Long-term suppression of hypermenorrhea by progesterone IUDs. *Am J Obstet Gynecol* 149:578, 1984

11. Cope E: Danazol in the treatment of menorrhagia. *Drugs* 19:342, 1980

12. Chimbria TH, Cope E, Anderson ABM, et al: Preliminary results in the treatment of menorrhagia with danazol. *J Int Med Res* 5:98, 1977

13. Chimbria TH, Cope E, Anderson ABM, et al: The effect of danazol on menorrhagia, coagulation mechanisms, haematological indices and body weight. *Br J Obstet Gynaecol* 86:46, 1979

14. Chimbria TH, Anderson ABM, Nash C, et al: Reduction of menstrual blood loss by danazol in unexplained menorrhagia: Lack of effect of placebo. *Br J Obstet Gynaecol* 87:1152, 1980

15. Lunstrom V, Green K, Svanborg K: Endogenous prostaglandins in dysmenorrhea and the effect of prostaglandin synthetase inhibitors (PGSI) on uterine contractility. *Acta Obstet Gynecol Scand Suppl* 87:51, 1979

16. Smith SK, Abel MH, Kelly RW, et al: Prostaglandin synthesis in the endometrium of women with ovular dysfunctional uterine bleeding. *Br J Obstet Gynaecol* 88:434, 1981

17. Lunstrom V, Green K: Endogenous levels of prostaglandin $F_{2\alpha}$ and its main metabolites in plasma and endometrium of normal and dysmenorrheic women. *Am J Obstet Gynecol* 130:640, 1978

18. Anderson ABM, Haynes PJ, Guillebaud J, et al: Reduction of menstrual blood loss by prostaglandin synthetase inhibitors. *Lancet* 1:774, 1976

19. Haynes PJ, Flint APF, Hodgson H, et al: Studies in menorrhagia: (a) mefenamic acid, (b) endometrial prostaglandin concentrations. *Int J Gynaecol Obstet* 17:567, 1980

20. Nygren K-G, Rybo G: Prostaglandins and menorrhagia. *Acta Obstet Gynecol Scand Suppl* 113:101, 1983

21. Callender ST, Warner GT, Cope E: Treatment of menorrhagia with tranexamic acid: A double-blind trial. *Br Med J* 4:214, 1970

22. Nilsson L, Rybo G: Treatment of menorrhagia. *Am J Obstet Gynecol* 110:713, 1971

23. Nilsson L, Rybo G: Treatment of menorrhagia with an antifibrinolytic agent, tranexamic acid (AMCA). A double-blind investigation. *Acta Obstet Gynecol Scand* 46:572, 1967

24. Goldrath MH, Fuller TA, Segal S: Laser photovaporization of endometrium for the treatment of menorrhagia. *Am J Obstet Gynecol* 140:14, 1981

Chapter 20

Premenstrual Syndrome

The Neuroendocrine Control of Mood and Behavior

Joyce M. Vargyas, M.D.

Introduction

As early as the 6th century BC, Semonides wrote of a woman whose disposition was like the sea, at times calm and innocent, and at other times turbulent. This truly must be the first description of the premenstrual syndrome some 2,500 years ago, although that precise term was not used. The first mention in a medical journal occurred in 1931, when Frank used the term "premenstrual tension" (PMT) and postulated that elevated estrogen levels were the major etiology. Since then, dozens of theories concerning the etiology of this syndrome have been published. Nonetheless, although its prevalence and importance are recognized, there remains little scientific evidence that might explain the underlying pathophysiology of this disorder.

Definition

The definition of the premenstrual syndrome is well recognized. It is considered a cyclic symptom complex that begins after ovulation, is unique to each patient in type and degree of symptomatology, and disappears with the onset of menses. Not only are the symptoms unique to each patient, but they also may vary from cycle to cycle, especially in severity. Most sufferers have relief of symptoms with menses. Dysmenorrhea is not considered a part of this syndrome.

Symptoms

It is necessary to decide at the outset whether all the reported symptoms apply to one entity with one pathophysiologic basis, or whether this syndrome has subcategories with different identifiable endocrinopathies and therefore several different treatment regimens.

Abraham, in 1980, described four categories of the premenstrual syndrome (Figure 20-1).[1] In the first, PMT-A, the predominant symptoms are tension, nervousness, mood swings, irritability, and anxiety. In the PMT-C category, predominant symptoms are those of hypoglycemic episodes: headaches, craving for sweets, and an increase in appetite. PMT-D symptoms consist primarily of depression, confusion, outbursts of crying, and forgetfulness. The systemic aspect of the premenstrual syndrome, PMT-H, comprises weight gain, swelling of the extremities, breast tenderness, and bloating. Certainly, it is possible that subgroups may ultimately be identified by biochemical measurements. Most patients fall into more than one category by

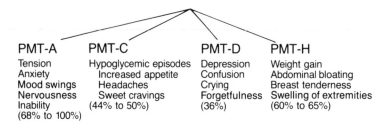

PMT-A	PMT-C	PMT-D	PMT-H
Tension	Hypoglycemic episodes	Depression	Weight gain
Anxiety	Increased appetite	Confusion	Abdominal bloating
Mood swings	Headaches	Crying	Breast tenderness
Nervousness	Sweet cravings	Forgetfulness	Swelling of extremities
Inability	(44% to 50%)	(36%)	(60% to 65%)
(68% to 100%)			

Figure 20-1

Premenstrual syndrome divided into categories according to major symptoms. Percentages represent incidence for each category.

Adapted from Abraham GE: Premenstrual tension. In Leventhal JM, Goldstein DP (eds): Current Problems in Obstetrics and Gynecology, *vol 3. Chicago, Year Book Medical Publishers, 1980, p 1. Used with permission.*

symptoms alone; considerable overlap exists. Ultimately, however, as studies are completed, subgroups will be more clearly defined and PMS probably will not be considered a simple single entity with one treatment regimen appropriate for all patients.

The quoted incidence of PMS varies from 3% to 90%, depending on the series reviewed. The large variation stems from the lack of consistency in definition. Surveys indicate that about 80% of women admit to some symptoms that are cyclic in nature and occur frequently during the premenstrual period.[2] However, severe debilitative symptoms are reported by only 20% to 40% of women.

The most commonly reported symptoms of PMS are anxiety and irritability.[2] Depending on the study, these two symptoms are reported in 68% to 100% of all PMS sufferers.[1] Somatic complaints of breast tenderness and weight gain—the second most common symptom complex—are reported in 60% to 65% of patients with PMS. Reports of symptoms associated with hypoglycemia, the third most common category, vary between 44% and 50%.[1] The most infrequent symptoms appear to be depression and withdrawal, with a reported incidence of 36%.[1] Women in this last category seem to experience the highest degree of incapacitation; some report suicidal ideation and attempts. They also report a high incidence of absenteeism from

work due to the confusion and withdrawal associated with severe depression.

The social and economic impact of the premenstrual syndrome has been described in the literature.[3] Increased absenteeism from work and an increased incidence of accidents, admission to hospitals, and suicide attempts during the premenstrual period are well documented.[4] One study also described the apparent influence of PMS on schoolgirls; their grade averages fell significantly during the luteal phase as compared with the follicular phase.[5] Another study reported that 36% of female factory workers sought sedation during the premenstrual week in order to continue working.[6] The most recognizable effect of PMS is its impact on the families of sufferers; both husband and children may be the objects of emotional lability.

Epidemiology

Epidemiologic studies agree that the incidence of PMS increases with age until the menopause.[7,8] The mean age of PMS sufferers in our patient population is 33. Prior childbirth also seems to predispose women to the symptoms of PMS.[3] The incidence appears to be higher in women with a history of preeclampsia or postpartum depression.[3] To date, there is no known increase in the incidence of PMS in women whose mothers had premenstrual symptoms.

Women with several types of disorders may

seek medical help for what they believe to be PMS. Some have serious underlying psychiatric disorders, such as manic-depressive illness or endogenous depression. Their symptoms may be exacerbated premenstrually, but basically they are present throughout the entire cycle. In many cases, such patients have had psychotherapy, but are looking for a new treatment for chronic problems.

A second group of women who commonly seek medical help for PMS have an exogenous source of stress with which they are unable to cope. Rather than address the real situational stress, they blame the resulting symptoms on PMS. Examples include women going through divorce or job change.

In contrast, women seeking medical attention who do indeed suffer from PMS may appear to have dual personalities. They are completely symptom-free during the follicular phase, but in the luteal phase they undergo a change in personality, manifesting various PMS symptoms.

Pathophysiology

Many theories have been proposed for the pathophysiology of PMS. Most treatments have been by-products of these theories. Some have been disproven and are discussed here to highlight their invalidity. Theories currently under investigation are presented in some detail.

Fluid imbalance
One of the earliest investigative approaches centered on fluid imbalance. Early observations indicated that most women gained from 3 to 6 pounds premenstrually. In 1934, it was reported that 70% of women gained less than 3 pounds before ovulation, but 30% gained more than 3 pounds premenstrually.[9] Later studies showed that it is very rare for any woman to gain more than 3 pounds above her mean weight during

the luteal phase.[10] Others have found no consistent alterations in weight associated with phase of the cycle in either symptomatic or asymptomatic women.[11,12]

Both angiotensin and aldosterone have been reported to be increased in the luteal phase, but not in the follicular phase, of the cycle.[13] Renin levels have also been found to be higher in the luteal phase than in the follicular phase in normal women.[14] Luteal phase aldosterone elevations have been substantiated by many studies. These investigators did not, however, compare levels of aldosterone, renin, or angio-

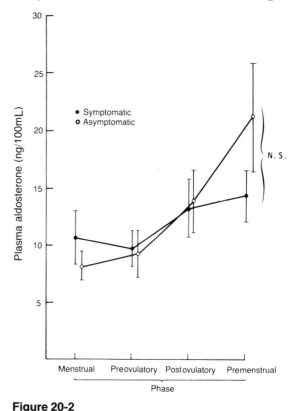

Figure 20-2
No significant difference in serum levels of aldosterone (mean ± SE) in symptomatic and asymptomatic women during all phases of the cycle.

Reproduced, with permission, from O'Brien PM, Craven D, Selby C, et al: Treatment of premenstrual syndrome by spironolactone. Br J Obstet Gynaecol 86:142, 1979.

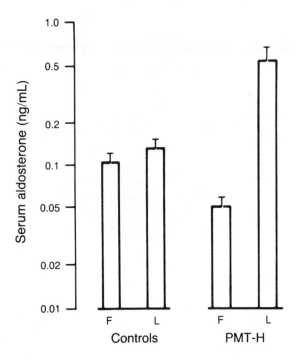

Figure 20-3
Elevated luteal phase (L) levels of serum aldosterone
(mean ± SE) in women with predominant symptoms of
weight gain and edema (PMT-H) compared with controls.
F, follicular phase.

*Reproduced, with permission, from Abraham GE: Premenstrual
tension. In Leventhal JM, Goldstein DP (eds): Current Problems in
Obstetrics and Gynecology, vol 3. Chicago, Year Book Medical
Publishers, 1980, p 1.*

tensin in patients with and without PMS symptoms. A 1979 study made such a comparison and found no significant difference in luteal phase aldosterone levels between 18 women with PMS and 10 controls (Figure 20-2).[15] But a study of women with edema and weight gain as the predominant complaints found that aldosterone levels were higher than in women who had no symptoms (Figure 20-3).[1]

It is difficult to attribute all the symptoms of PMS to fluid retention. Nonetheless, trials with spironolactone, which seems both to antagonize aldosterone and to have an inhibitory effect on steroidogenesis, appear to be promising. A 1980 report described a few women with PMS who

had a good response to spironolactone at a dosage of 25 mg twice a day, but there were no control subjects or placebo treatment.[16] In another study, 18 patients with PMS were given 25 mg of spironolactone four times daily for several cycles, and the results were compared with placebo administration. With spironolactone, but not with placebo, 80% of the subjects had a significant decrease in both physical and psychological symptoms.[15] It is difficult to attribute the success of spironolactone solely to its diuretic effect, since other diuretic agents such as bumetanide, chlorthalidone, and a thiazide have not been found more effective than placebo and/or other agents.[17,18]

Prolactin

A popular theory concerning the etiology and treatment of PMS suggested that elevated prolactin levels were the cause of symptoms. Studies in which prolactin levels were measured in patients both with and without PMS symptoms found no difference between the two groups (Figure 20-4).[19] When bromocriptine was used to treat PMS, it showed no distinct advantage over placebo in alleviating psychological symptoms. However, the drug did relieve the breast tenderness associated with this syndrome, and it has subsequently been used for treatment of severe cases of mastodynia.[17]

Prostaglandins

Because prostaglandins have been implicated in the etiology of depression and prostaglandin inhibitors appear to relieve symptoms of dysmenorrhea, prostaglandin inhibitors have been tried for treatment of PMS symptoms. An initial study in 1980 compared the effects of mefenamic acid and placebo on 37 patients.[20] It was conducted in double-blind, crossover fashion, with a control cycle preceding the treatment and placebo cycles. Mefenamic acid was given in a dosage of 500 mg three times a day (2 tablets after each meal), beginning with onset of PMS symptoms.

Abnormal endocrinology

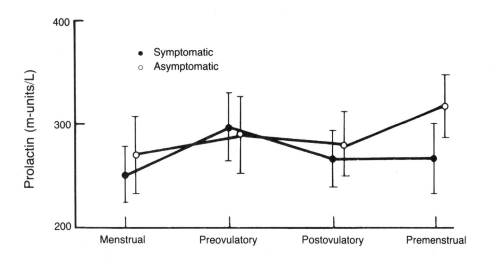

Figure 20-4
Similar serum prolactin levels (mean ± SE) in symptomatic and asymptomatic women throughout the menstrual cycle.

Reproduced, with permission, from O'Brien PM, Symonds EM: Prolactin levels in the premenstrual syndrome. Br J Obstet Gynaecol 89:306, 1982.

It was found that 23 patients experienced fewer and less severe symptoms with mefenamic acid. Although many symptoms persisted, the overall rating improved. However, mefenamic acid helped only the women who had both menstrual and premenstrual symptoms; those with premenstrual symptoms alone were not helped. These results show how important it is both to clarify the definition of premenstrual syndrome and to eliminate from consideration such menstrual symptoms as abdominal cramps, leg aches, backaches, and nausea.

A second trial was reported in 1983, using mefenamic acid and placebo in double-blind fashion.[21] A group of 43 women were given the drug 2 to 4 days prior to menses. Mefenamic acid alleviated only breast tenderness, abdominal bloating, edema, and dysmenorrhea—symptoms previously reported to improve during use of prostaglandin inhibitors. It thus appears that prostaglandin inhibitors are not effective in treating PMS as a whole but do relieve some of the physical symptoms associated with menses.

Nutrition

A nutritional etiology for PMS has been studied extensively and is still under investigation. In 1980, it was reported that women with PMS appeared to have a higher intake of salt and refined sugar and a lower intake of foods with higher nutritional value than women without PMS.[1,22] The investigators hypothesized that pyridoxine, or vitamin B_6, was one of the essential factors deficient in their patient population.

Currently, the use of B_6 for treatment of PMS is based on the following hypothesis: Patients with PMS are thought to have increased stress, with an increased need for glucose. It is thought that B_6 accelerates the hepatic breakdown of glycogen, thus inducing the liver to supply the needed glucose and preventing hypoglycemia. Moreover, it is now known that B_6 is a coenzyme in the biosynthesis of dopamine and serotonin. Variations in levels of both these neurotransmitters are thought to play a role in mood disorders. To date, there are no reported studies of serum B_6 levels in patients with PMS.

The data concerning the relation of magnesium to PMS are also unclear. In one study, mean red cell magnesium levels were found to be slightly lower in PMS patients than in controls, but no significant differences in serum magnesium levels were found.[23]

Other findings lend support to a nutritional etiology for the symptoms of PMS. As early as 1947, it was noticed that women in the luteal phase have an increase in carbohydrate tolerance.[24] Investigators have reported that the glucose tolerance curve is flattened during the luteal phase.[25] More recently, a decrease in insulin receptor concentration was detected in the monocytes of women in the luteal phase, as compared with the follicular phase.[26] This may be the physiologic basis for the carbohydrate aberration. The patients in these studies were women with normal cycles who were not tested for the presence or absence of premenstrual symptoms. It is still necessary to determine whether carbohydrate metabolism is altered more in PMS sufferers, particularly those with sweet cravings and hypoglycemic episodes, or is altered equally in all women during the luteal phase. The hypoglycemic episodes are thought to correlate with crying outbursts and sudden violent behavior, but this theory also needs to be substantiated.

No studies have tested the effect of changes in diet alone, but several have combined dietary alteration with vitamin supplementation. In a 1972 study, only four of 13 premenstrual subjects improved with 50 mg of B_6 per day, whereas five improved with placebo.[27] In a 1977 study that did not use placebo-treated controls, 50% of 70 PMS patients showed symptomatic improvement with 40 to 100 mg of B_6 daily.[28] Magnesium nitrate, at a daily dosage of 4.5 to 6.0 mg during the week preceding menses, was reported to have decreased the severity of premenstrual tension and edema in 192 women.[29] Unfortunately, there were no placebo or control cycles in this study—the only one using magnesium.

Two investigators administered 500 mg of B_6 per day to PMS patients during the luteal phase and compared resulting symptoms with those of placebo cycles.[22] Of the 25 patients in the study, 21 reported significant improvement in symptoms when B_6 was used, but no improvement during placebo cycles. The four patients who demonstrated no improvement during B_6 cycles had symptoms in the follicular phase as well as the luteal phase during screening cycles.

One of the investigators subsequently developed a multivitamin compound, Optivite, with 50 mg of B_6 and approximately 40 mg of magnesium.[30] To attain the therapeutic B_6 levels used in his studies, a woman must take 10 tablets per day—a cumbersome amount that also causes gastrointestinal side effects secondary to the high magnesium level. Other preparations now on the market, which give higher doses of B_6 per tablet, make compliance easier. More double-blind, crossover, placebo-controlled studies need to be performed with various nutritional agents in order to explore whatever roles they may play in the etiology and treatment of PMS.

Steroid imbalance

Another major area of interest is hormonal imbalance and its correction. Dalton proposed the original progesterone therapy and performed the first trials, but did not conduct controlled studies.[3] Nonetheless, treatment with natural progesterone has gained popularity in the US and is used in PMS clinics.

Natural-progesterone treatment is based on the theory that patients with PMS, as compared with controls, have decreased progesterone levels and increased estrogen levels during the luteal phase, with an overall increase in the estrogen/progesterone ratio. The literature on this subject is extremely controversial. In 1974, two investigators demonstrated a significant elevation in estrogen levels during premenstrual days 2 through 5 in PMS patients with anxiety symptoms, as compared with asymptomatic controls

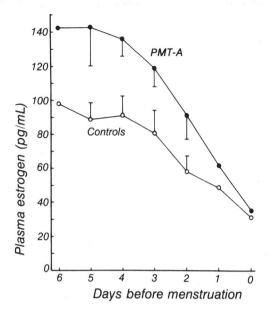

Figure 20-5
Significantly elevated estrogen levels in patients with predominant symptoms of anxiety (PMT-A) and asymptomatic control subjects on premenstrual days 5, 4, 3, and 2.

Reproduced, with permission, from Backstrom T, Carstensen H: Estrogen and progesterone in plasma in relation to premenstrual tension. J Steroid Biochem 5:257, 1974. Copyright 1974, Pergamon Press, Ltd.

(Figure 20-5).[31] They also found significantly lower progesterone levels during premenstrual days 4 through 6 in subjects with anxiety symptoms (Figure 20-6).[31] Another study reported increased estradiol levels during days 1 through 4 premenstrually, and significantly decreased progesterone levels on days 5 through 9 premenstrually.[32] This difference was found in only one-third of the patients—those who had the most severe symptoms, particularly anxiety. Interestingly, the 1974 study mentioned above found that patients complaining of symptoms of anxiety also had the most significant hormonal alterations (Table 20-1).[31]

Other investigators found no differences in luteal phase levels of either progesterone or estrogen between symptom-free controls and symptomatic subjects.[33,34] In our own initial prospective evaluation of patients with PMS symptoms, we also found no significant differences in progesterone or estrogen levels in comparison with a group of asymptomatic women.[35]

Because peripheral hormone measurements do not consistently show differences between symptomatic and asymptomatic women, a study was done measuring sex hormone-binding globulin (SHBG).[36] Although no differences were found in estrogen or testosterone levels, symptomatic subjects had a mean level of 31 nmol dihydrotestosterone bound per liter of SHBG, compared with 66 nmol in asymptomatic controls. The subjects were matched for age but not weight. This may have affected the results, since peripheral levels of SHBG are significantly lowered by obesity.[37] Nonetheless, the data are

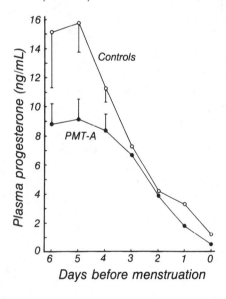

Figure 20-6
Significantly lowered progesterone levels in patients with predominant symptoms of anxiety (PMT-A) and asymptomatic control subjects on premenstrual days 6, 5, and 4.

Reproduced, with permission, from Backstrom T, Carstensen H: Estrogen and progesterone in plasma in relation to premenstrual tension. J Steroid Biochem 5:257, 1974. Copyright 1974, Pergamon Press, Ltd.

Table 20-1
Correlation between hormonal status
and premenstrual symptoms

Symptom	Estrogen (pg/mL)	Estrogen progesterone ratio	Progesterone (ng/mL)
Anxiety	0.729*	0.453	−0.042
Depression	0.486†	0.392	−0.081
Irritability	0.635‡	0.281	0.149
Swelling	0.259	0.104	−0.128
Anxiety and irritability	0.715*	0.383	0.062

*$P < 0.005$.   †$P < 0.05$.   ‡$P < 0.01$.

Values of estrogen and progesterone indicate variation from levels in asymptomatic controls during premenstrual days 2 through 5. Significant correlation was found between high estrogen and E/P ratios and anxiety, depression, and irritability. Estrogen and swelling show no significant correlation.

Adapted from Backstrom T, Carstensen H: Estrogen and progesterone in plasma in relation to premenstrual tension. J Steroid Biochem 5:257, 1974. Copyright 1974, Pergamon Press, Ltd.

interesting and may prove to be significant in weight-matched studies using not only the indirect assay but also the direct assay for SHBG.

Many treatment centers use the natural form of progesterone in vaginal or rectal suppositories, 100 to 400 mg twice a day. Treatment success has been reported anecdotally, but not demonstrated in well-controlled, double-blind, crossover studies. A study comparing the effects of 200 or 400 mg of progesterone twice a day against placebo[38] reported these results: At the 200-mg dose, 31% of 35 subjects preferred progesterone and 43% preferred placebo; at the 400-mg dose, 27% of 26 subjects preferred progesterone and 35% preferred placebo. It is apparent that if the natural progesterone suppositories are going to be used for treatment of PMS, randomized, prospective, double-blind studies from the centers now using this therapy must be done to prove that it is indeed effective.

Neurotransmitter alterations

Several authors have emphasized the possible role of the central nervous system in this disorder. Halbreich, Endicott, and colleagues distinguished two types of PMS, both secondary to endorphin abnormalities.[39] One, an atypical depressive type, they described as resulting from a decreased level of endorphins. The other, an anxious, agitated disorder, they postulated to be due to a disregulation of endorphins.

Similarly, Reid hypothesized that the symptoms of PMS result from fluctuations of opioid peptides under the influence of gonadal steroids.[40] He proposed that in the early luteal phase, when opioid activity is elevated, a decrease in dopamine and norepinephrine results in fatigue, depression, and constipation. He further proposed that in the late luteal phase, when endorphin levels start to decline, opioid withdrawal results in irritability and anxiety. This theory is attractive, but somewhat simplistic. Most women with PMS do not have a set time early in the luteal phase when they experience only fatigue and depression, which are then followed by irritability and anxiety. Most have varying degrees of all these symptoms throughout the luteal phase. It appears more likely that PMS patients have daily fluctuations of endorphin levels, rather than a set time in the luteal phase when they are overexposed and another when they have withdrawal.

The above hypotheses proposing central opioid abnormalities as the etiology of PMS might explain why progesterone seems effective in some women. Continual elevation of peripheral progesterone levels would result in stable, increased central endorphin levels, thus preventing the symptoms of opioid withdrawal, deficiency, and/or disregulation.

Diagnosis

In diagnosing PMS, any psychiatric disorder must first be identified. A careful history is also necessary to discover any personal problems that might be the source of anxiety or depression. It is essential that the patient record her basal body temperature so that the clinician can tell if and when ovulation occurs and define the length of the follicular and luteal phases. Finally, it is very important that each patient keep a "prospective" diary of symptoms. Since retrospective reporting is very inaccurate, the diary must precede the initiation of any treatment. Patients who truly have PMS will record a significantly higher symptom score during the luteal phase than during the follicular phase. Figure 20-7 is an example of a simple chart we have developed that clinicians may use for this purpose. Endicott and Halbreich developed a more complex form of assessment that is frequently used in clinical research of PMS.[41]

Treatment

No single form of therapy has been proven effective in all patients with PMS. Therefore, the major approach at this time is individualization of treatment. A good doctor-patient relationship is very important to the therapeutic process. The physician's recognition of the problem, an open and honest attitude, and a mutual approach to amelioration of syr therapeutic.

Candidates fc have significant symptom-free f underlying psy tional probler throughout the c, more appropriate care, as

Treatment candidates with ized symptoms who have not had previc of therapy should be started on a program of v. tamin B_6, 500 mg each day, combined with a daily exercise routine and reduced intake of salt and refined carbohydrates.

If these conservative measures are unsuccessful, it may be necessary to give medication during the symptomatic period of the luteal phase. If, for example, the predominant presenting complaint is physical discomfort due to edema, weight gain, and abdominal and breast swelling, spironolactone, 25 mg three times a day, may be given.

If careful history-taking and prospective symptom recording reveal that symptoms of prostaglandin excess (dysmenorrhea, low back pain, faintness, headache) are the major problems, prostaglandin inhibitors may be used during the symptomatic period. If breast tenderness and mastodynia are the major complaints, bromocriptine, 2.5 mg orally twice a day, may be all that is needed to keep the patient comfortable during the premenstruum.

In double-blind crossover trials using progesterone vaginal suppositories, progesterone has not been demonstrated to be more effective than placebo.[42,43] A recent report did however show some beneficial effects from the oral micronized form of progesterone, which has not yet been approved for use in this country.[44] There are retrospective uncontrolled reports of clinical effectiveness with the use of progesterone vaginal suppositories at 100, 200, or 400 mg twice daily. This form of treatment may be used

PREMENSTRUAL SYNDROME SYMPTOMATOLOGY QUESTIONNAIRE

Name _____

First Day of Last Menses _____

First Day of Present Menses _____

Grading Symptoms:

JOYCE M. VARGYAS, M.D.

0 = None	B = Bleeding
1 = Mild	S = Spotting
2 = Moderate	O = No Bleeding
3 = Severe	

LAC/USC Medical Center
Women's Hospital #L946
1240 North Mission Rd.
Los Angeles, CA 90033

HEIGHT: ____
WEIGHT: ____

AGE: ____

First day of period → Day of cycle	1	2	3	4	5	6	7	8	9	10	11	12	13	14	15	16	17	18	19	20	21	22	23	24	25	26	27	28	29	30	31
Month/date																															
Morning temp.																															
Bleeding																															
Nervous tension																															
Forgetfulness																															
Increased appetite																															
Abdominal bloating																															
Mood swings																															
Coordination loss																															
Headache																															
Depression																															
Fatigue																															
Crying																															
Insomnia																															
Hostility																															
Breast tenderness																															
Irritability																															
Craving for sweets																															
Decreased self-esteem																															
Irrational behavior																															
Confusion																															
Decreased libido																															
Anxiety																															
Total																															
Daily weight																															
Menstrual cramps																															

Figure 20-7

Premenstrual syndrome symptomatology questionnaire. Patients grade the degree of symptoms from 0 (none) to 3 (severe) daily throughout the cycle. Basal body temperature is noted for ovulatory status and timing of ovulation. Daily weight and severity of menstrual cramps are also noted.

Abnormal endocrinology

on a trial basis on selected patients who have been informed that it has not been proven effective for PMS. If progesterone is ineffective and a strong element of depression persists, an antidepressant may be tried in collaboration with a psychiatrist. The antidepressant is given on a daily basis throughout the cycle rather than in the luteal phase only as in progesterone treatment. An alternative may be an antianxiety agent such as alprazolam (0.5 mg three times daily during the symptomatic days of the luteal phase only), which has been found to be an effective antidepressant as well. Alprazolam therapy may prove useful for those patients with both anxiety and depression.

Future research

Ultimately, the interaction between the sex steroids and the central nervous system opioids and neurotransmitters may explain the pathophysiologic basis of PMS. Research in basic science appears to be moving toward this conclusion. The importance of the sex steroids on central nervous system levels of β-endorphins has been experimentally demonstrated. In a study in which the pituitary stalk of castrated female monkeys was transected and catheterized, the hypophyseal portal blood level of β-endorphin was measured after acute estradiol replacement as well as long-term physiologic estradiol replacement later supplemented with progesterone replacement. β-Endorphins were released into the portal blood only after the long-term progesterone treatment was added to the regimen. Although such an experimental design is impossible to implement in human subjects, studies such as this can point to possible avenues of human research and ultimately may help to explain how the variable neuroendocrine events of the menstrual cycle relate to alterations in personality.[45]

References

1. Abraha JM, Go and Gy Publish

2. Reid R Obstet C

3. Dalton Therapy

4. Dalton 2:1425

5. Dalton weekly

6. Bickers treatme

7. Morton study of premenstrual tension. Am J Obstet Gynecol 65:1182, 1953

8. Greene R, Dalton K: The premenstrual syndrome. Br Med J 1:1007, 1953

9. Sweeney JS: Menstrual edema. JAMA 103:234, 1934

10. Golub LJ, Menduhe H, Conly SS: Weight changes in college women during the menstrual cycle. Am J Obstet Gynecol 91:89, 1965

11. Chesley LC, Hellman LM: Variations in body weight and salivary sodium in the menstrual cycle. Am J Obstet Gynecol 74:582, 1957

12. Andersch B, Hahn L, Andersson M, et al: Body water and weight in patients with premenstrual tension. Br J Obstet Gynaecol 85:546, 1978

13. Sundsfjord JA, Aakvaag A: Plasma angiotensin II, and aldosterone excertion during the menstrual cycle. Acta Endocrinol 64:452, 1970

14. Michelakis AM, Yoshida H, Dormois JC: Plasma renin activity and plasma aldosterone during the normal menstrual cycle. Am J Obstet Gynecol 123:724, 1975

15. O'Brien PM, Craven D, Selby C, et al: Treatment of premenstrual syndrome by spironolactone. Br J Obstet Gynaecol 86:142, 1979

16. Hendler W: Spironolactone for premenstrual syndrome. Female Patient 5:17, 1980

17. Andersch B, Abrahamsson L, Wendestam C, et al: Hormone profile in premenstrual tension: Effect of bromocriptine and diuretics. Clin Endocrinol 2:657, 1979

18. Mattsson B, von Schoultz B: A comparison between lithium, placebo and a diuretic in premenstrual tension. Acta Psychiatr Scand (Suppl) 225:75, 1974

19. O'Brien PM, Symonds EM: Prolactin levels in the premenstrual syndrome. Br J Obstet Gynaecol 89:306, 1982

20. Wood D: The treatment of premenstrual syndrome symptoms with mefenamic acid. Br J Obstet Gynaecol 87:306, 1980

21. Budoff PW: The use of p the premenstrual synd

22. Abraham GE, Harg on premenstrual premenstrual t crossover stu

23. Abraham magnes tensi

24. B

...rostaglandin inhibitors for ...ome. *J Reprod Med* 28:469, 1983

...rove JT: Effect of vitamin B-6 ...ymptomatology in women with ...nsion syndrome: A double blind ...dy. *Infertility* 3:155, 1980

...GE, Lubran MM: Serum and red cell ...ium levels in patients with premenstrual ...n syndrome. *Am J Clin Nutr* 34:2364, 1981

...lig HE, Spaulding CA: Hyperinsulinism of menses. *Ind Med* 16:336, 1947

25. Tanett RJ, Graver HJ: Changes in oral glucose tolerance during the menstrual cycle. *Br Med J* 2:528, 1968

26. DePirro R, Fusco H, Bertoli A, et al: Insulin receptors during the menstrual cycle in normal women. *J Clin Endocrinol Metab* 47:1387, 1978

27. Stokes J, Mendels J: Pyridoxine and premenstrual tension. *Lancet* 1:1177, 1972

28. Kerr GD: The management of the premenstrual syndrome. *Curr Med Res Opin* 4:29, 1977

29. Nicholas A: Treatment of premenstrual syndrome and dysmenorrhea with magnesium. In *The First International Symposium on Magnesium Deficiency in Human Pathology.* Paris, Vittel, 1973

30. Goei GS, Abraham GE: Effect of a nutritional supplement, Optivite, on symptoms of premenstrual tension. *J Reprod Med* 28:527, 1983

31. Backstrom T, Carstensen H: Estrogen and progesterone in plasma in relation to premenstrual tension. *J Steroid Biochem* 5:257, 1974

32. Munday MR, Brush MG, Taylor RW: Correlations between progesterone, estradiol and aldosterone levels in the premenstrual syndrome. *Clin Endocrinol* 14:1, 1981

33. O'Brien PM, Selby C, Symonds EM: Progesterone, fluid, and electrolytes in the premenstrual syndrome. *Br Med J* 280:1161, 1980

34. Taylor JW: The timing of menstruation-related symptoms assessed by a daily symptom rating scale. *Acta Psychiatr Scand* 60:87, 1979

35. Vargyas J, Lobo R: The role of non-SHBG bound estradiol, total estradiol, progesterone and the E_2/P ratio in the premenstrual syndrome. *Soc Gynecol Invest* 307:65, 1983

36. Dalton M: Sex hormone-binding globulin concentrations in women with severe premenstrual syndrome. *Postgrad Med J* 57:560, 1981

37. Nisker JA, Hammond GL, Davidson BJ, et al: Serum sex hormone binding globulin capacity and the percentage of free estradiol in postmenopausal women with and without endometrial carcinoma. *Am J Obstet Gynecol* 138:637, 1980

38. Sampson GA: Premenstrual syndrome: A double-blind controlled trial of progesterone and placebo. *Br J Psychiatr* 135:209, 1979

39. Halbreich U, Endicott J, Schacht S, et al: The diversity of premenstrual changes as reflected in the Premenstrual Assessment Form. *Acta Psychiatr Scand* 65:46, 1982

40. Reid RL: Premenstrual syndrome: A therapeutic enigma. *Drug Ther* 12:65, 1982

41. Endicott J, Halbreich U: Psychobiology of premenstrual change. Retrospective report of premenstrual depressive changes: Factors affecting confirmation by daily ratings. *Psychopharmacol Bull* 18:109, 1982

42. Vargyas JM: The use of progesterone in the premenstrual syndrome. Presented at the American Fertility Society, Oct 2, 1985

43. Maddocks SE, Hahn PM, Moller F, et al: A double-blind placebo-controlled trial of progesterone vaginal suppositories in the treatment of premenstrual syndrome. Presented at the Society for Gynecologic Investigation, Phoenix, Arizona, March 20, 1985

44. Dennerstein L, Spencer-Gardner C, Gotts G, et al: Progesterone and the premenstrual syndrome double-blind crossover trial. *Br Med J* 390:1617, 1985

45. Wardlaw SL, Wehrenberg WB, Ferin M, et al: Effect of sex steroids on beta-endorphin in hypophyseal portal blood. *J Clin Endocrinol Metab* 55:877, 1982

Chapter 21

Dynamics of Hormone Testing

Rogerio A. Lobo, M.D.
Oscar A. Kletzky, M.D.

Clinicians can now test the dynamics of the hypothalamic-pituitary, thyroid, ovarian, and adrenal axes, because we have the ability to measure steroid and protein hormones accurately. We will confine our discussion to tests that have been shown to be helpful in the practice of reproductive endocrinology. Our list of tests is not exhaustive. We have deliberately omitted some clinical and research tests that have been used in the past.

Adrenocorticotropic hormone (ACTH)

ACTH-stimulation testing is indicated to rule out primary adrenal hypofunction (e.g., Addison's disease), as well as to help diagnose subtle adrenal enzymatic defects that result in adrenal hyperfunction. The protocols for the diagnoses of these opposite clinical situations are different and therefore will be discussed separately.

Adrenal hypofunction

Indications

If Addison's or adrenocortical hypofunction is suspected clinically because of anorexia, weight loss, weakness, hypotension, and hyperpigmentation, an ACTH test should be performed to establish the diagnosis. If the patient is acutely ill and hypotensive, it is best first to give dexamethasone (DEX), followed by a more prolonged infusion of ACTH (see below).

Another indication for ACTH-stimulation testing is to determine the ability of the adrenal to produce cortisol in patients with an abnormal serum cortisol response after an insulin tolerance test (ITT). The ITT tests the hypothalamic-pituitary response to stress, while the ACTH test determines if the adrenal itself is able to respond. Although the adrenal decreases in size when there is no endogenous ACTH stimulation, it does not lose its ability to respond to ACTH under normal circumstances. However, after many years of decreased endogenous

ACTH stimulation, the adrenal may require priming for an adequate response.

Procedure

As a quick test to rule out adrenal hypofunction, 250 μg (25 USP units) of cosyntropin are administered as an IV bolus. This test is not affected by time of day or food intake. The serum cortisol level should be measured three separate times— at baseline and 60 and 120 minutes following the bolus.[1] A 48-hour IV infusion test (80 units ACTH/24 hr) has also been suggested in order to test the time it takes for the adrenal to respond.[2] 17-Hydroxycorticosteroids (17-OHCS) are measured in 24-hour urine collections at baseline and after each 24 hours of infusion. The shorter test is sufficient for most diagnostic purposes.

If the patient is acutely ill, measurement of baseline serum cortisol should be performed, followed by IV administration of 4 mg of DEX. The urine collections should then begin together with the 48-hour ACTH infusion while the patient receives a maintenance dose of DEX. DEX does not interfere with the 17-OHCS measurements or the ACTH infusion.

Interpretation

After the rapid test, cortisol should increase above baseline by more than 7 μg/dL at 60 or 120 minutes or exceed 20 μg/dL.

If prolonged ACTH infusions are carried out, urinary 17-OHCS levels should be greater than 27 mg/24 hr after the first day and greater than 47 mg/24 hr after the second. Adrenal insufficiency should be diagnosed when urinary 17-OHCS levels are not greater than 4 mg/24 hr. If the adrenal is secondarily affected because of a defect in corticotropin-releasing factor (CRF) or ACTH secretion, 17-OHCS excretion will be in an intermediate range (4 to 10 mg/24 hr). Values significantly above 10 mg/24 hr are not diagnostic and require more intensive testing.

Side effects

Short-term studies cause no significant discomfort whatsoever. Prolonged ACTH infusions may result in some fluid retention.

Adrenal hyperfunction

Indications

An ACTH-stimulation test is indicated in a patient with an excess of adrenal androgen, when there is the possibility of an enzymatic defect such as congenital adrenal hyperplasia (CAH).

Procedure

For diagnosis of enzymatic defects resulting in adrenal hyperfunction, prior to ACTH stimulation, 1 mg of DEX is given at 11 PM the night before the test.[3] We and others have shown that the diagnostic sensitivity and reliability of the ACTH test are enhanced by the prior use of overnight DEX suppression. Blood is obtained at -15 and 0 minutes, followed by administration of an IV bolus of 0.25 mg of cosyntropin. Blood is then obtained for measurement of cortisol and 17-hydroxyprogesterone levels at $+30$ and $+60$ minutes. Other subtle enzymatic defects may also be uncovered by measuring blood levels of androstenedione, dehydroepiandrosterone (DHEA), DHEA sulfate (DHEA-S), and 17-hydroxypregnenolone. Samples at 120 minutes and 180 minutes post-ACTH are required if DHEA-S is measured, because the clearance of this steroid is extremely slow. 11-Deoxycortisol is measured only if the 17-hydroxyprogesterone response is elevated.

Food and activity do not affect the ACTH-stimulation test.

Interpretation

An increase in 17-hydroxyprogesterone of more than 20 ng/mL at either 30 or 60 minutes establishes the diagnosis of CAH (Figure 21-1).[3] For the diagnosis of 11β-hydroxylase deficiency, the

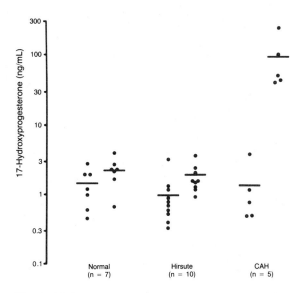

Figure 21-1
Serum 17-hydroxyprogesterone before and 60 minutes after the IV administration of a single bolus of 0.25 mg of ACTH to seven normal female controls and 10 hirsute oligomenorrheic women and to five patients with CAH.

Reproduced, with permission, from Lobo RA, Goebelsmann U: Adult manifestation of congenital adrenal hyperplasia due to incomplete 21-hydroxylase deficiency mimicking polycystic ovarian disease. Am J Obstet Gynecol 138:720, 1980.

11-deoxycortisol level should exceed 200 ng/dL 60 minutes after the administration of ACTH. Defects that are more subtle, such as deficiency of 3β-ol dehydrogenase, are uncovered by measuring other steroid intermediates such as androstenedione and DHEA. Pretreatment with DEX is imperative to establish an accurate diagnosis of adrenal hyperfunction.

Corticotropin-releasing factor (CRF)

CRF is a 41-amino-acid synthetic peptide that is not yet commercially available. Recently, CRF has been characterized by Vale,[4] and it has un-

dergone clinical testing for the evaluation of abnormalities in ACTH secretion such as occur in Cushing's syndrome.[5,6] Given as an IV bolus, 100 μg of CRF-41 (or a dose of 1 μg/kg) elicits an increase in ACTH and cortisol (Figure 21-2).[6] Plasma ACTH remains elevated fo 3 hours and has a biphasic curve because of the slow metabolic clearance rate of CRF. DEX abolishes the rise in cortisol after CRF administration. The use of CRF testing shows promise as an investigative tool for the diagnosis of abnormalities of the hypothalamic-pituitary-adrenal axis, and in the differential diagnosis of Cushing's syndrome. CRF appears to be very safe.

Dexamethasone (DEX) suppression test

Indications

As a single one-time overnight administration, DEX 1 mg given at 11 PM serves as a screening test for Cushing's syndrome and as an adjunct to ACTH testing. DEX pretreatment improves the diagnostic accuracy and sensitivity of ACTH testing for ruling out mild enzymatic blocks such as CAH. As a prolonged test (Liddle's),[7,8] it helps to differentiate a pituitary cause of Cushing's disease from an adrenal tumor. We do not advocate DEX suppression testing for the differential diagnosis of adrenal or ovarian androgen excess—as is sometimes advocated in the workup of hirsutism—because DEX can inhibit ovarian and gonadotropin secretion in addition to suppressing the adrenal.

Procedure

As a screen, 1 mg of DEX at 11 PM is followed by an 8 AM serum or plasma cortisol measurement. A baseline cortisol measurement is unnecessary.

For Liddle's test, 0.5 mg DEX every 6 hours for 48 hours is followed by 2 mg DEX every 6

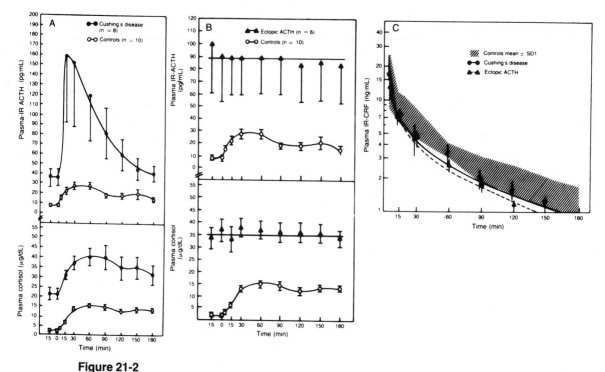

Figure 21-2

A and B. Responses of plasma immunoreactive (IR) ACTH and cortisol to corticotropin-releasing factor (mean ± SE) in eight untreated patients with Cushing's disease, six patients with Cushing's syndrome due to ectopic ACTH secretion, and 10 controls. C. Plasma disappearance curves for corticotropin-releasing factor (CRF) in eight untreated patients with Cushing's disease and six untreated patients with the ectopic ACTH syndrome. Here the normal curve (mean ± SD) is represented by the shaded area.

Reproduced, with permission, from Chrousos GP, Schulte HM, Oldfield EH, et al: The corticotropin-releasing factor stimulation test. N Engl J Med 310:622, 1984.

hours for 48 hours. Daily 24-hour urinary levels of 17-OHCS should be measured before and after DEX administration. Elevated urinary free cortisol measurements (normal: 20 to 90 μg/24 hr) have also proved useful in diagnosing adrenocortical hyperfunction.

Interpretation

As a screen, cortisol levels below 5 μg/dL effectively rule out Cushing's. If cortisol is greater than 5 μg/dL, this screening test is not diagnostic of Cushing's syndrome, and a Liddle suppression test is necessary. Stress itself, and altered DEX metabolism, may explain the lack of suppressibility. Cushing's may be ruled out using DEX suppression if a dose of 2 mg/day results in 17-OHCS levels less than 3 mg/24 hr or less than 50% of the basal 17-OHCS levels. Patients with Cushing's will fail to suppress on this dose (2 mg) but will suppress on 8 mg/day. On this higher dose, patients with Cushing's (ACTH-dependent adrenal hyperplasia) will show a 50% suppression of 17-OHCS, whereas patients with adrenal tumors will generally fail to suppress.

Severely stressed individuals and patients with psychological disturbances, but who otherwise have no endocrinopathy, may occasionally fail to suppress on 2 mg/day.

Abnormal endocrinology

Side effects

Short-duration administration of DEX, as used with both tests described above, is without marked side effects. Sodium retention effects are minimal.

Gonadotropin-releasing hormone (GnRH)

Indications

GnRH, as the synthetic decapeptide, is used to stimulate LH and FSH secretion. Although it was once thought that this simple test may differentiate between hypothalamic and pituitary defects in gonadotropin secretion, it has not proved to be of use in differentiating these disorders without prolonged GnRH priming. In hypogonadal states due to hypothalamic defects, GnRH priming of the pituitary is required for a normal response to be elicited if the initial test was abnormal. GnRH priming is accomplished by daily IM administration of 100 μg of GnRH for 1 week before testing. Using this approach, if the response remains abnormal, a rare patient may be found to have a true pituitary defect.

GnRH is useful in testing gonadotropic function after a known disease or injury[9-12] such as Sheehan's syndrome,[13] pituitary surgery, or irradiation.

In PCO patients, exaggerated responses of serum LH, but not of FSH, are found following the administration of GnRH. Postmenopausal women have exaggerated responses of both LH and FSH.

Although it was used in the past for such a purpose, GnRH testing cannot absolutely distinguish between physiological delay of puberty and a true gonadotropin-deficiency state. LH responses in these two disorders overlap.

Procedure

An IV 19- or 21-gauge Butterfly needle is used. At least two baseline samples are required 15 minutes apart before GnRH administration. Maximum responses have been found after 100 or 150 μg of IV GnRH. We administer 100 μg GnRH as an IV bolus over 30 seconds. Blood is usually obtained for LH and FSH measurement at +20, +30, +60, +90, and +120 minutes; however, in clinical practice, the +30- and +60-minute samples are all that are necessary.

Interpretation

Peak responses of LH after GnRH occur at +30 minutes. Peak FSH responses occur by 60 minutes. In normally ovulatory women, GnRH responses will vary according to the day of the menstrual cycle. Increased responses occur progressively toward midcycle.

Responses of normal women during the early follicular phase are a serum LH at 30 minutes of more than 20 mIU/mL and an FSH at 60 minutes of more than 5 mIU/mL. In Sheehan's syndrome, LH and FSH responses are absent (Figure 21-3).[13] In hypogonadal states, the FSH response is greater than that of LH—a response similar to that observed in puberty. Responses are not only affected by the day of the cycle but also by prior administration of estrogen or progesterone. An exaggerated response may be seen in hypothyroidism.

Side effects

Apart from vague, transient symptoms of nausea in a few patients, there are no immediate or long-term side effects from the administration of GnRH.

GnRH agonists

Although not available commercially, GnRH agonists have been used to down-regulate the secretion of pituitary gonadotropins.[14] Repeated daily subcutaneous injections will shut off gonadotropin secretion and, thereby, ovarian estrogen and androgen production. Adrenal steroid production does not appear to be affected. In this way, an ovarian source of hyperan-

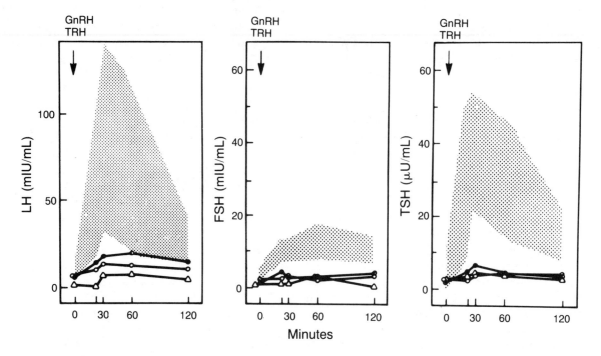

Figure 21-3
LH, FSH, and TSH responses to GnRH-TRH administration in the early follicular phase in control subjects (shaded area) and in three patients with Sheehan's syndrome.

Reproduced, with permission, from diZerega G, Kletzky OA, Mishell DR Jr: Diagnosis of Sheehan's syndrome using a sequential pituitary stimulation test. Am J Obstet Gynecol 132:348, 1978.

drogenism may be differentiated from an adrenal source (Figure 21-4).[14]

Insulin tolerance test (ITT)

Indications
The ITT remains one of the most valuable dynamic tests available for evaluating pituitary function. It is primarily useful for evaluation of growth hormone (GH) and ACTH or cortisol secretion. Combined with thyrotropin-releasing hormone (TRH) and GnRH, the sequential stimulation test[12] allows a more comprehensive testing of the pituitary such as that required to rule out Sheehan's syndrome (Figure 21-5).

Insulin induces hypoglycemia, the stress of which induces a hypothalamic response of growth hormone-releasing hormone (GH-RH) and CRF. These trigger the release of GH as well as of prolactin (PRL), β-endorphin (βEP), β-lipotropin (βLPH), and ACTH. The test, therefore, allows an evaluation of hypothalamic and pituitary function under stress. A cortisol response following hypoglycemia has been used to assess the adequacy of the pituitary-adrenal axis, although measurement of plasma ACTH is now being used more frequently.[15]

Procedure
After an overnight fast, regular insulin, 0.05 to 0.15 unit/kg of body weight, is infused over 1

Abnormal endocrinology

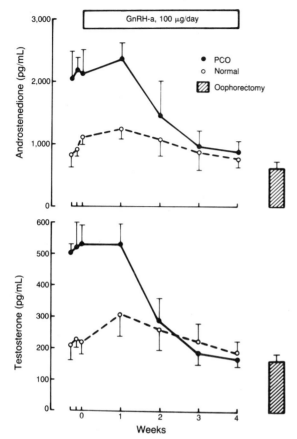

Figure 21-4
Mean serum androstenedione and testosterone concentrations in PCO and normal ovulatory subjects before and after GnRH agonist (GnRH-a) treatment and in oophorectomized women.

Reproduced, with permission, from Chang RJ, Laufer LR, Meldrum DR, et al: Steroid secretion in polycystic ovarian disease after ovarian suppression by a long-acting gonadotropin-releasing hormone agonist. J Clin Endocrinol Metab 56:897, 1983. © 1983, The Endocrine Society.

minute. Because a 50% reduction in glucose or a serum glucose lower than 40 mg/dL is necessary to evoke a stress response, we have used a dose of 0.15 unit/kg for the ITT without significant side effects. Blood is drawn at 20, 30, 45, 60, and 90 minutes after insulin administration, and glucose, GH, and ACTH or cortisol are measured.

A solution of 50% dextrose in water ($D_{50}W$) is required to be on hand to counteract severe hypoglycemic reactions. It is recommended that a physician stay with the patient at all times.

Interpretation

In a normal response, there is an increment in cortisol of 6 µg/dL above the baseline at 60 minutes. The level of GH should be 18 ng/mL above the baseline. ACTH, βEP, and βLPH responses are not as well standardized. The stimulatory response of opioid peptides is also of limited clinical usefulness.

While the finding of a blunted GH response is of limited diagnostic value in the adult, an evaluation of the ACTH-adrenal axis after hypoglycemia is extremely important, especially if GH and PRL responses are also blunted. Indeed, this test is the only sure way of evaluating adrenal response to stress. It has been shown that the response to hypoglycemia is superior to ACTH testing alone in detecting abnormal endogenous ACTH secretion (Figure 21-6).[16]

Side effects

Severe hypoglycemic reactions that may result in shock are to be avoided. An attendant physician should be ready to administer $D_{50}W$. Perspiration, light-headedness, thirst, and tachycardia may also occur.

Levodopa (L-dopa)

Indications

L-Dopa has been used to increase CNS dopamine and thereby decrease PRL and increase GH secretion.[17-20] Its lowering effect on PRL is of short duration and has not proved useful for the diagnosis of PRL-secreting pituitary adenomas, because of inconsistent results. However, L-dopa testing is helpful, taken together with such tests as the glucose tolerance test and argi-

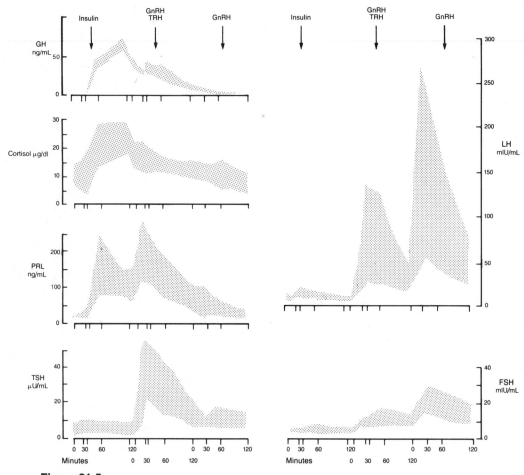

Figure 21-5
GH, cortisol, PRL, TSH, LH, and FSH responses to insulin, GnRH, and TRH. Normative data on this sequential stimulation test provided by data of Kletsky et al.

nine infusion studies, for diagnosis of abnormal GH secretion (e.g., acromegaly).

Procedure

L-Dopa, 500 mg, is given orally in the fasting state. Blood is obtained before and at 60 and 120 minutes after ingestion. The peak response occurs by 60 minutes. An indwelling catheter, left open with a heparin lock, can be used to diminish the number of venipunctures. If PRL responses are monitored, the test should be done after 8 AM, because before this time PRL is still undergoing its diurnal decline.

Interpretation

A normal PRL response is manifested by a decrement of 50% or more by 60 or 120 minutes. A normal GH response is manifested by an increment above baseline of at least 5 ng/mL and can be used to help rule out acromegaly (Figure 21-7). Deficient GH secretion may not be diagnosed on the basis of this test alone. Estrogen treatment enhances the GH response. Thus, an abnormal L-dopa test result in a hypoestrogenic patient should be repeated after 2 weeks of estrogen therapy.

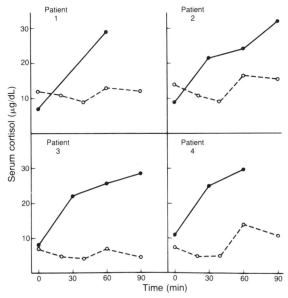

Figure 21-6
Responses of serum cortisol to injections of insulin (open circles) or ACTH (solid circles) in four patients with deficient ACTH secretion.

Reproduced, with permission, from Borst GC, Michenfelder HJ, O'Brian JT: Discordant cortisol response to exogenous ACTH and insulin-induced hypoglycemia in patients with pituitary disease. N Engl J Med 306:1462, 1982.

Side effects

Nausea and vomiting may occur in 30% to 40% of patients. There are no other major problems with this test, however.

Metoclopramide

Indications

Metoclopramide, a dopamine receptor antagonist, has been used to test central dopaminergic tone, specifically the ability of PRL to increase.[21,22] After its administration as an IV bolus to normal women, there is an increase of serum PRL only. There are no changes in serum LH or FSH (Figure 21-8).[21] It is potentially useful as a probe of dopaminergic function. It may help to diagnose a PRL-secreting pituitary adenoma by the finding of no increase in PRL in patients with tumor. However, the clinical usefulness of metoclopramide testing remains to be evaluated.

Procedure

Metoclopramide should be given as a 10-mg IV bolus, and both PRL and LH should be measured at − 15 and 0 minutes and at + 60, + 120, and + 180 minutes.

Interpretation

The PRL response after metoclopramide administration in normal cycling women varies, with greater responses occurring at midcycle than in the early follicular phase. In normal women, there is no LH or FSH response, but there is a PRL increment of 100 ng/mL by 60 or 120 minutes. In the hyperprolactinemic woman, the reverse occurs: an LH increment of 5 to 15 mIU/mL, and no increase in PRL. An increase in LH may also be noted in some patients with hypothalamic amenorrhea. While LH has been measured to assess the dopaminergic influence on LH secretion in amenorrheic patients, this is only a research protocol. Because the lack of PRL response in hyperprolactinemic patients with adenomas may not be absolute, metoclopramide testing is not being used at present in our management of hyperprolactinemia.

Side effects

There appear to be no particular problems with the use of metoclopramide. The drug has been marketed to increase gut motility.

Metyrapone

Indications

Metyrapone, which blocks 11β-hydroxylation, has been used to test ACTH release.[8,13,17,23] However, it tests only the steroid-suppressive

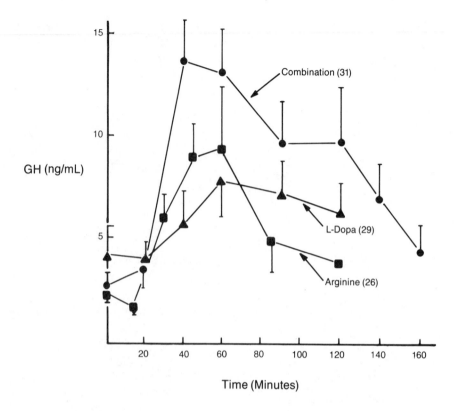

Figure 21-7
Changes in serum growth hormone (mean ± SE) after L-dopa and arginine.

Adapted from Weldon VV: J Pediatr 87:540, 1979.

control mechanism. ACTH may still be released in response to stress when metyrapone fails to produce a response. Metyrapone testing, therefore, is not as valuable as testing cortisol response with CRF, ITT, or ACTH. Metyrapone may result in falsely blunted responses in patients with thyroid disease, as well as in those taking oral contraceptives or phenytoin. A normal response is an increase in urinary 17-OHCS of 10 mg/24 hr or a doubling of the basal value. The increase in 11-deoxycortisol in serum or urine is a result of the block in 11β-hydroxylase activity. In serum, 11-deoxycortisol levels usually exceed 7 μg/dL after metyrapone.

Procedure

Baseline serum cortisol levels are measured at 8 AM and 4 PM, and at 8 AM the following day. Me-

Table 21-1
The metyrapone test

Day	Protocol
1	Control period; no medication; 24-hour urine collection for 17-hydroxycorticosteroids and 17-ketosteroids
2	Metyrapone 750 mg PO q4h × 6; 24-hour urine collection as above
3	No medication; 24-hour urine collection as above

tyrapone 750 mg is given orally after the second 8 AM blood sample is obtained. The same dose is administered every 4 hours for a total of 6 doses (Table 21-1). Urinary 17-OHCS are also measured before, during, and for 4 days after metyrapone.

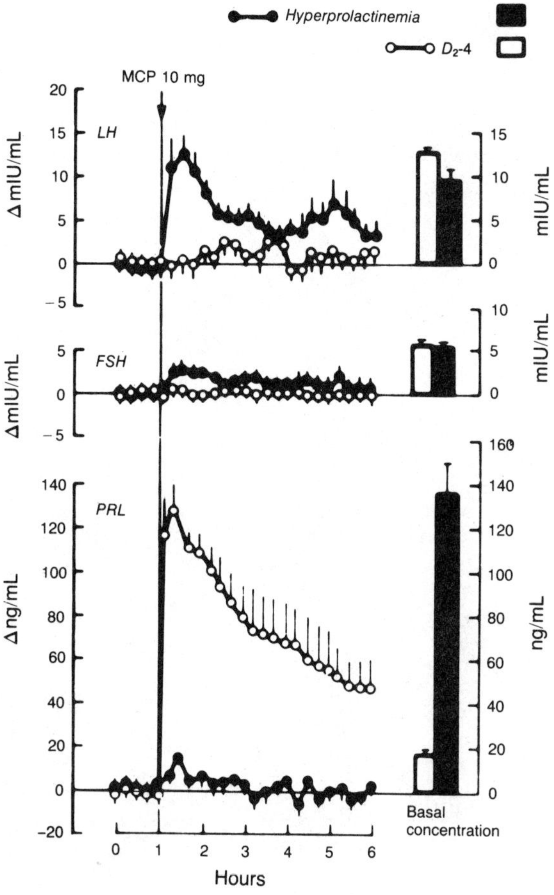

Figure 21-8

Mean (± SE) basal LH, FSH, and PRL levels (mean of five samples) and their Δ responses to IV bolus of 10 mg of metoclopramide (MCP) in five hyperprolactinemic patients with documented pituitary microadenoma and four cycling women on days 2 to 4 of their cycles.

Reproduced, with permission, from Quigley ME, Judd SJ, Gilliland GB, et al: Effects of a dopamine antagonist on the release of gonadotropin and prolactin in normal women and women with hyperprolactinemic anovulation. J Clin Endocrinol Metab 48:718, 1979. © 1979, The Endocrine Society.

tyrapone. An alternative method, which has been used effectively, is administration of a single oral dose of 3.5 g at 10 PM.

Interpretation

After metyrapone administration, the serum cortisol level should be less than 5 μg/dL, indicative of the 11β-hydroxylase blockade. The serum 11-deoxycortisol level (if measured) should rise (>7 μg/dL). A normal response is an increase in urinary 17-OHCS of 10 mg/24 hr or a doubling of the basal value. We do not regard metyrapone as a definitive test of ACTH response to stress.

Side effects

Nausea, as well as dizziness and abdominal discomfort, may occur.

Synthetic TRH (protirelin)

Indications

Protirelin (TRH), a synthetic tripeptide, is used for testing pituitary release of thyroid-stimulating hormone (TSH) and PRL.[24,25,26] The TRH-evoked TSH response is exaggerated in hypothyroid patients, and this serves as an extremely sensitive test for borderline primary hypothyroidism. In hyperthyroidism (Graves' disease), the TSH response is blunted. PRL is normally released after TRH, and a blunting of the normal response should make one suspect a PRL-secreting adenoma.

Procedure

An IV 19- or 21-gauge Butterfly needle is used. Synthetic TRH is administered (500 μg in 1 mL of normal saline) as an IV bolus over 30 seconds. Blood is obtained through the same line before (−30, −15 minutes) and after (+20, +30, +60 minutes) the bolus. TSH and PRL may both be measured. The peak responses for both hormones occur at $+20$ or $+30$ minutes. It is sufficient to obtain only one baseline sample, followed by another at 30 minutes. If desirable, GnRH may be administered simultaneously.

Interpretation

In a normal TSH response, the serum level of TSH at 30 minutes is at least 7 μU/mL and less than 28 μU/mL. However, an increase of at least 2 μU/mL should occur (Figure 21-9).[27] A normal PRL response is three times the basal level. The ingestion of thyroid hormone, corticoids, and tranquilizers may affect the TSH and PRL

responses after TRH. Endogenous depression may also blunt this response.

Side effects

A transient feeling of nausea frequently occurs. A feeling of warmth or flushing, an unusual taste in the mouth, or a slight urge to urinate may occur. These are all relatively mild symptoms. Transient hypertension may occur and may be relatively severe.[28] Baseline blood pressure should be measured in all patients, and if hypertension is marked, the test should not be performed.

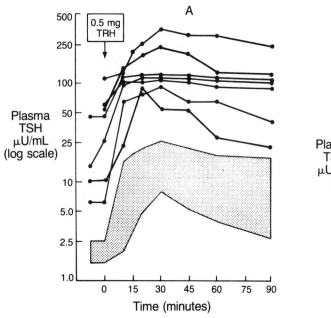
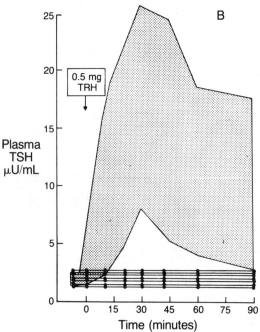

Figure 21-9
Plasma TSH responses to TRH in patients with primary hypothyroidism (A; note semilog scale) and with secondary hypothyroidism due to pituitary disease (B). Shaded areas represent normal ranges.

Reproduced, with permission, from Fleischer N, Lorente M, Kirkland J, et al: Synthetic thyrotropin releasing factor as a test of pituitary thyrotropin reserve. J Clin Endocrinol Metab 34:617, 1972. © 1972, The Endocrine Society.

Abnormal endocrinology

References

1. Melby JC: Assessment of adrenocortical function. *N Engl J Med* 285:735, 1971

2. Rose LI, Williams GH, Jagger PI, et al: The 48-hour adrenocorticotrophin infusion test for adrenocortical insufficiency. *Ann Intern Med* 73:49, 1970

3. Lobo RA, Goebelsmann U: Adult manifestation of congenital adrenal hyperplasia due to incomplete 21-hydroxylase deficiency mimicking polycystic ovarian disease. *Am J Obstet Gynecol* 138:720, 1980

4. Vale W, Spiess J, Rivier C, et al: Characterization of a 41-residue ovine hypothalamic peptide that stimulates secretion of corticotropin and β-endorphin. *Science* 213:1394, 1981

5. Lytras N, Grossman A, Perry L, et al: Corticotrophin releasing factor: Responses in normal subjects and patients with disorders of the hypothalamus and pituitary. *Clin Endocrinol* 20:71, 1984

6. Chrousos GP, Schulte HM, Oldfield EH, et al: The corticotropin-releasing factor stimulation test. *N Engl J Med* 310:622, 1984

7. Liddle GW: Tests of pituitary adrenal suppressibility in the diagnosis of Cushing's syndrome. *J Clin Endocrinol Metab* 20:1539, 1960

8. Liddle GW, Island D, Meador CK: Normal and abnormal regulation of corticotropin secretion in man. *Recent Prog Horm Res* 18:125, 1962

9. Rebar RW, Harman SM, Vaitukaitis JL: Differential responsiveness to LRF after estrogen therapy in women with hypothalamic amenorrhea. *J Clin Endocrinol Metab* 46:48, 1978

10. Rebar R, Yen SS, VandenBerg G, et al: Gonadotropin responses to synthetic LRF: Dose-response relationship in men. *J Clin Endocrinol Metab* 36:10, 1973

11. Yen SS, Rebar R, VandenBerg G, et al: Pituitary gonadotrophin responsiveness to synthetic LRF in subjects with normal and abnormal hypothalamic-pituitary-gonadal axis. *J Reprod Fertil* 20:137, 1973

12. Kletzky OA, Davajan V, Mishell DR Jr, et al: A sequential pituitary stimulation test in normal subjects and in patients with amenorrhea-galactorrhea with pituitary tumors. *J Clin Endocrinol Metab* 45:631, 1977

13. diZerega G, Kletzky OA, Mishell DR Jr: Diagnosis of Sheehan's syndrome using a sequential pituitary stimulation test. *Am J Obstet Gynecol* 132:348, 1978

14. Chang RJ, Laufer LR, Meldrum DR, et al: Steroid secretion in polycystic ovarian disease after ovarian suppression by a long-acting gonadotropin-releasing hormone agonist. *J Clin Endocrinol Metab* 56:897, 1983

15. Morente C, Kletzky OA: Pituitary response to insulin-induced hypoglycemia in patients with amenorrhea of different etiologies. *Am J Obstet Gynecol* 148:375, 1984

16. Borst GC, Michenfelder HJ, O'Brian JT: Discordant cortisol response to exogenous ACTH and insulin-induced hypoglycemia in patients with pituitary disease. *N Engl J Med* 306:1462, 1982

17. Eddy RL, Jones AL, Chakmakjian ZH, et al: Effect of levodopa (L-dopa) on human hypophyseal tropic hormone release. *J Clin Endocrinol Metab* 33:709, 1971

18. Eddy RL, Gilliland PF, Ibarra JD Jr, et al: Human growth hormone release: Comparison of provocative test procedures. *Am J Med* 56:179, 1974

19. Hayek A, Crawford JD: L-Dopa and pituitary hormone secretion. *J Clin Endocrinol Metab* 34:764, 1969

20. Lachelin GC, Leblanc H, Yen SS: The inhibitory effect of dopamine agonists on LH release in women. *J Clin Endocrinol Metab* 44:728, 1977

21. Quigley ME, Judd SJ, Gilliland GB, et al: Effects of a dopamine antagonist on the release of gonadotropin and prolactin in normal women and women with hyperprolactinemic anovulation. *J Clin Endocrinol Metab* 48:718, 1979

22. Quigley ME, Sheehan KL, Casper RF, et al: Evidence for increased dopaminergic and opioid activity in patients with hypothalamic hypogonadotropic amenorrhea. *J Clin Endocrinol Metab* 50:949, 1980

23. Keenan BS, Beitins IZ, Lee PA, et al: Estimation of ACTH reserve on normal and hypopituitary subjects: Comparison of oral and intravenous metyrapone with insulin hypoglycemia. *J Clin Endocrinol Metab* 37:540, 1973

24. Synder PJ, Utiger RD: Response to thyrotropin releasing hormone (TRH) in normal man. *J Clin Endocrinol Metab* 34:380, 1972

25. Marrs RP, Bertolli SJ, Kletzky OA: The use of thyrotropin-releasing hormone in distinguishing prolactin-secreting pituitary adenoma. *Am J Obstet Gynecol* 138:620, 1980

26. Hershman JM: Clinical application of thyrotropin-releasing hormone. *N Engl J Med* 290:886, 1974

27. Fleischer N, Lorente M, Kirkland J, et al: Synthetic thyrotropin releasing factor as a test of pituitary thyrotropin reserve. *J Clin Endocrinol Metab* 34:617, 1972

28. Borowski GD, Garofano CD, Rose LI, et al: Blood pressure response to thyrotropin releasing hormone in euthyroid subjects. *J Clin Endocrinol Metab* 58:197, 1984

Part III

Infertility

Chapter 22

Evaluation of the Infertile Couple

Val Davajan, M.D.
Daniel R. Mishell Jr., M.D.

The diagnosis of infertility is made when conception does not occur after 1 year of sexual exposure in a couple trying to achieve a pregnancy. The term "primary infertility" means that the couple has never achieved a pregnancy; "secondary infertility" implies that at least one previous conception has taken place. The term "sterility" should be used only if no therapy can correct the defect (for example, congenital absence of the uterus and ovaries, azoospermia).

Incidence of infertility

It has been estimated that 10% to 15% of all married couples in the US are infertile. Data obtained from the 1976 National Survey of Family Growth indicated that about 10% of all US couples in which the wives were aged 15 to 47 were infertile.[1] Although the exact incidence of infertility in the US among childless women of different ages is unknown, data from several sources indicate that fertility declines as a woman ages.

In 1982 Schwartz and Mayaux reported the incidence of pregnancy among 2,193 nulliparous French women who had azoospermic husbands and underwent artificial insemination at the Fédération CECOS.[2] Based on physical examinations and hysterosalpingography (HSG), all the women were presumed to be fertile. The percentage who conceived after 12 cycles of insemination declined after age 30 (Table 22-1).[2] It has been stated that the CECOS data may have overestimated the risk of infertility among childless women attempting to conceive at different ages, because of the reduced fertilizing capacity of frozen sperm and a possible unrepresentative sample of women. Nevertheless, the study excluded women who were infertile because of tubal blockage due to salpingitis as demonstrated by HSG. Since the chance of a woman developing salpingitis increases as she ages, the CECOS data may also underestimate the risks of infertility in the woman over 30.

Data obtained from the 1976 National Survey of Family Growth were used to calculate the percentage of currently married women aged 15 to 44 who would conceive during 12 months of unprotected intercourse. The pregnancy rates calculated (Table 22-2)[3] were very similar to the CECOS data, except for the 20- to 24-year age group. Studies of fertility rates in populations of women who do not practice contraception also reveal a substantial decline in fertility after age 30, with a greater decline after age 35.[4]

Table 22-1
Rates for success, loss to follow-up,
and dropping out, according to age group

Rate	Percentage			
	≤ 25 yr	26–30 yr	31–35 yr	> 35 yr (36–40)
Mean rate per cycle				
Successes	11.0	10.5	9.1	6.5 (6.5)
Losses to follow-up	2.8	2.5	2.4	2.4
Dropouts	4.0	4.0	4.7	4.9
Cumulative success rate after 12 cycles	73.0	74.1	61.5	53.6 (55.8)

From Schwartz D, Mayaux MJ: Female fecundity as a function of age: Results of artificial insemination in 2193 nulliparous women with azoospermic husbands. Fédération des Centres d'Etude et de Conservation du Sperme Humain. N Engl J Med 306:404, 1982.

Data from all these sources indicate that postponing childbearing until age 30 increases the chance that a woman will have difficulty in conceiving and that this problem will increase after age 35. As more women elect to postpone childbearing until after age 30, for financial reasons or to satisfy career goals, they must be made aware that this delay may increase the chance that they will have a problem with infertility.

Factors in infertility

The exact incidence of factors accounting for infertility varies among different populations and cannot be precisely determined. In general, however, 10% to 15% of infertility is due to failure of ovulation; 30% to 40% of infertility has been attributed to endometriosis, pelvic adhesions, or tubal disease (pelvic factor); about 30% to 40% of infertility is associated with such problems in the male reproductive system as oligoazoospermia, high viscosity of semen, low sperm motility, and low volume of semen (male factor); and an additional 10% to 15% of infertility is associated with abnormal sperm-cervical mucus penetration (cervical factor). At our medical center, about 5% of infertility is due to such uncommon causes as hypothyroidism, an immu-

nologic factor, inadequate luteal phase, or subclinical genital infections. With our current techniques, it is impossible to diagnose the cause of infertility in about 10% of couples.

Diagnosis

Initial evaluation

The diagnostic evaluation of infertility should be thorough and completed as rapidly as possible. At the initial interview, all the tests available and the reasons they are performed should be explained to patients. The available therapies and the prognosis for the various factors of in-

Table 22-2
Expected percentages of nonsterile
currently married women
who will conceive in 12 months
of unprotected intercourse

Age group	Conceiving in 12 months (%)
20–24	86
25–29	78
30–34	63
35–39	52

From Hendershot GE, Mosher WD, Pratt WF: Infertility and age: An unresolved issue. Fam Plan Perspect 14:287, 1982.

fertility should also be discussed. The patients should know that after a complete diagnostic infertility evaluation, in about 10% of cases the etiology for the infertility still cannot be defined. However, they should also be told that only a few years ago this was true for 30% of infertile couples. If medical science continues to advance, it may soon be possible to determine the cause of all infertility. Patients should be assured that as new diagnostic tests are developed, it is the physician's responsibility to make the new advances available.

Lab tests

All patients should have a complete history and physical examination. The initial laboratory tests should include a complete blood count, urine analysis, Pap smear, and a fasting blood glucose test. Measuring thyroid-stimulating hormone (TSH) and prolactin (PRL) at the initial visit is not cost effective. These tests are usually normal and should be delayed. Each couple should be instructed as to the optimum time for conception and should be encouraged to have frequent intercourse.

The most likely time for conception, as shown by correlation of a single successful artificial insemination with basal body temperature (BBT), is on the day before the rise of the BBT (Figure 22-1).[5] Data from the same study indicated that having intercourse more than 1 day after the luteal rise in BBT will not result in fer-

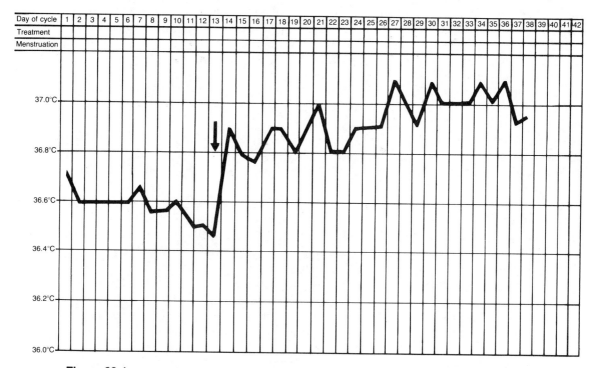

Figure 22-1
Pregnancy chart showing insemination (arrow) timed to fall on the day before the expected steep rise in the BBT.

From Newill RG, Katz M: The basal body temperature chart in artificial insemination by donor pregnancy cycles. Fertil Steril 38:431, 1982. Reproduced with permission of the publisher, The American Fertility Society.

Evaluation of the infertile couple

Table 22-3
Phase of cycle for performing tests

Test	Phase
Hysterosalpingogram ⎫ Laparoscopy ⎬ Hysteroscopy ⎭	Early follicular phase (postmenstrual)
Postcoital test	Preovulatory (before BBT shift)
Serum progesterone determination	Midluteal phase
Endometrial biopsy	Late luteal phase (premenstrual)

tilization. The couple should be instructed to have intercourse every other day throughout the midcycle, beginning soon after cessation of menses. Unless the husband has oligospermia, daily intercourse for 3 consecutive days at the exact midcycle should be encouraged. In some instances, women produce less than adequate amounts of vaginal lubricant. Some of the chemical lubricants used to improve coital satisfaction may interfere with sperm transport. Some men experience midcycle impotence because of the pressure of "command performance." In such cases, the intercourse schedule should be less rigorous. The couple should also be told that among fertile couples, there is only a 25% chance of conceiving in each ovulatory cycle.

The workup

The primary diagnostic steps to be followed in the workup of the infertile couple include: (1) documentation of ovulation (presumptive) by measurement of BBT or midluteal phase serum progesterone*; (2) semen analysis; (3) fractional postcoital test; (4) HSG; and (5) laparoscopy. These are performed in the order given above and at the specific times of the cycle shown in Table 22-3. This initial infertility evaluation

*Although only 3 to 5 ng/mL of progesterone has been reported to be indicative of ovulation, it has recently been reported in several studies that a level of at least 10 ng/mL of progesterone is found in the luteal phases of cycles during which conception occurred.[6]

should be performed within 2 to 3 months and not prolonged unnecessarily.

If an abnormality is found in one of the first (noninvasive) steps, that abnormality should be treated before proceeding with the more costly and invasive procedures. For example, if the woman has oligomenorrhea and does not ovulate each month, following a semen analysis, ovulation should be induced with clomiphene citrate before performing the other diagnostic measures. We have found that, provided they have no other infertility factors, most of the women (80% to 90%) with anovulation conceive following treatment that induces ovulation, and conception usually occurs during the first three ovulatory cycles. The prognosis for conception with the other causes of infertility varies, but is usually 20% to 40%.

Women with regular menses should record their BBT daily, at least through the cycle in which the postcoital test is performed. Although presumptive evidence of ovulation can also be established with a serum progesterone level or an endometrial biopsy, the BBT is less costly and has the added advantage of demonstrating the approximate time of ovulation. This information can then be used to instruct the couple about the optimal time for intercourse. A semen analysis should be performed concomitantly.

A postcoital test is the next step, and it should be scheduled for approximately 1 to 2 days before the expected rise in BBT. More recently, using serial ultrasonography and urine LH determinations, we have found that ovulation occurs most often after the BBT shift, usually during the upswing of the rise in temperature. This finding may indicate that sperm must be present in the fallopian tubes before ovulation. If all these tests are normal, an HSG should be done in the follicular phase of the next cycle. If only intrauterine lesions are demonstrated on the HSG, these should be treated with the use of a hysteroscope. If the HSG is normal, a laparoscopy should be performed in the follicular phase of a subsequent cycle. At least 3 months should elapse between HSG and laparoscopy, because an occasional patient does conceive following the HSG. It is unnecessary and inadvisable to perform a routine D&C at the time of laparoscopy. A concomitant hysteroscopy is necessary only if some type of uterine cavity defect has been observed on the previously obtained HSG.

Additional tests

If all the tests described so far are normal, the following additional laboratory procedures should be performed to try to establish the etiology of the infertility: (6) immunologic tests; (7) bacteriology (cultures of the cervical mucus and semen, including cultures for *Ureaplasma urealyticum*); (8) TSH and PRL; (9) a late luteal phase endometrial biopsy; and (10) a hamster egg penetration test.

If abnormalities are discovered in the initial five steps of the infertility evaluation, treatment should significantly increase the incidence of pregnancy, particularly if anovulation or total tubal obstruction are the etiologic factors. Treatment of abnormalities found in the last five diagnostic steps has not been documented to be more effective than withholding therapy. In a study of 47 couples whose infertility remained unsolved following laparoscopy (see below), no further treatment or investigation was per-

formed, and 65% conceived.[7] Thus, it must be demonstrated that treatment of abnormalities diagnosed in the last five steps results in a significantly better pregnancy rate than placebo or no treatment for the particular treatment to be considered beneficial. To date, no such studies have been performed.

Success rates

All infertile couples should be informed of the prognosis for curing their particular cause of infertility. Among 493 infertile couples who were followed up for 1 to 2 years, the chances of becoming pregnant were greater in women younger than 30 (52%) than in women older than 30 (37%).[8] In the same study, the success rate was higher in couples who had tried to conceive for less than 3 years prior to evaluation (63%) than in those who had tried for more than 3 years (34%). Of the patients who conceived, 90% of the pregnancies occurred within 1 year of the initial visit, and 96% before the second year. Thus, if a patient does not conceive within 2 years of her initial infertility evaluation, her chances of becoming pregnant are poor.

In the study mentioned above,[7] which followed 47 infertile couples with still-unexplained infertility after laparoscopy, the women had documented ovulation, and the husbands had normal semen analyses. Using life table techniques, it was found that the cumulative pregnancy rate for this population with undiagnosed and untreated infertility was 65% (Figure 22-2).[7] Of those pregnancies, 81% went to term. Expectation of pregnancy fell from 65% at the time of laparoscopy to 31% 12 months later and to 12% 2 years later. No pregnancies occurred after 30 months (Figure 22-3).[7] This study indicates that couples infertile for no apparent cause have a good chance of conception for about 2 years after laparoscopy, but a poor chance thereafter.

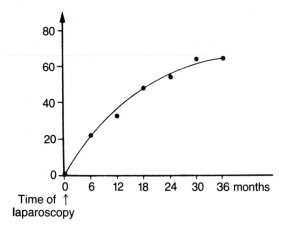

Figure 22-2
Cumulative pregnancy rate of all patients in the study population from the day of laparoscopy.

From Rousseau S, Lord J, Lepage Y, et al: The expectancy of pregnancy for "normal" infertile couples. Fertil Steril 40:768, 1983. Reproduced with permission of the publisher, The American Fertility Society.

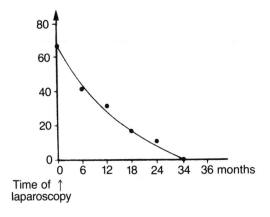

Figure 22-3
Expectation of pregnancy in the study population following laparoscopy.

From Rousseau S, Lord J, Lepage Y, et al: The expectancy of pregnancy for "normal" infertile couples. Fertil Steril 40:768, 1983. Reproduced with permission of the publisher, The American Fertility Society.

Spontaneous conception

Almost 120 years ago, Matthews Duncan of Edinburgh wrote: "a reputation for curing sterility is spoken of as if it were founded on substantial claims; . . . a coincidence has been regarded as a consequence." In a study published in 1969, 35% of 1,415 infertile patients conceived spontaneously without treatment, a finding similar to that reported in other series. In the same study, 7% of patients conceived after the initial interview and sperm count. An additional 4% conceived after the vaginal examination, where a cervical plug was removed; 17% of the conceptions occurred following the performance of a tubal patency test.

More recently, 2- to 7-year follow-up of 1,145 infertile couples showed that 246 (41%) pregnancies occurred in 597 couples treated for infertility; whereas 191 (35%) pregnancies occurred in a group of 548 untreated couples.[9] However, 75 (31%) of the 246 pregnancies in

the treated group occurred at least 3 months after the last medical treatment, or more than 12 months after adnexal surgery. Combining these 75 pregnancies with the 191 that occurred without any treatment, 61% of all the pregnancies occurred independently of treatment. Overall, 266 (23%) of the 1,145 infertile couples had a treatment-independent pregnancy. Thus, the chance that a spontaneous pregnancy will occur in an infertile couple is relatively high, and studies using untreated control groups, where ethically acceptable, must be done to evaluate all treatment modalities, especially those used to treat cervical factors, endometriosis, partial tubal disease, and moderate sperm defects. The study cited above[9] reported that more than 50% of the pregnancies in couples with those diagnoses occurred without treatment. In contrast, couples with anovulation and total tubal occlusion had higher fertility rates in the treated group. Nevertheless, until such controlled studies are performed, we recommend treatment for all women with infertility.

Other options

Finally, considerable confusion has existed in the past as to whether adoption increases the probability of pregnancy in infertile couples. Although studies have been published reporting a positive effect of adoption on subsequent fertility, these reports have been criticized because of the methods used for selecting the couples in the adopting and nonadopting groups. In a well-controlled study of 438 infertile couples, the pregnancy rates for the adopting and nonadopting couples were not significantly different (16.2% vs 18.2%).[10] Therefore, we believe that patients should be informed that adoption has not been proven beneficial in achieving a successful pregnancy.

In the following chapters, all the etiologies of infertility, the available tests, treatments, and prognoses will be discussed in detail. It is hoped that when the technique of in vitro fertilization becomes generally available, the prognosis for many infertile couples will be greatly improved.

References

1. Mosher WD: Infertility trends among U.S. couples: 1965-1976. *Fam Plan Perspect* 14:22, 1982

2. Schwartz D, Mayaux MJ: Female fecundity as a function of age: Results of artificial insemination in 2193 nulliparous women with azoospermic husbands. Fédération des Centres d'Etude et de Conservation du Sperme Humain. *N Engl J Med* 306:404, 1982

3. Hendershot GE, Mosher WD, Pratt WF: Infertility and age: An unresolved issue. *Fam Plan Perspect* 14:287, 1982

4. Tietze C: Reproductive span and rate of reproduction among Hutterite women. *Fertil Steril* 8:89, 1957

5. Newill RG, Katz M: The basal body temperature chart in artificial insemination by donor pregnancy cycles. *Fertil Steril* 38:431, 1982

6. Hull MGR, Savage PE, Bromham DR, et al: The value of a single serum progesterone measurement in the midluteal phase as a criterion of a potentially fertile cycle ("ovulation") derived from treated and untreated conception cycles. *Fertil Steril* 37:355, 1982

7. Rousseau S, Lord J, Lepage Y, et al: The expectancy of pregnancy for "normal" infertile couples. *Fertil Steril* 40:768, 1983

8. Kliger BE: Evaluation, therapy, and outcome in 493 infertile couples. *Fertil Steril* 41:40, 1982

9. Collins JA, Wrixon W, Janes LB, et al: Treatment-independent pregnancy among infertile couples. *N Engl J Med* 309:1201, 1983

10. Weir WC, Weir DR: Adoption and subsequent conceptions. *Fertil Steril* 17:283, 1966

Suggested reading

Seibel MM, Taymor ML: Emotional aspects of infertility. *Fertil Steril* 37:137, 1982

Vessey MP, Wright NH, McPherson K, et al: Fertility after stopping different methods of contraception. *Br Med J* 1:265, 1978

Chapter 23

Induction of Ovulation

Charles M. March, M.D.
Daniel R. Mishell Jr., M.D.

In the past, ovulation induction with pharmacologic agents has been restricted mainly to women with oligomenorrhea or those with amenorrhea without ovarian failure. More recently, these drugs have been used effectively to treat women with luteal phase defects, as well as to induce development of large numbers of follicles to facilitate recovery of multiple oocytes for in vitro fertilization and even to provide empiric therapy for unexplained infertility. This last indication must be considered investigational. In patients with oligomenorrhea, defined as menses occurring at intervals of more than 35 days, it is not important to determine whether the cycles are ovulatory or not. Ovulation should be induced monthly to increase the chance of conception. During any ovulatory cycle, the chance of conception is only 25%. Thus, all oligomenorrheic women who wish to conceive should be treated whether or not they occasionally ovulate spontaneously. Patients with primary or secondary amenorrhea and polycystic ovary (PCO) disease, hypothalamic-pituitary dysfunction, or hypothalamic-pituitary failure and who desire pregnancy should also be treated.

Clomiphene citrate

Pharmacology and physiology

The pharmacologic agent of choice for the induction of ovulation in most patients is clomiphene citrate (Clomid, Serophene), a synthetic weak estrogen with three benzene rings, available as 50-mg scored tablets. At present, there is no evidence that administration of clomiphene citrate to the infertile woman with normal ovulatory menstrual cycles increases the incidence of conception. Therefore, its use for such women is not advised. The use of clomiphene citrate obviates the need for surgical wedge resection of the ovary to induce ovulation in patients with PCO. And because clomiphene citrate is both safer and more effective than corticosteroids for ovulation induction, corticosteroid therapy should be limited to patients with either some form of congenital adrenal hyperplasia or adrenal androgen hyperfunction.

Clomiphene citrate acts by competing with endogenous circulating estrogens for estrogen-binding sites in the hypothalamus. Therefore, it blocks the normal negative feedback of the endogenous estrogens and permits release of gonadotropin-releasing hormone (GnRH). This hormone stimulates follicle-stimulating hormone (FSH) and luteinizing hormone (LH) release, with resultant oocyte maturation and an associated increase in estradiol (E_2) production. Clomiphene citrate is usually given daily for 5 consecutive days, beginning 5 days after a spontaneous menses or progesterone-induced withdrawal bleeding. While the drug is being administered, serum levels of FSH, LH, and E_2 rise (Figure 23-1). The rise in FSH causes follicular

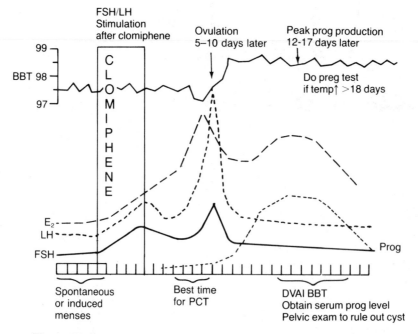

Figure 23-1
LH, FSH, estradiol (E$_2$), and progesterone (prog) levels before, during, and after
successful treatment with clomiphene citrate.

recruitment. When the drug is stopped, E$_2$ secretion continues and the rising endogenous E$_2$ levels produce a negative feedback action on the hypothalamic release of GnRH. This decreases gonadotropin output, and serum levels of FSH and LH fall. The patterns of hormone levels at this time are similar to those of the late follicular phase of the normal cycle. The exponential rise in the E$_2$ produced by the dominant follicle eventually has a positive feedback effect on the hypothalamus. GnRH release stimulates a surge of gonadotropin output, which, in turn, induces ovulation and follicular luteinization similar to that in the normal cycle.

Documentation of ovulation

Ovulation usually occurs within 5 to 9 days (mean, 7 days) after the last clomiphene tablet is taken. The time may vary in certain women and may be less than 5 or more than 9 days. There-

fore, it is best if women treated with this agent take their basal body temperatures (BBT) daily to provide a record of the approximate time of ovulation, as well as to document the fact that ovulation has occurred. Once ovulation occurs, menstruation takes place approximately 2 weeks later; that is, about 3 weeks after ingestion of the last tablet. In some instances, withdrawal bleeding will occur without being preceded by ovulation, because the increased E$_2$ production itself can induce endometrial growth. If ovulation does not occur, E$_2$ levels will eventually fall and withdrawal bleeding may take place. Thus, it is important to document by some indirect method that ovulation has occurred in each cycle.

Sustained elevation of BBT or a rise in serum progesterone concentration or pregnanediol excretion provides presumptive evidence of ovulation. Although BBT measurement is less expensive than a laboratory assay, it may be difficult or inconvenient for some women to take their temperatures daily throughout the cycle. If this is the case, the patient should be instructed to start taking her BBT on the day following ingestion of the last clomiphene tablet and to continue until the temperature shifts and the rise is sustained for 2 days. This mini-series of BBT determinations of 7 to 12 days provides the information necessary to document the occurrence as well as the time of ovulation.

If even these determinations cannot be carried out, a single serum progesterone level documents ovulation. A level of more than 3 ng/mL correlates well with the finding of secretory endometrium on an endometrial biopsy specimen, but is not necessarily diagnostic of ovulation, as the follicle may become luteinized without releasing an ovum. The progesterone measurement must be obtained between 4 and 11 days before the onset of the next menses, because the levels fall below 3 ng/mL 4 days before menses begin.[1] To coincide with the time when the serum progesterone is most likely to be elevated, the sample should be obtained about 2 weeks after the last clomiphene tablet. If the serum sample is obtained at the time of peak progesterone production, approximately 1 week after ovulation, it will usually exceed 15 ng/mL (Figure 23-2).[2] Levels of E_2 and progesterone are higher in clomiphene- or gonadotropin-stimulated cycles than after spontaneous ovulation, because multiple follicles mature and are luteinized. Patients who conceive without ovulation-inducing drugs have progesterone levels greater than 10 ng/mL; those who conceive after treatment with clomiphene or human menopausal gonadotropins (hMG) have progesterone levels exceeding 15 ng/mL—and a level of this magnitude is needed to provide presumptive evidence of ovulation.

Results of treatment

By 1965, complete case reports had been received on approximately 4,000 of the women who had been treated with clomiphene citrate in varying dosages and for varying time periods,

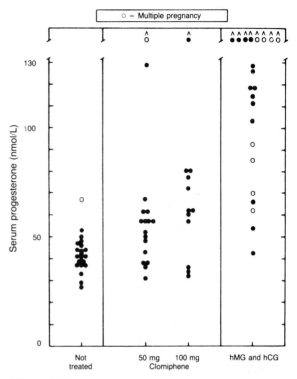

Figure 23-2
Midluteal serum progesterone concentration in conception cycles after treatment with clomiphene, in two different daily doses, or with gonadotropins, compared with untreated conception cycles. 1 ng/mL = 3.18 nmol/L.

From Hull MGR, Savage PE, Bromham DR, et al: The value of a single serum progesterone measurement in the midluteal phase as a criterion of a potentially fertile cycle ("ovulation") derived from treated and untreated conception cycles. Fertil Steril 37:355, 1982. Reproduced with permission of the publisher, The American Fertility Society.

many of which were greater than those used currently. Analysis of these premarketing studies revealed that the overall incidence of ovulation following treatment was about 72%, and the pregnancy rate was about 32%. The incidence of ovulation and pregnancy was found to be greater in women with oligomenorrhea than in those with amenorrhea. The incidence of ovulation (76% to 78%) and of pregnancy (33% to 34%) was similar to the overall incidence in patients with PCO and post-oral-contraceptive amenorrhea. Clomiphene citrate was not effective in patients who did not have a functioning hypothalamic-pituitary-ovarian axis.

The results of 2,369 pregnancies in which conception occurred after administration of clomiphene citrate were analyzed before the drug was marketed. Of these pregnancies, 19.2% were aborted spontaneously, 1.0% were stillbirths, and 1.2% were ectopic (Table 23-1). The incidence of these events was similar to the incidence in pregnancies occurring after spontaneous ovulation in other series of infertility patients. Of the 1,862 live births, 1,697 (91.1%) were singletons, and the neonatal death rate in this group was 1.9%. There were 165 (8.9%) multiple live births, with a neonatal death rate of 16.8%. This death rate is relatively low and reflects the predominance of twins who were carried to relatively late gestation. Of all the 2,369 pregnancies, 2,183 (92.1%) were single and 186 (7.9%) were multiple, with a distribution as follows: 6.9% twins, 0.5% triplets, 0.3% quadruplets, and 0.1% quintuplets.

The incidence of birth defects in infants born following clomiphene treatment is no greater than in the general population. Of these 2,369 pregnancies, 58 babies were born with congenital anomalies, for an overall incidence of 2.4% (Table 23-2). These anomalies were of

Table 23-1
Outcome after maternal treatment with clomiphene citrate (2,369 pregnancies)

Outcome of pregnancy	No. of cases	Percentage
All pregnancies (2,369)		
Abortions	455	19.2
Ectopics	28	1.2
Stillbirths	25	1.0
Total live births (1,862)		
Single live births	1,697	91.1
Neonatal deaths	33	1.9
Multiple live births	165*	8.9
Neonatal deaths	60/357†	16.8

*Number of pregnancies.   †Number of infants.

Data from Physician's Brochure for Clomiphene Citrate. Cincinnati, Merrell-National Laboratories.

Table 23-2
Birth defects following maternal treatment with clomiphene citrate (2,369 pregnancies)

Outcome of pregnancy	No. of patients	Percentage
Abortions/stillbirths	5*	0.8
Multiple gestations	14	3.9
Single gestations	39	2.3
Total	58	2.4

Data from Physician's Brochure for Clomiphene Citrate. Cincinnati, Merrell-National Laboratories.

*Includes aborted conjoined twins with anomalies.

many types, the majority being congenital heart defects, Down's syndrome, and anomalies of the skeleton and gastrointestinal tract. More recent studies have indicated that the risk of congenital anomalies does not increase as the dose of clomiphene is increased.[3]

When high doses of clomiphene, the equivalent of several times the human dose, were given to pregnant laboratory animals during the period of organogenesis, there was an increased incidence of congenital anomalies. Of a group of 158 women who had received clomiphene during the first 6 weeks following conception, eight (5.1%) had infants with congenital anomalies. This figure is higher, but not significantly, than the incidence of birth defects following spontaneous conception. At present, there is no evidence to indicate that clomiphene is teratogenic in humans. Thus, abortion is not recommended if a woman inadvertently ingests clomiphene during early pregnancy. However, because of the increased incidence of anomalies found in animal studies, care should be taken to avoid such use. It is important to document the occurrence of a normal menstrual period and decline in BBT to rule out pregnancy before each course of drug therapy. A pelvic examination should also be performed before each course of therapy to be certain there is neither uterine nor ovarian enlargement.

In the entire premarketing trials during which 8,029 anovulatory patients were treated with clomiphene citrate in various dosages and for varying durations, ovarian enlargement occurred in 13.6%, vasomotor symptoms in 10.4%, abdominal discomfort in 5.5%, and visual symptoms, mainly blurring, in 1.5%. An urticarial rash occurred in 0.6% and slight hair loss in 0.3%. It was found that the incidence of ovulation and pregnancy per cycle was similar with dosage regimens of either 50 or 100 mg/day for 5 days. The incidence of ovarian enlargement was likewise similar with these two dosages.[4] When a dosage of less than 50 mg/day for 5 days was administered, the incidence of ovulation and pregnancy per treatment course diminished; whereas with dosages greater than 100 mg/day, the incidence of ovarian enlargement increased. For these reasons, it was recommended in the physicians' brochure that only two dosages be used: either 50 mg or 100 mg/day for 5 days beginning 5 days after the onset of spontaneous menses or induced withdrawal bleeding. Furthermore, the brochure recommends that the drug be administered for only three cycles; if the patient does not conceive after three cycles, further treatment is not recommended.

Sequential graduated dosage regimen

For many years in our clinic, clomiphene citrate has been administered for more than three cycles. Patients cannot conceive if they do not ovulate, and most of these patients will not ovulate without ovulation-inducing drug treatment. Certain patients are also treated with higher than recommended dosage. Before instituting therapy with clomiphene, a semen analysis is obtained to rule out a concomitant male cause of infertility. No other laboratory investigations are needed in the patient who has oligomenorrhea without galactorrhea. All anovulatory patients who have galactorrhea should be evaluated to rule out the presence of a pituitary adenoma before receiving ovulatory drugs.

All women who have primary or secondary amenorrhea should receive an injection of 100 mg of progesterone in oil before treatment with clomiphene. If withdrawal bleeding occurs, fur-

ther investigation is not necessary before treatment. If the patient fails to have withdrawal bleeding, a serum FSH level should be obtained. Those women without withdrawal bleeding, who have low or normal FSH levels, have hypothalamic-pituitary failure and further diagnostic studies should be obtained. A markedly elevated serum FSH level, more than 40 mIU/mL, correlates well with the absence of ovarian follicles. Patients with an elevated FSH have premature ovarian failure and should not be treated with ovulation-inducing drugs because they will not respond to therapy.

We use and advocate a sequential graduated dosage regimen, starting with an initial dose of 50 mg/day for 5 days.[5] Treatment is begun on the fifth day of a spontaneous or induced menstrual period. If ovulation occurs, but the patient does not conceive, this dose is continued in subsequent cycles. If conception fails to occur after three ovulatory cycles, further infertility evaluation is initiated. If the patient does not ovulate following treatment with this dose, 100 mg/day for 5 days is prescribed. If ovulation occurs, this dose is maintained. Otherwise, the dosage is sequentially increased to 150 mg, then 200 mg, and finally 250 mg/day for 5 days.

If, following any of these dosages, ovulation is induced, the patient is maintained on her individualized ovulatory dosage. We have not seen a difference in response if the daily medication is taken in one dose or in divided doses. If 250 mg/day does not cause ovulation, it is repeated in the next cycle and followed approximately 1 week later by 5,000 IU of human chorionic gonadotropin (hCG) to possibly increase the chances of inducing ovulation by simulating the LH surge. If hCG is given, the day of administration is determined by following a rise in the patient's cervical score, an indirect index of the rising E_2 levels that accompany follicular maturity, or by ovarian ultrasound.[6] The hCG should be administered when the cervical score is 8 and/or when one follicle is at least 20 mm in diameter. Evidence of ovulation should be obtained in

Table 23-3
Response to clomiphene citrate

Category	Total	Ovulated		Conceived	
		No.	%	No.	%
Oligomenorrhea	330	307	93.0	157	51.1
Amenorrhea					
Polycystic ovary disease	29	18	62.1	12	66.7
Hypothalamic-pituitary dysfunction	39	30	76.9	9	30.0
Hypothalamic-pituitary failure	10	0	0	0	0
Amenorrhea/galactorrhea					
Prog (+)*	10	9	90	5	55.6
Prog (−)†	10	1	10	0	0
All amenorrheic patients	98	58	59.1	26	44.8
Total	428	365	85.3	183	50.1

*Prog (+), withdrawal bleeding after IM progesterone.

†Prog (−), no progesterone-induced uterine bleeding.

Adapted from Gysler M, March CM, Mishell DR Jr, et al: A decade's experience with an individualized clomiphene treatment regimen including its effect on the post-coital test. Fertil Steril 37:161, 1982. Reproduced with permission of the publisher, The American Fertility Society.

every treatment cycle by either a biphasic BBT curve or midluteal rise in the serum progesterone concentration. The presence of menstrual bleeding a few weeks after clomiphene treatment is not presumptive evidence of ovulation, because this bleeding may result from falling estrogen levels without ovulation.

Experience at LAC/USC Medical Center

We analyzed our experience with this treatment regimen from May 1970 to May 1980.[5] During this time, more than 5,000 new patients were seen in the infertility clinic at LAC/USC Medical Center. Of these, 863 had oligomenorrhea or amenorrhea and 753 of these were treated with clomiphene citrate. It was possible to perform adequate follow-up, consisting of treatment for three or more ovulatory cycles, a fractional post-coital test, hysterosalpingography (HSG), and laparoscopy and semen analysis of the partners for 428 of these 753 women. All tests, except the semen analyses, were delayed until three ovulatory cycles were achieved. Of these 428, 330 had oligomenorrhea, and 98 had amenorrhea. The overall incidence of ovulation was 85.3% and of pregnancy was 50.1% (Table 23-3).[5] The incidence of ovulation was highest among those who had oligomenorrhea and extremely low among estrogen-deficient amenorrheic women.

Treatment plan

Slightly more than half of the 365 patients who eventually ovulated did so when treated with the 50-mg dose, and an additional 22% ovulated with the 100-mg dose (Table 23-4).[5] A total of 74% of the patients who ovulated did so following the recommended 50- or 100-mg dosage regimen. Of the patients who conceived, almost 74% did so following treatment with these dosages. Thus, about 26% of both patients who ovulated and patients who conceived following treatment with clomiphene did so only with higher dosages than recommended in the physicians' brochure. It should be noted that all of this group of patients failed to ovulate at the lower (recommended) treatment dosage before the higher dosage was given.

Results of treatment

When duration of use was analyzed, 84.5% of the conceptions occurred in the first three ovulatory cycles. However, some women did not conceive until after the sixth ovulatory cycle, and one woman conceived only after 29 cycles of treatment. Overall, of the 193 patients who conceived in this series, 81 (41.9%) did so only with higher dosages and/or longer treatment than recommended in the drug brochure.

Use of hysterosalpingography (HSG)

In our clinic, the infertility workup, except for a semen analysis, is not carried further until a patient has ovulated three times with clomiphene citrate. The vast majority of patients who have no other causes of infertility will have conceived by this time, and it is unnecessary to perform an expensive and uncomfortable HSG or laparoscopy. This practice is not followed in patients whose history or examination indicates that other factors, such as salpingitis, are likely to be present. These women should have an HSG before the third ovulatory treatment cycle. After three ovulatory treatment cycles, further infertility evaluation takes place. It was found that in those 195 patients who had no other demonstrable cause for infertility, 172 conceived after treatment with clomiphene citrate for a corrected pregnancy rate of 88.2%. The only cause for these patients' infertility was ovulatory failure. If the patients had such problems as poor cervical mucus, tubal disease, or oligospermia, the incidence of conception was markedly less, being less than 15% in each of these categories.

Postcoital testing

Clomiphene citrate may act to inhibit the action of estrogen on the cervical mucus. However, the incidence of poor cervical mucus among the patients who had a postcoital test was 15% (34 of 227). In our study group, 163 patients conceived within the first three ovulatory cycles and did not have a postcoital test performed. If we presume that these 163 patients did not have hostile cervical mucus, the incidence of poor-quality mucus would fall to 10.6%. Because the overall incidence of poor cervical mucus is approximately 10% to 15% among infertility patients treated at our clinic for factors other than anovulation, it is doubtful that clomiphene has a clinically significant antiestrogenic effect on cervical mucus. Most of these women probably have an unrelated cervical factor. Nevertheless, if the

Table 23-4
Dose-related response to clomiphene citrate

Dose (mg)	Treated	Ovulated			Pregnancies		
		No.	%	% total	No.	%	% total
50	428	190	44.4	52.1	102	53.9	52.8
100	238	80	33.6	21.9	40	50.0	20.7
150	158	45	28.5	12.3	19	42.2	9.8
200	113	25	22.1	6.9	17	68.0	8.8
250	88	18	20.5	4.9	12	66.7	6.2
250 + hCG*	70	7	10.0	1.9	3	42.9	1.6

*hCG, 10,000 IU of human chorionic gonadotropin.

The percentages indicate the proportion of the total number of ovulations (or pregnancies) that were achieved at each dose.

Adapted from Gysler M, March CM, Mishell DR Jr, et al: A decade's experience with an individualized clomiphene treatment regimen including its effect on the post-coital test. Fertil Steril 37:161, 1982. Reproduced with permission of the publisher, The American Fertility Society.

postcoital test is poor because of abnormal cervical mucus, exogenous estrogen is given, usually 0.1 or 0.2 mg of diethylstilbestrol (DES) daily for 10 days, beginning the day after the last tablet of clomiphene citrate is ingested. Of 34 patients treated in this manner, four conceived. An alternative effective method of treatment for infertility caused by hostile cervical mucus is intrauterine insemination with washed semen. Higher doses of DES or doses of conjugated estrogens above 0.3 mg or any dose of ethinylestradiol may delay or inhibit ovulation.

Luteal phase defects

The claim made by some authors that clomiphene induces corpus luteum inadequacy cannot be supported. Endometrial biopsies are in phase during clomiphene treatment and progesterone levels are either within the normal range or higher during clomiphene-induced ovulations, compared with those achieved during spontaneous cycles.[2] Moreover, correlation between the dosage of clomiphene and increased serum progesterone concentrations following stimulated ovarian steroidogenesis has been demonstrated. In the few patients who have a biphasic BBT and no other cause of infertility, who do not conceive, and whose cycles are accompanied by either peak serum progesterone levels below 15 ng/mL or histologic evidence of an inadequate luteal phase, the dose of clomiphene should be increased. Instead of interpreting the insufficient response as luteal phase inadequacy induced by clomiphene, the clinician should assume that the problem of anovulation has been corrected only partially. A higher dose of clomiphene is required. In some women treated with clomiphene, the endometrial biopsy reveals a discrepancy between the degree of maturation of the glands and stroma. If this abnormality is repetitive, clomiphene should be discontinued and treatment with hMG begun.

Pregnancy rate and outcomes

Using this individualized graduated treatment regimen, 193 pregnancies occurred in 183 patients in the 10-year series in our clinic. The outcome of these pregnancies is shown in Table 23-5.[5] Of the 193 pregnancies, 14 patients were lost to follow-up during the first trimester. Also during the first trimester, 25 spontaneous abortions occurred in 19 patients (14.0%), confirming that the incidence of abortion is not increased in conceptions occurring after clomiphene treatment. There were six ectopic pregnancies in five patients (3.4%). This rate is not significantly higher than the rate of ectopic pregnancy in our general patient population. There were only seven multiple gestations (all twins) among the 147 pregnancies (4.8%) that advanced beyond the first trimester. There was one neonatal death, secondary to multiple congenital anomalies. The perinatal mortality was 33.3, which is elevated but not significantly so. Three other infants had a congenital anomaly: one heart defect, one club foot, and one renal defect. The incidence of anomalies (2.6%) is not higher than that which occurs after spontaneous conception—in agreement with other published reports.[3,4]

It has been recommended that some patients not attempt to conceive in the first induced ovulatory cycle, because the incidence of

Table 23-5
Outcome of 193
clomiphene-induced pregnancies

Term living singleton	130
Premature living singleton	6
Twins	7
Term stillborn	4
Term neonatal death	1
First-trimester abortion	25
Ectopic pregnancy	6
Unknown	14
Congenital anomaly	4/155 (2.6%)

Adapted from Gysler M, March CM, Mishell DR Jr, et al: A decade's experience with an individualized clomiphene treatment regimen including its effect on the post-coital test. Fertil Steril 37:161, 1982. Reproduced with permission of the publisher, The American Fertility Society.

spontaneous abortion was thought to be greater than normal in this cycle. A higher abortion rate did not occur in conceptions following the first treatment cycle in an earlier study by us.[7] Thus, we recommend that patients attempt to conceive in the first treatment cycle. Nor were abortions more common following conception induced with the higher dosage regimens.

Ovarian cysts

During one or more courses of therapy, ovarian cysts occurred in 22 patients (5.1%), only one of whom had bilateral ovarian enlargement. These cysts were small (5 to 9 cm), and none required operative intervention. They all regressed spontaneously in 2 to 4 weeks. The incidence of ovarian cysts in this series was less than the incidence of 13.6% reported in the original premarketing experience, possibly related to the individualized dosage regimen. Cysts were noted during the first course of treatment in three patients, and in treatment cycles 2 to 17 in the others. Cyst formation occurred following treatment with each of the prescribed doses, but the incidence was not greater following higher doses. Recurrent cyst formation in subsequent treatment cycles, using the same dose of clomiphene, was uncommon. However, because cysts can occur in subsequent treatment cycles and in any treatment cycle, and not just the first at a particular dosage, it is imperative to do a pelvic examination every month before prescribing the drug. If an ovarian cyst is present, further treatment should not be given until the cyst regresses spontaneously. In this way, further stimulation and further ovarian enlargement that might require operative intervention can be avoided.

Ovulation induction

The incidence of induced ovulation was greater than 85% among all anovulatory patients treated with clomiphene citrate in our clinic (Table 23-3). About 77% of these patients had oligomenorrhea, and 93% of the oligomenorrheic women ovulated. The ovulation rate in the group of 98 women with primary or secondary amenorrhea, treated with the individualized graduated therapeutic regimen, was 59%, significantly lower ($P < 0.001$). The results of clomiphene therapy in 78 patients with amenorrhea and 20 with amenorrhea and galactorrhea are listed in Table 23-3. Further inspection of these data revealed two populations of amenorrheic patients: (1) those with circulating E_2 levels above 40 pg/mL, who had withdrawal uterine bleeding following IM progesterone administration, and of whom 73% had ovulation induced, and (2) those with very low E_2 levels (<40 pg/mL), who did not have withdrawal bleeding, and in whom ovulation could be induced in only one of 20 patients. Thus, the administration of progesterone in oil may be used to select patients with secondary amenorrhea who are very unlikely to respond to clomiphene and who will require therapy with hMG. However, hMG treatment is expensive and inconvenient. Because there is a remote possibility that ovulation may be induced with clomiphene, those women who are estrogen deficient should be treated with one course of clomiphene citrate in a high dosage (250 mg daily for 5 days), followed by 5,000 IU of hCG 1 week later. If ovulation does not occur, the patient should be treated with hMG.

New protocols

A few patients who do not ovulate on the regimen of 250 mg/day of clomiphene plus hCG just described may ovulate following treatment with one of three recently described therapeutic protocols. Each of these adds a new dimension to the treatment of anovulatory women. Candidates for one of these may be selected by one laboratory test; the other two regimens involve merely higher doses of clomiphene.

Many anovulatory women have clinical and laboratory features of androgen excess. Although most of these women do ovulate when treated with clomiphene according to the regimen outlined, resistant patients with levels of dehydroepiandrosterone sulfate (DHEA-S) above 2.8 µg/mL may respond to a combined regimen of dexamethasone and clomiphene.

Dexamethasone (DEX) is prescribed using a dose of 0.5 mg nightly. After 2 weeks, the DHEA-S measurement is repeated to verify that it has decreased to normal. Nightly DEX is continued at the same dosage, and after another 2 weeks, progesterone in oil, 100 mg, is given IM. After withdrawal bleeding ensues, clomiphene 250 mg/day is given on days 5 through 9. DEX is continued, and hCG 5,000 IU is given 5 to 10 days after stopping the clomiphene. Approximately 50% of women with elevated DHEA-S levels will ovulate when treated with this regimen.[8] DEX is discontinued when pregnancy is confirmed.

Women who have normal DHEA-S levels will not benefit from combined dexamethasone-clomiphene treatment, but may respond to an increased dose and/or prolonged clomiphene treatment. One proven regimen is the use of a daily clomiphene dose of 250 mg for 8 days, followed by 10,000 IU of hCG 6 days after stopping the clomiphene.[9] Other regimens have consisted of higher daily doses and/or prolongation of treatment to 10 or more days. The goal of these various regimens is to provide therapy that is cheaper and more convenient than hMG. One difficulty with these newer protocols is that, in order to maximize their efficacy, the dose and duration of clomiphene and the day of hCG administration must be individualized. Thus, the same monitoring techniques used with hMG treatment, including serum or urinary estrogens and ovarian ultrasound, are needed.

One new treatment regimen uses both modern methods of judging response to ovulatory agents and a more rapid method of finding the dose of clomiphene needed to cause ovulation.[10] As shown above, almost three-quarters of women who ovulate when treated with clomiphene will do so on daily doses of 50 or 100 mg. For those who do not respond, the stepwise regimen we use requires a few months to reach the high-er dose needed, or 5 or more months to decide that the patient is resistant to clomiphene and will need other therapy. O'Herlihy and co-workers[10] start clomiphene treatment with a daily dose of 50 mg for 5 days. Total urinary estrogens are measured before treatment and on day 5 of clomiphene. If the urinary estrogens increase by 20 µg/24 hr or more, clomiphene is discontinued. If not, clomiphene is continued, using 100 mg/day for 5 days, and urinary estrogens are obtained again on the last day of treatment. If still unchanged, the daily dose is increased in increments of 50 mg/day every 5 days up to a maximum dose of 250 mg/day and 25 days of continuous therapy. After reaching the dose that causes a 20 µg/24 hr rise in urinary estrogens, clomiphene is discontinued and further monitoring is done by measuring urinary estrogens and performing daily ovarian ultrasonography. When the largest follicle reaches 18 mm in greatest diameter, ovulation is induced with 3,000 to 5,000 IU of hCG. This regimen permits more precise monitoring of response and allows a patient who might be resistant to be treated with the ideal dose more rapidly. However, it is also more costly. Because most patients ovulate and conceive when lower doses are prescribed, monitoring such as described by O'Herlihy's group is probably best reserved for those whose responses are atypical and those who require more complex treatment regimens. Table 23-6 summarizes the overall results that may be expected with clomiphene citrate therapy.

Bromocriptine

The ergot alkaloid 2-bromo-α-ergocryptine (CB-154, Parlodel) has been approved for marketing in the US for the treatment of amenorrhea-galactorrhea, ovulation induction, and suppression of puerperal lactation. Bromocriptine is most useful for patients with amenorrhea, galactorrhea, and hyperprolactinemia. Most of these women have very low serum estrogen lev-

Table 23-6
Typical overall results following clomiphene citrate therapy

Ovulation	
Oligomenorrhea	>90%
Secondary amenorrhea	67%
Pregnancy (overall)	50%
Pregnancy (no other infertility factors)	85%
Twins	5%
Abortion	20%
Other side effects	3%
Teratogenicity	No ↑

els and therefore are unlikely to ovulate when treated with clomiphene. It has been suggested that elevated prolactin (PRL) levels interfere with the normal cyclic discharge of gonadotropins from intact gonadotropin-releasing cells and result in amenorrhea and low production of estrogen.

Serum levels of PRL increase minimally, or not at all, following administration of both insulin and thyrotropin-releasing hormone (TRH) to most women with hyperprolactinemic amenorrhea and galactorrhea.[11] This finding suggests that this endocrinopathy is at least partially of pituitary origin. Bromocriptine exerts a direct effect on the pituitary gland to lower serum PRL levels, thus removing the block to FSH and LH release. Therefore, it acts specifically at the site of the endocrinologic defect. This dopaminergic drug also works through receptors in the hypothalamus, possibly to stimulate the release of prolactin-inhibiting factor. In women with amenorrhea, galactorrhea, and hyperprolactinemia, bromocriptine lowers PRL levels, suppresses lactation, and induces ovulatory menstrual cycles in over 80% of patients.

The results of 1,385 pregnancies occurring throughout the world after bromocriptine therapy are listed in Table 23-7.[12] No increase in the incidence of multiple gestations, abortions, or congenital abnormalities has been noted. Nausea, usually mild and transient, occurs in over

half of patients. This symptom may be minimized by taking the medication with meals and starting with a dosage of 1 (2.5-mg) tablet per day. The dosage should be increased slowly, by 1 tablet per day, only if the lower dosage is tolerated. Other GI side effects include occasional abdominal pain, vomiting, diarrhea, or constipation. Headache, dizziness, light-headedness, and nasal congestion have also been reported. In a published series of 75 hyperprolactinemic women, bromocriptine treatment was given for 5 to 7 years.[13] Dosage was maintained at the lowest amount needed to keep serum PRL levels in the normal range. No complications or side effects other than those noted with short-term treatment occurred, even in 16 patients with macroadenomas and 49 who had microadenomas.

Because most of these subjects are hypoestrogenic and therefore unlikely to ovulate when treated with clomiphene, the use of bromocriptine may reduce the number who eventually require treatment with hMG. Bromocriptine has also been reported occasionally to induce ovulation in amenorrheic women without galactorrhea and in those with normal serum PRL levels. However, the number of these patients who respond is very low. In contrast to studies with clomiphene, the results are no better than for treatment with placebo. Successful ovulation induction and pregnancies in women with PRL-

Table 23-7
Outcome of bromocriptine-induced pregnancies (1,385)

Live births, singleton	1,182
Live births, twin	24
Live births, triplet	2
Stillborn	5
Spontaneous abortion	160
Ectopic pregnancy	12
Congenital malformations	
major	12/1,241 (1.0%)
minor	31/1,241 (2.5%)

From Turkalj I, Braun P, Krupp P: Surveillance of bromocriptine in pregnancy. JAMA 247:1589, 1982.

Table 23-8
Typical overall results following bromocriptine therapy

Ovulation	90%
Pregnancy (overall)	50%
Pregnancy (no other infertility factor)	80%
Twins	No ↑
Abortion	20%
Persistent side effects	25%
Teratogenicity	No ↑?

secreting pituitary adenomas have been reported.[14] Bromocriptine can reduce the size of both microadenomas and macroadenomas and reverse visual field defects.

Dosages of 20 to 30 mg/day are often required in patients with prolactinomas. Bromocriptine both inhibits PRL secretion and reduces tumor size. Treatment is continued until pregnancy is confirmed at which time it is stopped. On occasion, tumor expansion occurs during pregnancy, and retreatment with bromocriptine is necessary. Bromocriptine has been used during all trimesters. Surgical intervention for expanding adenomas is usually reserved for the first or second trimester. In late pregnancy, glucocorticoids and/or premature delivery may be used to stop growth of the tumor. Following delivery, women with prolactinomas may nurse. However, if they choose not to breast-feed, estrogenic compounds should not be used to suppress lactation, because they may cause marked tumor expansion. Table 23-8 summarizes the results that may be achieved with bromocriptine therapy.

Human menopausal gonadotropins (hMG)

If the patient fails to ovulate with clomiphene citrate or bromocriptine, treatment with hMG should be used. This extract of urine from postmenopausal women contains FSH and LH in a ratio of 1:1. It can cause severe adverse reactions unless proper safeguards are used. Complications include superovulation, multiple pregnancy, and the hyperstimulation syndrome. The last consists of rapid ovarian enlargement, ascites, pleural effusion, and thromboembolic phenomena due to hemoconcentration.

The only indication for hMG treatment is anovulatory infertility in patients who do not ovulate normally following treatment with clomiphene citrate or bromocriptine or who have serious side effects when these drugs are prescribed. Patients enrolled in IVF (in vitro fertilization) programs are also given the drug. Contraindications to hMG therapy include ovarian failure and marked ovarian enlargement. The presence of other infertility factors will reduce the number of pregnancies following gonadotropin treatment. Therefore, a complete infertility workup, including laparoscopy, should be performed before treatment. If other abnormalities are present, these should be corrected before treatment with hMG is attempted, and the couple should be advised of the reduced chance of success. Infants born following gonadotropin-induced pregnancies do not have a higher rate of congenital anomalies than those born after spontaneous conception.[15]

Each patient responds individually to hMG.[16] The amount of medication and the duration of therapy vary not only in different patients but also in different treatment cycles in the same patient. Therefore, it is imperative to monitor the patient carefully to determine when a mature preovulatory follicle has developed. Measurement of either urinary total estrogens or serum estrogens is satisfactory (Figure 23-3), but measuring estrogenicity by vaginal smears or cervical mucus is not sufficiently precise to be reliable.[17] Once it has begun, the process of follicular maturation proceeds rapidly. In women with normal ovulatory menstrual cycles, the estrogen peak in serum precedes that in urine by 1 day; thus, serum levels more accurately reflect the exponential rise in estrogen production by

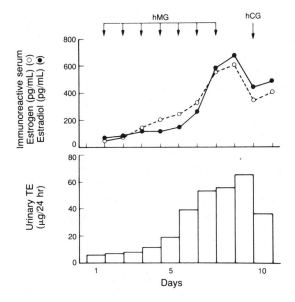

Figure 23-3
Example of normal ovulatory estrogen levels during hMG therapy. Three different methods were used for determining estrogen levels. FSH, 150 IU, was given for 7 days, followed by hCG 10,000 IU, on day 9. TE, total estrogen.

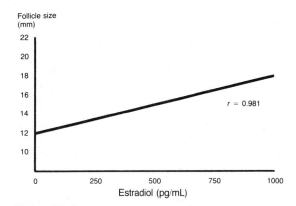

Figure 23-4
Correlation between serum estradiol concentration and dominant follicle maximal diameter.

Reproduced, with permission, from Marrs RP, Vargyas JM, March CM: Correlation of ultrasonic and endocrinologic measurements in human menopausal gonadotropin therapy. Am J Obstet Gynecol 145:417, 1983.

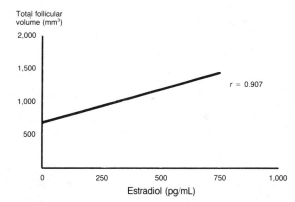

Figure 23-5
Correlation between serum estradiol concentration and total follicular volume.

Reproduced, with permission, from Marrs RP, Vargyas JM, March CM: Correlation of ultrasonic and endocrinologic measurements in human menopausal gonadotropin therapy. Am J Obstet Gynecol 145:417, 1983.

the developing follicle. For this reason, we use serum estrogen levels in our clinic to monitor therapy with hMG.

It has been determined that in hypoestrogenic women the optimal time to induce ovulation with hCG occurs when urinary estrogen levels are between 50 and 100 μg/24 hr or serum estrogen levels are between 500 and 1,000 pg/mL. If estrogen levels are lower, the incidence of ovulation diminishes; when higher, the incidence of hyperstimulation increases. There is an excellent correlation between maximal diameter of the dominant follicle and the serum E_2 level (Figure 23-4).[18] The total volume of all developing follicles also correlates with the E_2 concentration (Figure 23-5).[18] One mature preovulatory follicle will be detected in association with a serum E_2 level of approximately 450 pg/mL. In two-thirds of treatment cycles, estrogen-deficient women will have only one dominant follicle achieve maturity. Thus, among these women, serum E_2 concentrations of 1,000 pg/mL may be presumed to indicate that at least one or two follicles have reached preovulatory status.

Although E_2 levels can be used to assess follicular maturity satisfactorily among estrogen-deficient women, the same is not true for normoestrogenic patients, such as those with PCO or oligomenorrhea. Among these women, two or more follicles mature and reach a preovulatory size of 16 mm or greater in 70% of treatment cycles. Because all follicles, both large and small, contribute to the serum E_2 concentration, it is difficult to predict that even one follicle is mature if the E_2 level is approximately 1,000 pg/mL. If 2,000 pg/mL of E_2 are present in the serum, the physician cannot be certain that an excessive number of mature follicles are present. If there are many mature follicles, marked ovarian enlargement and/or a multiple gestation of high number is likely. Although the mean E_2 level at the time when at least one mature follicle is identified by ultrasound is 1,600 pg/mL among this group of patients, we have found only one preovulatory follicle with levels as low as 650 pg/mL and as high as 2,750 pg/mL. Thus, monitoring follicular development by frequent ultrasound studies is a critical aspect of gauging response to hMG in normoestrogenic women. It is also helpful in estrogen-deficient women.

Since ultrasound has been used to monitor hMG therapy, the pregnancy rate in our center has doubled among normoestrogenic women. At the same time, the mean E_2 level reached at the time of hCG administration is twice the mean level reached when hCG was administered in the years before the use of ovarian scanning, when only serum E_2 levels were used to judge response. Thus, it is likely that in the past many patients received hCG before developing a mature preovulatory follicle. Figure 23-6 shows the progressive follicular enlargement in one patient treated with hMG, which correlated with her serum E_2 levels.

Protocol and experience at LAC/USC Medical Center

Before starting treatment, we obtain a baseline serum E_2 level and do ovarian imaging using a real-time sector scanner. In all patients, following spontaneous menses or induced withdrawal bleeding, treatment with hMG is begun with an initial dose of 2 ampules (150 units FSH and 150 units LH). This same dose is maintained daily. After 3 days, the serum E_2 is repeated. If the baseline concentration has doubled, the same dose of hMG is continued. If the E_2 level is unchanged, the daily dose of hMG is increased by 50% and the E_2 level is measured 3 days later. If the E_2 remains similar to the baseline level, this sequence of increasing the dose by 50% and repeating the E_2 level every 3 days is continued until a response occurs. Whenever the E_2 level has doubled, this new dose is maintained. During all subsequent treatment cycles, therapy will begin at this level.

Once there is a significant increase in the level of E_2, ovarian scanning is repeated. If both ovaries can be seen clearly, further monitoring is done by ultrasound alone. Scanning is repeated every 2 to 3 days until the largest diameter of the dominant follicle reaches or exceeds 14 mm. From this point on, scanning is performed daily. Whenever a follicle that is 16 mm in diameter or larger is identified, hMG is discontinued and hCG is given 24 hours later to cause ovum release. Among normoestrogenic women, an hCG dosage of 5,000 IU is used. Estrogen-deficient women receive 10,000 IU. In order to maintain the corpus luteum in hypoestrogenic women, a dose of 3,000 IU is given 7 days after the initial injection. If there is ovarian enlargement or tenderness, these supplemental doses are withheld.

In addition to monitoring by E_2 levels and ultrasound, patients are examined before receiving hCG. The cervical score is determined[6] and a postcoital test performed. If the cervical mucus is scanty and/or if sperm survival is inadequate, artificial inseminations are performed with the husband's semen 24 hours and 48 hours after the hCG is given. Either the cervical cup or intrauterine insemination technique is used. Intrauterine inseminations are performed if cervical mucus is inadequate.

With the above protocol in the 11 years from 1973 to 1984 (scanning was introduced in 1981), the rate of ovulation in our center has

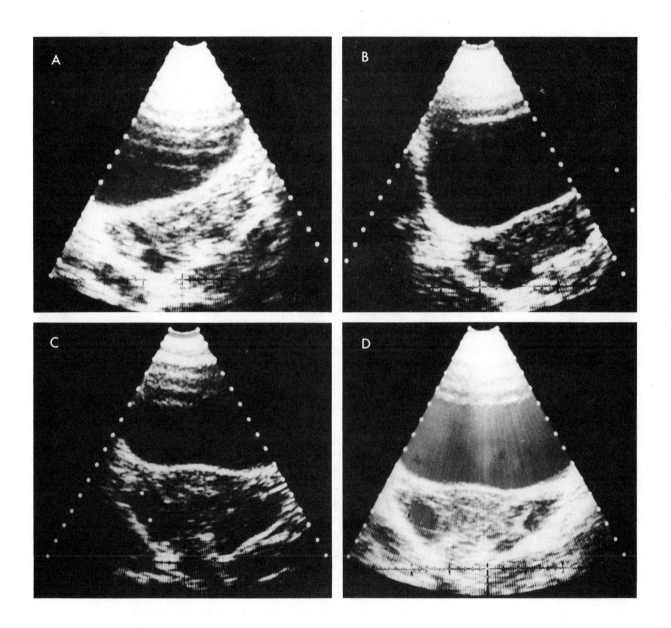

Figure 23-6
Progressive rise in serum E_2 levels and enlargement of dominant follicle during treatment with human menopausal gonadotropins. A. Serum E_2, 229 pg/mL; follicle, 11 x 12 mm. B. Serum E_2, 379 pg/mL; follicle, 13 x 15 mm. C. Serum E_2, 505 pg/mL; follicle, 16 x 18 mm. D. Serum E_2, 890 pg/mL; follicle, 17 x 19 mm.

been more than 99%, and 58% of the patients have conceived. The pregnancy rate per cycle has been 22%, and the mean number of treatment cycles necessary to achieve pregnancy has been 2.7. The abortion rate has remained at 33%, and 8% of the pregnancies have been multiple. Minimal ovarian enlargement occurred in 8% of the treatment cycles. Therefore, the chance of conceiving in one of these treatment cycles is only about 20%, and the incidence of spontaneous abortion after conception is high. The reason for the high abortion rate is unknown. Because of the intensive laboratory monitoring of these patients, some of the abortions are diagnosed by measurement of hCG levels alone, but even if these subclinical abortions are eliminated, the abortion rate is above that following spontaneous conception. Table 23-9 summarizes the results that may be achieved during properly monitored hMG therapy.

Combination hMG regimens

Pregnancies were achieved in 20 of 27 patients using combined DEX and hMG/hCG.[19] All the women had PCO and hyperandrogenism. Earlier therapy with hMG/hCG had resulted in ovulation in only two-thirds of these women, and none conceived. More studies are needed before the ultimate value of this combination therapy will be known. Simultaneous estrogen and

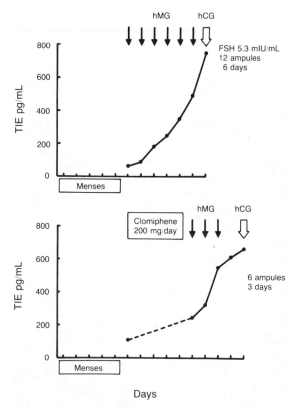

Figure 23-7
Effect of clomiphene pretreatment on total immunoreactive estrogens (TIE) and hMG requirements in a patient with a normal serum FSH who bled after IM progesterone.

Reproduced, with permission, from March CM, Tredway DR, Mishell DR Jr: Effect of clomiphene citrate upon amount and duration of human menopausal gonadotropin therapy. Am J Obstet Gynecol 125:699, 1976.

hMG/hCG therapy has not proven efficacious, nor has simultaneous clomiphene-hMG treatment. Too little is known at this time about combination GnRH-hMG therapy.

Clomiphene citrate pretreatment
In 1976, we reported the effect of treatment with clomiphene citrate before therapy with hMG.[20] In the 10 patients studied, we found that clomiphene pretreatment at 200 mg/day for 5 days could significantly reduce the amount

Table 23-9
Typical overall results following human menopausal gonadotropin therapy

Ovulation	>99%
Pregnancy	60%
Multiple gestation (3/4 twins)	10%
Abortion	25%
Ovarian enlargement	5%
Hyperstimulation syndrome	<0.1%
Teratogenicity	No ↑

and duration of hMG treatment only in patients who had withdrawal bleeding following IM progesterone and a normal serum FSH. In these patients, partial follicular maturation was achieved during clomiphene pretreatment, as evidenced by increasing estrogen levels (Figure 23-7).[20] For the five patients who did not have withdrawal bleeding after progesterone and who had low FSH, the amount of hMG necessary to induce ovulation and the length of treatment were no different with or without clomiphene pretreatment. In this group, estrogen levels were unchanged during clomiphene pretreatment (Figure 23-8).[20] It was concluded that pretreatment with clomiphene citrate reduces both the duration and the amount of hMG only in patients who have withdrawal bleeding after IM progesterone. Therefore, clomiphene pretreatment should be given to this group of patients, as hMG therapy is expensive and time-consuming. A reduced multiple gestation rate in women treated with sequential clomiphene-hMG-hCG has been reported.[21] If confirmed by other studies, this finding is an additional benefit of this regimen.

Estrogen pretreatment

Estrogen-deficient women with hypothalamic-pituitary failure respond promptly to hMG by maturing one or more follicles, as evidenced by elevations in serum E_2 concentrations two or three times higher than those achieved in spontaneous ovulatory cycles. However, cervical mucus production often remains scanty and endometrial histology abnormal. These discrepancies may be caused by chronic estrogen deprivation. Thus, before the first course of hMG, estrogen-deficient patients receive conjugated estrogens, 1.25 mg daily for 25 days. During the last 5 days of estrogen treatment, medroxyprogesterone acetate, 10 mg/day, is added. This sequential estrogen-progestin regimen is prescribed for 2 months before beginning hMG. It "primes" the endocervix and endometrium and has significantly increased the pregnancy rate in our clinic

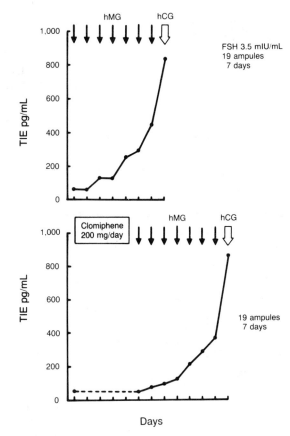

Figure 23-8
Effect of clomiphene pretreatment on total immunoreactive estrogens (TIE) and hMG requirements in a patient with a low serum FSH who did not bleed after IM progesterone.

Reproduced, with permission, from March CM, Tredway DR, Mishell DR Jr: Effect of clomiphene citrate upon amount and duration of human menopausal gonadotropin therapy. Am J Obstet Gynecol 125:699, 1976.

during the first treatment cycle for estrogen-deficient women, compared with the results without such pretreatment.

Selection of agent for induction

For all patients with oligomenorrhea, and for amenorrheic patients who have withdrawal bleeding after progesterone administration, initial treatment should be clomiphene citrate given according to the individualized graduated regimen outlined above. Clomiphene is the first choice of therapy whether or not the patient has hyperprolactinemia. A high ovulation rate has been achieved in amenorrheic patients with and without hyperprolactinemia if they had progesterone-induced withdrawal bleeding.[22] Therefore, normal estrogen status is the key to predicting a probable ovulatory response during clomiphene therapy.

Bromocriptine has resulted in high ovulatory rates in women with hyperprolactinemia. Almost all therapeutic regimens have included daily treatment until pregnancy was documented. Although bromocriptine has not been found to be teratogenic in humans, its ingestion during the period of embryogenesis is not justified if an equally effective agent without this harmful potential is available. Recently, excellent results have been reported with cyclic bromocriptine therapy, but more studies of its efficacy are needed. Until these confirmatory studies are available, clomiphene citrate should be used to induce ovulation in the normoestrogenic patient with amenorrhea and hyperprolactinemia. Other advantages of clomiphene include lower cost and fewer side effects. Although clomiphene therapy is associated with multiple gestations and, therefore, prematurity, twins predominate and the perinatal complications are few.

The low-estrogen patient with amenorrhea and hyperprolactinemia is best treated with bromocriptine. Although the theoretical disadvantage of drug ingestion during early gestation also applies to these patients, the only alternative is hMG therapy. The use of hMG is more complex, expensive, and potentially hazardous without careful monitoring. Successful induction of ovulation with bromocriptine in amenorrheic patients without hyperprolactinemia is rare.

At the present time, however, hMG should be given to patients who do not ovulate despite adequate therapy with clomiphene. hMG is also indicated for the treatment of amenorrheic patients who are estrogen-deficient with or without hyperprolactinemia. It is rare for such patients to ovulate with the use of clomiphene. Many months of unsuccessful clomiphene therapy are expensive, time-consuming, and frustrating for both patient and physician. Treatment with hMG should be undertaken only if rapid estrogen assays and real-time ovarian ultrasound can be obtained daily. By observing this protocol, hMG may be used safely. The ovulation rate should be almost 100%, and a pregnancy rate of about 60%, with a low rate of multiple gestations and complications, should be expected.

Ovulation may be readily and safely induced in almost all amenorrheic patients, except those with ovarian failure. Categorization by estrogen status and by the presence or absence of hyperprolactinemia allows the selection of the most effective drug, thus facilitating therapy.

New preparations

New gonadotropin preparations have been developed in an attempt to improve the pregnancy rate. Preparations with an FSH/LH ratio of 3:1 and 9:1 have had some success.[23] These preparations might be ideal for the woman with PCO who has more than adequate LH production by her own pituitary gland. The use of "pure" FSH to induce ovulation and pregnancy has also been reported in women with PCO.[24]

Another drug, tamoxifen citrate, has been used successfully for induction of ovulation in Europe, but is not approved for this use in the US, and is unlikely to be in the near future. With rare exceptions, glucocorticoids alone should not be prescribed for the treatment of anovulation. These drugs are potentially dangerous and should be given only to patients who have proven adult-onset congenital adrenal hyperplasia with a DHEA-S level of 5 μg/mL or greater.

Gonadotropin-releasing hormone (GnRH)

The effects of GnRH on the release of LH and FSH were first reported in 1969, and the first pregnancy was reported 2 years later. The IV or IM administration of this decapeptide leads to a prompt release of both LH and FSH. The absolute amount of LH released exceeds that of FSH. A dose-response relationship has been demonstrated, and the maximal stimulation occurs after treatment with 400 to 500 μg. Among normally menstruating women, the greatest release of LH and FSH occurs when GnRH is administered at the time of the preovulatory 17β-estradiol peak. Among amenorrheic women, those with normal follicular-phase 17β-estradiol levels have a greater response than do estrogen-deficient women.

The control of FSH and LH release by GnRH was demonstrated by Knobil, who treated GnRH-deficient rhesus monkeys. He showed that pulsatile replacement with exogenous GnRH resulted in LH/FSH release that mimicked that of spontaneously ovulating animals in promoting oocyte maturation, ovulation, and corpus luteum function.[25]

In contrast, continuous GnRH administration results in the inhibition of LH and FSH release after an initial discharge of both hormones. The pulsatile administration of GnRH should remain at a level amount in order to mimic the permissive effect of endogenous GnRH in maintaining normal positive and negative feedback relations between the pituitary and ovaries. Some authors have suggested that because the pituitary-ovarian axis remains intact, the frequency of multiple gestations and other signs of hyperstimulation should approximate that following spontaneous ovulation. Although preliminary results have not confirmed these speculations, the multiple-birth rate may be lower than that following clomiphene or gonadotropin therapy.

Early studies indicated that the administration of GnRH to anovulatory women has resulted in pregnancies only occasionally. In a summary of 333 patients, it was reported that only 46 conceived.[26] Because of the very brief half-life of GnRH, treatment has been given by multiple daily injections. Leyendecker and colleagues reported the induction of ovulation in patients with hypothalamic amenorrhea following IV administration of a bolus of GnRH every 90 minutes using an automatic portable pump.[27] In this group of women, corpus luteum function was maintained by hCG injections during the luteal phase. The need for postovulatory support by hCG or more GnRH has not been proved.

Various dosages, frequencies, and routes of administration have been employed. The doses for IV administration have been between 1 and 20 μg per pulse, and pulse intervals of 60 to 180 minutes have been used. The dose is dependent primarily upon the route of administration. IV administration is less costly because lower doses are employed. The response to IV GnRH is more predictable; thus rate of ovulation has been higher than those achieved with subcutaneous administration (Table 23-10).[28] However, the subcutaneous route is easier for most patients than having to maintain a patent peripheral vein, cannot result in phlebitis or vascular thrombosis, and does have many proponents (Table 23-11).[28,38,39]

Reid and co-workers have demonstrated that subcutaneous GnRH treatment can lead to irregular absorption patterns that cause an LH/FSH response typical of that seen in women with PCO.[42] In addition, some patients who fail to respond to subcutaneous therapy do respond to IV administration. However, some proponents of subcutaneous therapy have reported excellent results.[40]

Most patients will respond to doses of 0.075 μg/kg IV or 0.3 μg/kg subcutaneously. The pulse interval should be 90 minutes. Despite suggestions to the contrary, monitoring by serum E_2 determinations and/or ultrasound scans

Table 23-10
Results of intravenous GnRH therapy from multiple studies

Author	μg/pulse	Interval (min)	Cycles	Ovulation	Pregnancy
Leyendecker[29,30]	2.5–20	90	123	123	38
Schoemaker[31]	10–20	90–120	24	21	6
Miller[32]	1–5	62, 96, 120	23	20	7
Goerzen[33]	10	120	6	6	4
Menon[34]	10	90	20	16	4
Liu[35]	1–10	96–180	45	37	11
Reid[36]	2.5–5	90–120	8	7	1
Loucopoulos[37]	2–30	90–180	25	10	2
			274	240 (88%)	73 (27%)

From March CM: New methods for the induction of ovulation. In Sciarra JJ (ed): Gynecology and Obstetrics, vol 5, ch 70. Philadelphia, Harper & Row, 1985.

of the ovaries is helpful to reduce the frequency of hyperstimulation. If GnRH is discontinued after ovulation, most authors advise that hCG (1,000 to 2,500 IU) be given every 3 to 4 days to maintain the corpus luteum.

Women with severe hypothalamic amenorrhea may require high doses of GnRH to initiate and maintain oocyte maturation. In this group of patients, IV doses up to 20 μg of GnRH every 90 minutes have been utilized. Pumps to administer the GnRH vary greatly in size, weight, cost, variability of dose administered, and pulse intervals. Only after the most appropriate treatment regimen has been found will we know which pump is preferred. Some authors have suggested that prolonged high-dose therapy is likely to

be successful. When Hammond and associates treated 13 patients with 1 mg of GnRH 2 or 3 times per day, eight of the 13 women ovulated and five conceived.[43]

Improving efficacy

Two other approaches have been advocated to improve rates of ovulation and pregnancy. The intranasal route is a convenient method of prolonging therapy; however, larger doses of medication are required than when IM or IV administration is used. Another method of prolonging the action of GnRH is the use of the very potent and long-acting analogs. These substituted peptides may be useful as adjunctive agents for inducing ovulation.

Table 23-11
Results of subcutaneous GnRH therapy from multiple studies

Author	μg/pulse	Interval (min)	Cycles	Ovulation	Pregnancy
Mason[38]	10–25	90	89	83	30
Weinstein[39]	12–20	120	7	7	0
Hurley[40]	5–15	90	36	30	13
Skarin[41]	1–20	90	NR	36	8
Menon[34]	5–20	90	8	1	0
Leyendecker[30]	2.5–20	90	21	13	5
Reid[36]	2–20	120–240	11	2	0
Loucopoulos[37]	2–20	90–180	14	0	0
			186+	136+ (73%)	48+ (26%)

NR = Not reported.
From March CM: New methods for the induction of ovulation. In Sciarra JJ (ed): Gynecology and Obstetrics, vol 5, ch 70. Philadelphia, Harper & Row, 1985.

Because GnRH can stimulate the release of both gonadotropins, it is useful in all steps of the ovulatory process: initial follicular development, final follicular maturation, ovum release, and corpus luteum maintenance. Thus, alone or in various combinations, GnRH or its analogs may achieve widespread use.

One such combination is that of GnRH and clomiphene. This combined regimen may be applicable to women in the same category as those who respond to sequential clomiphene-hMG-hCG. Sequential clomiphene with intranasal GnRH has resulted in pregnancies in a few patients.[44] Thus, partial follicular development would be achieved by clomiphene, and GnRH would then be added to complete the maturation process. For estrogen-deficient women, GnRH might be given initially. After follicular development begins and 17β-estradiol levels rise, the hypothalamus and pituitary would be more sensitive to clomiphene stimulation.

Although GnRH more closely mimics the physiologic mechanism involved in spontaneous ovulation than other ovulation-inducing agents, more studies are needed before the ideal dose, frequency, and route of administration, as well as method of monitoring therapy are known. Only then will GnRH find an appropriate place in our therapeutic armamentarium.

Ovarian wedge resection

With the excellent results obtained with medical therapy, ovarian wedge resection should not be used for treatment of anovulatory infertility. Reported rates of ovulation following this surgical procedure vary and are below those achieved with the medical regimens. If ovulatory cycles are induced after wedge resection, this effect is often transient, and the previous anovulatory pattern is usually resumed. Alterations in gonadotropin and steroid levels following surgery are also short-lived. Peritubal and periovarian adhesions have been reported to occur fre-

quently following ovarian wedge resection, thereby introducing another etiology for infertility. For these reasons, ovarian wedge resection should not be performed.

References

1. Israel R, Mishell DR Jr, Stone SC, et al: Single luteal phase serum progesterone assay as an indicator of ovulation. *Am J Obstet Gynecol* 112:1043, 1972

2. Hull MGR, Savage PE, Bromham DR, et al: The value of a single serum progesterone measurement in the midluteal phase as a criterion of a potentially fertile cycle ("ovulation") derived from treated and untreated conception cycles. *Fertil Steril* 37:355, 1982

3. Kurachi K, Aono T, Minagawa J, et al: Congenital malformations of newborn infants after clomiphene-induced ovulation. *Fertil Steril* 40:187, 1983

4. MacGregor AH, Johnson JE, Bunde CA: Further clinical experience with clomiphene citrate. *Fertil Steril* 19:616, 1968

5. Gysler M, March CM, Mishell DR Jr, et al: A decade's experience with an individualized clomiphene treatment regimen including its effect on the post-coital test. *Fertil Steril* 37:161, 1982

6. Insler V, Melmed H, Eichenbrenner I, et al: The cervical score: A simple semiquantitative method for monitoring of the menstrual cycle. *Int J Gynecol Obstet* 10:233, 1972

7. Rust LA, Israel R, Mishell DR Jr: An individualized graduated therapeutic regimen for clomiphene citrate. *Am J Obstet Gynecol* 120:785, 1974

8. Lobo RA, Paul W, March CM, et al: Clomiphene and dexamethasone in women unresponsive to clomiphene alone. *Obstet Gynecol* 60:497, 1982

9. Lobo RA, Granger LR, Davajan V, et al: An extended regimen of clomiphene citrate in women unresponsive to standard therapy. *Fertil Steril* 37:762, 1982

10. O'Herlihy C, Pepperell JR, Brown JB, et al: Incremental clomiphene therapy: A new method for treating persistent anovulation. *Obstet Gynecol* 58:535, 1981

11. March CM, Kletzky OA, Davajan V: Clinical response to CB-154 and the pituitary response to thyrotropin-releasing hormone-gonadotropin-releasing hormone in patients with galactorrhea-amenorrhea. *Fertil Steril* 28:521, 1977

12. Turkalj I, Braun P, Krupp P: Surveillance of bromocriptine in pregnancy. *JAMA* 247:1589, 1982

13. Corenblum B, Taylor PJ: Long-term follow-up of hyperprolactinemic women treated with bromocriptine. *Fertil Steril* 40:596, 1983

14. Kletzky OA, Marrs RP, Davajan V: Management of patients with hyperprolactinemia and normal or abnormal tomograms. *Am J Obstet Gynecol* 147:528, 1983

15. March CM: Complications of gonadotropin therapy. *J Reprod Med* 21:208, 1978

16. March CM: Therapeutic regimens and monitoring techniques for human menopausal gonadotropin administration. *J Reprod Med* 21:198, 1978

17. Jensen MR, Kaplan BJ, Marrs RP, et al: Maturation value as an indicator of the serum estrogen concentration during treatment with gonadotropins. *Acta Cytologica* 25:251, 1981

18. Marrs RP, Vargyas JM, March CM: Correlation of ultrasonic and endocrinologic measurements in human menopausal gonadotropin therapy. *Am J Obstet Gynecol* 145:417, 1983

19. Evron S, Narot D, Laufer N, et al: Induction of ovulation with combined human gonadotropins and dexamethasone in women with polycystic ovarian disease. *Fertil Steril* 40:183, 1983

20. March CM, Tredway DR, Mishell DR Jr: Effect of clomiphene citrate upon amount and duration of human menopausal gonadotropin therapy. *Am J Obstet Gynecol* 125:699, 1976

21. Robertson S, Birrell W, Grant A: A reduction in multiple pregnancies following the use of a clomiphene citrate: human gonadotropin sequence. *Acta Eur Fert* 7:83, 1976

22. March CM, Davajan V, Mishell DR Jr: Ovulation induction in amenorrheic women. *Obstet Gynecol* 53:8, 1979

23. Rosemberg E, Lee SG, Butler PS: Induction of ovulation. In Saxena BB, Beling CG, Gandy HM (eds): *Gonadotropins*. New York: Wiley Interscience, 1972, p 704

24. Kamrava MM, Seibel MM, Berger MJ, et al: Reversal of persistent anovulation in polycystic ovarian disease by administration of chronic low-dose follicle-stimulating hormone. *Fertil Steril* 37:520, 1982

25. Knobil E: The neuroendocrine control of the menstrual cycle. *Rec Prog Horm Res* 36:53, 1980

26. Zarate A, Canales E, Soria J, et al: Therapeutic use of gonadoliberin (follicle stimulating hormone/luteinizing hormone-releasing hormone). *Fertil Steril* 27:1233, 1976

27. Leyendecker G, Struve T, Plotz EJ: Induction of ovulation with chronic intermittent (pulsatile) administration of LH-RH in women with hypothalamic and hyperprolactinemic amenorrhea. *Arch Gynecol* 229:177, 1980

28. March CM: New methods for the induction of ovulation. In Sciarra JJ (ed): *Gynecology and Obstetrics*, vol 5, ch 70. Philadelphia, Harper & Row, 1985

29. Leyendecker G, Wildt L, Hausmann M: Pregnancies following chronic intermittent (pulsatile) administration of GnRH by means of a portable pump (Zyklomat): A new approach in the treatment of infertility in hypothalamic amenorrhea. *J Clin Endocrinol Metab* 51:1214, 1980

30. Leyendecker G: Induction of ovulation with pulsatile LH-RH in hypothalamic amenorrhea. *Upsala J Med Sci* 89:19, 1984

31. Schoemaker J, Simons AHM, von Osnabrugge GJC, et al: Pregnancy after prolonged pulsatile administration of luteinizing hormone-releasing hormone in a patient with clomiphene-resistant secondary amenorrhea. *J Clin Endocrinol Metab* 52:882, 1981

32. Miller DS, Reid RL, Cetel NS, et al: Pulsatile administration of low-dose gonadotropin releasing hormone. *JAMA* 250:2937, 1983

33. Goerzen J, Corenblum B, Wiseman DA, et al: Ovulation induction and pregnancy in hypothalamic amenorrhea using self-administered intravenous gonadotropin-releasing hormone. *Fertil Steril* 41:319, 1984

34. Menon V, Butt WR, Clayton RN, et al: Pulsatile treatment of hypogonadotropic hypogonadism. *Clin Endocrinol* 21:223, 1984

35. Liu JH, Yen SSC: The use of gonadotropin-releasing hormone for the induction of ovulation. *Clin Obstet Gynecol* 27:975, 1984

36. Reid RL, Sauerbrei E: Evaluation of techniques for induction of ovulation in outpatients employing pulsatile gonadotropin-releasing hormone. *Am J Obstet Gynecol* 148:648, 1984

37. Loucopoulos A, Ferin M, Vande Wiele RL, et al: Pulsatile administration of gonadotropin-releasing hormone for induction of ovulation. *Am J Obstet Gynecol* 148:895, 1984

38. Mason P, Adams J, Morris DV, et al: Induction of ovulation using pulsatile luteinizing hormone-releasing hormone. *Br Med J* 288:181, 1984

39. Weinstein FG, Seibel MM, Taymor ML: Ovulation induction with subcutaneous pulsatile gonadotropin-releasing hormone: The role of supplemental human chorionic gonadotropin in the luteal phase. *Fertil Steril* 41:546, 1984

40. Hurley DM, Brian R, Outch K, et al: Induction of ovulation and fertility in amenorrheic women by pulsatile low-dose gonadotropin-releasing hormone treatment of anovulatory infertility. *Fertil Steril* 40:575, 1983

41. Skarin G, Nillius SJ, Wide L: Pulsatile subcutaneous low-dose gonadotropin-releasing hormone treatment of anovulatory infertility. *Fertil Steril* 40:454, 1983

42. Reid RL, Leopold GR, Yen SSC: Induction of ovulation and pregnancy with pulsatile luteinizing hormone-releasing factor: Dosage and mode of delivery. *Fertil Steril* 36:553, 1981

43. Hammond CB, Weibe RB, Haney AF, et al: Ovulation induction with luteinizing hormone-releasing hormone in amenorrheic infertile women. *Am J Obstet Gynecol* 135:924, 1979

44. Phansey SA, Barnes MA, Williamson HO, et al: Combined use of clomiphene and intranasal luteinizing hormone-releasing hormone for induction of ovulation in chronically anovulatory women. *Fertil Steril* 34:448, 1980

Suggested reading

Ben-Rafael Z, Dor J, Mashiach S, et al: Abortion rate in pregnancies following ovulation induced by human menopausal gonadotropin/human chorionic gonadotropin. *Fertil Steril* 39:157, 1983

Daly DC, Walters CA, Soto-Albors CE, et al: A randomized study of dexamethasone in ovulation induction with clomiphene citrate. *Fertil Steril* 41:844, 1984

Ory SJ: Clinical uses of luteinizing hormone-releasing hormone. *Fertil Steril* 39:577, 1983

Yen SSC: Clinical applications of gonadotropin-releasing hormone and gonadotropin-releasing hormone analogs. *Fertil Steril* 39:257, 1983

Chapter 24

Postcoital Testing

The Cervical Factor as a Cause of Infertility

Val Davajan, M.D.

The exact incidence of infertility secondary to abnormal midcycle cervical mucus-spermatozoa interaction is unknown, but has been estimated to be about 10%. Specimens of postcoital cervical mucus obtained from a substantial number of infertile patients, when examined under the microscope, reveal either few or no sperm, or in some cases only immobilized sperm. It has been assumed, but never absolutely proven, that these findings are incompatible with normal reproductive processes.[1]

In the evaluation of infertility, the postcoital test (PCT) is the only in vivo test that brings together both partners in a testing system. In vitro methods of evaluating sperm-cervical mucus interaction have not been routinely used at this medical center, because we consider an in vivo method more accurate in evaluating what occurs following normal intercourse. The most popular methods of in vitro testing are the slide test of Miller and Kurzrok,[2] the capillary tube method described by Kremer,[3] and more recently, the in vitro cervical mucus penetration test (CMPT) using bovine mucus.[4]

In vitro tests

Slide test

In 1932, Miller and Kurzrok[2] evaluated the ability of spermatozoa to penetrate cervical mucus by placing a quantity of semen and cervical mu-

cus on a clean glass slide and covering the separated specimens with a coverslip. The interface between the specimens results when the specimens come into contact and form the "phase-line." The preparation is then observed under a microscope for penetration of fingerlike projections of semen into the cervical mucus. Under normal conditions, these sperm-containing protrusions gradually increase in size and depth of penetration into the mucus. The sperm finally break through the seminal plasma environment and disseminate into the cervical mucus.

This test is not used clinically any longer because its validity has been shown to be unreliable. Inert carbon particles have been reported to pass freely into the phalanges and across all contact zones, proving that sperm transport is not unique and not due to a chemotactic phenomenon.[5] Reverse migration from cervical mucus into seminal plasma has also been reported.[6]

Capillary tube testing system

The capillary tube testing system has been used by numerous investigators to study the sperm-cervical mucus interaction. The method described here, one of the most commonly used, was devised in 1965 by Kremer.[3]

The cervical mucus is drawn into a capillary tube. One end of the tube is placed in a small reservoir containing semen. The entire apparatus is then placed under a microscope set on low power, and sperm penetration from the reservoir into the cervical mucus is observed directly. Kremer found that immobilized sperm did not penetrate the cervical mucus-filled capillary tubes, thus demonstrating that sperm penetration is not a passive phenomenon. Under normal conditions at midcycle, sperm are found to penetrate the mucus in one direction only, demonstrating that cervical mucus has structural design that helps direct the sperm toward the upper genital tract.

The capillary tube test is a valid and useful tool for evaluating sperm-cervical mucus interaction. However, it is an in vitro testing method and more difficult to perform than an in vivo postcoital test.

CMPT

This test uses in vitro bovine cervical mucus prepared in commercially available flat capillary tubes. The semen is exposed to the mucus sample and microscopically evaluated for sperm penetration. This test method is gaining popularity. However, we feel that more data must be evaluated before the CMPT can be a viable replacement for the in vivo PCT.

The in vivo fractional postcoital test technique

To perform the postcoital test (PCT), the cervix should first be cleansed with a saline-moistened sponge before the cervical mucus is aspirated. To provide adequate suction, a large (20-mL) syringe is attached to polyethylene tubing. The size of tubing should be customized to the size of the cervical os, which usually measures 10 to 12 French. The catheter is grasped 2.5 cm from the distal end with an atraumatic cervical clamp (a large Allis clamp can be used). The aspiration must begin just as the beveled tip of the catheter is inserted into the external os. A constant negative pressure is maintained with the syringe as the catheter is advanced to the internal os level

at approximately 2.5 cm (Figure 24-1). The aspiration should then be terminated, and the clamp closed completely (Figure 24-2). The catheter is slowly withdrawn from the endocervical canal and the trailing mucus cut free from the catheter with scissors. This procedure is essential to avoid dragging the mucus sample in the catheter out into the vagina. The catheter segment containing the mucus is then cut into three smaller segments (Figure 24-3). The segment from the tip of the catheter contains mucus from the internal os level, and the segment closest to the grasping jaws (atragrip) of the clamp contains the mucus from the level closest to the external os.[7] A smear from the posterior vaginal fornix should also be obtained with a moistened cotton-tipped swab, to make sure that spermatozoa were deposited in the vaginal vault.

The PCT should be performed within 2 to 2½ hours following coitus, because it has been shown that the number of sperm in the cervical canal is maximal during that time. The test should be scheduled 1 to 3 days before the expected rise in basal body temperature (BBT). This is best determined by reviewing a temperature graph from the previous month. A "mini-BBT," taken from the end of menses until the BBT has been elevated for at least 3 days, should be performed in every cycle in which a PCT is performed. If the PCT is abnormal, it should be repeated every 2 days until there is a temperature rise. This assures that the test is performed during the time of maximal estrogen stimulation of cervical mucus, which occurs 1 to 3 days before the rise in BBT. Before each PCT, the couple should observe their usual period of sexual abstinence so that the test reflects an accurate evaluation of sperm transport based on the usual frequency of intercourse for the couple.

A normal test should have at least five actively motile sperm per high-power field at the internal os level.[7-9] The spinnbarkeit measured in the same mucus sample should be no less than 6 cm (Table 24-1). In order to evaluate its biophysical characteristics, the mucus from one seg-

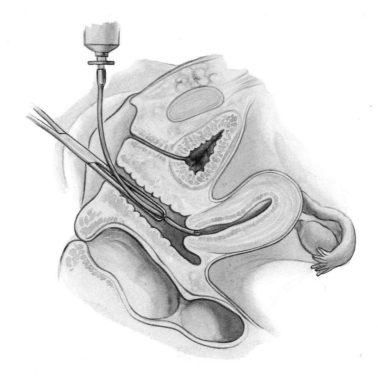

Figure 24-1
A syringe attached to a polyethylene suction catheter is used in aspiration of cervical mucus. The tubing is stabilized by grasping it 2.5 cm from the distal end with a clamp. The atragrip of the clamp should be adjusted so that when the clamp is set at the first ratchet, the tube is partially but not totally occluded. Aspiration must be initiated just as the tip of the catheter is inserted into the external os.

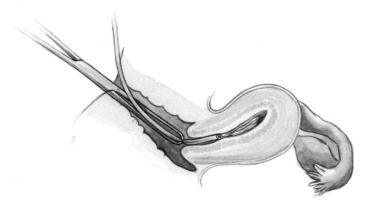

Figure 24-2
Aspiration is terminated when the catheter is inserted to the internal os level. The atragrip should then be completely closed.

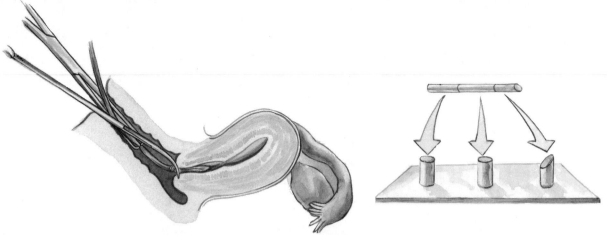

Figure 24-3
The catheter should be gently withdrawn and the trailing mucus cut away with scissors. The catheter segment is then cut into three smaller segments. The distal segment (beveled end) contains mucus collected from the internal os level, and the most proximal segment (closest to the atragrip) contains mucus collected from the level of the external os.

ment of the catheter should be stretched out on a microscopic slide, and a coverslip placed over a portion of it (Figure 24-4). The mucus beneath the coverslip, when dried, slowly forms linear crystals in parallel alignment (Figure 24-4A). In contrast to this slow-drying mucus phenomenon, when normal mucus is allowed to dry rapidly without a coverslip (Figure 24-4B), it is distorted rapidly, forming the fern pattern.[10]

A discussion of the principal causes of abnormal PCTs (see Table 24-2) follows.

Abnormal PCT
with anatomic defects

Cervical stenosis
Conization of the cervix is still the most common etiology of cervical stenosis. If conization must

be performed in a young woman, it should be as shallow as possible in order to leave behind as much of the mucus-producing endocervical cells as possible.[11] Stenosis is diagnosed when attempts to pass a 5 French catheter into the endocervical canal encounter resistance. Neither estrogen therapy nor attempts to recanalize the endocervix with dilators or cryosurgery have been very successful. Small *Laminaria* have been used in our clinic, and an occasional pregnancy has been achieved. More recently, intrauterine insemination using a washed sperm specimen has been extensively evaluated for treatment of this disorder. The washed sperm techniques are described later in this chapter.

Varicosities of the
hypoplastic endocervical canal
In some patients, even the gentlest attempt to

Table 24-1
Normal postcoital test

Days of abstinence	Usual pattern of abstinence
Day of exam	1–3 days before BBT rise
Hours from coitus to exam	2–2½
Sperm/high-power field (×400), internal os level	≥5
Spinnbarkeit	≥6 cm

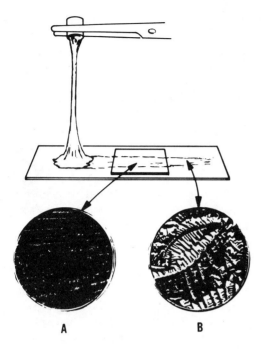

Figure 24-4
The mucus from mid catheter segment is stretched out longitudinally on a microscopic slide, and a coverslip is placed over a portion of it. A. Photomicrograph of normal midcycle cervical mucus dried under a coverslip shows formation of linear crystals in parallel alignment. B. Photomicrograph of normal midcycle mucus dried without a coverslip illustrates the classic fern.

A   B

Abnormal PCT with abnormal cervical mucus

Poor quality of mucus

Many infertile patients secrete very thick, cellular cervical mucus at midcycle. In some, a daily dose of 0.1 mg diethylstilbestrol (DES) given on days 5 to 15 of a 28-day menstrual cycle improves the quality of mucus and results in a normal PCT. If there is no improvement, the DES dose should be increased to 0.2 mg/day. With the use of DES, pregnancies have been reported in the range of 15% to 20%.[12]

DES treatment should result in an improved PCT. Therefore, all treatment efforts should be evaluated by performing a repeat PCT during a treatment cycle. If the PCT does not improve, the abnormal mucus should be removed by aspiration. If clear mucus trails behind the thick mucus, the thick mucus should be cut away from the clear mucus and the clear mucus allowed to remain in the canal. After this "unplugging" procedure, the patient should be instructed to return home to have intercourse.

In our institution, we have recently been using intrauterine washed sperm inseminations in

collect cervical mucus causes immediate cervical bleeding.[12] These patients have a very fragile and thinly developed columnar epithelium with numerous superficial varicosities. This diagnosis can be made only by colposcopy. In the past, the treatment of these superficial varicosities has been by cryosurgery, and in a small number of patients this therapy has improved the lining epithelium and the microvaricosities have disappeared. A newer technique, using laser cautery,[13] has also been attempted, but no published information is available as to its efficacy. At this institution, these patients are currently being treated with intrauterine insemination using washed sperm.

Table 24-2
Categorization of causes of abnormal PCT

Anatomic defects
Cervical stenosis
Varicosities of the hypoplastic endocervical canal

Abnormal cervical mucus
Poor quality
Low quantity

Abnormal PCT with normal cervical mucus
Faulty coital technique
Vaginal factor or weak sperm factor
Oligospermia and/or low motility
Low semen volume
Immobilized sperm in endocervical canal
Large semen volume
Highly viscous semen

lieu of DES or other estrogen treatment. The preliminary results have been encouraging. In a group of patients with abnormal cervical mucus, we achieved a 46% pregnancy rate this way. This is almost three times higher than the pregnancy rate reported following estrogen treatment.[12]

If washed sperm insemination is not available, conjugated estrogens, 1.25 to 5 mg/day, can be given to patients in whom the DES therapy is ineffective. However, doses in the range of 2.5 to 5 mg/day may suppress or delay ovulation. Therefore, all patients receiving high doses of conjugated estrogens should be encouraged to keep a BBT graph. If ovulation is suppressed, clomiphene citrate can be prescribed.

Low quantity of mucus

Some infertile patients secrete only minimal amounts of essentially normal mucus at midcycle. These patients are also sometimes helped by the use of DES therapy (0.1 mg/day on days 5 to 15 of a 28-day cycle). The PCT should be repeated at midcycle to see if there is improvement in mucus production with DES. If the repeat PCT test becomes normal, the therapy should be continued for at least 1 year or until a pregnancy occurs. In unresponsive patients, the dose of DES should be increased to 0.2 mg/day. If mucus production does not improve at this dose level, the higher dose of conjugated estrogens described above should be prescribed. Pregnancy rates of only 15% have been reported in patients with this diagnosis.[12]

Intrauterine insemination may also be used in these patients as an alternative to estrogen treatment.

Abnormal PCT with normal cervical mucus

Faulty coital technique

In some infertile patients, no spermatozoa are seen in the cervical mucus following intercourse. A faulty coital technique must be suspected if a smear taken from the posterior vaginal fornix also contains no sperm and the man is known to have sperm in his semen. At this institution, we found that the partners of a few extremely obese women were unable to penetrate the vagina. A review of coital technique or artificial insemination will usually correct the problem. On rare occasions, failure of intravaginal ejaculation has been diagnosed as the cause of an abnormal PCT. In one instance, the woman was completely unaware of the problem. Male partners in these cases should be referred to licensed sex counselors or psychiatrists trained specifically in dealing with sexual dysfunction.

Vaginal factor or weak sperm factor

If the semen analysis is normal and no sperm are seen in the cervical mucus but are found in the vagina, cervical cup insemination (Figure 24-5) followed by a PCT in 1 hour can be used to rule out a "hostile vaginal factor." A specially designed plastic cup (Milex Products, Los Angeles) is placed on the cervix. The cups come in various sizes, labeled in millimeters. The correct size is selected by visual estimation. Semen is introduced through the stem into the cup and exposed to the cervix for 1 hour. The cup is then removed, the cervix cleansed, and an in vivo PCT performed. If motile sperm are seen at the internal os level after this technique, the procedure can be used as therapy in ensuing cycles.

The exact etiology of the vaginal factor, or weak sperm factor, has not yet been established. Recently, washed sperm intrauterine inseminations have been substituted for the cupping technique. However, not enough patients have been inseminated to determine the efficacy of this treatment for this specific type of abnormality. At our institution, the vaginal factor does not appear to be related to immunologic factors, as circulating agglutinating or immobilizing antibodies have not been detected in these women.

Oligospermia and/or low motility

Oligospermia describes a semen specimen with a

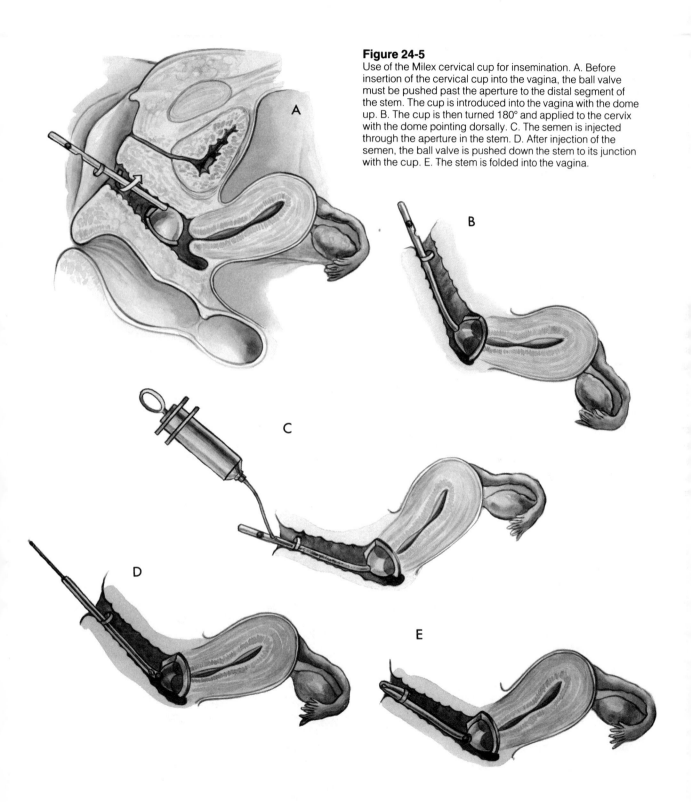

Figure 24-5
Use of the Milex cervical cup for insemination. A. Before insertion of the cervical cup into the vagina, the ball valve must be pushed past the aperture to the distal segment of the stem. The cup is introduced into the vagina with the dome up. B. The cup is then turned 180° and applied to the cervix with the dome pointing dorsally. C. The semen is injected through the aperture in the stem. D. After injection of the semen, the ball valve is pushed down the stem to its junction with the cup. E. The stem is folded into the vagina.

concentration of less than 20 million/mL. When sperm motility in the specimen is 40% or less, low motility is diagnosed. If an abnormal PCT is due to oligospermia or low motility, cervical cup insemination as outlined above should be used. If an improvement of the PCT is noted, cup therapy can be used for at least four cycles. If no improvement is noted, washed sperm intrauterine insemination should be performed; if possible, for at least four to six cycles. The best days for performing inseminations are the day prior to the BBT rise (when there is usually a nadir) and the day following the nadir. Both cupping[12] and intrauterine washed sperm insemination yield pregnancy rates of approximately 30%.

Low semen volume
In some couples, the abnormal PCT may be due to an abnormally low volume of semen (less than 2 mL). If semen specimens are consistently less than 2 mL, cervical cup insemination can be tried as therapy. As stated previously, it is essential to perform a PCT 1 hour following the first cup insemination, in order to determine the efficacy of such therapy. If the cup method does not improve the PCT, washed sperm intrauterine insemination should be done. At this institution, the primary method of therapy is now washed sperm insemination, but the results are too preliminary to quote success rates.

Immobilized sperm in the endocervical canal
An abnormal PCT may be due to immobilization of sperm in the cervical mucus. Immunologic tests (Kibrick, Isojima) should be done in these patients, although in most instances there is no correlation between positive immunologic tests and sperm immobilization in cervical mucus. Immobilization may be due to some as yet undetermined factors or to locally secreted antibodies not detected by the Kibrick or Isojima tests. Because *Mycoplasma (Ureaplasma urealyticum)* and other organisms in either the semen or cervical mucus may play a role in sperm immobilization,

cervical and semen cultures should be obtained. If immunologic tests and cultures are both negative, cup insemination can be attempted. If the postcup PCT shows motile sperm at the internal os level, the cup technique or intrauterine insemination should be tried as therapy for at least four to six cycles.

Large volume of semen
If a PCT is normal and the only finding is a large volume of semen (more than 8 mL), a split ejaculate specimen should be collected and cup insemination performed using the first 2 mL of ejaculate. If the PCT 1 hour later is normal, cup inseminations should be continued for at least four cycles. An alternative is to perform washed sperm intrauterine inseminations using sperm obtained from the entire specimen.

High-viscosity semen (incomplete liquefaction)
A substantial number of patients have abnormal PCTs where the only finding is failure of the semen to liquefy completely. The etiology of high semen viscosity is most likely an enzyme deficiency or abnormality. With the washed sperm technique, almost all semen specimens can now be liquefied adequately and intrauterine insemination attempted. Occasionally the semen specimen resists even vigorous washing and remains in a semiliquid state. If the supernatant is discarded, the entire specimen will be lost, because no real precipitate forms at the bottom of the centrifuge tube. In such cases, it is better to aspirate the supernatant layered just above the "gel" found at the bottom of the tube. The aspirate should then be centrifuged and the bottom 0.5 mL in the centrifuge tube used as the insemination specimen.

Preparing spermatozoa for intrauterine insemination
Washed sperm techniques
A semen specimen is collected by masturbation

with ejaculation into a sterile jar. The specimen is transferred to a sterile, tapered centrifuge tube and washed by one of two methods, depending on the density of sperm.

Method 1 (for normal semen)

If the semen specimen has a concentration of 20 million sperm/mL or more, the volume is tripled by adding Ham's F-10 solution (an electrolyte and amino acid solution; available in 500-mL containers from Gibco, Santa Clara, CA, and Nova Laboratories, Sherman Oaks, CA) at 37°C. The solution should be stored at 4°C. The specimen is first mixed on a Vortex mixer at a reading of 4, then centrifuged for 5 minutes at 300 × g. The supernatant is poured out, and 1 mL of Ham's F-10 solution is added to the concentrate of sperm found at the bottom of the centrifuge tube. The specimen is mixed again on the Vortex mixer and then centrifuged for 3 minutes at 300 × g. The supernatant is discarded again, and 0.5 mL of F-10 solution is added to the concentrate. The specimen is mixed again and drawn up in a sterile 3-mL syringe. An 8 or 5 French feeding tube is most often adequate for proper insemination. With severe cervical stenosis, a metal 1-mm cannula (Hevesy Medical Instruments, Anaheim, CA) can be used. The portio vaginalis is then cleaned with a dry swab, and the specimen is gradually deposited high in the fundus of the uterus, using a sterile ring forceps to hold the catheter. Following the deposition, approximately 0.5 to 1.0 mL of air is gently pushed through the catheter to make sure that the entire specimen is cleared out.

Method 2 (for oligospermia or low motility)

If the semen specimen has a concentration of less than 20 million sperm/mL or motility of less than 40%, a fractional method of washing is used. The semen specimen is divided into three 0.5- to 1.0-mL aliquots, and each is centrifuged at 300 × g for 5 minutes. Each of the pellets formed is then resuspended in 1.0 mL of Ham's F-10 solution and centrifuged at 300 × g for 3

minutes. The supernatant is discarded, and the pellet from each tube is resuspended in the same 0.5 mL of F-10 solution. After mixing, the specimen is placed high in the uterine fundus.

At our institution, antibiotics are not routinely given to the recipient of the insemination, nor is the husband given prophylactic antibiotics. The Ham's F-10 solution can have antibiotic added to it, although in most of our inseminations we have not used antibiotic-treated wash media. If the semen specimen is noted to have an abnormal number of leukocytes, the semen should be cultured for both aerobic and anaerobic bacteria.

Sperm selection techniques

Percoll technique (discontinuous gradient)

This technique separates motile sperm from immobilized and defective sperm, WBCs, and seminal plasma debris. It is used to treat the semen of patients with abnormal results on the hamster-egg penetration test (see Chapter 25). The procedure was first described in 1981[14] and modified in 1983.[15] The initial (or continuous gradient) technique involved a two-step Percoll gradient that was found effective in separating motile sperm; the separated sperm had a greater capacity for penetrating zona-free hamster ova. But because the original method required the use of a high-speed centrifuge and rotor, it was modified to a one-step discontinuous Percoll gradient. The modification has been found both easier to perform and more effective in separating motile sperm.[16]

METHOD. Hypertonic Percoll solution (Pharmacia Labs, Uppsala, Sweden) is made isotonic by mixing 9 parts Percoll with 1 part modified Ham's F-10 (10 ×). The solution is further diluted with 1-part quantities of Ham's F-10 to obtain densities of 90%, 80%, 70%, 55%, and 40%. Discontinuous gradients are made in 16 × 125 mm tissue culture tubes (Falcon 3033) by pipetting and layering 1.5 mL each of 100%, 90%, 80%,

70%, and 55% Percoll, in a manner that shows interface between the layers.

On top of the 55% layer, 2 mL of 40% Percoll are added. A 1-mL specimen of semen is layered on top of the 40% gradient, and the entire tube is centrifuged for 20 minutes at 300 × g. The semen and the 40%, 55%, and 70% layers are removed with a pipette and discarded. The 80%, 90%, and 100% layers are then combined and diluted with 2 volumes of Ham's F-10. The solution is divided into two tubes, which are centrifuged at 160 × g for 10 minutes. The supernatant is discarded. The pellets formed at the bottom of the tubes are resuspended in 1 mL of F-10 containing 10% serum and recentrifuged.

The specimen can then be used for intrauterine inseminations, hamster-egg penetration tests, or in vitro fertilization.

Swim-up technique

This is a rather easily performed technique that is also used for separating motile sperm from immobilized sperm, WBCs, RBCs, and seminal plasma debris.[16] An aliquot of 0.5 mL of semen is layered beneath 2 mL of Ham's F-10 solution in a 12 × 75 mm culture tube. After 60 minutes, the upper 1-mL layer is aspirated carefully with a Pasteur pipette and discarded. After an additional hour, the upper interface is aspirated and washed twice in serum-supplemented F-10 medium. The separated spermatozoa are then used to perform intrauterine inseminations.

Intrauterine insemination: Special concerns

Approximately two-thirds of our first 200 patients undergoing intrauterine inseminations had no complaints, and another one-fifth complained of minimal uterine cramps lasting less than 10 minutes. About 10% reported moderate uterine cramps lasting about an hour. Severe cramps for more than an hour occurred in 2%. Two patients had a mild temperature elevation (<100° F). Both were given antibiotic therapy

(tetracycline) and were afebrile within 14 hours following the insemination.

We pretreat patients with a history of "irritable uterus" with antiprostaglandin medication; we have found it effective in most cases. A very rare patient may require not only the antiprostaglandin pretreatment, but also a triple wash of the semen instead of the double-wash technique described above.

References

1. Davajan V, Kharma K, Nakamura RM: Spermatozoa transport in cervical mucus. *Obstet Gynecol Surv* 25:1, 1970

2. Miller EG Jr, Kurzrok R: Biochemical studies of human semen. *Am J Obstet Gynecol* 24:19, 1932

3. Kremer J: A simple sperm penetration test. *Int J Fertil* 10:209, 1965

4. Alexander JA: Evaluation of male infertility with an in vitro cervical mucus penetration test. *Fertil Steril* 36:201, 1981

5. Perloff WH, Steinberger E: In vivo penetration of cervical mucus by sperm. *Fertil Steril* 14:231, 1963

6. Moghissi KS: Mechanism of sperm migration. *Fertil Steril* 15:15, 1964

7. Davajan V, Kunitake GM: Fractional in vivo and in vitro examination of post-coital cervical mucus in the human. *Fertil Steril* 20:197, 1969

8. Kunitake G, Davajan V: A new method of evaluating infertility due to cervical mucus-spermatozoa incompatibility. *Fertil Steril* 21:706, 1970

9. Tredway DR, Settlage DS, Nakamura RM, et al: The significance of timing for the postcoital evaluation of cervical mucus. *Am J Obstet Gynecol* 121:387, 1975

10. Davajan V, Nakamura RM, Mishell DR Jr: A simplified technique for evaluation of the biophysical properties of cervical mucus. *Am J Obstet Gynecol* 109:1042, 1971

11. Boddington MM, Spriggs AI: Cervical cone biopsy and fertility. *Br Med J* 2:271, 1974

12. Scott JZ, Nakamura RM, Mutch J, et al: The cervical factor in infertility. Diagnosis and treatment. *Fertil Steril* 28:1289, 1977

13. Townsend D, personal communication

14. Gorus FK, Pipeleers DG: A rapid method for the fractionation of human spermatozoa according to their progressive motility. *Fertil Steril* 35:662, 1981

15. Forster MS, Smith WD, Lee WI, et al: Selection of human spermatozoa according to their relative motility and interaction with zona free hamster eggs. *Fertil Steril* 40:655, 1983

16. Berger T, Marrs RP, Moyer DL: Comparison of techniques for selection of motile spermatozoa. *Fertil Steril* 43:268, 1985

Chapter 25

Male Factor in Infertility

Gerald S. Bernstein, Ph.D., M.D.

It is important to consider the couple as a unit when the problem of infertility occurs. Both partners must be evaluated and the interaction between male and female factors considered. The gynecologist dealing with infertility should understand male reproduction well enough to interpret a semen analysis and understand the significance of the functional properties of spermatozoa and the prognosis of disorders that lead to abnormal semen. The gynecologist must also be ready to provide counsel about the application of artificial insemination with either the husband's (AIH) or donor's (AID) semen. In this chapter, special attention will be given to the interpretation of the semen analysis and tests of spermatozoan functional properties. In addition, this chapter offers a brief, practical guide to the evaluation and treatment of the male with abnormal semen.

Requirements for male fertility

To cause a pregnancy, a man must deposit an adequate number of functional spermatozoa in his partner's vagina. Therefore, he must have the following: endocrine function sufficient to support spermatogenesis; testes able to respond to endocrine influence to produce spermatozoa;

an intact ductal system to carry spermatozoa away from the testes to eventually reach the urethra; normal epididymal function to allow maturation of sperm; functional accessory glands to produce seminal plasma; and an intact nervous system that will permit penile erection and normal ejaculation.

Once the semen reaches the vagina, the next steps depend on the functional properties of the spermatozoa: motility, ability to migrate through cervical mucus into the upper female genital tract, and ability to penetrate and activate the ovum.

Semen quality, including sperm motility, is ascertained by the semen analysis. The other functional properties are tested by other means. The postcoital and in vitro sperm penetration tests are used for evaluating the ability of sperm to migrate through cervical mucus. In vitro tests with zona-free golden hamster eggs or human ova are used to evaluate fertilizing capacity.

Male reproductive physiology

The testes contain two distinct but interrelated parts: the seminiferous tubules, lined with Sertoli cells and containing developing sperm cells; and the interstitial tissue, containing interstitial or Leydig cells that produce androgens. Spermatogenesis involves a series of steps in which diploid spermatogonia each develop into four haploid spermatozoa.

Endocrinology

Testicular function is controlled by the pituitary gonadotropins: luteinizing hormone (LH) and follicle-stimulating hormone (FSH). Both are secreted in rhythmic pulses in response to gonadotropin-releasing hormone (GnRH) emanating from the hypothalamus. GnRH is influenced by neurotransmitters and peptides from hypothalamic and extrahypothalamic neurons.

It has generally been believed that LH binds to receptors in the Leydig cells to induce and maintain the production of testosterone (T), and that FSH binds to receptors in the Sertoli cells and initiates the synthesis of an androgen-binding protein (ABP) and a polypeptide, inhibin. The interacting effects of the gonadotropins initiate spermatogenesis. There is negative feedback between T and LH and between inhibin and FSH, such that LH levels increase as the level of T decreases, and FSH levels increase when the Sertoli cells are damaged.

While these concepts are basically correct, the system is far more complicated. LH also induces the production of estradiol (E_2) in Leydig cells through aromatization of T. Some E_2 is also produced by the same mechanism in the liver and by peripheral aromatization of androstenedione to estrone, which subsequently is converted to E_2. Some LH feedback may be modulated by the conversion of T to E_2 in the hypothalamus (Figure 25-1).[1]

T supports the function of the prostate and seminal vesicles and maintains libido. It is also secreted in a pulsatile manner in response to LH. There is a diurnal variation in T levels, with higher levels occurring in the early morning. In blood, the major portion of T is bound to sex hormone-binding globulin (SHBG). Only the unbound portion is biologically available. In some target tissues, T is converted to dihydrotestosterone (DHT) by the enzyme 5α-reductase.

There are FSH receptors in Leydig cells as well as in Sertoli cells. FSH increases the number of LH receptors in the Leydig cells and thereby enhances the effect of LH on steroidogenesis. LH itself will decrease the number of its receptors, in a down-regulation process. FSH also induces the formation of a small amount of E_2 in the Sertoli cells by aromatization of T.

Both T and E_2 probably play a role in regulating the level of FSH, but inhibin has a more potent effect. Inhibin has not been isolated from men, but there is presumptive evidence for its presence. It has been detected in semen and serum by radioimmunoassay (RIA). A peptide with inhibin-like activity has recently been isolated from human seminal plasma.[2]

The endocrine control of spermatogenesis is still poorly understood. T is necessary for some steps in the process, but other steps do not appear to be under hormonal control. There is some evidence that FSH may be required only for initiating spermatogenesis. Thus, if the testes are allowed to become quiescent in a hypophysectomized animal, both FSH and LH are necessary to initiate spermatogenesis. However, once started, sperm production can be maintained by LH alone.

A very high level of intratesticular T is required to support spermatogenesis. In men, it is impossible to achieve this level by giving exogenous T. It is necessary to induce endogenous production of T by the Leydig cells. When large amounts of T are administered to a man with an intact pituitary, spermatogenesis is suppressed, because LH levels drop and the intratesticular level of T decreases, although blood levels are maintained. Large amounts of T also suppress FSH secretion.

Time relationships

The process of spermatogenesis begins with the proliferation of the stem cells or spermatogonia. There are at least four types of spermatogonia in the human (Figure 25-2).[1] The type B sper-

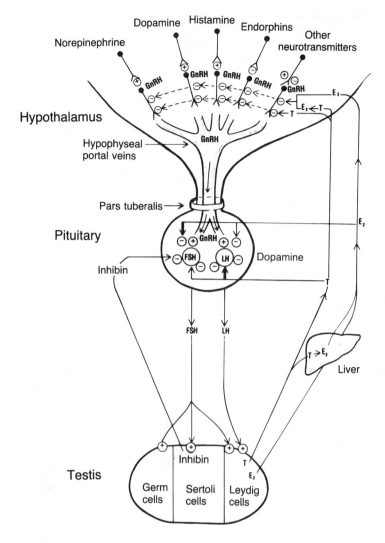

Figure 25-1
Schematic representation of the endocrine relationships among the hypothalamus, pituitary, and testis. GnRH, gonadotropin-releasing hormone; T, testosterone; E_2, estradiol; LH, luteinizing hormone, FSH, follicle-stimulating hormone.

Reproduced, with permission, from Vigersky RA: Pituitary-testicular axis. In Lipshultz LI, Howards SS (eds): Infertility in the Male. *New York, Churchill Livingstone, 1983, p 20.*

matogonia differentiate into the preleptotene spermatocytes, which undergo meiotic division to produce haploid spermatids. The spermatids differentiate into mature spermatozoa through a series of changes called spermiogenesis.

The time required for spermatogenesis in the human can only be approximated, because the early stages of the process have not been completely elucidated. Approximately 74 days are required for spermatozoa to be produced,

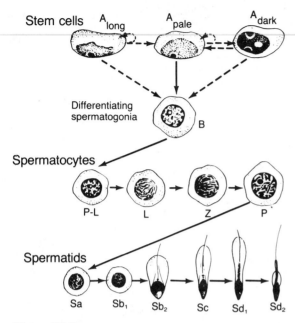

Figure 25-2
Sequence of germ cell development in man. The dashed
lines represent uncertain relationships between the various
types of A spermatogonia and the methods by which stem
cells are renewed. P, L, and Z refer to pachytene, leptotene,
and zygotene spermatocytes. Sa, Sb$_1$, Sb$_2$, etc., refer to
spermatids in various stages of differentiation.

*Reproduced, with permission, from Huckins C: Adult
spermatogenesis: Characteristics, kinetics, and control. In Lipshultz
LI, Howards SS (eds): Infertility in the Male. New York, Churchill
Livingstone, 1983, p 108.*

once spermatogonial differentiation begins. The
length of the spermatogonial differentiation
phase is unknown, but spermatocyte maturation
occurs over a period of 25 days and spermiogenesis requires approximately 22 days.

Additional time is required for passage of
sperm into and through the epididymis. It requires an average of 12 days, and sometimes as
long as 26 days, for sperm to appear in the ejaculate after leaving the testes. This time depends,
in part, on the frequency of ejaculation.

The semen analysis thus represents events
that were initiated some 3 or more months before the specimen was collected. If spermato-

genesis is interrupted at some point in its cycle,
there will be a lag period before the effect is noted in the semen analysis. There will be a similar
delay before the semen returns to normal after
the inhibition is removed. The length of the lag
time depends on the stage of spermatogenesis
that is affected.

The epididymis and sperm maturation

The epididymis is a reservoir for sperm storage
and the site of sperm maturation. When sperm
enter the epididymis from the testis, they are
functionally inactive. They are unable to achieve
progressive motility or fertilize ova. During passage through the epididymis, the spermatozoa
undergo a series of biochemical and morphologic changes. There are also changes in the fluid
surrounding the sperm. By the time the sperm
reach the vas deferens, they are capable of progressive motility upon ejaculation and have the
ability to fertilize eggs. It is unclear whether
abnormal epididymal function is a factor in
some cases of male infertility.

Ejaculation

As the vasa deferentia approach the prostate,
they are joined by the ducts of the seminal vesicles to form the ejaculatory ducts, which carry
sperm and seminal vesicular fluid through the
prostate into the urethra (Figure 25-3). The
openings of the prostatic glands enter the urethra separately from the ejaculatory ducts. Because of this, an ejaculate of prostatic fluid
is possible, even if the ejaculatory ducts are
blocked or the vasa deferentia and seminal vesicles are congenitally absent.

The neurophysiology of erection, orgasm,
and ejaculation is clinically important. Erection
is controlled by the parasympathetic nervous
system. Outflow from sympathetic spinal gan-
glia from T_{12} to L_3 causes contractions of the vas
deferens, prostate, and seminal vesicles, forcing
sperm and glandular secretions into the posteri-
or urethra (seminal emission) and initiating par-

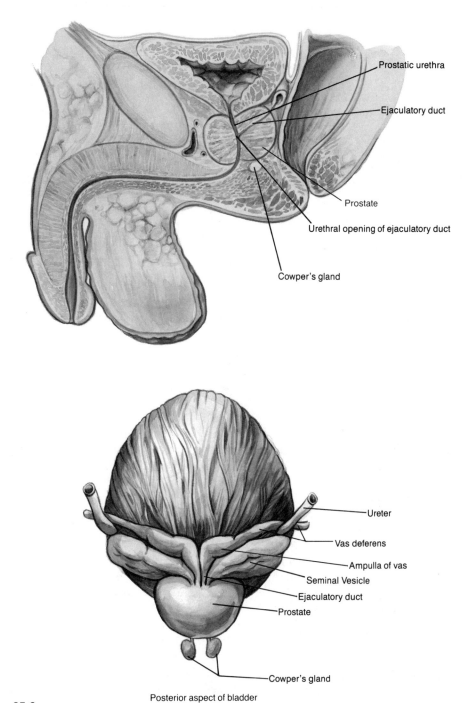

Prostatic urethra

Ejaculatory duct

Prostate

Urethral opening of ejaculatory duct

Cowper's gland

Ureter

Vas deferens

Ampulla of vas

Seminal Vesicle

Ejaculatory duct

Prostate

Cowper's gland

Posterior aspect of bladder

Figure 25-3
Relationship of vas deferens, seminal vesicles, ejaculatory ducts, and urethra and bladder in men.

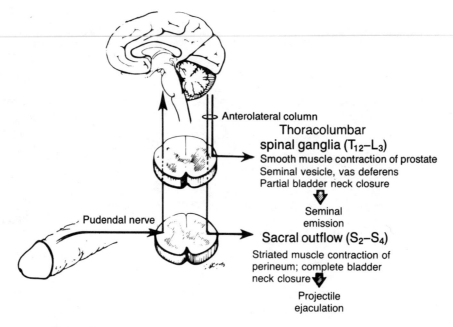

Figure 25-4

The physiology of ejaculation, shown schematically.

Reproduced, with permission, from Kedia K, Markland C: Effect of sympathectomy and drugs on ejaculation. In Sciarra JJ, Markland C, Speidel JJ (eds): Control of Male Fertility. Hagerstown, MD, Harper & Row, 1975, p 244.

tial closure of the bladder neck (Figure 25-4).[3] Ejaculation is completed by contractions of the bulbocavernous and ischiocavernous muscles. These muscles are controlled by the parasympathetic nerves, which are also responsible for complete closure of the bladder neck.

If the bladder neck does not close completely, as occurs in conditions such as diabetic neuropathy or after surgery of the bladder neck, the semen is partially or totally ejected into the bladder rather than through the penile urethra (retrograde ejaculation), and little or no visible ejaculate is produced. If the sympathetic pathway is interrupted by T_{12} to L_3 sympathectomy or by the action of a ganglionic blocking drug such as guanethidine, no semen at all may be produced (ejaculatory failure), because of lack of contraction of the vas deferens, prostate, and seminal vesicles. Erection occurs, however, and the sen-

sation of orgasm is retained owing to the contraction of the pelvic striated muscles.

Ejaculation is a sequential event. First, the prostatic fluid and contents of the distal vas deferens are ejected, followed by release of seminal vesicular secretions. If the ejaculate is carefully collected in two parts (split ejaculate), the first portion will usually contain primarily prostatic fluid and most of the spermatozoa; the second portion will contain primarily seminal vesicular fluid and relatively few sperm.

Semen

The semen consists of spermatozoa suspended in seminal plasma, which is composed mostly of secretions from the prostate and seminal vesicles, with some contribution from the proximal reproductive tract and bulbourethral (Cowper's) glands. The seminal plasma contains a number of chemical constituents—secreted largely by the seminal vesicles (fructose) or the prostate (acid phosphatase, citric acid, and zinc)—that can be measured to determine the relative contribution of these glands to the ejaculate. Seminal plasma has a regulatory effect on sperm metabolism and motility.[4,5] Alterations in its composition, because of infection or other factors, may immobilize the sperm or reduce their motility.

Semen coagulates during ejaculation, but usually liquefies within 15 to 30 minutes because of proteolytic enzymes in prostatic fluid. Liquefaction may be incomplete or fail to occur at all, and this may be associated with infertility.

Semen analysis

The semen analysis is a critical test in the evaluation of male fertility. Because the gametes of the male, unlike those of the female, are readily available for observation, considerable information can be obtained from a properly performed analysis. What follows is a discussion of various aspects of the semen analysis and a description of some of the techniques that are used. More detailed descriptions are given by Belsey and co-authors and Eliasson.[6,7]

Procedure

Timing
The period of abstinence required to obtain an optimal semen analysis is debatable. Some andrologists recommend as long as 5 to 7 days, but we usually allow a more practical interval of 2 to 3 days. If the sexual history reveals frequent emissions from coitus or masturbation, a comparison should be made between samples collected at the patient's usual ejaculatory frequency and after several days of abstinence. Frequent ejaculations will reduce the sperm count in some men. In such cases, semen quality can be improved by decreasing ejaculatory frequency.

Because the sperm count may vary widely with time, it is important to obtain more than one semen analysis. If the count is low or borderline, at least three samples should be analyzed to determine the trend of semen quality. We prefer to obtain analyses at monthly intervals, because a short-term illness may cause a transient decrease in sperm count.

Collection
The specimen should be collected by masturbation into a clean, wide-mouthed jar. The container does not have to be sterile, unless cultures are to be taken. Care should be used to collect the entire specimen. It should not be collected by coitus interruptus, because part of the sample may be lost or contaminated by material from the vagina.

If masturbation is unacceptable to the patient, the specimen may be collected with a polyethylene condom. Ordinary condoms should not be used because they may contain chemicals that immobilize sperm. The patient should be instructed to wipe the outside of the condom before removing it, invert it over the collection jar, and milk the entire specimen into the container.

Part of the specimen should be observed to assess sperm motility as soon as possible after liquefaction, which usually occurs 15 to 30 minutes after ejaculation. Ideally, semen should be collected in the office or laboratory to permit rapid observation. If this is not possible, the sample should be observed for sperm motility within 2 hours and preferably within 1 hour after collection. Sperm motility normally begins to decline after 2 hours.

Semen should not be exposed to extreme changes in temperature before analysis. If the semen is collected at home during cold weather, the specimen should be kept warm during transport to the laboratory. The patient can do this by placing the sample jar inside the waistband of his or his partner's clothing, so that the jar is held against the body. The sample should be evaluated as soon as it is delivered.

Observations and techniques

The initial part of the semen analysis can be performed in a short time. After the semen has liquefied, it is mixed by gentle rotary motion, and a wet mount is made by placing a drop of semen on a slide and covering it with a coverslip. This is examined at once to evaluate sperm motility as described below. The technician then transfers the specimen into a graduated centrifuge tube by means of a Pasteur pipette or draws it into a calibrated syringe to determine its volume. This should be done gently to avoid foaming. The viscosity is noted when the specimen is transferred, and the semen remaining on the tip of the pipette or syringe is placed on indicator paper to determine the pH. Then the specimen is mixed again, and 0.1 mL is drawn into a calibrated pipette and transferred to a 2-mL volumetric flask to be diluted with 1% formalin for the sperm count. A small drop of semen is transferred to a slide and a thin smear is made. The smear is air-dried and used to evaluate sperm morphology.

Viscosity

Viscosity is rated subjectively as either well liquefied (flows freely from pipette or syringe), moderately viscous, or very viscous (specimen tends to remain in one piece and cannot be pipetted).

Motility

Sperm motility is evaluated in terms of proportion of motile sperm and quality of motility. The wet mount is scanned at $100\times$ magnification to gain a general impression of sperm density and motility and to observe agglutination and the presence of extraneous cells or material. The percentage of motile sperm is estimated by observing five to 10 fields at $400\times$ magnification.

Quality of sperm motility refers to the rapidity of sperm movements and the presence or absence of progressive motility. A number of rating systems are used. In our laboratory, very rapid forward motility is rated 4+; rapid forward motility, 3+; sluggish forward motility or rapid tailbeat without forward motility, 2+; and sluggish tailbeat without forward motility, 1+.

A second wet mount is examined after the specimen is 4 hours old to determine whether sperm motility has rapidly declined or delayed agglutination has occurred. This second observation is valuable, because such changes may indicate the presence of infected semen, sperm antibodies, or other abnormalities of the spermatozoa or seminal plasma.

Live-dead stain

If fewer than 50% of the sperm are motile at the time the specimen is initially evaluated, a live-dead stain is performed (modified after the technique of Eliasson[8]) to determine whether the nonmotile sperm are alive or dead. One drop of eosin Y (50 mg in 10 mL of 0.15 M phosphate buffer, pH 7.4) is mixed with a drop of semen in a depression tray or small tube, and a sample is examined at $400\times$ magnification with a phase-contrast microscope. The stained sperm are considered to be dead. Live sperm, whether motile or nonmotile, do not take up the stain.

Sperm count

A portion of the sample is diluted to an appropriate volume, and the sperm are counted in a counting chamber. Alternatively, the sample may be directly counted without dilution in a Makler chamber.[9]

In the dilution method, a 0.1-mL sample of semen is diluted with 1% formalin in distilled water in a 2-mL volumetric flask. The flask is shaken well and a sample placed into a hemacytometer. After the sperm have settled onto the grid, they are counted in the five squares used to count red blood cells. When the semen has been diluted 1:20, the number of sperm in the five squares is multiplied by 10^6 to determine the number of sperm per cubic milliliter.

Viscous specimens may be difficult to pipette accurately. In most instances, the viscosity can be reduced by forcibly ejecting the ejaculate two or three times from a syringe fitted with a 21-gauge needle, or the sample can be placed in a test tube and agitated on a vortex mixer.

Table 25-1
Criteria for morphologic evaluation of human spermatozoa

Parameter	Length (μm)	Width (μm)	Remarks
Normal dimensions			
Head	3.0–5.0	2.0–3.0	Regular oval shape; borderline forms must be counted as normal
Midpiece	5.0–7.0	≈1.0	
Tail	≈45.0		
Abnormal heads			
Too large	>5.0	>3.0	As long as shape approximates oval, count primarily according to size (large, small, tapering)
Too small	<3.0	<2.0	
Tapering	>5.0	<3.0	
	<5.0	<2.0	
Amorphous			
Duplicate			
"Pear-shaped"			Counted as amorphous or tapering; regard borderline forms as normal
Abnormal midpiece		>2.0	Cytoplasmic droplet is included here when it is larger than half the sperm head; broken midpieces are abnormal
Tail defects			For example, broken or coiled tail (not bent nor asymmetric insertion)

From Eliasson R: Standards for investigation of human semen. Andrologie 3:49, 1971.

Sperm morphology

Various stains are recommended for semen smears. Papanicolaou's is excellent, but Wright's stain is sufficient for office use. In our institution, 100 to 200 cells are examined at 1,000× magnification and are classified (Table 25-1)[7] according to a modification of the systems of MacLeod[10] and Eliasson.[7] (See also Belsey.[6]) Sperm that appear abnormally large or small can be measured with an ocular micrometer.

Chemical studies

Seminal plasma is a complex mixture of chemical components from various parts of the male reproductive tract, as well as metabolites from spermatozoa. There have been many studies of the chemical composition of seminal plasma from humans and animals,[11] but there is little information about the significance of these measurements for the evaluation of male infertility.

Evaluation of relative amounts of fructose and acid phosphatase (or one of the other chem-

ical markers of prostatic fluid) may be helpful in diagnosing prostatitis or partial obstruction of the ejaculatory ducts. In azoospermia, the absence of fructose in the ejaculate suggests obstruction of the ejaculatory ducts or absence of the seminal vesicles. It has been suggested that levels of transferrin in seminal plasma reflect, in part, Sertoli-cell activity,[12] and that poor sperm motility may result from the absence or reduced activity of enzymes in the seminal plasma.

Chemical studies of the semen, apart from fructose measurement, are not usually done for other than research purposes. But there is promise that biochemical analyses of semen may eventually aid in the diagnosis and management of the infertile male.

Interpretation

There have been numerous efforts to define the normal limits of semen quality. Tables 25-2 and 25-3 show some recommendations.[13] There is a basic problem in dealing with semen-analysis

Table 25-2
Definitions recommended by the International Society of Andrology

-spermia	Referring to semen volume
Aspermia	No semen
Hypospermia	Volume < 2 mL
Hyperspermia	Volume > 6 mL
-zoospermia	Referring to spermatozoa in semen
Azoospermia	No spermatozoa in semen
Oligozoospermia	<40 million spermatozoa/mL
Polyzoospermia	>250 million spermatozoa/mL
Asthenozoospermia	Decreased motility of spermatozoa
Teratozoospermia	>40% abnormal spermatozoa

Table 25-3
Recommended standards for semen analysis

Parameter	Recommended normal value
Volume	2–6 mL
Viscosity	Full liquefaction within 60 minutes
Sperm density	†20–250 million/mL
Sperm motility	
Progressive	Good to very good*
Quantitation	First hour ≥60%, 2–3 hr ≥50%
Vital staining	≤35% dead cells
Sperm morphology	≥60% within normal configuration

*3–4+ quality in the USC laboratory.

†20 million/mL is low normal, USC lab in contrast to 40 million/mL, Int. Soc. of Andrology.

Modified from Eliasson R: Parameters of male fertility. In Hafez ESE, Evans TN (eds): Human Reproduction. New York, Harper & Row, 1973.

data that does not occur with other laboratory tests. Clinicians use laboratory tests to determine whether an organ or system is functioning normally. In semen evaluation, it is important not only to detect abnormal function but also to estimate fertility potential. At present, there is no agreement about whether the limits of normality should coincide with the limits of fertility or with the limits of normal function as usually determined by statistics from population studies.

The picture is further complicated by several factors related to the defining of fertility: (1) Fertility is a function of both partners and not the male alone. (2) There may be wide fluctuations in semen quality over a period of time, and the nature of the ejaculate that causes pregnancy usually is not known. (3) Fertility is a relative term applied not only to whether pregnancy is achieved, but also to the time required to achieve it. (4) The semen analysis does not measure all of the functional properties of spermatozoa. The following should be read with these considerations in mind.

Semen quality and male fertility

Sperm count and motility
Statistical data and clinical experience indicate that a count of 20 million sperm/mL is the lower limit for "normal fertility," provided that sperm motility is good. Yet there is a reasonable probability of conception with good motility even when the count is as low as 10 million/mL. Motility is an important factor, because nonmotile sperm do not enter the cervical mucus and do not penetrate the ovum.

Morphology
There is no definite proportion of abnormal forms associated with infertility, but with greater than 40% abnormal forms, fertility is probably reduced. Abnormal spermatozoa do not penetrate cervical mucus well, because the mucus is organized into channels that are too small to admit grossly enlarged or deformed sperm. Abnormal spermatozoa most commonly seen in the cervical mucus are those with very small or round rather than oval heads. These sperm are considered incapable of fertilizing eggs because they lack acrosomes. Abnormal morphology is frequently, but not always, associated with low sperm counts and poor sperm motility. It may also be a primary factor when other measurements are normal.

Volume
Very small or very large semen volume may be associated with infertility. However, this finding is not necessarily a causal factor.

Immature forms

Immature spermatozoa (spermatogonia, spermatocytes, or spermatids) in the ejaculate indicate a disorder in spermatogenesis in which the developing germ cells are sloughed prematurely from the germinal epithelium.

Other cells

The presence of white blood cells (pyospermia) or red blood cells (hemospermia) in the semen may indicate infection of the prostate or other portions of the male tract.

Agglutination

Spontaneous agglutination suggests that there are sperm-agglutinating antibodies in the seminal plasma or that the semen is infected. Agglutination of small numbers of sperm, particularly around clumps of cells or debris or in very dense suspensions, is usually not a significant finding.

Live-dead stain

When all or most of the sperm in an ejaculate are nonmotile, it is important to determine whether the nonmotile sperm are alive (akinesis) or dead (necrozoospermia). It may be possible to reactivate the live nonmotile sperm.

Viscosity

In some instances, semen may fail to liquefy and will remain highly viscous. High-viscosity seminal plasma slows sperm motility and may impair the movement of sperm into the cervical mucus. The importance of this factor as a cause of infertility is not known, but the viscosity can be altered if no other abnormality is present.

In general, sperm with normal morphology and good, progressive motility have the best chance of penetrating cervical mucus and eventually fertilizing an ovum. In this respect, the most important factor in the semen analysis is the number of sperm with normal motility and morphology.

Other functional properties of spermatozoa

The following discussion deals with functional properties of spermatozoa that cannot be evaluated by the semen analysis.

Sperm-cervical mucus interaction

Several in vitro tests can evaluate the ability of spermatozoa to migrate through cervical mucus. For clinical evaluation, the most commonly used test is the fractional postcoital test (PCT). The PCT is an important adjunct to the semen analysis. Its outcome depends on semen quality and the inherent ability of the sperm to enter and move through the mucus, as well as the state of the mucus. Male factors that may contribute to a poor PCT are azoo- or oligozoospermia, teratozoospermia, poor sperm motility, low semen volume, infection, sperm antibodies, ejaculatory disturbances, or faulty coital technique.

Assuming that the cervical mucus is of good quality and the test is performed at the appropriate time of the menstrual cycle, the relationship between the PCT and the semen analysis may be interpreted as follows:

GOOD PCT AND NORMAL SEMEN ANALYSIS. This is the expected result. If pregnancy does not occur, there may be an undiagnosed female factor or the fertilizing capacity of the spermatozoa may be impaired.

GOOD PCT AND POOR SEMEN ANALYSIS. One cause of this outcome is a variable sperm count; there may have been adequate numbers of sperm on the day of the PCT, but poor semen quality at most other times. The PCT may be adequate with counts as low as 10 to 20 million sperm/mL, or even less, if sperm motility is good.

It is important to note the morphology of the sperm in the cervical mucus. If there are large numbers of spermatozoa with round or pin heads, the test should be considered abnormal, because these sperm are incapable of fertilizing ova.

POOR PCT AND POOR SEMEN ANALYSIS. The male partner should be evaluated and treated as indicated below. AIH may be useful.

POOR PCT AND NORMAL SEMEN ANALYSIS. This may be due to a male or female factor. Either partner may have sperm antibodies. Occasionally, a man with sperm antibodies may have normal-appearing semen, with a poor PCT as the only sign of the problem. Acid cervical mucus can also cause poor sperm migration. Diagnostic tests include sperm antibody studies and measurement of the pH of the mucus. If these are normal, crossed in vitro testing (husband's sperm versus donor mucus and donor sperm versus wife's mucus) may be necessary to determine whether the problem lies with the sperm or the cervical mucus.

Fertilizing capacity

The development of techniques for acquiring human ova and performing in vitro fertilization (IVF) has made it possible to evaluate the interaction between human gametes. At present, it is not practical to use these techniques for routine testing of fertilizing capacity of human sperm. It is possible, however, to estimate fertilizing capacity by means of an assay using eggs from the golden hamster instead of human ova.[14] Normal human sperm will penetrate ova from these animals after the zona pellucida has been removed. The test is performed in the USC laboratories[15] in the following manner:

Semen samples are washed twice by centrifugation for 10 minutes at $160 \times g$ in two volumes of modified Ham's F-10 culture medium (HF-10). Sperm are resuspended to a concentration of 10^7 motile cells/mL in HF-10 and are incubated for 3 hours in 5% CO_2 in air at 37°C before being added to the ova.

Eggs are obtained by superovulating the animals and dissecting the cumulus masses from the oviducts. The cumulus cells are dispersed with hyaluronidase (0.1% for 5 minutes). The eggs are washed twice in HF-10, and the zonae pellucidae are removed with trypsin (0.1% for 1.5 to 2 minutes). The eggs are then washed three times in HF-10 and transferred in a volume of 15 μL to a small (15 × 35 mm) tissue culture dish. Then 100 μL of washed sperm are added and the gametes are incubated for 5 hours in 5% CO_2 in air at 37°C.

After incubation, the ova are washed twice, placed on slides, and compressed by a coverslip mounted on a support of Vaseline-paraffin. The ova are fixed, stained, and examined microscopically (400×, phase-contrast optics) for evidence of sperm penetration. In the USC laboratory, the minimum proportion of eggs penetrated by sperm from fertile donors is 15%.

A number of variables can influence the outcome of the test (Table 25-4). However, when appropriate techniques are used, differences are apparent when sperm from fertile and infertile men are tested. There is reasonable, but not perfect, correlation between the outcome of this test and the ability of sperm to actually fertilize human ova in vitro.

An abnormal hamster-egg penetration test suggests a defect of the spermatozoa or an abnormality of the seminal plasma. At present, this test is primarily useful for: (1) helping to determine, in some cases, the etiology of otherwise unexplained infertility; and (2) influencing decisions on performing or repeating AIH. Many abnormal assays cannot yet be explained, but the test should become more useful for diagnosis and management when more data are collected.

Table 25-4
Factors influencing outcome
of sperm penetration assay

Time of sperm preincubation
Time of incubation of sperm with ova
Sperm concentration
Time sperm reside in seminal plasma before first washing
Presence of leukocytes in semen

Etiology of male infertility

A number of schemes have been proposed to categorize the etiologic factors in male infertility. One scheme, described below, identifies anatomic, endocrine, genetic, inflammatory, idiopathic, immunologic, and exogenous factors.

Anatomic factors include varicocele (varicosities or incompetence of the spermatic veins), cryptorchidism, and congenital anomalies. Common congenital anomalies include hypospadias, epispadias, congenital testicular hypoplasia or aplasia, partial or total absence of the vas deferens, failure of the vas to join the epididymis, and localized atresia of the vas. A spermatocele (an intrascrotal sperm-containing cyst) can partially obstruct the tubular system.

Endocrine factors in male infertility include such hypogonadotropic states as gigantism or dwarfism, acromegaly, Cushing's disease, isolated gonadotropin deficiency, pituitary tumor or pituitary failure, and hypogonadotropic hypogonadism. Hypothyroidism or hyperthyroidism may also be involved. Testicular failure may be idiopathic in "hypergonadotropic" states or secondary (genetic, posttraumatic, or postinflammatory). A case of an enzymatic defect in T synthesis has been reported.[16] Androgen receptor deficiency may also be an etiologic factor.

Among the genetic factors, abnormalities in sex chromatin, including Klinefelter's syndrome (47,XXY), may be present. Not all patients with 47,XXY have the clinical findings of Klinefelter's syndrome. Other genetic anomalies associated with infertility include XXXY, XXXXY, XXYY, XX/XXY, and XY/XXY patterns. Autosomal translocations should also be considered.

Inflammatory conditions may cause infertility. Orchitis may be the result of mumps, tuberculosis, syphilis, or pancreatitis. Epididymitis from tuberculosis, gonorrhea, *Chlamydia trachomatis*, and other bacterial or nonbacterial inflammations should be considered. Prostatitis can be caused by a variety of bacteria and possibly other agents. Seminal vesiculitis can result from tuberculosis, *Trichomonas vaginalis,* and other organisms. Urethritis may be caused by gonorrhea, *T. vaginalis, Ureaplasma urealyticum, C. trachomatis,* and other organisms. Elevation of temperature from any cause can produce a transient suppression of spermatogenesis.

The possibility of idiopathic infertility factors—Sertoli-cell-only syndrome (germinal-cell aplasia), maturation arrest, and hypospermatogenesis—should not be overlooked. The last two are histologic diagnoses and are discussed later in this chapter.

Immunologic factors, i.e., autoimmune reactions, may be involved. The seminal plasma and blood may contain sperm-agglutinating or sperm-immobilizing antibodies. Immune reactions against testicular tissue may also occur, as in leprosy.

Exogenous factors are known to cause infertility. Many drugs have been implicated: antihypertensives, including thiazide diuretics and α- and β-adrenergic receptor-blocking agents; cimetidine; antipsychotic drugs; tricyclic antidepressants; CNS depressants, including cannabis and heroin; hormones (T, estrogen, and progestational agents); nitrofurantoin; and anticancer drugs.[17] Sources of radiation, including x-rays, isotopes, and microwaves, and toxic substances, such as metals and dyes, may be involved. Alcohol may have an indirect effect by altering hepatic metabolism of steroid hormones. It may also have a direct toxic effect on the testes.

Mechanical damage, such as trauma or torsion of the testes, injuries to the vas deferens or spermatic artery during hernia repair, or disruption of nerves and ejaculatory ducts during prostatectomy, may result in sexual dysfunction.

Other factors may produce ejaculatory dysfunction. Retrograde ejaculation (i.e., ejaculation of semen into the urinary bladder) may be secondary to diabetic neuropathy, or may follow prostatectomy or surgery of the bladder neck. Ejaculatory failure (orgasm without ejaculation and without evidence of retrograde ejaculation)

Table 25-5
Etiology of semen abnormalities

Finding	Etiology
Abnormal count	
Azoospermia	Klinefelter's syndrome or other genetic disorders
	Sertoli-cell-only syndrome
	Seminiferous tubule or Leydig cell failure
	Hypogonadotropic hypogonadism
	Ductal obstruction, including Young's syndrome[18]
	Varicocele
	Exogenous factors
Oligozoospermia	Genetic disorder
	Endocrinopathies, including androgen receptor defects[19]
	Varicocele and other anatomic disorders
	Maturation arrest
	Hypospermatogenesis
	Exogenous factors
Abnormal volume	
No ejaculate	Ductal obstruction
	Retrograde ejaculation
	Ejaculatory failure
	Hypogonadism
Low volume	Obstruction of ejaculatory ducts
	Absence of seminal vesicles and vas deferens
	Partial retrograde ejaculation
	Infection
High volume	Unknown factors
Abnormal motility	Immunologic factors
	Infection
	Varicocele
	Defects in sperm structure[20]
	Metabolic or anatomic abnormalities of sperm
	Poor liquefaction of semen
Abnormal viscosity	Etiology unknown
Abnormal morphology	Varicocele
	Stress
	Infection
	Exogenous factors
	Unknown factors
Extraneous cells	Infection or inflammation
	Shedding of immature sperm

can be due to sympathectomy, lymphadenectomy, or ganglionic blocking drugs.

Psychological factors may be the cause of impotence, premature ejaculation, and stress. Faulty coital technique may also be a factor in infertility. Infrequent or too frequent coitus, poor coital timing, and lack of vaginal penetration may all impair fertility. The use of lubricants or postcoital douching may also affect fertility. The relationship between semen abnormalities and the disorders described above is shown in Table 25-5.

Patient evaluation

The evaluation of the male infertility patient includes a history, physical examination, semen analysis, and various other laboratory tests. These procedures are incorporated into a step-by-step systematic workup as shown in Figure 25-5. Such a scheme is helpful when explaining the steps in the evaluation and the possible therapies to the patient. It is also useful for the physician in categorizing patients and following the progress of workups. The scheme divides patients into three groups, depending upon when the diagnosis can be made. Patients diagnosed on the basis of the initial evaluation are in group I; those diagnosed after a laboratory test series are in group II; those requiring testicular biopsy and possibly a vasogram are in group III. Each group is subdivided further according to available therapeutic measures—specific or nonspecific—or lack of currently available treatment.

History

The history should include information about the patient's general health and problems specifically related to the genitourinary tract. The patient should be asked about past reproductive performance and the fertility of his current and past sex partners, sexual history, age at puberty, history of exposure to radiation or other toxic factors, genitourinary or other surgery, testicular trauma, and urogenital anomalies or infection. Past and present illnesses, use of medications, and smoking and drinking habits should also be ascertained.

Physical examination

This should include a general examination and evaluation of the secondary sexual characteristics, hair distribution, gynecomastia, and measurement of height, span, and body weight.

Examination of the genitalia

The testes should be measured with calipers or with a device that estimates testicular volume. The normal testis is at least 3.5 cm in length (range, 3.5 to 5.5) × 2.6 cm (range, 2.1 to 3.2) from side to side. Care should be taken not to include the epididymis in the measurement. The consistency, shape, and location of the testes should also be noted.

The epididymides should be palpated for evidence of thickening, tenderness, or masses. The cord should be observed and palpated for a varicocele. A large varicocele should be visible, but a small one can sometimes be seen or felt only when the patient performs a Valsalva maneuver. The vas should also be palpated.

The penis should be observed for size, skin lesions, position of urethral meatus, evidence of poor hygiene, and urethral discharge. The prostate should be examined for size, consistency, shape, and tenderness, then massaged to obtain secretions for microscopic examination.

The seminal vesicles, located cephalad to the prostate, are not ordinarily palpable unless they are diseased. To evaluate these glands, the examiner should reach above the prostate with the rectal finger while elevating the bladder by means of the other hand on the abdomen.

Laboratory studies

These can be divided into general tests; tests for endocrine, genetic, and immunologic factors; microbiologic studies; and other, special purpose studies. General laboratory tests are done for almost all patients; the other tests should be used selectively, as discussed below. Table 25-6 gives a brief summary of some indications for the various types of tests.[21]

General tests

The general laboratory tests include: complete blood count, urinalysis, serologic test for syphilis, and a biochemical profile including liver function tests.

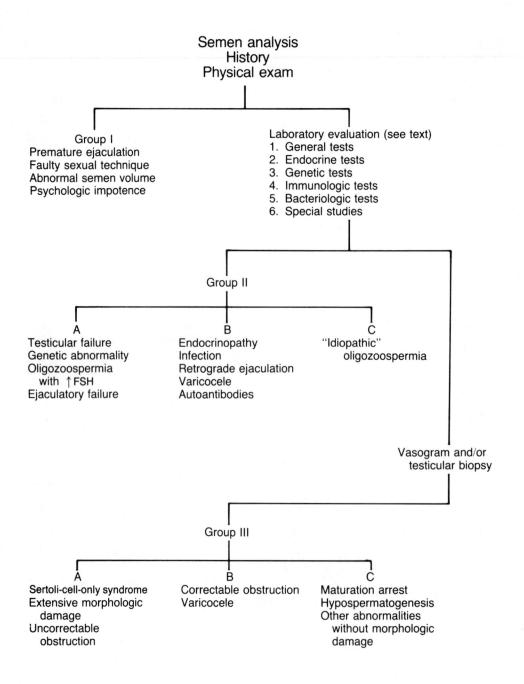

Figure 25-5
Systematic approach to evaluation of the male infertility patient. Subgroups: A, no therapy currently available to restore fertility; B, specific therapy can be used to correct pathology; C, only nonspecific therapy currently available.

Table 25-6
Indications for various types of diagnostic tests

Findings	Recommended tests
Most patients	General laboratory evaluation
Sperm count $< 40 \times 10^6$/mL	Endocrine evaluation
Sperm count $< 20 \times 10^6$/mL Teratozoospermia Partner has recurrent abortion	Genetic studies
Sperm agglutination Poor motility Poor cervical mucus penetration	Immunologic studies Microbiologic studies
Inflammatory or red blood cells in semen	Bacteriologic studies

Modified from Eliasson R: Semen analysis and laboratory work-up. In Cockett ATK, Urry RL (eds): Male Infertility: Work-up, Treatment, and Research. *New York, Grune and Stratton, 1977.*

Endocrine tests

The endocrine tests include TSH for the evaluation of subclinical hypothyroidism; serum T for testicular function; and serum FSH, LH, and prolactin for pituitary function. Other tests should be done as clinically indicated.

The endocrine evaluation should be done on all patients with either oligozoospermia or azoospermia—even if other pathology is present that could be responsible for the abnormal semen analysis. For example, a patient with a varicocele should be carefully evaluated before it is assumed that the varicocele is causing the seminal abnormality. The same is true for a patient with prostatitis whose semen does not improve after antibiotic therapy.

If any test suggests abnormal function of the hypothalamus, pituitary, or testes, further evaluation is required. To evaluate the status of T and the gonadotropins critically, more than one blood sample is needed. Otherwise, errors may occur because of the pulsatile release of the hormones. A simple method is to draw three blood samples 10 to 20 minutes apart and determine the hormone levels in a pool made of aliquots from all three specimens. More extensive laboratory testing, such as with GnRH and human chorionic gonadotropin (hCG) stimulation, may be needed in some cases but is not indicated in the initial evaluation. The androgen receptor assay may be of value in detecting the cause of some cases of "idiopathic" oligozoospermia, as discussed below.

Genetic studies

A karyotype should be done when the patient's sperm count is consistently below 10 million/mL, there is severe teratozoospermia, or the patient's partner has a history of recurrent abortion. The karyotype should include chromosome banding to detect translocations and other subtle structural abnormalities.

Immunologic studies

We use the gelatin agglutination (Kibrick) test and the sperm immobilization (Isojima) test to screen for sperm antibodies. Indications for the tests are poor sperm motility, sperm agglutination, or sperm that demonstrate a rapid decline in motility or poor ability to penetrate cervical mucus. Men who have had a vasectomy and a subsequent vasovasostomy should also be evaluated for sperm antibodies. About 60% to 70% of vasectomized men develop sperm-agglutinating and/or sperm-immobilizing antibodies. While the amount of antibody may decline with time, enough may remain after reconstructive surgery to impair sperm function.

Microbiologic studies

The patient's semen should be cultured if there is any suggestion of infection in the semen analysis. Patients with prostatitis may be asymptomatic; the first diagnostic clue may be the semen analysis and not the clinical history. If any prostatic fluid is obtained during examination of the prostate gland, it should also be cultured. There is generally good agreement between the results of cultures obtained from semen and those obtained from prostatic fluid, but occasionally one site may be positive while the other is negative. One negative culture does not rule out infection; multiple cultures may be needed for a diagnosis.

The semen should be cultured initially for aerobic organisms and *Neisseria gonorrhoeae*. Many other organisms may infect the male tract, including *T. vaginalis, U. urealyticum, Gardnerella vaginalis, C. trachomatis,* and possibly anaerobic organisms. It is not feasible to culture for all of these initially, because of the expense. However, if the patient has a history of nongonococcal urethritis, the semen should be evaluated for the presence of *Chlamydia* and *Ureaplasma,* since these organisms are frequently involved.

It is also important to evaluate the patient's partner, because she may harbor the same organism as he carries in his semen. In fact, if she has vaginitis, the findings may provide a clue to the male's problem. Most types of vaginitis can be sexually transmitted. If both partners are infected, both must be treated to achieve a cure.

Other tests

Examination of the urine for spermatozoa (associated with retrograde ejaculation) and in vitro cervical mucus penetration tests should be performed when indicated. Some andrologists recommend that studies such as venography or ul-trasonography be used to diagnose subclinical varicoceles. The current consensus is that these and similar studies have not yet been proven useful in clinical management.

Testicular biopsy and vasography

These two studies should be performed in cases of azoospermia or severe oligozoospermia when a diagnosis cannot be made from the initial examinations and laboratory tests. Both testes should be sampled by open biopsy. During the procedure, the epididymis should be examined for any evidence of partial obstruction due to epididymitis. If the patient is azoospermic, the surgeon must make certain that the vas deferens is continuous with the epididymis. A vasogram should be done in all cases of azoospermia or persistent, severe oligozoospermia ($<20 \times 10^6$ cells/mL) requiring testicular biopsy.

The classification scheme for testicular biopsies used in our institution is shown in Table 25-7. Other patterns may also occur, including thickening of the basement membrane of the seminiferous tubules, premature sloughing of the germinal epithelium, and focal abnormalities in an otherwise normal testis.

Patient management

Group I patients

Patients are placed in group I (Figure 25-5) if they have premature ejaculation, faulty sexual technique, high or low semen volume that can be managed by AIH, or a congenital anomaly that prevents deposition of semen into the vagina. Patients with psychological impotence can also be placed in this group. However, since impotence may also result from hypogonadism secondary to a pituitary tumor, some endocrine evaluation is required to rule out an organic lesion. Patients in group I require counseling or psychiatric care, AIH, or surgical repair of the anatomic abnormality.

Table 25-7
Classification of testicular biopsies

Normal testes: Suggests obstruction of duct system distal to testis

Hypospermatogenesis: All elements of germinal epithelium are present, but uniformly reduced in quantity

Germinal cell or maturation arrest: Spermatogenesis proceeds up to particular cell types, and few cells develop beyond that point

Sertoli-cell-only (germinal cell aplasia): Seminiferous tubules lined only by Sertoli cells; other elements of germinal epithelium absent

Seminiferous tubule hyalinization

Immature testes: Pattern seen in hypogonadotropic hypogonadism or in prepubertal testis

Group II patients

Patients in group II are divided into subgroups A, B, and C, depending on the type of therapy available to manage their problem (Figure 25-5).

Group IIA

There is no treatment available that will achieve fertility for men in this group, who have azoospermia or persistent oligozoospermia and cannot achieve a pregnancy by AIH or IVF. AID is required for pregnancy in these cases; although if any normal, motile sperm are present, the patient should not be considered sterile.

Group IIB

A patient is placed in this group if specific therapy is available for his problem. Thyroid disease and treatable gonadal or pituitary disorders are relatively rare causes of male infertility, but specific therapy is available for these conditions. Infection can be treated with antibiotics as indicated by culture and sensitivity tests.

The sulfamethoxazole-trimethoprim combination (one double-strength tablet twice daily until cultures are negative) is excellent for the treatment of most cases of prostatitis caused by gram-negative enteric organisms, but the sensitivity of the infecting organism must be considered. Patients should be treated until the semen culture is negative. This may require treatment for 10 days to 6 weeks or longer with sulfamethoxazole-trimethoprim, and for as long as several

months with other antibiotics. The semen quality may not improve until a month or more after treatment is stopped. Permanent obstruction of the ejaculatory ducts secondary to infection may have to be treated surgically.

In cases of retrograde ejaculation, sperm may be recovered from the bladder and used for AIH. Medical therapy with sympathomimetic drugs has been used for this condition, but there are insufficient data to indicate its effectiveness.

A varicocele should be treated by high ligation of the internal spermatic vein, if it is considered to be the etiologic factor for the abnormal semen analysis.

Several types of treatment have been used for men with autoantibodies. Suppression of spermatogenesis with high doses of T (100 mg of testosterone propionate or cypionate IM once a week for 20 weeks) has been used to reduce the antigenic stimulus. Although some pregnancies have occurred after cessation of therapy, it is unclear whether they were due to the treatment or occurred by chance. This mode of therapy has been abandoned. At present, the most commonly used treatment regimen is oral administration of a high dose (96 mg) of methylprednisolone daily for 7 to 10 days. Pregnancies have also occurred with this treatment, but the drug has not been tested in randomized, double-blind trials.

The initial laboratory and other evaluations do not always reveal the etiology of seminal abnormality. In some cases, testicular biopsy and vasography will result in a definitive diagnosis, but in others they will not provide information useful for selecting a treatment method. For example, oligozoospermic patients with elevated FSH most likely have untreatable damage to the germinal epithelium and Sertoli cells. With our present state of knowledge, biopsy is generally not recommended for these patients. The use of testicular biopsy for patients with oligozoospermia and an otherwise normal laboratory evaluation is discussed below.

Group IIC

Evaluations of oligozoospermic men often fail to reveal the cause of the abnormal semen. This reflects the current lack of basic information on spermatogenesis and the mechanisms controlling the process. As often happens in such situations, a large number of treatment regimens have been devised, including therapy with various medications as well as AIH. Pregnancies have occurred during or after various treatments, but in most cases a causal relationship has not been proven. Most of the treatment modalities have not been tested in controlled, double-blind studies, and their efficacy is unknown. Pregnancy rates seldom exceed 25% to 30%—no better than the spontaneous pregnancy rate among couples with oligozoospermia as the apparent major infertility factor. The spontaneous pregnancy rate may be improved without any medication if the couples are given reassurance and are instructed to have coitus more frequently near the time of ovulation.

When improvement in sperm count is used as an end point, normal variations in the semen analysis make it difficult to assess the results of therapy. More critical work is required to evaluate the various types of treatment adequately.

We manage patients with idiopathic oligozoospermia as follows: Artificial insemination is performed as described below. If pregnancy does not occur, the patient is offered nonspecific medical therapy, preferably after a testicular biopsy has been performed.

Artificial insemination, homologous (AIH)

We use artificial insemination with the husband's (homologous) semen as the initial nonspecific management in cases of oligozoospermia. The methods that can be used are: cup insemination, intracervical insemination, and intrauterine insemination (IUI). In the past we have favored the insemination cup, but we now use IUI with washed sperm in almost all cases.

Cup insemination

If this method is used, a PCT should be done at the initial insemination after the cup has been in place for about 2 hours. The PCT will demonstrate whether the cup insemination procedure improves sperm transport.

Intracervical insemination

Sperm are deposited in the endocervical canal in this procedure. The sperm may be concentrated by centrifugation, with or without washing, or the first part of a split ejaculate may be used.

Intrauterine insemination (IUI)

We now use IUI with washed sperm as the method of choice for dealing with suboptimal semen. This technique permits the concentration of spermatozoa into a small volume so that all the sperm harvested by centrifugation can be placed within the uterus.

With this technique, little seminal plasma is placed into the uterine cavity, thereby minimizing the chance of uterine cramping or immunization against seminal proteins. The Ham's F-10 medium, in which the spermatozoa are suspended, often improves sperm motility. Centrifugation must be done under carefully controlled conditions, because sperm may be traumatized by high centrifugal forces. It is also important to ascertain whether sperm will sediment with the technique used.

Other measures in AIH

Theoretically, it should be possible to accumulate sperm from oligozoospermic men by freezing cells from a number of samples. Generally, these sperm do not tolerate the freezing procedure very well, and the techniques currently in use have given disappointing results.

Management of other idiopathic disorders

Disorders of volume

If the volume of the ejaculate is low (<2 mL) without apparent cause, AIH cup insemination or IUI may be used. In some instances, bethanechol (10 mg four times daily) may increase semen volume.[22]

Disorders of viscosity

There is no known treatment for an ejaculate that remains so thick that it can be picked up with forceps. If a specimen is partially liquefied, it is usually possible to reduce its viscosity by aspirating it into a 5-mL syringe and forcibly ejecting it once or twice through a 21-gauge needle, but this may have an adverse effect on sperm motility. Viscosity may also be reduced by allowing the semen to pass through a column of glass wool or by placing the sample in a test tube and agitating it on a vortex mixer. The sample may then be used for AIH.

Disorders of motility

The patient should be carefully evaluated for underlying causes of abnormal motility, such as infection or sperm antibodies. Other causes may be metabolic or ultrastructural abnormalities of the spermatozoa or abnormalities of the seminal plasma. Special facilities are required for the biochemical testing and electron microscopy required to detect these problems.

In some instances, motility may be improved by the addition of chemical stimulants, such as caffeine, arginine, or kinins, to the semen specimen, but the safety of these agents for clinical use has not been demonstrated. It is sometimes possible to concentrate sperm with good motility by one of various methods, such as collecting a split ejaculate, passing the semen through a column of glass wool, separating motile sperm in a density gradient, or separating the sperm from seminal plasma and resuspending them in Ham's F-10 solution as described above. The sperm can then be used for IUI. If washing does improve motility, this procedure should be used because of its simplicity.

Group III patients

Oligozoospermic or azoospermic patients with tissue damage are placed in group IIIA (Figure 25-5). A few patients with Sertoli-cell-only syndrome are also in this group. Generally, a presumptive diagnosis of Sertoli-cell-only syndrome can be made after physical examination (normal testes), laboratory evaluation (azoospermia, elevated FSH), and a careful history (no radiation exposure, chemotherapy, or other exogenous factors). In some cases, however, patients with this problem have a normal FSH and the diagnosis can be made only by biopsy. AID is the treatment of choice for patients in group IIIA, as it is for those in group IIA.

Group IIIB consists of patients with surgically correctable obstructions and also the rare patient with azoospermia due to a varicocele.

Patients are considered for inclusion in group IIIC if they have idiopathic oligozoospermia that cannot be managed by AIH. Our present regimen is to perform testicular biopsy and vasography on these patients. Medical therapy can be offered, as discussed below, if the testicular biopsy reveals maturation arrest, hypospermatogenesis, or other histologic abnormalities without evidence of tissue damage, and if the exploration and vasogram do not show any obstruction in the male tract. At present, the biopsy does not provide information about the type of medical therapy that might be successful. However, it does help determine when treatment is not indicated because of extensive tissue damage. Generally, when there is damage to the germinal epithelium, the FSH level is elevated, but this is not always the case.

Nonspecific medical therapy of idiopathic oligozoospermia

Many medications have been used for nonspecific treatment of oligozoospermia: clomiphene citrate, hMG, hCG, low doses of testosterone, high doses of testosterone (to induce azoospermia with the hope of a subsequent rebound increase in sperm count), adrenal corticosteroids, arginine, kinins, tamoxifen, testolactone, and other modalities.[23-25]

At present, none of these treatments has been proven effective by double-blind studies, and there are no criteria for selecting any one of them. Pregnancy rates as high as 50% have been obtained without any treatment in couples with an oligozoospermic male partner; thus, when a pregnancy does occur it is difficult to attribute it to treatment. For this reason, and because the drugs are expensive and may sometimes depress sperm production, it is recommended that nonspecific therapy be used only after complete evaluation of the patient and his partner and with close monitoring. The patient should be aware that there is no assurance the treatment will be effective. To properly evaluate their effects, the medications should be taken for at least 3 months. The agents used most often today are hCG, clomiphene citrate,[23] tamoxifen,[24] and testolactone.[25]

Clomiphene is a weak estrogen that may increase LH and FSH secretion, because of its ability to block the negative feedback of estrogen on the hypothalamus and pituitary. At doses of 50 or 25 mg daily, this drug may cause substantial increases in the gonadotropins and T, but not necessarily in the sperm count. Tamoxifen also blocks estrogen receptors, but is not estrogenic. It has an effect somewhat similar to clomiphene.

Testolactone is an aromatase inhibitor that reduces the production of E_2 by blocking the aromatization of T. The rationale for its use is the supposition that some infertile men may have increased levels of E_2 in the hypothalamus and/or testes and that treatment may alleviate this abnormality.

We offer clomiphene or tamoxifen to patients when they have requested medical therapy. While there have been some improvements in sperm counts and some pregnancies during therapy, it is difficult to become enthusiastic about nonspecific therapy without better evidence for its effectiveness. It is important to stress to the patients that use of these drugs for the treatment of male infertility is experimental.

A more promising approach is to develop techniques to find causes of oligozoospermia in cases now considered idiopathic. One lead is the finding that some men with very low counts or azoospermia have a reduction in androgen receptors (determined by measuring receptors in cultures of fibroblasts obtained from scrotal skin).[19] Some of these men had increased levels of T, LH, and, in some cases, E_2, but more than 40% of them had normal endocrine evaluations. Although the medical management of oligozoospermic men is not very satisfactory, research of this type promises some hope for the future. At present, IUI with washed sperm appears to be a more satisfactory approach.

The couple as a unit

Because fertility depends on the status of both partners, it is important not to abandon the evaluation of the female partner when the male is found to have a low sperm count or other semen abnormality. She may have unsuspected tubal disease, ovulatory dysfunction, or some other problem that, when corrected, will enhance the fertility potential of the couple—even when the semen is subnormal.[26] Occasionally, a cervical factor will be overlooked because a poor PCT will be attributed to the male.

Artificial insemination with donor semen (AID)

AID should be offered when the male partner has azoospermia, oligozoospermia, or other semen abnormalities that do not respond to therapy. When physicians discuss AID with patients, they must be certain that the male has been evaluated sufficiently to rule out a treatable cause of infertility. The attitudes of both partners toward AID and the state of the marital relationship are important factors to consider during counseling.

Donors

We generally recruit college students, interns and resident physicians, and other professionals of proven intelligence as semen donors. The donor must be in good health and have no family history of genetic diseases. He should not have had homosexual relationships because of the risk of transmitting acquired immune deficiency syndrome (AIDS). There is some variation in the extent of the workup for screening prospective donors. The minimum should include a medical and genetic history, a semen analysis, ABO/Rh blood type, serologic tests for syphilis and hepatitis-associated antigen, tests for antibodies to HTLV III (human T lymphocyte virus III), and semen culture for gonorrhea. Karyotyping with banding and more extensive microbiologic testing of the semen have also been recommended.

The donor is selected on the basis of race, resemblance to the male partner, and blood type to avoid the possibility of Rh incompatibility between mother and fetus. The couple is consulted regarding preferences for a donor of a particular religion or ethnic group. In some instances, a donor of the same blood group as the husband is requested, so the paternity of the child cannot be readily determined by blood typing, or there may be other specific requests.

The identities of the donor and couple are kept confidential, and they must remain unknown to each other for both medicolegal and ethical reasons.

Techniques

Either fresh or frozen semen may be used for insemination. Generally, fewer insemination cycles are needed to achieve a pregnancy when fresh semen is used. Nevertheless, most patients who readily conceive do so by the fourth insemination cycle, regardless of whether fresh or frozen semen is used. We prefer to use fresh semen, but frozen semen is convenient when logistic problems make it impossible to have both donor and patient available at the proper time.

Usually, the woman has had some evaluation before the male partner was tested. She should have a normal pelvic exam and demonstrate presumptive evidence of ovulation before AID. We do not evaluate the oviducts unless the patient's history or physical exam suggests tubal disease or if she fails to become pregnant after three or four properly timed insemination cycles. Additional testing should be done if the hysterosalpingogram is normal. If the patient is anovulatory or has irregular menses, she is given clomiphene to induce ovulation or make her menstrual cycles more predictable.

The patient is requested to record her basal body temperature (BBT) for two menstrual cycles, and insemination is timed for 1 or 2 days before the expected temperature rise. Insemination is repeated every second day until and including the day of the temperature rise. Usually, good timing can be achieved by using the BBT alone, but in some cases it is necessary to monitor follicle growth by ultrasound in order to determine the appropriate insemination time.

INSEMINATION WITH FRESH SEMEN. The insemination can be done with an insemination cup or by IUI with washed sperm. Most patients prefer IUI, because the other technique requires wearing a cup for several hours, then removing and cleaning it. If the IUI method will be used, the sperm should be washed soon after collection, because fertilizing capacity is maintained better in Ham's solution than in seminal plasma. With the cup technique, insemination should be done as soon as possible after the sample is collected and preferably within 1 hour. Otherwise, the fertilizing capacity of the sperm may decline.

If a cup is used, the adequacy of sperm transport should be determined at the first insemination by removing the cup after 1 or 2 hours and performing a PCT. This does not have an adverse effect; some patients become pregnant in the cycle in which the test is done. In subsequent inseminations, the patient wears the cup for about 4 hours and removes it at home.

INSEMINATION WITH FROZEN SEMEN. We prefer the freezing technique described by Steinberger and Smith, with some modifications, because of its simplicity and convenience.[27] The semen is transferred into a flask after a small sample is examined to assure it is normal. Glycerol is added to a final concentration of 10%, and the mixture is allowed to equilibrate for 10 minutes. The mixture is then put into screw-top plastic (Nunc) vials, with 0.3 to 0.5 mL in each. For 15 minutes, the vials are exposed to liquid nitrogen vapor by suspension above the fluid level in a liquid nitrogen storage tank. Then they are stored in the liquid nitrogen until the semen is needed. Before use, the vials are thawed at room temperature or 37°C, and a sample is observed for satisfactory recovery of sperm motility. Then, 1 mL of the semen is drawn into a syringe and discharged against the cervix. The cervix is allowed to bathe for 20 to 30 minutes in the seminal pool formed by the posterior blade of a speculum. Alternatively, the semen may be put into an insemination cup or into the endocervical canal.

Medicolegal issues

The status of children conceived by means of AID is regulated by the individual states and should be investigated at the state level. Both partners should sign an informed consent form. Many clinicians do not perform AID for unmarried women because of the potential for legal complications should the mother die, or because of their own ethical views. The donor and the recipient should remain anonymous, and care should be taken to prevent them from meeting by chance in the office. If a couple requests a designated donor (someone they know), legal contracts should be drawn to define the rights and responsibilities of the parties involved.

References

1. Lipshultz LI, Howards SS (eds): *Infertility in the Male.* New York, Churchill Livingstone, 1983

2. Ramasharna K, Sairan MR, Seidah NG, et al: Isolation, structure, and synthesis of a human seminal plasma peptide with inhibin-like activity. *Science* 223:1199, 1984

3. Sciarra JJ, Markland C, Speidel JJ (eds): *Control of Male Fertility.* Hagerstown, MD, Harper & Row, 1975

4. Trifunic NP, Bernstein GS: Inhibition of the oxidative metabolism of human spermatozoa by a heat-labile factor in seminal plasma. *Fertil Steril* 27:1295, 1976

5. Eliasson R, Johnson O, Lindholmer C: Effects of seminal plasma on some functional properties of human spermatozoa. In Mancini RE, Martini L (eds): *Male Infertility and Sterility.* New York, Academic Press, 1974, p 107

6. Belsey MA, Eliasson R, Gallegos AJ, et al (eds): *Laboratory Manual for the Examination of Human Semen and Semen-Cervical Mucus Interaction.* Singapore, Press Concern, 1980

7. Eliasson R: Standards for investigation of human semen. *Andrologia* 3:49, 1971

8. Eliasson R: Supravital staining of human spermatozoa. *Fertil Steril* 28:1257, 1977

9. Makler A: A new chamber for rapid sperm count and motility estimation. *Fertil Steril* 30:313, 1978

10. MacLeod J: The parameters of male fertility. *Hospital Practice* 8:43, 1973

11. Mann T, Lutwak-Mann C (eds): *Male Reproductive Function and Semen. Themes and Trends in Physiology, Biochemistry, and Investigational Andrology.* Berlin, Springer-Verlag, 1981

12. Holmes SD, Lipshultz LI, Smith RG: Transferrin and gonadal dysfunction in man. *Fertil Steril* 38:600, 1982

13. Eliasson R: Parameters of male fertility. In Hafez ESE, Evans TN (eds): *Human Reproduction.* New York, Harper & Row, 1973

14. Yanagimachi R, Yanagimachi H, Rogers BT: The use of zona-free animal ova as a test system for the assessment of the fertilizing capacity of human spermatozoa. *Biol Reprod* 15:471, 1976

15. Berger T, Marrs R, Saito H, et al: Factors affecting human sperm penetration of zona free hamster ova. *Am J Obstet Gynecol* 145:397, 1983

16. Steinberger E, Fisher M, Smith KD: An enzymatic defect in androgen biosynthesis in human testis: A case report and response to therapy. *Andrologia* 6:59, 1974

17. Drugs that cause sexual dysfunction. *Med Lett* 25:73, 1983

18. Handelsman DJ, Conway AJ, Boylan LM, et al: Young's syndrome. Obstructive azoospermia and chronic sinopulmonary infections. *N Engl J Med* 310:3, 1984

19. Aiman J, Griffin JE: The frequency of androgen receptor deficiency in infertile men. *J Clin Endocrinol Metab* 54:725, 1982

20. Eliasson R, Mussberg B, Camner P, et al: The immotile-cilia syndrome. *N Engl J Med* 297:1, 1977

21. Cockett ATK, Urry RL (eds): *Male Infertility: Work-up, Treatment, and Research.* New York, Grune and Stratton, 1977

22. Winer J: personal communication, 1983

23. Paulson DF: Clomiphene citrate in the management of male hypofertility: Predictors for treatment selection. *Fertil Steril* 28:1226, 1977

24. Vermeulen A, Comhaire F: Hormonal effects of an antiestrogen, tamoxifen, in normal and oligospermic men. *Fertil Steril* 29:320, 1978

25. Vigersky RA, Glass AR: The effect of testolactone (Teslac) on the pituitary-testicular axis in oligospermic men. *J Clin Endocrinol Metab* 52:897, 1981

26. Steinberger E, Rodriquez-Rigan LJ, Smith KD: The interaction between the fertility potentials of the two members of an infertile couple. In Frajese G, Hafez ESE, Conti C, et al (eds): *Oligozoospermia: Recent Progress in Andrology.* New York, Raven Press, 1981

27. Steinberger E, Smith KD: Artificial insemination with fresh or frozen semen. *JAMA* 223:778, 1973

Suggested reading

Bain J, Schill W-B, Schwartzstein L (eds): *Treatment of Male Infertility.* Berlin, Springer-Verlag, 1982

Bardin CW, Paulsen CA: The testes. In Williams RH (ed): *Textbook of Endocrinology.* Philadelphia, WB Saunders, 1981

Burger H, Dekretser D (eds): *The Testis.* New York, Raven Press, 1981

Hamilton DW, Greep RO (eds): *Handbook of Physiology,* vol V: *Male Reproductive System,* sec 7: *Endocrinology.* Washington DC, American Physiological Society, 1975

Jecht EW, Zeitler E (eds): *Varicocele and Male Infertility.* Berlin, Springer-Verlag, 1982

Negro-Vilar A (ed): *Male Reproduction and Fertility.* New York, Raven Press, 1983

Steinberger A, Steinberger E (eds): *Testicular Development, Structure, and Function.* New York, Raven Press, 1980

Troen P, Nankin HR (eds): *The Testis in Normal and Infertile Men.* New York, Raven Press, 1977

White RD: *Aspects of Male Infertility.* Baltimore, Williams & Wilkins, 1982

Chapter 26

Hysterosalpingography

John A. Richmond, M.D.

A hysterosalpingogram (HSG) is a radiographic examination of the endocervical canal, endometrial cavity, and the lumina of the fallopian tubes using a radiopaque contrast medium. The indications of the HSG are outlined in Table 26-1.

The HSG should be performed during the week following the last day of the menstrual period to avoid the possibility of irradiating an unsuspected pregnancy. A pelvic examination should immediately precede the HSG. If pelvic tenderness is present, the HSG should be delayed until after the patient has received a course of antibiotic therapy and the tenderness has resolved. This will help prevent an acute exacerbation of chronic salpingitis, which is the most important complication of the procedure. In the absence of the screening pelvic examination, the incidence of reactivating chronic salpingitis may be as high as 3.5%.[1] A course of doxycycline, 100 mg twice daily for 7 days, is recommended for treatment of pelvic tenderness. If tenderness persists after the antibiotic therapy, the patient should be evaluated with hysteroscopy and laparoscopy in lieu of the HSG.

In the patient with a previous history of salpingitis and no tenderness on pelvic examination, prophylactic treatment with doxycycline, 100 mg twice daily for 5 days, is recommended beginning 2 days before the scheduled HSG. If dilated fallopian tubes are demonstrated on the HSG, antibiotic prophylaxis has been found to be effective in reducing the incidence of acute salpingitis following the procedure.[2] A course of doxycycline, 100 mg twice daily for 5 days, is recommended as prophylactic treatment for dilated fallopian tubes.

The HSG should not be a prolonged or painful procedure. The use of a tenaculum should be avoided, and the speculum should be removed before the contrast medium is injected. We have successfully employed the Vacuum Uterine Cannula[3] for HSG procedures. However, this cannula is relatively expensive and must be carefully maintained to be used successfully. An inexpensive and disposable vacuum cannula is now available and is recommended for routine use. The new device, like the older one, is comfortable for the patient and produces no cervical trauma.

The vacuum cannula provides a satisfactory seal of the external os and allows the patient to change position easily. Occasionally, a metal cannula, pediatric Foley catheter, or other alternative device will be necessary. An infant feeding tube or an embryo transfer catheter can be used when cervical stenosis is present.

The examination should be performed using image-intensified fluoroscopy, which allows control in injecting the appropriate amount of contrast medium. Spot radiographs can then be obtained during early filling of the endometrial cavity and during filling of the fallopian tubes,

Table 26-1
Indications for the HSG

Infertility evaluation
Uterine factors (endometrial adhesions, polyps, submucous leiomyomas)
Tubal factors (chronic salpingitis, tuberculosis, tubal obstruction, salpingitis isthmica nodosa)

Evaluation of previous uterine or tubal surgery
Postoperative myomectomy or metroplasty, posthysteroscopic lysis of endometrial adhesions
Postoperative tubal reanastomosis or reimplantation, efficacy of tubal sterilization, postoperative salpingostomy, determination of proximal tubal length prior to tubal reanastomosis

Evaluation of abnormal uterine bleeding
Menometrorrhagia or menorrhagia (submucous leiomyomas, endometrial polyps, adenomyosis)
Hypomenorrhea or amenorrhea (Asherman's syndrome, endometrial tuberculosis)

Evaluation of recurrent abortion
Delineation of known uterine anomaly
Localization of intrauterine device

before intraperitoneal spill of the contrast medium. This technique ensures visualizing optimal detail of the endometrial cavity and fallopian tubes. Overhead radiographs are then obtained in anteroposterior and lateral projections to complete the study.

A water-soluble contrast medium is recommended, because this provides satisfactory delineation of the endometrial and tubal mucosa. This is particularly important in evaluating a patient with distal tubal obstruction. Besides the degree of tubal dilation, there is evidence that preservation of the mucosal folds (endosalpingeal plicae) in the distal portion of the tube is a factor in the success of subsequent surgery.[4] When an oil-based contrast medium is used, the tubal mucosa is obscured. There is also the possible complication of pulmonary oil embolization.[5] An increased pregnancy rate in infertile patients has been described following use of an oil-soluble contrast medium, as compared to use of a water-soluble medium.[6] However, the au-

thors of the report recommend use of the water-soluble medium for the diagnostic purpose of the HSG, followed by injection of the oily medium for an enhanced therapeutic effect.

The following series of HSGs demonstrates normal anatomy and a spectrum of pathologic conditions. All of the examinations were performed using Sinografin.

Normal radiographic anatomy

The endocervical canal may be relatively smooth or may contain prominent mucosal folds, the plicae palmatae.[7] The endometrial cavity is usually triangular, but occasionally may exhibit a T-shaped configuration. The fallopian tube consists of a thin proximal portion, which represents the interstitial segment and isthmus, and a more distended distal portion, representing the ampulla and fimbriated end. The distal portion contains longitudinal mucosal folds, the endosalpingeal plicae. Figure 26-1 shows many of the normal anatomic features.

Uterine lesions

Adhesions, submucous leiomyomas, and polyps are demonstrated by endocervical or endometrial filling defects in the contrast medium. Filling defects produced by localized adhesions are usually linear or irregular in configuration, and generally are not altered by increasing distension of the endometrial cavity by the injected contrast medium. With more advanced fibrosis, the endometrial cavity will be deformed and contracted and may be completely obliterated. Previous uterine surgery (endometrial curettage, myomectomy, and, occasionally, cesarean section) and endometrial tuberculosis are causes of adhesions. Adhesions and deformity of the endometrial cavity may also be seen in association with antenatal diethylstilbestrol exposure.[8]

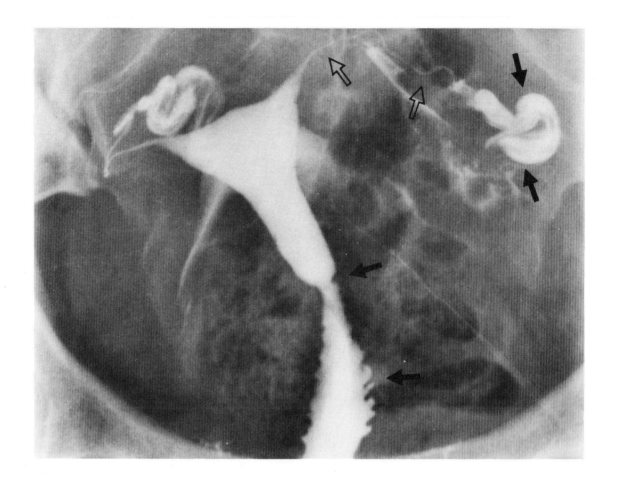

Figure 26-1
Normal hysterosalpingogram. The serrated appearance of the endocervical canal (lower solid arrow) represents normal mucosal folds, the plicae palmatae. The internal os (upper solid arrow) is at the junction of the endocervical canal and the triangular endometrial cavity. The thin proximal portion of the fallopian tube (open arrows) represents the interstitial segment and the isthmus. The more distended distal portion (solid arrows) represents the ampulla, which terminates in the fimbriated end and contains longitudinal mucosal folds, the endosalpingeal plicae.

Figures 26-2 and 26-3 are examples of endometrial adhesions.

Submucous leiomyomas produce round or lobulated filling defects of varying size on the HSG and may be indistinguishable from endometrial polyps. Occasionally, the normal endometrial mucosa may have a polypoid appearance,[9] which may be confused with small submucous myomas or polyps. Unlike adhesions, a small submucous myoma may become effaced and obscured with increased filling of the endometrial cavity with contrast medium. A spot radiograph obtained during early filling of the endometrial cavity may provide the only evidence

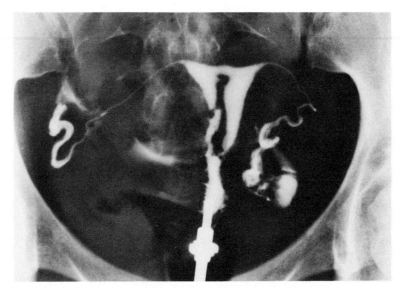

Figure 26-2
Endometrial adhesions. The patient was a 23-year-old gravida 5, para 0, spontaneous abortus 4, ectopic 1 (G5 P0 SAB4 ECT1), with previous left linear salpingostomy, being evaluated for recurrent abortion. The irregular, linear filling defect represents adhesions between the anterior and posterior walls of the endometrial cavity, extending from the internal os to a level near the fundus.

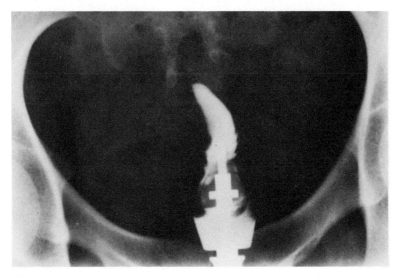

Figure 26-3
Asherman's syndrome. The patient (33-year-old G3 P0 TAB3) had been amenorrheic for 6 months after dilatation and curettage for her most recent therapeutic abortion (TAB). Filling of the endocervical canal and nonvisualization of the endometrial cavity are consistent with complete obliteration of the cavity by adhesions or with obstruction at the internal os level by adhesions in the lower endometrial cavity. This appearance may also be seen with advanced endometrial tuberculosis.

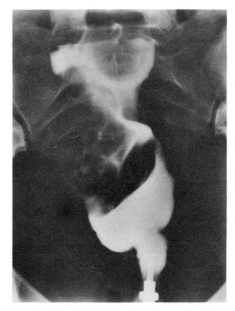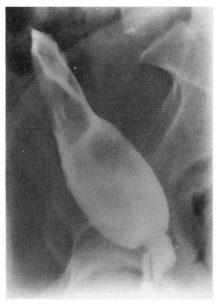

Figure 26-4
Multiple submucous leiomyomas. The patient was a 23-year-old woman (G0) with menometrorrhagia and a 16-week size fibroid uterus on physical examination. Expanded and elongated endometrial cavity has multiple, large filling defects. (Left) AP view; (Right) lateral view.

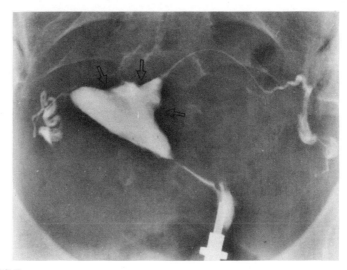

Figure 26-5
Submucous and intramural leiomyomas in a 31-year-old woman with a history of second-trimester spontaneous abortion and a 12-week-size uterus on physical examination. Small filling defects (arrows) represent submucous myomas on the fundal and left lateral aspects of the endometrial cavity. A large intramural myoma has produced stretching of the interstitial segment and isthmus of the left fallopian tube.

of such a lesion. Large submucous leiomyomas may expand and elongate the endometrial cavity and can cause cornual obstruction of the fallopian tube. Large intramural myomas may elongate or deviate the endometrial cavity and may stretch the proximal portion of the fallopian tube. Figures 26-4 and 26-5 illustrate submucous and intramural leiomyomas.

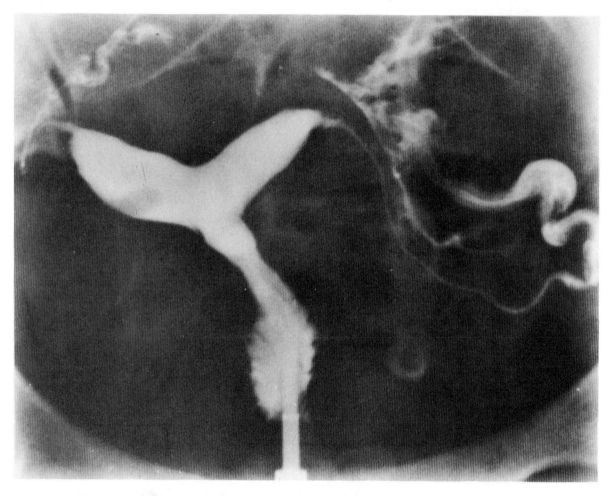

Figure 26-6
Arcuate uterus in a 31-year-old woman with primary infertility. The central depression in the fundus of the endometrial cavity was subsequently verified as arcuate uterus during hysteroscopy and laparotomy. A small filling defect may be seen on the right side of the endometrial cavity, representing a small submucous myoma or polyp.

Infertility

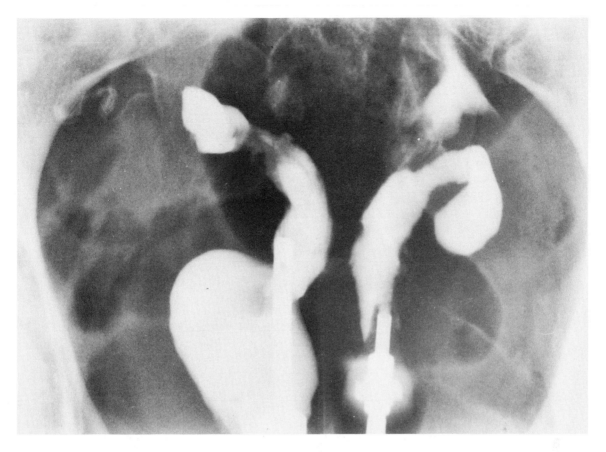

Figure 26-7
Uterus didelphys in a 33-year-old woman (G3 P0 SAB3) being evaluated for recurrent abortion. Vaginal examination revealed a double cervix and midline septum to the introitus. A vacuum cannula was applied to the left cervix and a Jarcho cannula was inserted into the right cervix. Oblong endometrial cavities are shown above duplicated endocervical canals. Reflux of contrast medium is noted filling the right vagina.

Uterine anomalies

A uterine anomaly may be discovered on the HSG during evaluation for recurrent abortion or incidentally, during examination for some other indication. If evidence of an anomaly is discovered on vaginal examination, an HSG will provide more precise information concerning uterine anatomy. Figures 26-6 and 26-7 are examples of uterine anomalies.

Localization of intrauterine device

If the initial clinical evaluation for a "lost" intrauterine device (IUD) is negative, a single radiograph of the abdomen and pelvis should then be obtained. This will determine whether the IUD has been expelled, is in the pelvis, or has migrated into the abdomen. If the IUD is in the pelvis, an HSG will provide the necessary anatomic information concerning its precise location with

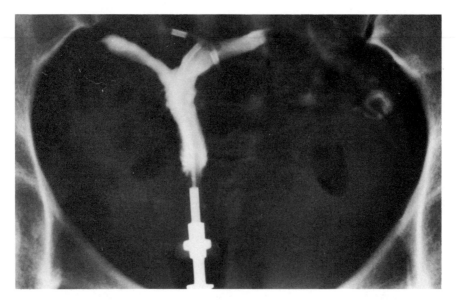

Figure 26-8
Horizontal arm of a copper-T IUD embedded in the fundus of a subseptate uterus.

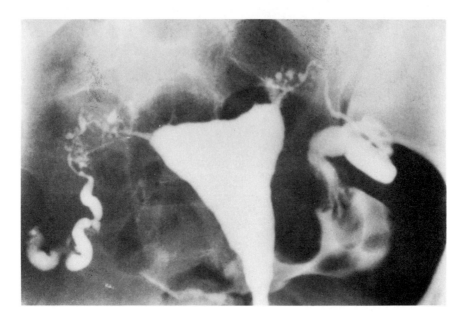

Figure 26-9
Bilateral salpingitis isthmica nodosa in a 28-year-old woman (G2 P1 ECT1) with previous segmental right salpingectomy and secondary infertility of 10 years' duration. Multiple diverticula may be seen along the proximal portions of the tubes bilaterally, with a few diverticula adjacent to the right ampulla. The right tube is occluded distally because of the previous segmental salpingectomy.

Infertility

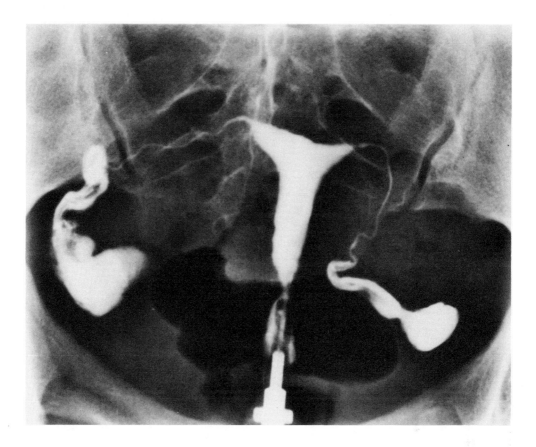

Figure 26-10
HSG showing bilateral hydrosalpinges with dilation, clubbing, and obstruction at the fimbriated ends. The patient was a 32-year-old woman with a 10-year history of primary infertility.

respect to the endometrial cavity. It may then be possible to remove it through a hysteroscope or laparoscope. Figure 26-8 shows an IUD embedded in the fundus of a subseptate uterus.

Fallopian tube lesions

Salpingitis isthmica nodosa (SIN) consists of localized or numerous diverticula along the interstitial segment and/or isthmus of the fallopian tube. Pathologically and radiographically, this condition can be found in an otherwise normal fallopian tube or in association with chronic salpingitis. The tubal diverticula are readily demonstrated on the HSG (Figure 26-9).

Radiographic manifestations of chronic salpingitis predominantly involve the distal fallopian tube. These include elongation and dilation of the ampulla, clubbing and contour irregularity of the fimbriated end, hydrosalpinx, and loss of mucosal folds. Occasionally, a cornual or isthmic obstruction may be produced. Figures 26-10 and 26-11 are examples of chronic salpingitis.

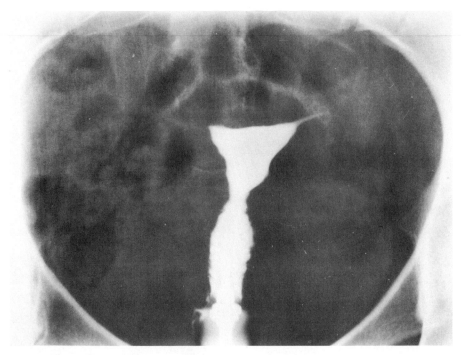

Figure 26-11
Right cornual and left isthmic obstructions in a 26-year-old woman (G3 P0 SAB1 TAB2) with secondary infertility. An obstruction is demonstrated in the left isthmus, and the right tube cannot be visualized, perhaps because of a cornual obstruction or tubal spasm. At laparotomy, the obstruction in the left isthmus was confirmed, and there was a left hydrosalpinx distal to this. The right tubal lumen was obliterated, so that an infant feeding tube could not be passed beyond the right fimbria.

The radiographic features of tuberculous salpingitis have been previously described in detail.[10] Although tuberculosis can produce hydrosalpinx and other changes seen with chronic salpingitis, distinctive radiographic findings are frequently demonstrated that are virtually diagnostic of tuberculosis. These include: (1) calcified lymph nodes or granulomas in the pelvis; (2) tubal obstruction in the distal isthmus or proximal ampulla, sometimes resulting in a "pipe-stem" configuration of the tube proximal to the obstruction; (3) multiple strictures along the course of the tube; (4) irregularity to the contour of the ampulla; and (5) deformity or obliteration of the endometrial cavity, in the absence of a previous curettage. Some of these features are shown in Figure 26-12.

HSG findings

Hysterosalpingography can be used to evaluate a variety of conditions. Endocervical and endometrial lesions can be identified, then definitively treated with hysteroscopy. The HSG provides the most accurate method for localization of a lost IUD. Information that would not be evident with laparoscopy can be obtained concerning the fallopian tube. Mucosal detail of the ampulla in chronic salpingitis and SIN of the interstitial segment are examples. This information will complement laparoscopy. Finally, the HSG is an excellent screening procedure for pelvic tuberculosis, as diagnostic features are frequently demonstrated.

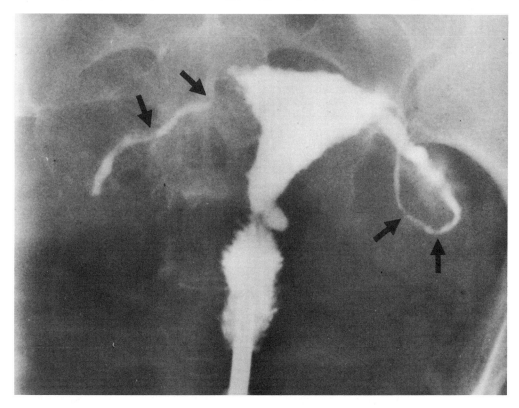

Figure 26-12
Tuberculous salpingitis in a 37-year-old nulligravida with primary infertility for 15 years. The right tube is obstructed in the zone of transition between the isthmus and ampulla. Arrows indicate multiple strictures in both tubes. The nodular contour of the endometrial cavity may also be related to tuberculosis and is analogous to a pattern that has been found in the ampulla in other cases. The small diverticulum near the internal os probably represents adenomyosis. The diagnosis of tuberculosis was confirmed by a positive endometrial culture.

References

1. Stumpf PG, March CM: Febrile morbidity following hysterosalpingography: Identification of risk factors and recommendations for prophylaxis. *Fertil Steril* 33:487, 1980

2. Pittaway DE, Winfield AC, Maxson W, et al: Prevention of acute pelvic inflammatory disease after hysterosalpingography: Efficacy of doxycycline prophylaxis. *Am J Obstet Gynecol* 147:623, 1983

3. Malmström T: A vacuum uterine cannula. *Obstet Gynecol* 18:773, 1961

4. Özaras H: The value of plastic operations on the fallopian tubes in the treatment of female infertility. A clinical and radiological study. *Acta Obstet Gynecol Scand* 47:489, 1968

5. Siegler AM: Dangers of hysterosalpingography. *Obstet Gynecol Surv* 22:284, 1967

6. De Cherney AH, Kort H, Barney JB, et al: Increased pregnancy rate with oil soluble hysterosalpingography dye. *Fertil Steril* 33:407, 1980

7. Asplund J: The uterine cervix and isthmus under normal and pathological conditions. *Acta Radiol (Suppl)* 91, 1952

8. Kaufman RH, Adam E: Genital tract anomalies associated with *in utero* exposure to diethylstilbestrol. *Isr J Med Sci* 14:353, 1978

9. Slezak P, Tillinger KG: Hysterographic evidence of polypoid filling defects in the uterine cavity. *Radiology* 115:79, 1975

10. Ekengren K, Rydén ABV: Roentgen diagnosis of tuberculous salpingitis. *Acta Radiol* 34:193, 1950

Chapter 27

Hysteroscopy and the Uterine Factor in Infertility

Charles M. March, M.D.

The exact incidence of infertility caused by endometrial and structural uterine abnormalities is unknown, but it is thought to be 5% to 10%. Endometritis secondary to infection with the gonococcus, the tubercle bacillus, and *Ureaplasma urealyticum* (T-mycoplasma) has been associated with reproductive failure. However, other infective organisms may also play a role. Infertility due to gonococcal infection is most frequently caused by inflammation and resultant changes in the oviduct. *U. urealyticum* infections may cause infertility and/or repeated abortion. These two types of infection are discussed in other chapters.

Tuberculosis

Pelvic tuberculosis (almost always of hematogenous origin) is seldom encountered in the US, but internationally and in Central and South American and Middle Eastern populations residing here, this disease is not uncommon. There are many reviews of the pathogenesis, natural history, and treatment of pelvic tuberculosis (TB). Relatively little information, however,

is available about methods of diagnosing infertility due to TB.

Pelvic TB is diagnosed in approximately five women among the 500 new patients seen each year in our endocrine-infertility clinic. Most have no history of earlier tuberculous infection, and pelvic examinations are usually normal. Although the diagnosis is substantiated in most patients by endometrial or menstrual cultures and/or by endometrial biopsies, the single most valuable diagnostic study is the hysterosalpingogram (HSG).

Only 50% of women with pelvic TB have endometrial infection. In many patients, the disease is focal, with only scattered tubercles containing epithelial cells and giant cells surrounded by zones of lymphocytes. Tubercles are most likely to be identified during the premenstrual phase of the cycle, following maximal hormonal stimulation of the endometrium. When the tuberculous process is extensive, the endometrium is destroyed and replaced by hyalinized connective tissue, thereby obliterating the cavity. Most of these patients are amenorrheic.

Pelvic TB originates by hematogenous spread and begins in the fallopian tube. It is very destructive. The pathognomonic changes often present on the HSG are: (1) rigid "pipestem" tubes (best seen during fluoroscopy), (2) ragged tubal contours (irregular strictures, fistulas), (3) small terminal tubal dilatations, (4) calcified pelvic lymph nodes, and (5) partial or complete obliteration of the endometrial cavity (see Chapter 26, Figure 26-12).

Among our patients with pelvic TB, the HSG was always abnormal and, in most, characteristic of pelvic TB. Generally, pelvic TB was initially suspected following review of the HSG, and subsequent studies confirmed the diagnosis. The great value of the HSG lies in its revelation of the characteristic radiographic changes that are diagnostic. Once the diagnosis is made, therapy should be instituted rapidly, the infertility investigation terminated, and reconstructive infertility surgery avoided.

Patients with TB of the upper genital tract and tubal obstruction are sterile and will not benefit from conservative tubal surgery. Treatment should be triple drug therapy [isoniazid hydrochloride (INH), ethambutol, and streptomycin] for 6 months, and INH and ethambutol for an additional 18 months. Tests of liver function, visual acuity, and hearing should be performed before beginning therapy, after 1 month of treatment, and then at 6-month intervals thereafter.

biopsy is required to establish the diagnosis with certainty. The histologist must be careful to distinguish the pathologic presence of plasma cells from the normal premenstrual leukocyte infiltration. Patients with endometritis may be asymptomatic or may have intermenstrual spotting or hypermenorrhea. Broad-spectrum antibiotic therapy should be administered for 2 weeks and the endometrial biopsy repeated. If the condition persists, a curettage is required to eradicate the infection. The infection usually clears but the effect on fertility is less certain, because this entity remains a partial enigma.

Intrauterine adhesions

Intrauterine adhesions (IUA) that cause infertility had been difficult to treat prior to the advent of hysteroscopy. In the past 11 years, hysteroscopic diagnosis of IUA has been confirmed in 175 patients referred to the LAC/USC Medical Center. Those with endometrial obliteration secondary to TB have been excluded from this series.

Etiology

The factors antecedent to IUA in these 175 patients are listed in Table 27-1. Most adhesions occurred following endometrial curettage dur-

Infections by other organisms

Staphylococci, aerobic and anaerobic streptococci, *Escherichia coli*, Aerobacter, *Bacteroides fragilis*, and Proteus are the bacteria commonly responsible. Infections may be puerperal, postabortal, or secondary to such procedures as endometrial biopsy, HSG, uterotubal insufflation, and IUD insertion. Infertility may occur following acute endometritis with suppuration. When chronic endometritis is present, the influence on fertility is less certain. Careful review of the endometrial

Table 27-1
Antecedent factors in 175 patients with intrauterine adhesions

Factor	No. of patients
Dilatation and curettage	
Elective first-trimester abortion	74
Spontaneous incomplete abortion	70
Postpartum hemorrhage	14
Diagnostic	6
Hydatidiform mole	2
Cesarean section	4
Metroplasty	2
Unknown	3

ing or shortly after pregnancy. IUA have also been reported following the evacuation of a hydatidiform mole, cesarean section, myomectomy, diagnostic curettage, and pelvic irradiation. Endometrial TB and septic abortion are also predisposing factors. Although the combination of pelvic infection and endometrial curettage has been reported to be the most common etiology of adhesions, that has not been our experience. In our series, elective first-trimester abortion by aspiration was the most common cause. A postpartum curettage is most likely to result in adhesions if it is performed between the second and fourth weeks after delivery. Concomitant breast-feeding increases the risk of adhesion formation. Women who nurse remain amenorrheic and estrogen deficient for a prolonged time. The use of depo-medroxyprogesterone acetate following evacuation of a molar pregnancy is an analogous situation and should be avoided. Recent data suggest that adhesions occur more often after curettage for a missed abortion than after curettage for a spontaneous incomplete abortion. Adhesions were found after curettage in 13 (30.9%) of 42 women who had a missed abortion, compared with only five (6.4%) of 78 who had an "early" abortion.[1]

The development of IUA after a diagnostic D&C has important implications for management of the infertile patient. The routine use of curettage at the time of diagnostic laparoscopy is unwarranted and may cause adhesions. If the laparoscopy is performed in the follicular phase of the cycle, endometrial histology serves no purpose; if performed in the luteal phase, an endometrial biopsy will provide the necessary information and be less traumatic.

Presenting symptoms and diagnosis

Patients with IUA may present with menstrual disturbances, infertility, or recurrent abortion or they may be symptom-free. The menstrual patterns of the 175 patients studied at USC are listed in Table 27-2. In patients with normal menses, hysteroscopy was performed because a cavity defect had been discovered by an HSG obtained during an infertility investigation.

A relationship was observed between the menstrual pattern and the antecedent factor among these patients. Elective first-trimester abortion, usually performed by an aspiration technique, was followed by amenorrhea in 62 of 74 patients. However, menstrual periods were normal in 35 of 70 patients with intrauterine synechiae that were diagnosed after curettage was performed because of spontaneous incomplete abortion.

The menstrual pattern correlates well—but not completely—with the extent of intrauterine scarring (Table 27-2). Although amenorrhea is the most commonly observed menstrual aberration, 37 (21%) of these 175 patients had cyclic, painless menses of normal flow and duration. Therefore, IUA cannot be excluded in such patients, nor in those amenorrheic patients who have bleeding after gestagen or sequential estrogen-gestagen administration. The key to the

Table 27-2
Correlation between presenting menstrual pattern and extent of adhesions at hysteroscopy

Menstrual pattern	No. of patients	Extent of intrauterine adhesions		
		Severe	Moderate	Minimal
Amenorrhea	105	54	37	14
Hypomenorrhea	28	8	17	3
Oligomenorrhea	5	1	1	3
Normal menses	37	4	8	25

Table 27-3
Correlation between HSG findings and extent of adhesions at hysteroscopy in 134 patients

HSG findings	No. of patients	Hysteroscopy findings		
		Severe	Moderate	Minimal
Severe	80	53	23	4
Moderate	25	0	20	5
Minimal	29	0	0	29

diagnosis is careful attention to patients with a history of previous intrauterine trauma (especially curettage associated with pregnancy).

When traditional diagnostic signs and methods (failure to bleed following sex steroid administration, inability to sound the uterine cavity, HSG) indicate that IUA are present in an amenorrheic patient, the diagnosis is relatively certain.

Hysterosalpingography remains the principal study used to diagnose IUA. Classically, single or multiple lacunar-shaped filling defects of variable size are seen within the endometrial cavity (Figures 26-2 and 26-3). These may be centrally or peripherally located, are irregularly shaped, and must be present on each film (to enable differentiation from polyps). The cavity may be completely obliterated in some patients. Technical problems precluding adequate uterine distension may give either a false-positive study or the impression of extensive scar formation when, in fact, the process is quite limited (Table 27-3). The slow instillation of the contrast medium by the gynecologist who is familiar with the patient's history and physical findings and visualization by fluoroscopy with image intensification will increase the value of the HSG immeasurably.

Hysteroscopy

Hysteroscopy has a number of advantages over hysterosalpingography. It allows direct inspection of the uterine cavity with assessment of both the extent and the location of scar formation. Table 27-4 presents a classification of IUA that permits meaningful comparisons between various hysteroscopic therapeutic techniques.[2] The value of adjunctive therapeutic measures used in the management of intrauterine synechiae can also be assessed more precisely if the original lesions are classified according to location and extent. Lysis of adhesions can be performed under direct vision, using local anesthesia, on an outpatient basis. Transcervical endoscopy is a relatively new technique, with many applications to reproductive problems.

Procedure

Except during menses, hysteroscopy may be performed anytime in the menstrual cycle. However, visualization is best within 2 to 3 days after the cessation of menstrual flow. The endometrium is thin early in the cycle, but later the tubal ostia may become obscured by endometrial growth. If hysteroscopy is performed during the luteal phase, it is necessary for the patient to be using adequate contraception. No special preoperative instructions are needed, except limited dietary intake before the procedure. For brief procedures, patients are given premedication with 600 mg of ibuprofen. If a longer or more

Table 27-4
Classification of IUA by hysteroscopic findings

Class	Findings
Severe	More than three-fourths of uterine cavity involved; agglutination of walls or thick bands; ostial areas and upper cavity occluded
Moderate	One-fourth to three-fourths of uterine cavity involved; no agglutination of walls, adhesions only; ostial areas and upper fundus only partially occluded
Minimal	Less than one-fourth of uterine cavity involved; thin or filmy adhesions; ostial areas and upper fundus minimally involved or clear

From March CM, Israel R, March AD: Hysteroscopic management of intrauterine adhesions. Am J Obstet Gynecol 130:653, 1978.

difficult hysteroscopy is anticipated, sedation consisting of 50 mg of meperidine or 5 to 10 mg of diazepam should be given IV. Hysteroscopy may be performed safely in the office. If general anesthesia is necessary, an outpatient surgical unit provides an adequate setting and the patient may be discharged in a few hours.

Following the introduction of a paracervical block (injection of 10 mL of 1% lidocaine without epinephrine into the uterosacral ligaments), the uterine cavity is sounded, the cervix is dilated to No. 6 Hegar, and the hysteroscope is introduced. Because the anterior and posterior walls of the uterus are in apposition, the cavity must be distended by one of three different types of media to ensure proper visualization. After systematic inspection of the cavity, accessory instruments may be introduced through the operating channel of the hysteroscope for biopsy; resection of synechiae, polyps, or myomas; incision of a septum; or IUD removal.

Media

Dextrose solution

Five percent glucose in water is a readily available and inexpensive medium. It is instilled via a one-liter IV infusion bottle to which a hand pump is attached. Constant high pressure is applied to instill the solution. The high-volume, high-flow-rate system of delivery increases pain during the examination. Another disadvantage of this medium is that it mixes with blood, thus obscuring vision. Normal saline may also be used for hysteroscopy and has the same attributes as glucose in water.

Carbon dioxide

A special insufflator is required (the CO_2 insufflator used to create the pneumoperitoneum for laparoscopy must not be used). CO_2 is instilled at a flow rate of up to 100 mL/minute at a maximum pressure of 200 mm Hg. The visualization is not as good as with dextran. There is less magnification due to the lower index of refraction compared with glucose in water or dextran. The cervical adaptors used to prevent CO_2 leakage to ensure adequate uterine distension are not suitably designed for use in all patients. Many procedures require up to 500 mL of CO_2 to compensate for both absorption and spillage into the peritoneal cavity. The latter will cause shoulder pain when the patient resumes an erect position. This medium is very neat and is perfectly suited for diagnostic procedures in the office.

Dextran

Dextran, being immiscible with blood, provides excellent visualization. It is instilled via a 50-mL syringe attached to infusion tubing 5 mm in diameter. Intermittent delivery of 5- to 10-mL volumes to enhance visualization results in less uterine cramping. This medium is very difficult to remove from instruments; thus, instruments should be rinsed immediately after the procedure with copious amounts of hot water. Two forms of dextran have been used for hysteroscopy: The first, Rheomacrodex, is a 10% dextran solution, molecular weight 40,000, in 5% glucose in water. The second, Hyskon Hysteroscopy Fluid, is a 32% dextran solution, molecular weight 70,000, in 10% glucose in water. This medium was developed specifically for use in hysteroscopy. Almost all examinations may be completed using one 100-mL bottle. The excellent clarity and minimal equipment needed make Hyskon the medium of choice.

Indications

Intrauterine pathology

Hysteroscopy is used to establish definitively the presence of intrauterine pathology in the following conditions:
1. Endometrial polyps may be differentiated from submucous leiomyomas, which is not always possible with the HSG (Figure 27-1). The polyps should be excised under direct vision and then their bases should be curetted.

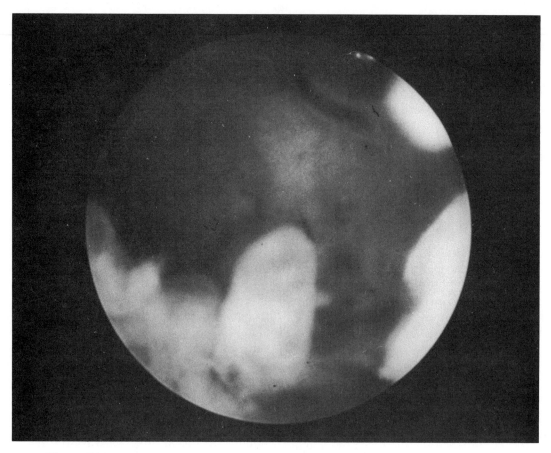

Figure 27-1
Hysteroscopic view of an endometrial polyp. A feathery appearance and transillumination distinguish a polyp from a myoma.

2. Submucous leiomyomas may be differentiated from polyps, their extent evaluated, and they may be biopsied, resected, or excised (if pedunculated) (Figure 27-2).

3. IUA may be definitively diagnosed, and their extent evaluated. Synechiae may be lysed under direct vision, and the success of treatment evaluated by repeat hysteroscopy (or HSG) at a later date.

4. The extent of congenital anomalies of the uterus may be accurately defined, treatment planned, and subsequent results assessed. The septate uterus may be unified.

5. Embedded IUDs may be visualized and removed under direct vision, thereby reducing endometrial trauma.

6. In cases of abnormal bleeding, structural abnormalities of the uterine cavity may be evaluated or ruled out so that appropriate medical or surgical treatment can take place. Malignancies occasionally missed by curettage may be diagnosed. Endometrial carcinoma may be staged more accurately than by fractional curettage.

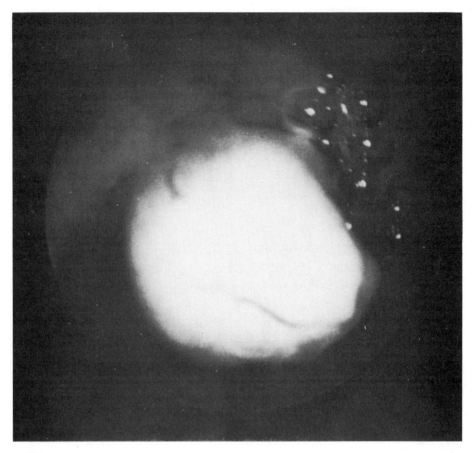

Figure 27-2
Pedunculated submucous leiomyoma visualized with the hysteroscope. Myomas appear white and glistening. Bubbles are commonly present when a dextran medium is used.

Unexplained infertility and recurrent abortion

The exact role of hysteroscopy in the investigation and management of the couple with repeated pregnancy wastage or unexplained infertility is uncertain. Asymptomatic polyps, submucous myomas, or synechiae that may be responsible for unexplained infertility or recurrent abortion, and that have not been seen on an HSG, may be diagnosed by hysteroscopy. However, of more than 500 infertile patients as well as 50 with recurrent abortion, all of whom had normal HSGs and subsequently underwent hysterosco-py, none had a cavity defect diagnosed hysteroscopically. Our study indicates that a carefully performed HSG demonstrating a normal cavity obviates the need for hysteroscopy. Thus, the routine use of hysteroscopy at the time of laparoscopy for infertility is not indicated if the patient's HSG is normal.

Contraindications

Absolute contraindications to hysteroscopy are acute pelvic infection and uterine perforation. Active uterine bleeding, uterine cancer, and pregnancy are relative contraindications. If Hyskon is used to distend the uterine cavity, the examination can usually be completed satisfactorily, even if the patient is bleeding heavily. The contact hysteroscope (Figure 27-3) has been used to examine pregnant patients in the first trimester without ill effects. Although hysteroscopy may be used to diagnose and stage cancer, the potential for tumor dissemination has prevented its widespread use. This theoretical objection does not apply if contact hysteroscopy is performed.

Complications

Complications have been infrequent in the more than 3,000 hysteroscopies we have performed. Most have been mild.

Pain

Pain usually is mild to moderate during hysteroscopy. Most hysteroscopies can be performed on an outpatient basis using a paracervical block. Meperidine, diazepam, or a prostaglandin synthetase inhibitor may be used to supplement the paracervical block. Cramps increase substantially if operating time exceeds 20 to 30 minutes. Following hysteroscopy, mild cramping may persist for a few hours and is easily controlled with aspirin.

Bleeding

Bleeding has occurred in nine patients and was secondary to a cervical laceration at the site of tenaculum placement in six. In two women, a branch of the uterine artery was severed and tamponade using an intrauterine balloon was used to control the bleeding. In the last patient, heavy bleeding necessitating transfusion occurred after IUD placement following incision of a uterine septum. Bleeding may also occur following extensive dissection of synechiae or resection of polyps or a submucous myoma.

Infection

Three patients have developed infections after hysteroscopy. Both had histories of salpingitis. Broad-spectrum antibiotic therapy, including an agent effective against anaerobic organisms, should be instituted immediately if symptoms of infection develop. We have not used prophylactic antibiotic therapy routinely for hysteroscopy.

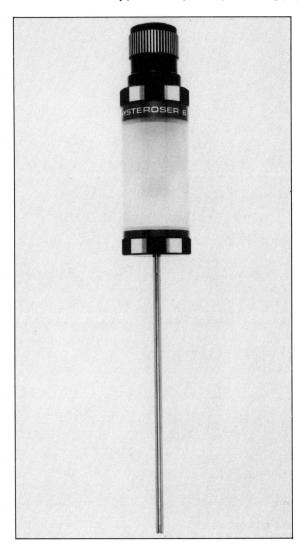

Figure 27-3
Contact hysteroscope manufactured by M.T.O. Company, Paris, France; distributed by Advanced Biomedical Instruments, Woburn, Massachusetts.

Uterine perforation

This is a rare complication of hysteroscopy and usually occurs only in the most severe cases of IUA. If the dissection proves to be extremely difficult, the procedure should be terminated and repeated on another occasion under general anesthesia, with simultaneous laparoscopy to reduce the chance of uterine perforation. Central perforations may be managed by observation only. Antibiotics are not used and hospitalization is unnecessary.

Endometrial dislocation

The subsequent development of endometrial implants on peritoneal surfaces is a theoretical complication. It is unlikely that displaced endometrial cells can survive in the high-molecular-weight dextran solution that we recommend. Avoidance of hysteroscopy during menses further reduces the risk of this complication.

Anesthetic accidents

The rare anesthetic complications are related to the agents used rather than to the hysteroscopic procedure itself.

Complications related to the medium

Allergic reactions to dextran occur rarely. If a large amount of dextran enters the venous circulation, circulatory overload is possible. A symptom complex consisting of acute noncardiogenic pulmonary edema and disseminated intravascular coagulation has occurred in four of our patients. All required large volumes (500 to 800 mL) of Hyskon and had extensive dissection of their endometrial surfaces. It is advisable to limit the amount of Hyskon used to 300 mL or less, in order to avoid this serious complication.[3] Acute fluid overload has also been reported when large volumes of glucose in water or saline have been used. In some patients, potent diuretics have been used prophylactically. CO_2 acidosis and arrhythmias are probably only theoretical complications.

Value of hysteroscopy

During hysteroscopy, numerous intrauterine findings can be detected, although the significance of some is yet to be determined. The hysteroscope may provide better insight into endometrial growth and development. It may also help to define defects in the preimplantation and early postimplantation phases of human conception.[4] As instrumentation is improved, more extensive transcervical surgery will become a reality. The recently developed contact hysteroscope is a valuable office instrument (Figure 27-3).

The hallmark of contact hysteroscopy is simplicity. Equipment such as a light source or distending medium is not necessary. Two instruments are available: one with a 6-mm diameter and one of 8 mm. The former is most suited to office use, because it requires less cervical dilation. There is also a biopsy/grasping forceps that fits over the 6-mm endoscope and can be used to remove embedded IUDs. A focusing device that increases the depth of field can be attached.

Because the contact hysteroscope does not provide a panoramic view of the cavity, learning to use it is more difficult than with the operating hysteroscope. Complete inspection of the cavity requires discipline and patience. The instrument can also be used for amnioscopy, and has been successful in identifying meconium staining and fetal anomalies. It has been used to improve staging of endometrial cancer and even for examination of the urinary bladder.

Treatment of IUA

Lysis of adhesions under direct vision is safer and more complete than blind curettage or hysterotomy. With the hysteroscope, it is possible to cut scar tissue only and not traumatize normal endometrium. Each adhesive band is identified and divided with miniature scissors (Figure 27-4). In women with extensive scarring, complete lysis of adhesions can be achieved. If the dissection is unusually difficult, the procedure should

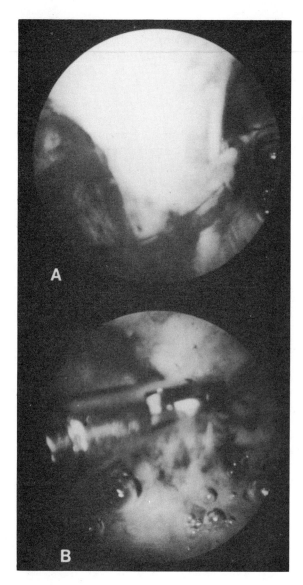

Figure 27-4
A. Intrauterine scar as seen through the hysteroscope.
B. Division of scar using miniature scissors.

and retained for 2 months. Postoperative use of an IUD may reduce the chances that the raw, dissected surfaces will readhere to one another.[5] If an IUD cannot be inserted, an 8 French Foley catheter with a 3-mL balloon can be used. The balloon is inflated, the catheter remains for 1 week, and a broad-spectrum antibiotic is prescribed for that time.

Conjugated estrogens, using a daily dose of 5 mg, are given to all patients for 60 days, and medroxyprogesterone acetate, 10 mg, is added during the last 5 days of estrogen therapy.[2] High-dose, sequential estrogen-progestin treatment maximally stimulates the endometrium so that the scarred surfaces are reepithelialized. The adequacy of therapy should be assessed accurately by repeat hysteroscopy or by HSG following the steroid-induced withdrawal bleeding. If the HSG is normal, complete resolution may be presumed. An abnormal HSG, however, does not definitively indicate persistent adhesions and the hysteroscopy should be repeated.

The results of this approach to IUA at our institution are summarized in Table 27-5. Of the 105 patients who originally presented with secondary amenorrhea, 100 have cyclic, spontaneous, painless menses of normal flow and duration, four have hypomenorrhea, and one has remained amenorrheic. Of the 28 who had hypomenorrhea before therapy, all have normal menses. After one hysteroscopic treatment, 90% of patients have had a normal follow-up hysteroscopy or HSG. Although most of the others have needed only a second procedure to restore normal uterine architecture, a few women have needed three to five operations.

The pregnancy results are excellent and surpass other types of treatment regimens[6] (Table 27-5). Of these 175 patients, 69 wished to conceive and had no other known infertility factors. Fifty-two (75%) conceived 62 times, and 54 (87%) of the 62 pregnancies have gone to term. Two patients have had placenta previa and one required manual removal of the placenta. These results are superior to those achieved by outdated treatment modalities (Table 27-6).

be terminated. To reduce the risk of uterine perforation, the dissection is resumed under general anesthesia using simultaneous laparoscopy for additional safety. As large a loop IUD as possible is then placed in the uterine cavity

Table 27-5
Results of lysis of IUA using hysteroscope

Before		After	
Findings	No. of patients	Findings	No. of patients
Amenorrhea	105	Normal menses	100
		Hypomenorrhea	4
		Amenorrhea	1
Hypomenorrhea	28	Normal menses	28
Infertile	69	Delivered or currently pregnant	54

Table 27-6
Gestational outcome after treatment for IUA*

Method	No. of pregnancies	First- or second-trimester losses	Term
Traditional*	369	104 (28%)	147 (40%)
USC†	62	8 (13%)	54 (87%)

*Includes blind disruption of adhesions and is gathered from the literature.

†University of Southern California data have been corrected to eliminate losses from known causes (e.g., elective abortion, cervical incompetence).

From Jewelewicz R, Khalaf S, Neuwirth RS, Vande Wiele RL: Obstetric complications after treatment of intrauterine synechiae (Asherman's syndrome). Obstet Gynecol 47:701-705, 1976. Reprinted with permission from The American College of Obstetricians and Gynecologists.

Structural defects

Congenital anomalies
This section deals with the influence of uterine defects on reproduction in patients who are phenotypically and genotypically female. Uterine anomalies are found in 1% to 2% of all women, in 4% of infertile women, and in 10% to 15% of women with recurrent abortion[7] (Figure 27-5).

Classification
Congenital uterine anomalies may be classified as follows:
1. Unicornuate anomaly. There is complete developmental arrest of one müllerian duct.
2. Didelphic anomaly. Uterus didelphys entails a complete lack of fusion, with duplication of corpus and cervix. The duplication may extend into the vagina. It is not associated with

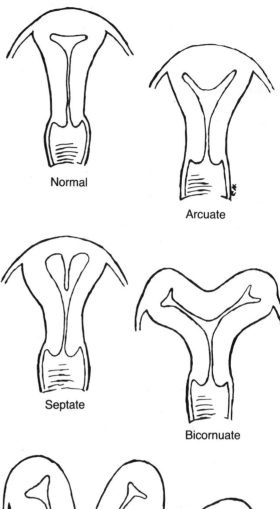

Normal

Arcuate

Septate

Bicornuate

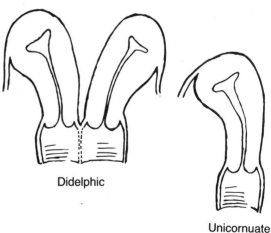

Didelphic

Unicornuate

Figure 27-5
Normal uterine configuration and various congenital anomalies.

recurrent abortion, but rather with premature delivery and abnormal presentations.

3. Bicornuate anomaly. There is partial lack of fusion of varying degrees associated with a single cervix. The defect is manifested externally and internally. This is the most common anomaly and is manifested by malpresentations and premature delivery.

4. Septate uterus. There is a partial lack of fusion of varying degrees that is manifested internally only. This is the anomaly most often associated with reproductive problems, primarily with recurrent abortions.

5. Arcuate anomaly. This is a very mild, asymptomatic form of septate uterus. It is a hystero-graphic or hysteroscopic diagnosis only, and has no reproductive consequences.

6. Rudimentary horn. There is incomplete development of one horn. The horn may be either communicating or noncommunicating. The latter is more common.

Symptoms

Reproductive failure is the most common symptom in patients with uterine anomalies. Uterine defects rarely cause primary infertility. More common symptoms are premature labor and abnormal fetal presentations. Although two-thirds of pregnancies in women with uterine duplication progress to term, abortion has been report-

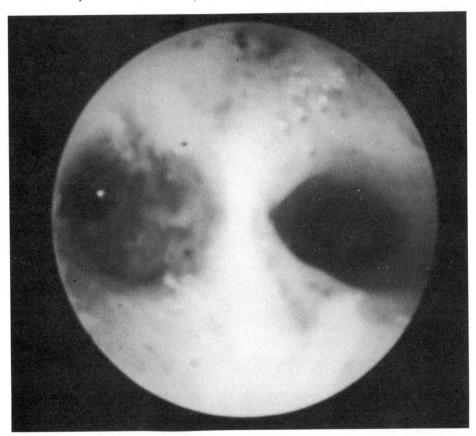

Figure 27-6
Hysteroscopic view of uterine septum.

Infertility

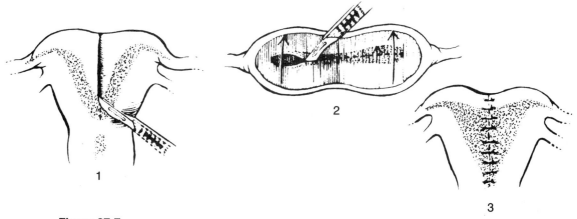

Figure 27-7
Tompkins's metroplasty.

Adapted from Rock JA, Jones HW Jr: The clinical management of the double uterus. Fertil Steril 28:798, 1977. Used with permission of the publisher, The American Fertility Society.

ed to occur in as many as 90% of pregnancies in women with septate uteri. If the endometrium present in a noncommunicating rudimentary horn is functional, recurrent abdominal pain, hematometra, and even rupture simulating an ectopic pregnancy may occur.

Evaluation and treatment

HSG and hysteroscopy (Figure 27-6) can be used to delineate uterine defects and serve as a baseline prior to treatment. However, the HSG also provides information regarding tubal patency and may be combined with a pneumogynogram to provide information about the external configuration of the uterus.

A complete infertility investigation is mandatory before surgical intervention for a uterine anomaly, so that other infertility factors can be ruled out. Depending on the severity of the defect, 10% to 35% of women who have a uterine anomaly also have a urinary tract anomaly.[8] Thus, an IV pyelogram should be performed.

The only type of uterine anomaly (other than that related to in utero DES exposure) definitely associated with reproductive failure is a uterine septum, which is a cause of recurrent

abortion. A uterine septum is not usually an indication for surgery in infertile patients because it rarely causes infertility. Laparotomy with uterine unification and incision or excision of the septum was formerly the procedure of choice for women with this anomaly and a history of recurrent abortion. The procedure advocated by Tompkins spares more uterine tissue than does that of Jones. In the Tompkins procedure (Figure 27-7),[9] which uses a midline uterine incision, the nonfunctional endometrium overlying the fibromuscular septum is removed and the cornual portions of the uterus are avoided.

More recently, hysteroscopy has been used not only to assess the size and extent of the septum but also to treat the anomaly.[10] Simultaneous laparoscopy is needed to verify that the uterus is unified externally and also to provide guidance for the hysteroscopist. Flexible scissors are passed through the operating channel of the hysteroscope, and the central portion of the septum is incised. The fibroelastic band of tissue retracts immediately and does not bleed. The dissection is carried cephalad, until the septum is incised completely and the uterine architecture is normalized.[11] If a loop IUD is placed, it is re-

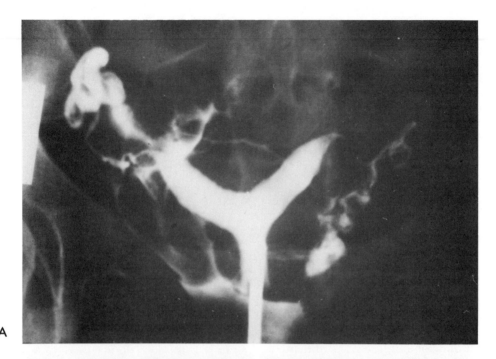

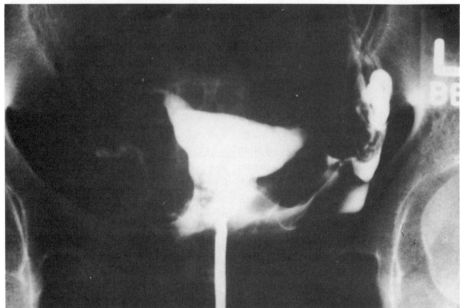

Figure 27-8
Preoperative (A) and postoperative (B) hysterograms in a patient with repeated first-trimester
abortion. View B was obtained 1 month after incision of a septum under hysteroscopic control.

Table 27-7
Comparison of abdominal metroplasty
and hysteroscopic incision of uterine septum

	Abdominal metroplasty	Hysteroscopic incision
Hospitalization	Yes	No
Surgery	Major	Minor
Avoid pregnancy	3–6 months	1 month
Delivery route	Cesarean section	Vaginal

tained for 25 days. The need for any intrauterine splint is controversial, but we do not believe that it is necessary.

The patient may be discharged from the surgery unit a few hours after the procedure is finished. To epithelialize the area of the septum, conjugated estrogens, 1.25 mg, are prescribed for 25 days. Medroxyprogesterone acetate, 10 mg daily, is given during the last 5 days of the estrogen treatment. If an IUD is placed, it is removed during the withdrawal menses. The patient may attempt to conceive immediately thereafter.

Preoperative and postoperative HSGs of a patient treated by hysteroscopic incision are shown in Figure 27-8. Outcomes are excellent in three series of hysteroscopic treatment of patients with uterine septa and histories of recurrent abortion.[10,11,12] The rates of abortion were reduced from 90% (pretreatment) to 10% (post-treatment). Transfundal and transcervical treatments of the septate uterus are compared in Table 27-7. The multiple advantages of hysteroscopic therapy make it the method of choice for treating uterine septa. In fact, because this method of treatment is so easy and safe, it may permit us to expand the indications for treating patients with uterine septa. For example, it may be used before complex therapy such as ovulation induction with gonadotropins, or even for patients with unexplained infertility. The value of hysteroscopic treatment of uterine septa for these "expanded" indications remains uncertain. However, its value for those with reproduc-

tive failure is unquestioned. This operation has made abdominal metroplasty obsolete.

If hysteroscopic treatment is unavailable and abdominal metroplasty is considered, it must be remembered that the presence of other factors associated with recurrent abortion or infertility markedly worsens the prognosis for term pregnancy in a patient with a septate uterus. Therefore, complex, combined treatment regimens involving metroplasty and tuboplasty are usually ill-advised.

Following incision of the septum, an HSG or hysteroscopy should be repeated three months postoperatively to assess results of the surgery. Patients may attempt pregnancy six months after abdominal metroplasty. Term pregnancies after metroplasty have been reported to be in the range of 80% of patients.[9] Delivery should be performed by cesarean section before the onset of labor. Women with bicornuate uteri may have abnormal presentations or premature labor. For those with repeated second- and third-trimester wastage, a Strassman procedure should be performed. Delivery by cesarean section is mandatory after any type of abdominal metroplasty.

Associated conditions

A transverse vaginal septum or an imperforate hymen may be associated with many uterine anomalies. A complete septum or an imperforate hymen will lead to cyclic abdominal pain, hematocolpos, and hematometra in the menstruating woman.

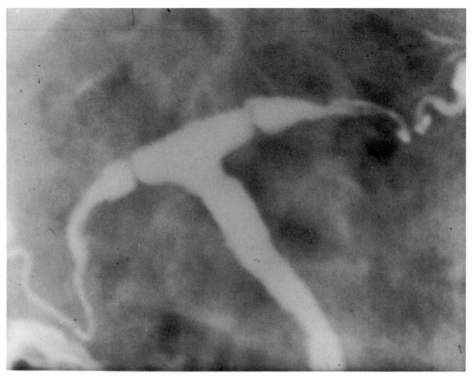

Figure 27-9
Typical hysterographic changes after in utero exposure to diethylstilbestrol.

Diethylstilbestrol-related anomalies

Currently, the most common müllerian anomaly is that following in utero exposure to diethylstilbestrol (DES). From a series of 267 patients who were exposed to DES in utero, typical changes were noted on the HSG in 69% (Figure 27-9).[13] These findings include a "T" shape with cornual constriction bands and pretubal bulges, lower uterine segment dilatation, and small cavities with irregular borders resembling intrauterine adhesions. These findings occur in over 80% of women who have typical DES changes in the cervix or vagina, compared with about 50% of DES-exposed women with normal cervices and normal vaginas.[13]

The gestational outcome after DES exposure is summarized in Table 27-8. Approximately 30% of all pregnancies terminate in spontaneous abortion or ectopic pregnancy, and another 15% end in premature delivery. Overall, two-thirds of pregnancies result in an infant who survives. Of those patients who conceive, 20% never have an infant who survives. As a general

Table 27-8
Gestational outcome after DES exposure in utero

Abortion rate doubled
Prematurity rate tripled
Term pregnancy rate 55%
Survival in 67% of pregnancies
Survival in 80% of women
Upper-tract abnormalities critical
Ectopic pregnancies more common
Cervical incompetence possibly increased

Infertility

Table 27-9
Correlation between hysterographic findings and gestational outcome in DES-exposed women

HSG	Normal	Abnormal	Total
Women (No.)	32	44	76
Abortion only	5 (10%)	12 (27%)	17 (22%)
Ectopic only	0	3 (7%)	3 (4%)
Premature only	6 (19%)	7 (16%)	13 (17%)
Term only	16 (50%)	13 (29%)	29 (38%)
Term ever	21 (66%)	20 (46%)	41 (54%)
Term never	11 (34%)	24 (54%)	35 (46%)

Adapted from Kaufman RH, Adam E, Binder GL, et al: Upper genital tract changes and pregnancy outcome in offspring exposed in utero to diethylstilbestrol. Am J Obstet Gynecol 137:299, 1980.

rule, those who deliver prematurely had been exposed to a higher dose of DES, given earlier in pregnancy, and taken for a longer time. There is an excellent correlation between the HSG findings and the gestational outcome (Table 27-9).[13] Although the prognosis is not good for any DES-exposed woman, those who have normal HSGs are much more likely to have an infant who survives than are those with abnormal uteri.[13]

Ectopic pregnancies occur five to six times more frequently in women exposed to DES in utero than in control populations who were not DES exposed. The etiology is uncertain, however. These patients have foreshortened, convoluted tubes with sacculations, pinpoint ostia, and constricted fimbriae.[14] Because the fallopian tube is also a müllerian structure, it is reasonable to expect that influences affecting the corpus also affect the tube. The influence of DES on cervical competence is less certain. Although some investigators have reported that cervical incompetence may occur in up to 10% of DES-exposed women, more careful studies have not substantiated these claims.[13,15] Thus, in the absence of historical data or cervical effacement/dilatation, prophylactic cerclage is not indicated in the patient with DES-associated anomalies and a previous abortion. If premature labor occurs, tocolytic agents should be used.

Overall, as many as 2 million women in the US have had in utero DES exposure. At this time, no data have proven an increased rate of infertility among these women. During the 1980s, peak numbers of these women will be in their reproductive years. It is likely that more information regarding fertility, reproductive outcome, mechanisms of reproductive failure, and therapy will be generated in the near future.

Leiomyomata uteri

The effect of myomas on reproduction, like that of uterine anomalies, is difficult to assess. Infertility, abortion (during either the first or second trimester), premature labor, and abnormal presentations have all been associated with the presence of submucous myomas.[16] Rarely, a cervical myoma may markedly distort the endocervix or displace the cervical os, thereby excluding it from the seminal pool. Both effects will interfere with sperm transport.

Submucous myomas may hinder endometrial nutrition and afford a poor implantation site (resulting in abortion or infertility). Large intramural myomas may cause enlargement of the endometrial cavity (possibly resulting in poor sperm transport) and may, on occasion, occlude the intramural portion of the tube(s). Both types, but particularly the submucous variety, may not allow normal uterine enlargement during pregnancy, and thus lead to abortion and premature labor.

Diagnosis

The diagnosis of intramural myomas is usually made at the time of bimanual examination. The presence of submucous tumors may be suspected during curettage, but HSG is necessary for confirmation. Smooth, circular, or crescent-shaped defects persisting after the entire cavity is filled suggest submucous myomas (Figure 26-4). Occasionally, it is impossible to differentiate the defect caused by a myoma from that of an

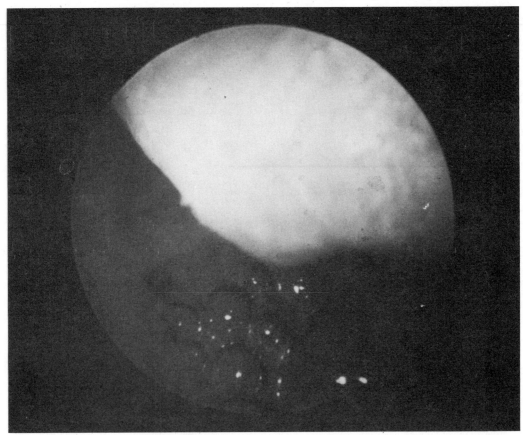

Figure 27-10
Broad-based submucous myoma on anterior uterine wall.

endometrial polyp or a gestational sac. By performing an HSG before myomectomy, the gynecologist knows whether or not the endometrial cavity should be entered. Routine exploration of the cavity is not recommended. The HSG also gives prognostic information, because marked tubal disease would contraindicate conservative surgery in almost all cases.

The definitive diagnosis of a submucosal myoma is made by hysteroscopy. Direct visualization can establish the nature of the defect(s) more accurately and pinpoint the location, size, and relation to the tubal ostia and internal os (Figure 27-10).

Myomectomy

Indications for myomectomy are: (1) to conserve the uterus in a woman with large or symptomatic myomas and (2) to improve reproductive potential. Before performing a myomectomy to improve reproductive potential, a complete infertility investigation must be carried out to place the role of the myoma(s) in proper perspective. Additional infertility factor(s) should be corrected if possible prior to surgery. Subsequent pregnancy rates are reduced if myomectomy is performed in patients with multifactorial infertility.

Smaller myomas (less than 5 cm) may be resected or, if pedunculated, may be excised under hysteroscopic control. Two types of instruments have been used. A standard operating hysteroscope with scissors has been used to resect submucosal myomas. The line of resection follows that of the adjacent normal endometrial surface. This technique is most suitable for myomas in the center of the endometrial cavity and has been used to resect solitary or multiple myomas of up to 7 cm in diameter. After resection, the mass must be morcellated to permit removal via the cervical os.

Another approach is that of using a resectoscope and "shaving" the myoma gradually to a point even with the normal endometrial surface.[17] This technique requires simultaneous laparoscopy and may be used for myomas that are more eccentrically placed. Although the number of procedures performed was small, Neuwirth reported that two-thirds to three-fourths of all patients had no recurrence of bleeding over 1 to 7 years of follow-up. Many conceived and delivered uneventfully.

If abdominal myomectomy is planned, a preoperative HSG (or preferably hysteroscopy) is mandatory to assess the nature and location of any submucosal lesions. The patient must be informed that intraoperative findings may necessitate hysterectomy. A dilute vasopressin solution is injected along the line of uterine incision to reduce intraoperative loss of blood. Twenty units of vasopressin are dissolved in 20 to 40 mL of saline. Blood loss during the operative procedure will be reduced further by placing a tourniquet around the uterine vessels; however, this technique is rarely needed if vasopressin is used. The uterine incision(s) should be vertical and confined to the anterior fundal wall, if possible. This reduces the chance of subsequent bowel or adnexal adherence. To minimize the total number of myometrial incisions, as many myomas as possible should be excised through each. The endometrial cavity should be entered only if a submucous myoma is present. Pregnancy may be attempted 3 to 6 months after the surgery.

The results of myomectomy were studied in 75 patients who had been infertile for 1 to 18 years (mean, 3.9 years).[18] Although 49% of the patients conceived following surgery, the age of the patient significantly influenced the incidence of success. As with most types of infertility surgery, most pregnancies occurred soon after the procedure.

If multiple uterine incisions are made, or if the endometrial cavity is entered, subsequent delivery should be by cesarean section. If a cervical myomectomy has been performed, elective cervical cerclage in the second trimester should be considered.

Recurrence of myomas following conservative surgery has been reported in 20% to 50% of women.[18] Most of these patients eventually require a hysterectomy.

References

1. Adoni A, Palti Z, Milwidsky A, et al: The incidence of intrauterine adhesions following spontaneous abortion. *Int J Fertil* 27:117, 1982

2. March CM, Israel R, March AD: Hysteroscopic management of intrauterine adhesions. *Am J Obstet Gynecol* 130:653, 1978

3. Zbella EA, Moise J, Carson SA: Noncardiogenic pulmonary edema secondary to intrauterine instillation of 32% dextran 70. *Fertil Steril* 43:479, 1985

4. Edstrom K, Fernstrom I: The diagnostic possibilities of a modified hysteroscopic technique. *Acta Obstet Gynecol Scand* 49:327, 1970

5. March CM, Israel R: Intrauterine adhesions secondary to elective abortion: Hysteroscopic diagnosis and management. *Obstet Gynecol* 48:422, 1976

6. March CM, Israel R: Gestational outcome following hysteroscopic lysis of adhesions. *Fertil Steril* 36:455, 1981

7. Buttram VC, Gibbons WE: Mullerian anomalies: A proposed classification (an analysis of 144 cases). *Fertil Steril* 32:40, 1979

8. Semmens JP: Congenital anomalies of female genital tract. *Obstet Gynecol* 19:328, 1962

9. Rock JA, Jones HW Jr: The clinical management of the double uterus. *Fertil Steril* 28:798, 1977

10. Daly DC, Walters CA, Soto-Albors CE, et al: Hysteroscopic metroplasty: Surgical technique and obstetric outcome. *Fertil Steril* 39:623, 1983

11. Israel R, March CM: Hysteroscopic incision of the septate uterus. *Am J Obstet Gynecol* 149:66, 1984

12. DeCherney A, Polan ML: Hysteroscopic management of intrauterine lesions and intractable uterine bleeding. *Obstet Gynecol* 61:392, 1983

13. Kaufman RH, Adam E, Binder GL, et al: Upper genital tract changes and pregnancy outcome in offspring exposed in utero to diethylstilbestrol. *Am J Obstet Gynecol* 137:299, 1980

14. DeCherney AH, Cholst I, Naftolin F: Structure and function of the fallopian tubes following exposure to diethylstilbestrol (DES) during gestation. *Fertil Steril* 36:741, 1981

15. Barnes AB, Colton T, Gunderson J, et al: Fertility and outcome of pregnancy in women exposed in utero to diethylstilbestrol. *N Engl J Med* 302:609, 1980

16. Buttram VC, Reiter RC: Uterine leiomyomata: Etiology, symptomatology and management. *Fertil Steril* 36:433, 1981

17. Neuwirth RS: A new technique for and additional experience with hysteroscopic resection of submucous fibroids. *Am J Obstet Gynecol* 131:91, 1978

18. Malone MJ, Ingersol FM: Myomectomy in infertility. In Behrman SJ, Kistner RW (eds): *Progress in Infertility,* ed 2. Boston, Little, Brown, 1975

Suggested reading

Jones HW Jr, Jones GES: Double uterus as an etiological factor of repeated abortion: Indication for surgical repair. *Am J Obstet Gynecol* 65:325, 1953

Schenker JG, Margalioth EJ: Intrauterine adhesions: An updated appraisal. *Fertil Steril* 37:593, 1982

Chapter 28

Tubal Surgery

Richard P. Marrs, M.D.

The incidence of infertility secondary to tubal disease has increased in the US during the past 10 years. The reason appears to be an increased incidence of salpingitis. Women with damaged oviducts who wish to become pregnant must either have surgical correction or use in vitro fertilization (IVF). It is impossible to surgically normalize the intraluminal portion of the oviduct, which is usually damaged after one or more episodes of salpingitis.

In evaluating patients with tubal factor infertility, it is of the utmost importance to determine the anatomic status of the fallopian tubes before attempting any surgery. An estimation of the prognosis for successful pregnancy should be attempted, and a detailed discussion should be undertaken with the couple before surgical intervention. Alternatives to tubal surgery, such as IVF with embryo replacement, are resulting in an ever increasing rate of pregnancy success. Therefore, these options must be considered and discussed before attempting surgical reconstruction of the oviduct.

Hysterosalpingography

To assess tubal damage accurately, both the tubal lumen and its exterior must be evaluated. The hysterosalpingogram (HSG) is of great benefit in evaluating the luminal environment of the fal-

lopian tube. As discussed in Chapter 26, a water-based contrast medium, such as Sinografin, is best for demonstrating mucosal folds and rugal markings within the tubal lumen. The appearance of these markings is extremely important in determining the extent of intraluminal damage (the more apparent the markings, the less severe the damage). Oil-based contrast material has been advocated as possibly enhancing fertility in patients with open tubes, but it does not provide as good intraluminal demarcation in patients with distal obstruction.[1]

A bimanual pelvic examination should be performed before the contrast material is injected, because in the presence of an active inflammatory process, an HSG may worsen the extent of damage. An HSG should never be performed when there is adnexal tenderness. Furthermore, at least 6 months should elapse from an episode of acute salpingitis before an HSG is done. A study from this institution revealed that 14 (3.1%) of 448 patients undergoing HSG developed acute salpingitis within 24 hours after the procedure. It appears that patients with a positive history for previous pelvic inflammatory disease (PID) have a higher risk of inflammatory reaction following HSG.[2]

Measurement of white blood cell count and sedimentation rate may be helpful when the presence of adnexal tenderness is questionable. All patients undergoing HSG require broad-spectrum antibiotic coverage. We give doxycycline, 100 mg twice daily for 5 days, beginning 2 days before the scheduled HSG. If an allergy to tetracycline is present, ampicillin, 250 mg four times a day, may be used. The Rubin test, or carbon dioxide insufflation, has been used in the past to determine tubal patency, but it is of no value for prognostic evaluation of fallopian tube function. In the best of circumstances, the Rubin test can demonstrate only whether fallopian tubes are patent. No estimation of intraluminal damage can be gained by this technique.

Laparoscopy

The second major technique used to identify tubal damage is laparoscopy. Using laparoscopy, an evaluation can be made of the external environment and appearance of the fallopian tubes, ovaries, and the rest of the pelvic cavity. When laparoscopy is combined with HSG, the pelvic reparative surgeon can better estimate pregnancy prognosis before surgical intervention. Laparoscopy should be performed in the follicular phase of the menstrual cycle, when the endometrial lining is minimal, so that dye instillation will be unobstructed through the interstitial segment of the fallopian tube.

Closed laparoscopy, using a Veress needle insufflation before trocar placement (see Figure 29-3), is used in most procedures. Risk of injury to major blood vessels or bowel is approximately 1/1,000 procedures.[3] In patients who have had previous surgery through a midline incision or a history of severe intraabdominal adhesions, an open laparoscopy approach should be used (see Figure 29-4). A subumbilical incision is made through the skin and fascia. The peritoneum is opened and the blunt laparoscopy cannula is placed intraperitoneally under direct visualization. When the cannula is sutured to the fascia, it creates an airtight seal for gas insufflation. Intrauterine injection of indigo carmine (1 ampule in 500 cc normal saline) is performed with a Conn or Huey cannula or a 10 French pediatric Foley catheter placed in the uterine cavity. The use of a rigid cannula attached to a tenaculum, which is attached to the cervix, is preferable, because the uterus can be moved by the surgeon or assistant. Determination of the integrity and patency of the fallopian tube, under direct laparoscopic visualization, is carried out by instilling the indigo carmine solution and observing spill from the distal ends of the fallopian tubes.

The laparoscopic evaluation of tubal status may be immediately followed by laparotomy in patients with surgically treatable distal tubal disease or those undergoing sterilization reversal. The combined procedures need only a single anesthetic. Some practitioners, however, prefer to perform the laparoscopy at a separate time from the laparotomy. This gives them a chance to explain the prognosis fully to the patient before they attempt the tubal reconstructive surgery.

This chapter discusses the clinical presentations of tubal disease, as well as the prognosis for pregnancy after their correction. Basic surgical approaches—microsurgical versus conventional macrosurgical techniques—are compared. Complications of tubal surgery, namely, ectopic tubal pregnancies, and their surgical treatment are also discussed.

Distal tubal disease

The most common etiology for distal tubal disease is an inflammatory insult, due primarily to bacterial infection within the pelvic cavity. Distal tubal disease or intraluminal disease secondary to pelvic tuberculosis (TB) is rare in the US. The HSG appearance of tubal disease from an inflammatory process is mainly one of hydrosalpinx or distal tubal closure (see Figure 26-10). The HSG will reveal a filling of the fallopian tube and a closed-off or sacculated terminal end of the tube. Before the fallopian tube is closed completely, phimosis, or narrowing, can be seen. During HSG, this appears as a narrowing of the distal aspect of the tube with dilitation (Figure 28-1A) and dye spillage into the pelvic cavity (Figure 28-1B). Of great importance at the time of HSG is the appearance of the mucosal folds and the rugal patterns after injection of contrast. The HSG should ideally be performed by the tubal surgeon, because these patterns are best visualized before dye filling causes marked tubal distension.

The characteristic appearance of tubal damage from pelvic TB includes rigid, fixed fallopian tubes, so-called "lead pipe tubes," or a "tobacco pouch" appearance. The tube is patent, but has a marked narrowing at the terminal aspect and proximal dilation (see Figure 26-12). The diagnosis should be confirmed by appearance of granuloma in an endometrial biopsy performed between cycle days 24 and 27 or by successful culture of menstrual blood revealing acid-fast organisms.

Treatment should include isoniazid and rifampin. If active or widespread disease is evident, ethambutol should be given with the other two drugs. One to 2 years of treatment are necessary to clear the disease. The pregnancy prognosis is essentially nil after treatment for pelvic TB; thus, patients should be counseled accordingly. Surgical procedures to correct the tubal status of patients with a history of pelvic TB are unwarranted; therefore, these patients should be referred for an IVF procedure if the endometrial cavity is free of disease.

Laparoscopy should be the second step in the evaluation of distal tubal disease to determine what the overall prognosis will be after surgical correction. The appearance of the fallopian tube in the nondistended state at the time of laparoscopy is important in judging its integrity. The amount of muscularis and the amount of dilation of the hydrosalpinx before injection of indigo carmine are important prognostic indications. If, with injection of dye, the tube appears

to have an extremely thin wall with no adequate surrounding muscular coat, the prognosis for pregnancy is poor and surgical correction should not be attempted. The severity of pelvic adhesion formation should also be considered at laparoscopy, because severe intraabdominal adhesions involving the adnexal structures decrease the chances of successful surgery for distal tubal disease. Distal hydrosalpinges less than 2 cm in diameter usually have a prognosis for pregnancy success of approximately 30% to 35% after surgical opening.[3-6]

The usual surgical approach for correcting distal tubal occlusion has been through a laparotomy incision, with reconstruction of the fimbrial opening. The macrosurgical technique uses no magnification; the fallopian tube is merely opened in a stellate fashion and a new ostium is created by suturing back the open end of the tube with nonreactive suture material (Figure 28-2). Recently, most surgeons have been using a microsurgical approach that includes atraumatic tissue handling, constant irrigation throughout the operative procedure, pinpoint electrocoagulation for hemostasis, use of magnification, and very fine (6-0) nonreactive suture material.[1,5,6]

Essentially the same type of tubal opening is performed with microsurgery as with macrosurgery. With the use of magnification, however, avascular areas can be identified and the occluded end of the tube can be opened between islands of healthy mucosa within the tubal lumen. This approach conserves healthy intraluminal mucosa where it is present. The carbon dioxide laser, either handheld or manipulated by a joystick through the operating microscope, has also been used with a laparotomy incision for treating distal tubal disease. To date, no significant improvement in pregnancy outcome has been demonstrated with this technique.[7,8] A CO_2 laser has been used through an operating laparoscope to perform cuff salpingostomy procedures in patients with distal tubal occlusions.[9]

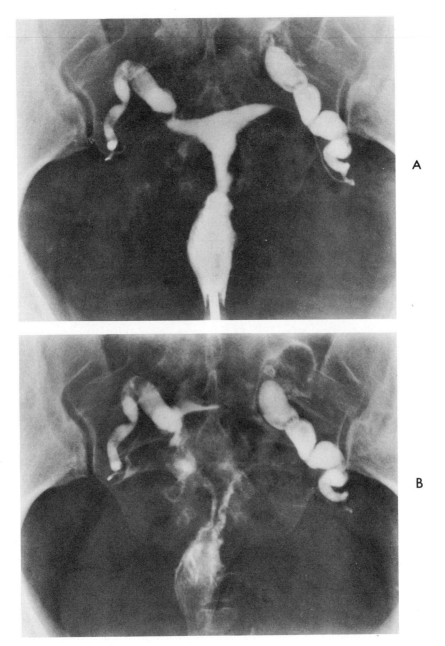

A

B

Figure 28-1
Bilateral chronic salpingitis with tubal patency in a 21-year-old woman (gravida 3, para 1) with 1½ years of secondary infertility. A. Elongation and dilation of the ampullae, clubbing at the fimbriated ends, and destruction of the mucosal folds. B. Bilateral tubal spill, seen more easily after removal of the cannula and drainage of contrast medium from the endometrial cavity. Extensive pelvic adhesions were seen at laparoscopy, retracting the tubes into the cul-de-sac.

Infertility

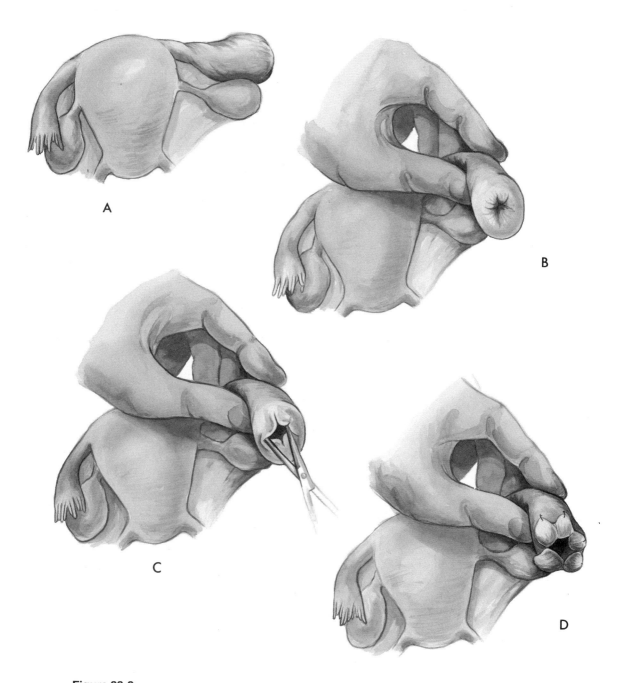

Figure 28-2
Macrosurgical cuff salpingostomy. A. Right hydrosalpinx after dye insufflation. B. Avascular dimple of the distal tube, which is incised. C. Further opening in a stellate fashion. D. Suturing of the distal tubal opening.

Table 28-1
Pregnancy results after macrosurgical or microsurgical cuff salpingostomy

Surgeon	Technique	Intrauterine pregnancy	Ectopic pregnancy
O'Brien	Macro	25%	2%
Cognat	Macro	24%	4%
Grant	Macro	41%	0
Siegler	Macro	7%	0
Swolin	Micro	24%	18%
Winston	Micro	18%	9.5%
Gomel	Micro	31%	9%

The number of patients treated is extremely small, so the ultimate feasibility of this procedure is still unknown.

Overall pregnancy rates following distal tubal opening have varied. With conventional macrosurgical approaches, intrauterine pregnancy rates have been reported to range between 20% and 35%. The incidence of tubal pregnancy has ranged from 4% to as high as 20%.[1,5] The ectopic pregnancy rate appears to be directly proportional to the amount of intraluminal tubal disease present at the time of surgical correction. It is not directly associated with the surgeon's technical ability. The 24% to 40% pregnancy rates with microsurgical techniques are not a marked improvement compared to those obtained with conventional macrosurgery. Moreover, ectopic pregnancy rates have been in the same general range as those reported with conventional surgery (Table 28-1).

Optimal candidates for cuff salpingostomy should have a minimal dilation of the distal fallopian tube on the HSG, with good healthy rugal markings indicating a fairly healthy mucosal pattern intraluminally. At laparoscopy, the tube should be able to be visualized. Optimally, there should be minimal or no adhesions in the pelvic cavity and only minimal dilation of the distal tube. When the indigo carmine is instilled, good muscularis should be visualized surrounding the tube. In such circumstances, with gentle tissue handling and a modified microsurgical approach, the chance of intrauterine pregnancy should be approximately 30%. However, there is up to a 20% chance of an ectopic pregnancy. With increasing amounts of tubal damage, the chances of successful pregnancy diminish and the chances of tubal pregnancy increase. Patients found to have large (>2 cm) thin-walled hydrosalpinges, with visible ovaries, should consider utilizing IVF rather than cuff salpingostomy. The pregnancy success with tubal surgery is equivalent to, or less than, the success with IVF, and the risk of ectopic pregnancy is markedly less with IVF.[10]

Techniques such as fimbrioplasty should not be confused with cuff salpingostomy. Fimbrioplasty is the removal of fimbrial bridges or adhesions in a tube that is patent; cuff salpingostomy is the reopening of a closed distal tube. Fimbrioplasty is used for patients who have a narrowing of the fimbrial opening, secondary to bridges between individual fimbriae. These bridges are easily lysed with microsurgical techniques, and 40% to 50% of patients so treated are reported to subsequently achieve intrauterine pregnancy[11,11a] (Table 28-2). Severe tubal phimosis is primarily treated in a fashion similar to that for total occlusion (cuff salpingostomy). However, by definition, a cuff salpingostomy is not performed, because the tube is minimally open at the time of surgical correction.

Table 28-2
Pregnancy results after microsurgical fimbrioplasty

Author	No. of cases	Term pregnancy rates	Ectopic pregnancy rates
Siegler and Koutopoulos	9	5/9 (56%)	1/6 (11%)
Patton	35	21/35 (60%)	1/22 (3%)

Proximal tubal blockage

The most common etiology for proximal tubal disease or interstitial tubal blockage is thought to be an inflammatory insult, most commonly salpingitis isthmica nodosa (SIN). SIN is a pathologic diagnosis that can be made only after the oviduct is examined histologically, but it can be suspected by HSG before it causes tubal occlusion. On the HSG, SIN appears as diverticula within the tubal lumen (see Figure 26-9). Even though there is tubal patency, the pregnancy prognosis is poor and the risk of ectopic pregnancy is increased. Rarely, endometriosis within the tubal lumen can be the causative factor.

The diagnosis of proximal tubal blockage should be entertained when the HSG reveals nonfilling of the fallopian tubes. This process can be differentiated from interstitial tubal spasm on the HSG by visualization of part or all of the interstitial segment of the tube (see Figure 26-11). If no filling occurs in any portion of the interstitial segment bilaterally, then the possibility of tubal spasm should be considered.

Laparoscopy is necessary to confirm the diagnosis of this type of tubal blockage. Under general anesthesia, interstitial spasm should not be encountered and, if interstitial patency is present, tubal spill of dye will occur. Moreover, laparoscopy is important for visualizing the distal aspect of the tubes, because the combination of proximal block and distal disease (hydrosalpinx) has a very poor prognosis (<5% pregnancy rate) after surgical correction.[1] Surgery should not be attempted with bipolar tubal disease. If, at the time of laparoscopy, the pelvic cavity is free of adhesions and the fallopian tubes and fimbriae appear to be normal and healthy, with a block in the proximal tubal aspect, pregnancy prognosis ranges from 30% to 50%, depending on the type of corrective procedure performed (Table 28-3).[12-15]

The types of surgical correction for proxi-

Table 28-3
Success of various surgical techniques to treat proximal tubal obstruction

Procedure	No. of cases	Ectopic pregnancy	Term pregnancy
Reimplantation			
Kistner and Patton	646		204/646 (32%)
Siegel and Perez	124	2/23 (7%)	21/124 (17%)
Palmer	118		52/118 (44%)
Rock	52	2/15 (13%)	13/52 (25%)
Peterson et al	16		8/16 (50%)
Reanastomosis (tubocornual)			
Gomel	38	2	20/38 (53%)

mal tubal disease have varied over the years. Initially, interstitial or cornual block was treated solely by closed or open cornual reimplantation procedures. In the closed procedure, the cornual aspect of each tube was resected and the proximal portion of each remaining oviduct was placed through a cornual opening into the endometrial cavity[14] (Figure 28-3). Alternatively, the uterine fundus was opened in a Strassman-like procedure and the proximal portion of each tube was fish-mouthed and sutured to the endometrial lining. Then, the fundus was closed in layers (Figure 28-4).

In the past few years, these cornual reimplantation procedures have been replaced by a procedure originally described in 1977.[12] A posterior fundal incision is performed, and the fallopian tubes are placed in the posterior fundal aspect of the uterus. In 1977, Winston described a tubal-cornual reanastomosis procedure that does not require reimplantation (Figure 28-5).[13] The myometrium of the interstitial aspect of each tube is shaved serially, until a patent canal into the endometrial cavity can be demonstrated. This is done by instillation of dye into the uterus via an indwelling pediatric Foley catheter. Serial shaving of the myometrium is continued until dye flows freely from the uterine cavi-

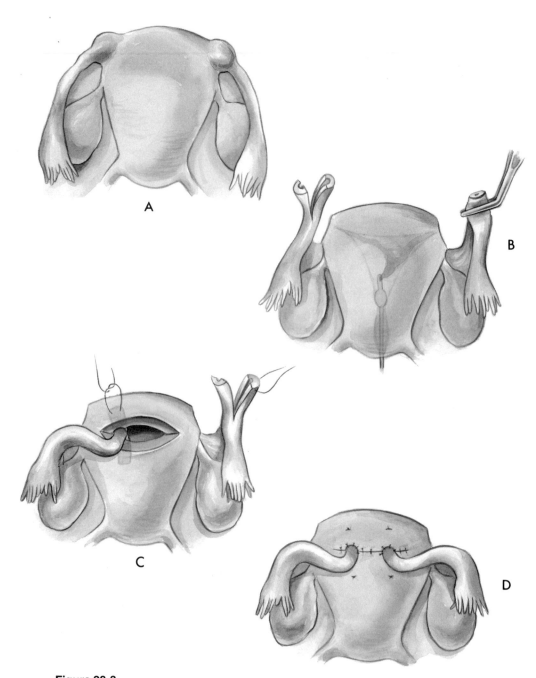

Figure 28-3
Posterior tubal reimplantation, closed procedure. A. Bilateral isthmic obstruction. B. Tubal division distal to the obstructive area and fish-mouthing of the proximal tubal ends. C. Incision of the posterior myometrium at the level of the utero-ovarian suspensory ligament and suturing of the proximal tubal flaps within the endometrial cavity. D. Closure of the myometrium in layers.

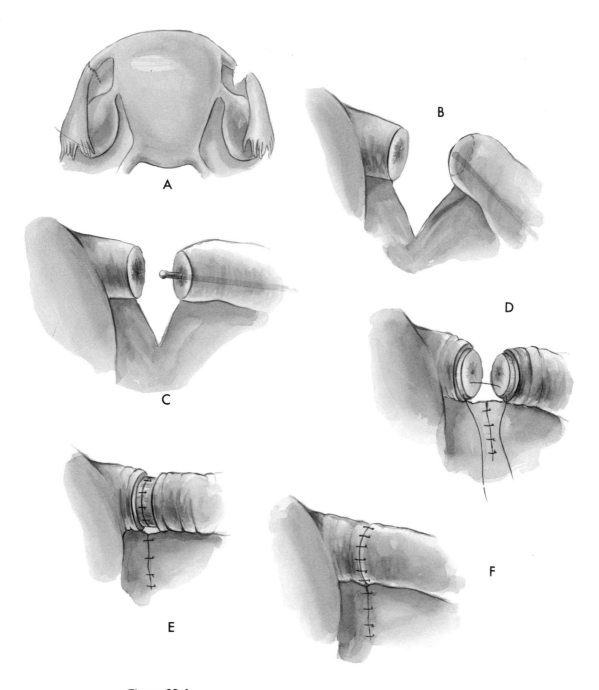

Figure 28-4
End-to-end reanastomosis, open procedure. A. Right tube before procedure. B and C. Preparation of the proximal and distal segments. D and E. Approximation of the muscularis layers. F. Closure of the serosal layers.

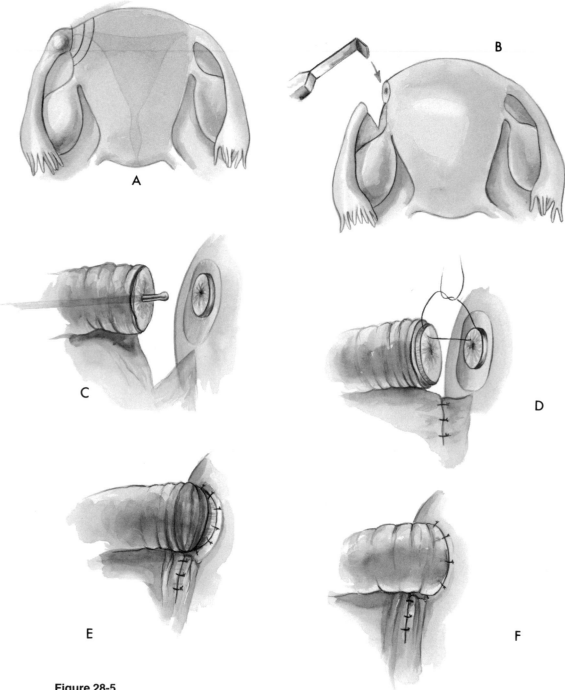

Figure 28-5
Tubal-cornual reanastomosis. A. Planes of myometrial shaving. B. Shaving to establish a patent interstitial segment. C. Opening of the proximal end of the distal tubal segment. D and E. Placement of cardinal sutures for approximation of the muscularis layers. F. Approximation of the serosal layers.

Infertility

ty. Then, dye is instilled in retrograde fashion from the tubal fimbriated end, and the tubal isthmic portion is serially sectioned until a flow of dye is seen. The muscularis of the isthmic portion is then approximated with 8-0 sutures to the muscularis of the interstitial portion at cardinal points (6, 9, 12, and 3 o'clock). The tubal serosa and the uterus are approximated with 6-0 sutures. Reinstillation of dye through the uterus should demonstrate patency without leakage at the anastomotic site.

With this type of tubal disease, the current therapy of choice is the tubal-cornual reanastomosis technique. With this technique, pregnancy success has been reported to range between 50% and 60%.[13,15] The posterior reimplantation procedure[12] is reported to have a 40% to 50% intrauterine pregnancy rate. However, this latter procedure requires cesarean delivery, as does any reimplantation procedure. There is also a risk of asymptomatic uterine dehiscence in approximately 10% to 15% of patients who become pregnant.[12]

Sterilization reversal

The most encouraging and satisfying type of tubal reparative surgery is reversal of a previous tubal sterilization procedure. The difference between this type of reconstructive procedure and those discussed above is that with the former, the fallopian tubes are healthy, both proximally and distally. Thus, tubal function results in better pregnancy outcome. Even though women who undergo this type of procedure have become pregnant in the past, a full fertility evaluation of both partners should be undertaken before attempting surgical sterilization reversal. Two important preoperative procedures, besides evaluation of the male factor and female ovulatory function, are an HSG and laparoscopy. The HSG is important to pinpoint proximal tubal segments and determine their length.

Laparoscopy is the only way to evaluate the length and condition of the distal tubal segment.

A composite measurement of the proximal and distal segments must be made before entering the abdomen for an attempt of tubal reanastomosis. The overall tubal length after reanastomosis, as well as which areas of the tube are involved in the surgical procedure are important determinants for prognosis. Tubal reanastomosis after tubal sterilization involves either a tubal-tubal or tubal-cornual reapproximation. Tubal-tubal reanastomosis is reapproximation of the isthmic-ampullary, isthmic-isthmic, or ampullary-ampullary portions of the fallopian tube. In contrast, a tubal-cornual reanastomosis is required when the proximal tube is absent. A reapproximation of the distal tube with the interstitial segment is performed as described above for proximal tubal blockage.

For tubal-tubal reanastomosis, the closed proximal and distal segments are opened under magnification by removing each fibrotic end with microscissors. Hemostasis is obtained by a microtipped bovie instrument. Approximation of the mesosalpinx is performed with interrupted 6-0 sutures. Approximation of the muscularis of the proximal and distal segments is then performed with 8-0 single sutures at the 12, 3, 6, and 9 o'clock positions. The serosa is approximated with 6-0 sutures. Dye instillation through the uterus should demonstrate tubal patency without leakage at the anastomotic site. Reimplantation procedures for sterilization reversal are necessary on rare occasions when tubal cautery has been performed. Interstitial segments may not be patent after proximal tubal segment coagulation.

As mentioned above, tubal length is an important factor in the prognosis for pregnancy. Patients who have in excess of 4 cm of fallopian tube following anastomosis have a pregnancy success rate in the range of 50% or better. Pregnancy success is markedly diminished if postanastomosis tubal length is less than 4 cm. Pa-

Table 28-4
Effect of postoperative tubal length on pregnancy success following tubal reanastomosis

Author	Postoperative length	Pregnancy rate (%)
Silber and Cohen	<3 cm	0/7
	3–4 cm	3/7 (43%)
	>4 cm	11/11 (100%)
Winston	<4 cm	4/11 (36%)
	4–6 cm	8/15 (53%)
	>6 cm	7/9 (78%)

Table 28-5
Effect of site of anastomosis on pregnancy rate following reanastomosis

Site of anastomosis	Pregnancy rate (%)
Isthmic-cornual	14/20 (70%)
Isthmic-isthmic	24/38 (63%)
Isthmic-ampullary	7/11 (64%)
Ampullary-ampullary	2/4 (50%)

Modified from Seiler JC: Factors influencing the outcome of microsurgical tubal ligation reversal. Am J Obstet Gynecol 146:292, 1983.

Table 28-6
Pregnancy results after macrosurgical or microsurgical sterilization reversal

Surgeon	Technique	Intrauterine pregnancy (%)	Ectopic pregnancy (%)
Siegler	Macro	22	4
Rock et al	Macro	42	0
Winston	Micro	58	2
Gomel	Micro	65	1

tients whose postsurgical tubal length will be that small should be counseled against undergoing a reanastomosis procedure, because they may be more successfully treated by IVF. As the length of the fallopian tubes approaches 6 cm or more, 60% to 70% of patients will achieve an intrauterine pregnancy[1,16-18a] (Table 28-4).

The pregnancy prognosis also depends on the site of anastomosis. The highest incidence of pregnancies occurs with isthmic-isthmic and isthmic-cornual reanastomosis; the lowest, with ampullary-ampullary reanastomosis (approximately 50%; Table 28-5).[17] With microsurgical techniques, there is a low incidence of ectopic pregnancy (3% to 6%) following surgical sterilization reversal.[1,16-18]

Microsurgical techniques appear to improve the surgical outcome, when compared with conventional macrosurgical techniques. A comparison of several different reports of conventional and microsurgical therapy is shown in Table 28-6. Of the three types of surgical correction for tubal disease that have been discussed, the results of tubal reanastomosis appear to be most improved by microsurgical techniques.

Ectopic pregnancy

In the general population, the incidence of tubal ectopic pregnancies ranges from one in every 300 deliveries to as high as one in every 30 deliveries. One of the factors that definitely increases the incidence of ectopic gestation is tubal reconstructive surgery. The highest incidence of ectopic pregnancies (approximately 20%) occurs among patients who have had previous distal tubal surgery, because these patients tend to have the largest amount of intraluminal damage from the previous inflammatory process. The lowest incidence of ectopic pregnancies after tubal surgery (3% to 6%) is seen in those patients who have had a microsurgical reversal of a previous sterilization procedure.[1,16-18]

Certainly, the evaluation and diagnosis of a suspected ectopic pregnancy have improved in the past few years. This is due primarily to the use of rapid sensitive pregnancy tests. Irregular bleeding, abdominal discomfort, and a positive pregnancy test should suggest the possibility of a tubal gestation, especially if the woman has had prior tubal surgery. The diagnosis may also be improved by using ultrasound to identify an intrauterine or an extrauterine pregnancy. Culdocentesis can determine the presence of intraperitoneal blood. Laparoscopy is the ultimate technique for diagnosing an ectopic pregnancy.

The finding of an ectopic pregnancy involves the patient and physician in a decision-making process. It is no longer acceptable merely to remove the affected fallopian tube. For the past 15 years, a conservative surgical approach for the treatment of ectopic pregnancy has been increasingly favored. Conservation of the fallopian tube does not appear to increase the overall risk of a second ectopic pregnancy.

Recent reports have shown that linear salpingostomies for removal of ectopic gestations have not increased the risk of a second ectopic in comparison with surgical removal of the affected fallopian tube[19,20] (Table 28-7). Moreover, in a recent report of the outcome in 15 patients who had single remaining fallopian tubes and had conservative operations to remove ectopic pregnancies, there was only a 20% incidence of repeat ectopic pregnancy. Over 50% of the patients had subsequent pregnancies that proceeded to normal term delivery (Table 28-7).[20] Thus, the primary conservative therapy for an unruptured ectopic pregnancy is linear salpingostomy.

The procedure is most often performed in patients with an early diagnosis of unruptured tubal gestation. The fallopian tube is opened over the area of the ectopic pregnancy on the surface opposite the mesosalpinx. The ectopic pregnancy is shelled out, bleeders are electrocoagulated, and the tube is left open and allowed to heal by secondary intention (Figure 28-6). Tubal patency rates are good, and repeat ectopic rates range between 15% and 18%.[19,20] This incidence is not statistically different from that seen when the involved fallopian tube is removed (Table 28-7).

Tubal closure is not recommended at the time of linear salpingostomy, because this may cause a constriction at the suture line, or blood or serum may collect and create an area of obstruction. With secondary healing, the salpingostomy site can drain, if necessary, and usually

Table 28-7
Conservative treatment of ectopic pregnancy

Surgeon	No. of patients	Intrauterine pregnancy (%)	Ectopic pregnancy (%)
Suchet	14	57	15
Timonen and Nieminen	240	38	16
Jarvruen	10	60	30
Stromme	45	71	15
DeCherney et al	49	40	12
DeCherney*	15	53	20

*Ectopic in only remaining tube.

closes spontaneously 3 to 4 weeks following surgery. If, after linear salpingostomy and removal of the gestational material, bleeding persists at the mesenteric side of the tube, interrupted 2-0 or 3-0 sutures are placed in the mesosalpinx to control bleeding from the tubal bed. If bleeding into the tubal lumen continues, a segmental resection should be performed by placing a single 3-0 nylon suture through the mesosalpinx and ligating the tube proximal and distal to the site of the salpingostomy. The segment between the sutures is then sharply removed, and bleeding in the mesosalpinx can be controlled by coagulation or suture ligation. With this technique, a major portion of the tube can be salvaged. If necessary, in the future, an end-to-end reanastomosis can be performed to create tubal patency.

The most recent method for treating unruptured tubal pregnancy is laparoscopic removal. This technique is used primarily for ampullary ectopic pregnancies. The fallopian tube can be opened, the ectopic pregnancy removed, and bleeding points cauterized by laparoscopic instrumentation (Figure 28-7). This technique can be performed in selected patients by physicians with expertise in laparoscopic surgery. If a tubal abortion or fimbrial ectopic pregnancy is apparent at laparoscopy, the products of conception can usually be removed and bleeders can usually be coagulated through the laparoscope. This avoids the necessity for laparotomy.

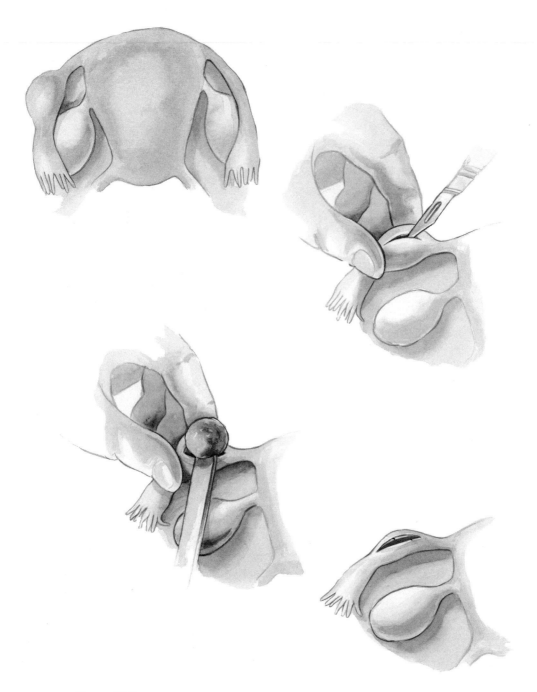

Figure 28-6
Linear salpingostomy via laparotomy, with the salpingostomy site left open at the end of the
procedure.

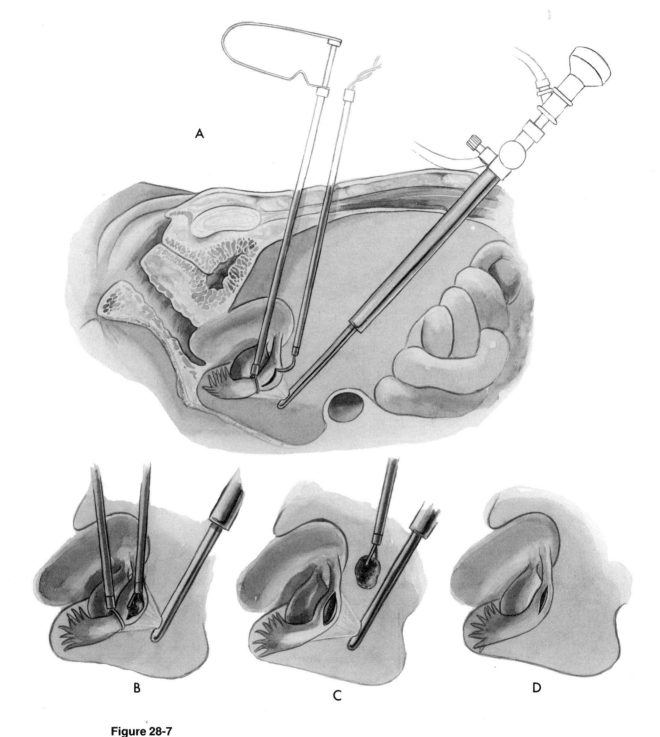

Figure 28-7
A. Laparoscopic linear salpingostomy. A cutting electrocurrent is used to make the tubal opening over the site of an unruptured tubal gestation. B and C. The gestational products are then removed with grasping forceps. D. The salpingostomy site is left open, and bleeding points are coagulated.

Tubal surgery

Adjunctive therapy
with tubal reconstructive surgery

For several decades, the use of hydrotubation after tubal surgery has been thought to help maintain tubal patency and decrease intraabdominal adhesions. To date, no prospective studies have been done to compare the results of distal tubal surgery with and without hydrotubation. Currently, after distal tubal surgery, our approach is to perform only one hydrotubation after microsurgical opening of distal tubal blockage. Over 90% of the tubes will maintain patency without additional hydrotubations. Tubal stints or hoods are no longer used; these devices may maintain patency, but they also damage the mucosal lining of the oviduct.

Following reanastomosis procedures, the use of intraluminal stints does not improve tubal patency or rates of pregnancy. Intraluminal stints do cause erosive changes within the tubal mucosa. Hydrotubations are not needed after tubal-cornual or tubal-tubal reanastomosis or after tubal reimplantation procedures. They might adversely affect the early healing of the anastomotic site. In cases where hydrotubations are used (distal tubal surgery), broad-spectrum antibiotic coverage (doxycycline, 100 mg twice daily) begins 2 days before and extends for 5 days. Various solutions can be used: normal saline, saline with 100 mg hydrocortisone, or dextran-40. A 30-mL instillation is adequate. If hydrotubation is used, we perform it on the third, fourth, or fifth postoperative day with 30 mL of dextran-40.

There is also controversy about methods used for postoperative adhesion prophylaxis following tubal reconstructive procedures. Several approaches have been described. The intraperitoneal use of dextran-70 (Hyskon), a high-molecular-weight dextran solution, has been advocated to diminish intraabdominal adhesions.[21] Dextran-70 works primarily by providing a flo-

tation mechanism for the pelvic structures. It acts as an osmotic gradient that draws fluid into the abdominal cavity, creating a mild ascites that keeps the adnexal structures in a floating environment for 7 to 10 days. By separating the serosal surfaces during this time, this method is thought to decrease the chances of adhesion formation. Preliminary studies, in animals as well as humans, have shown a potential decrease in adhesions with intraperitoneal dextran-70.[21]

In our practice, between 100 and 200 mL of dextran-70 are placed intraperitoneally before wound closure. Intraabdominal intraperitoneal corticosteroid instillation at the completion of the procedure, either in saline or in dextran-70, has also been used in combination with systemic corticosteroid therapy in an attempt to decrease the inflammatory reaction seen during normal healing.[22] One suggested protocol includes placing 100 to 200 mL of dextran-70 in the peritoneal cavity just prior to closure of the anterior peritoneum. Postsurgically, the patient receives 4 mg of dexamethasone IV push every 4 hours for a total of 12 doses over the first 48 hours. In addition, promethazine (Phenergan) 25 mg is given IM every 6 hours for 8 doses over 48 hours. Promethazine, an antihistamine, is combined with systemic steroid therapy because it has been theorized that a histaminic response plays a part in scar formation.[22]

This combined approach, using systemic steroid therapy to reduce inflammation and the antihistamine to block histamine release, was first reported by Replogle and co-authors.[22] It was concluded in a nonrandomized study that adhesion formation was reduced. Our patients are also maintained on a broad-spectrum antibiotic (doxycycline, 100 mg IV every 12 hours for 48 hours), which is instituted at the beginning of surgery. It must be realized, however, that there is no evidence in any randomized study that any of these pharmaceutical agents reduce the incidence of adhesion formation.[23]

Probably the most important way to retard

adhesions is the surgical technique itself. Much emphasis must be placed on atraumatic tissue handling, fine atraumatic instrumentation, and fine nonreactive suture material.[24] The abdominal contents should be packed with nonabrasive material, and the surgeon should handle tissues gently. Of the utmost importance is continuous irrigation with a solution of Ringer's lactate containing heparin 5,000 to 10,000 units/L. The irrigation keeps the serosal surfaces constantly moist throughout the operative procedure, and the heparin may also help retard formation of adhesions.

A final approach to decrease scar formation following surgery is through second-look laparoscopy (SLL). Some have advocated that this procedure be performed in the first 2 to 6 weeks postoperatively. The object is to lyse adhesions as they form, before they become dense and well vascularized. The advantage of this has not yet been proven, but the disadvantages are clear. The earlier in the postoperative period the SLL is performed, the greater the likelihood of bleeding. Moreover, the increased risk of another anesthetic and the increased cost to the patient cannot offset the lack of evidence of improved pregnancy results from the procedure. SLL is not a current standard practice.

Following reconstructive surgery of the oviduct, pregnancy should be avoided for 8 weeks. This allows healing of muscularis and serosal surfaces, so that normal tubal function can occur. In cases of tubal reimplantation, 3 months are adequate time for uterine healing before attempts at conception. If conception does not occur after proximal or distal tubal surgery, an HSG should be performed 6 months postoperatively. If the postoperative HSG reveals recurrent tubal occlusion, a repeat surgical procedure is not recommended, because pregnancy success is generally below 10%.[25] If tubal patency is present, pregnancy should continue to be attempted. If no conception occurs within the first 12 months after proximal tubal surgery, or within 24 to 36 months after distal tubal surgery, laparoscopic evaluation of the pelvis should be undertaken. (It has been reported that most pregnancies occur within the first 12 months following proximal tubal surgery versus 24 to 36 months following distal tubal surgery.[26,27])

Conclusion

Overall, the presence of tubal disease has a discouraging prognosis for fertility. Distal tubal disease carries a worse prognosis than proximal tubal disease or sterilization reversal procedures. In the past 5 years, the ability to bypass fallopian tube function by the IVF embryo replacement (ER) technique has provided an alternative for some patients who have irreparable tubal damage. It must be considered in cases of severe tubal damage, because tubal reconstructive surgery should not be performed if the prognosis for pregnancy is less than 20%. The rate of pregnancy following IVF procedures currently exceeds this figure in several centers. This alternative should be discussed with the couple. IVF procedures carry much less risk of ectopic pregnancy and, certainly, involve much less operative manipulation for the patient. The incidence of pregnancy success for certain types of tubal disease with IVF-ER can be identical to or better than microsurgical reconstruction of the oviduct. Patients with large hydrosalpinges or with recurrent hydrosalpinges following previous surgical correction should utilize IVF.

References

1. Gomel V: *Microsurgery in Female Infertility.* Boston, Little, Brown, 1983
2. Stumpf PG, March CM: Febrile morbidity following hysterosalpingography: Identification of risk factors and recommendations for prophylaxis. *Fertil Steril* 33:487, 1980
3. Israel R, March CM: Diagnostic laparoscopy: A prognostic aid in the surgical management of infertility. *Am J Obstet Gynecol* 125:969, 1976

4. Winston RM: Microsurgery of the fallopian tube: From fantasy to reality. *Fertil Steril* 34:521, 1980

5. Gomel V: Salpingostomy by microsurgery. *Fertil Steril* 29:380, 1978

6. Swolin K: Electromicrosurgery and salpingostomy: Long-term results. *Am J Obstet Gynecol* 121:418, 1975

7. Kelly RW, Roberts DK: Experience with the carbon dioxide laser in gynecologic microsurgery. *Am J Obstet Gynecol* 146:585, 1983

8. Fayez JA, Jobson VW, Lentz SS, et al: Tubal microsurgery with the carbon dioxide laser. *Am J Obstet Gynecol* 146:371, 1983

9. Daniell JF, Herbert CM: Laparoscopic salpingostomy utilizing the CO_2 laser. *Fertil Steril* 41:558, 1984

10. Vargyas JM, Yee B, Serafini P, et al: The use of single or combination agents for ovarian stimulation to induce multiple follicle development for human in vitro fertilization. *Infertility,* in press

11. Patton GW Jr: Pregnancy outcome following microsurgical fimbrioplasty. *Fertil Steril* 37:150, 1982

11a. Siegler AM, Koutopoulous V: An analysis of macrosurgical and microsurgical techniques in the management of the tuboperitoneal factor in infertility. *Fertil Steril* 32:377, 1979

12. Peterson EP, Musich JR, Behrman SJ: Uterotubal implantation and obstetric outcome after previous sterilization. *Am J Obstet Gynecol* 128:662, 1977

13. Winston RM: Microsurgical tubocornual anastomosis for reversal of sterilization. *Lancet* 1:284, 1977

14. Rock JA, Katayama KP, Martin EJ, et al: Pregnancy outcome following uterotubal implantation: A comparison of the reamer and sharp cornual wedge excision techniques. *Fertil Steril* 31:634, 1979

15. Levinson CJ: Implantation procedures for intramural obstruction: Pure bilateral implantation in 35 patients. *J Reprod Med* 26:347, 1981

16. Gomel V: Microsurgical reversal of female sterilization: A reappraisal. *Fertil Steril* 33:587, 1980

17. Seiler JC: Factors influencing the outcome of microsurgical tubal ligation reversal. *Am J Obstet Gynecol* 146:292, 1983

18. Gomel V: Tubal reanastomosis by microsurgery. *Fertil Steril* 28:59, 1977

18a. Silber SJ, Cohen R: Microsurgical reversal of female sterilization: The role of tubal length. *Fertil Steril* 33:598, 1980

19. DeCherney AH, Romero R, Naftolin F: Surgical management of unruptured ectopic pregnancy. *Fertil Steril* 35:21, 1981

20. DeCherney AH, Maheaux R, Naftolin F: Salpingostomy for ectopic pregnancy in the sole patent oviduct: Reproductive outcome. *Fertil Steril* 37:619, 1982

21. Neuwirth RS, Khalaf SM: Effect of thirty-two per cent dextran 70 on peritoneal adhesion formation. *Am J Obstet Gynecol* 121:420, 1975

22. Replogle RL, Johnson R, Gross RE: Prevention of postoperative intestinal adhesions with combined promethazine and dexamethasone therapy: Experimental and clinical studies. *Ann Surgery* 163:580, 1966

23. Luciano AA, Hauser KS, Benda J: Evaluation of commonly used adjuvants in the prevention of postoperative adhesions. *Am J Obstet Gynecol* 146:88, 1983

24. Holtz G, Kling OR: Effect of surgical technique on peritoneal adhesion reformation after lysis. *Fertil Steril* 37:494, 1982

25. Lauritsen JG, Pagel JD, Vangsted P, et al: Results of repeated tuboplasties. *Fertil Steril* 37:68, 1982

26. Katayama KP, Ju KS, Manuel M, et al: Computer analysis of etiology and pregnancy rate in 636 cases of primary infertility. *Am J Obstet Gynecol* 135:207, 1979

27. Umezaki C, Katayama KP, Jones HW Jr: Pregnancy rates after reconstructive surgery on the fallopian tubes. *Obstet Gynecol* 43:418, 1974

Chapter 29

Pelvic Endometriosis

Richard P. Marrs, M.D.
Joyce M. Vargyas, M.D.

For many years, endometriosis has been known to be associated with reproductive problems in women. Endometriosis is a disease characterized by viable endometrial-like tissue found in aberrant or ectopic locations. Most commonly, the surfaces of the ovary and the serosal surfaces of the pelvic cavity, including the bowel and bladder, are involved. It is uncommon for endometriosis to invade the mucosal lining of the bowel or bladder. Widespread dissemination has been seen in the pleural cavities and nasopharynx.

Sampson proposed the first theory to explain the phenomenon of pelvic endometriosis.[1] His theory states that pelvic endometriosis is due to reflex menstruation or retrograde menstruation. This theory is supported by the fact that in pelvic endometriosis, ovarian surfaces and the most dependent portion of the pelvic cavity, the posterior cul-de-sac, are the areas most frequently involved with endometrial implants. Other theories that have been reported to explain widespread or disseminated endometriosis include lymphatic spread and mechanical transport. Endometriosis, which has been found in most organ systems of the human female, probably occurs by each of these mechanisms. Overall, in women of reproductive age, the incidence of endometriosis has been reported to vary from 4% to 32%, with a mean of 7% to 8%. Endometriosis is found in 40% to 50% of women evaluated for infertility.[2]

The mechanism whereby endometriosis produces infertility is incompletely understood. Certainly, no mechanical processes can be attributed to this infertile state unless tubal adhesions are present, but it has been thought that hormonal aberrations may occur because of the endometriosis. Several years ago, it was reported that increased concentrations of prostaglandins were found in the peritoneal fluid, as well as in the peripheral serum, of these patients.[3] However, this has been negated somewhat more recently. A recent study found no difference in peritoneal prostaglandin content in infertile women, with or without endometriosis.[4] There is, however, an increase in pelvic and tubal macrophage content that appears to be phagocytic for human sperm in patients with endometriosis.[4,5] This increased macrophage activity might play a part in the mechanism of infertility in patients with mild endometriosis. More information is needed on both prostaglandin function and macrophage activity in women with pelvic endometriosis.

Diagnosis

The symptoms of pelvic endometriosis are fairly characteristic and complex. Most often, affected women complain of secondary dysmenorrhea, which usually is a slowly progressing process. In about 20% to 30% of patients with endometriosis, this symptom becomes so severe that bed rest and narcotic analgesics are necessary for the first 2 days of menses. Pain is associated not only with menstrual bleeding or the time immediately before its onset, but also with intercourse. Dyspareunia is present in about one-fourth of patients with endometriosis. This symptom is found in all phases of the disease, whether it is mild or severe. In severe cases, chronic pelvic pain may be the complaint that brings the patient into the physician's office. Anovulatory cycles or menstrual irregularities do not seem to be increased in women with endometriosis, compared with the population in general. Spontaneous abortion and early pregnancy wastage are no higher in women with endometriosis.[2]

Physical findings can be helpful in making the preliminary diagnosis of endometriosis. These include unilateral ovarian enlargement, with a somewhat cystic consistency, and minimal ovarian mobility. Uterosacral nodularity, cul-de-sac nodularity, or visualization of endometrial implants on the cervical or vaginal mucosa are characteristic findings of pelvic endometriosis.

The diagnosis of pelvic endometriosis is best established by a direct view of the pelvic cavity. This can be performed at the time of laparotomy for indicated reasons, but usually the diagnosis is made by laparoscopy. In evaluating the existence and/or the extent of endometriosis in the pelvic cavity, a two-puncture technique should be used. This technique allows an unobstructed view and ease in manipulating the adnexal structures to observe the undersurfaces (Figures 29-1 to 29-4).

Characteristic findings at laparoscopy include so-called "powder-burn" lesions on the serosal surfaces within the peritoneal cavity. These are opaque, bluish or brownish spots on the peritoneum. Endometrial implants are characteristically large, firm, and fibrous nodules that may be reddish-yellow with yellowish, firm reactive tissues surrounding them. These surrounding areas are actually islands of endometrial tis-

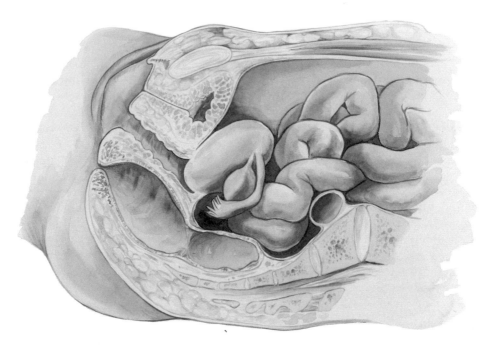

Figure 29-1
Sagittal view of normal female pelvis.

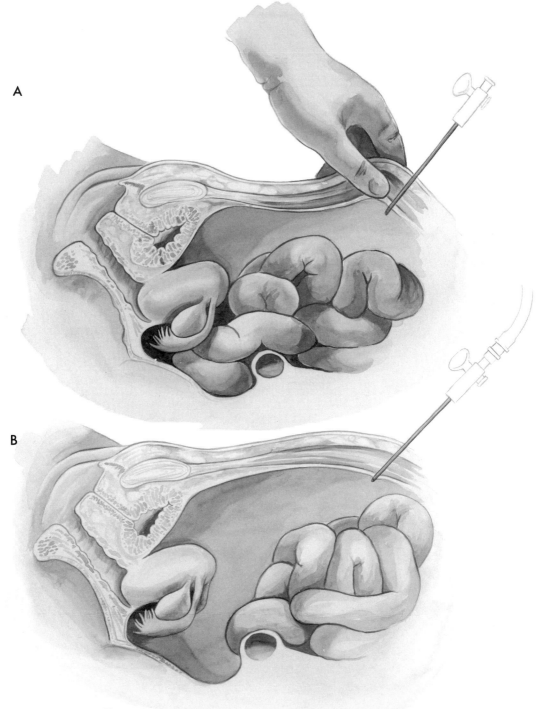

Figure 29-2
A. Placement of the Veress needle. B. Insufflation of the pelvic cavity.

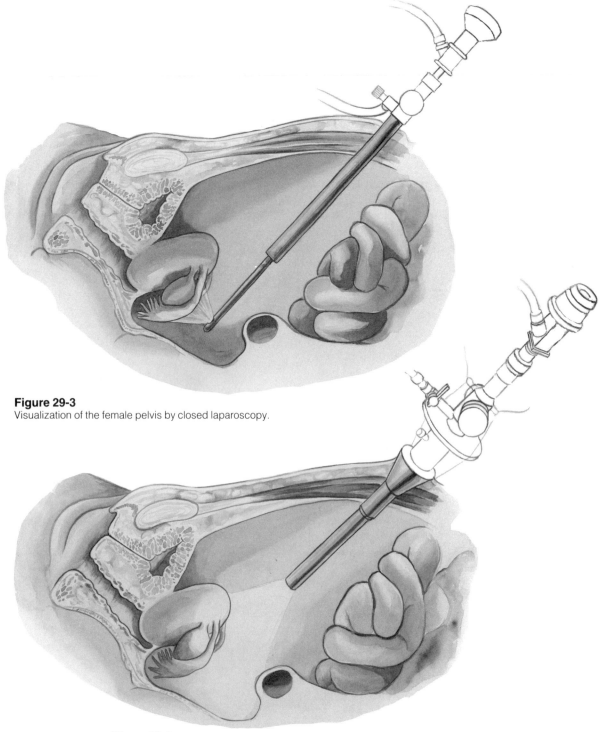

Figure 29-3
Visualization of the female pelvis by closed laparoscopy.

Figure 29-4
Cannula placement and visualization of the pelvic cavity by open laparoscopy.

sue that have set up an inflammatory reaction and have become fibrotic and firm (Figure 29-5). Endometriomas, sometimes visible within the ovarian capsule, have a characteristic bluish appearance, rather than a clear, fluid-filled cystic structure (Figure 29-6). Most often, the ovaries involved in endometriosis have surface lesions or may be fixed to the posterior, lateral pelvic side wall. In rare cases, the ovaries adhere to each other—the so-called "kissing ovaries," which are smooth in appearance and fixed in the posterior cul-de-sac as well as to each other (Figure 29-7). It is important at the time of diagnostic evaluation that an investigation of the entire intraabdominal cavity be performed. The serosal surfaces of the bowel, bladder, uterus, tubes, ovaries, cul-de-sac, and broad ligament should be examined. In this way, the extent as well as the severity of the disease can be established.

It is important to use a classification system when staging the disease. This will help determine prognosis and the best form of therapy for the patient. The two most common schemes are those of Acosta and associates (Table 29-1)[6] and the American Fertility Society (Figure 29-8). One of these classifications should be used. At the diagnostic evaluation, it is usually not necessary to take biopsies of lesions for histologic confirmation, unless the lesions appear atypical. Then, a laparoscopic biopsy of the affected area can be accomplished, and histologic confirmation can be made. The differentiation of mild versus moderate disease is based upon the presence of adhesions and/or small endometriomas. If these are seen, the stage of disease becomes at least moderate.

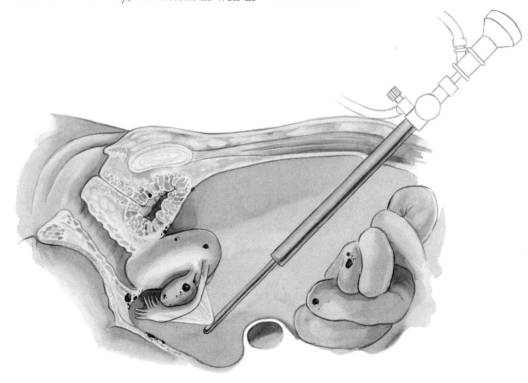

Figure 29-5
Common areas of involvement with endometriosis as viewed laparoscopically.

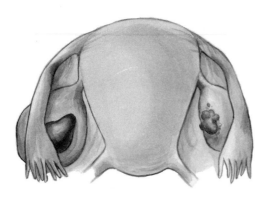

Figure 29-6
Endometrioma involving the left ovary and surface implants
of endometriosis on the right ovary.

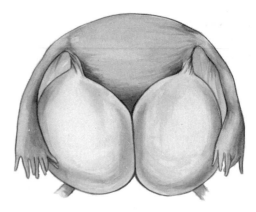

Figure 29-7
Ovaries enlarged bilaterally by ovarian endometriomas,
which have fixed the ovarian surfaces to the pelvic side wall
and cul-de-sac.

Table 29-1
Acosta-Buttram classification of pelvic endometriosis

Classification	Characteristics
Mild	1. Scattered, fresh lesions (i.e., implants not associated with scarring or retraction of the peritoneum) in the anterior or posterior cul-de-sac or pelvic peritoneum 2. Rare surface implant on ovary, with no endometrioma, without surface scarring and retraction and without periovarian adhesions 3. No peritubular adhesions
Moderate	1. Endometriosis involving one or both ovaries, with several surface lesions, with scarring and retraction, or small endometriomas 2. Minimal periovarian adhesions associated with ovarian lesions described 3. Minimal peritubular adhesions associated with ovarian lesions described 4. Superficial implants in the anterior and/or posterior cul-de-sac with scarring and retraction. Some adhesions, but not sigmoid invasion
Severe	1. Endometriosis involving one or both ovaries with endometrioma >2 × 2 cm (usually both) 2. One or both ovaries bound down by adhesions associated with endometriosis, with or without tubal adhesions to ovaries 3. One or both tubes bound down or obstructed by endometriosis; associated adhesions or lesions 4. Obliteration of the cul-de-sac from adhesions or lesions associated with endometriosis 5. Thickening of the uterosacral ligaments and cul-de-sac lesions from invasive endometriosis with obliteration of the cul-de-sac 6. Significant bowel or urinary tract involvement

*From Acosta AA, Buttram VC Jr, Besch PK, et al: A proposed classification of pelvic endometriosis. Obstet
Gynecol 42:19, 1972. Reprinted with permission from The American College of Obstetricians and Gynecologists.*

Patient's Name ______________________ Date ______________________

Stage I (Minimal) - 1-5
Stage II (Mild) - 6-15
Stage III (Moderate) - 16-40
Stage IV (Severe) - >40

Total ______________

Laparoscopy ________ Laparotomy ________ Photography ________

Recommended Treatment ______________________

____

Prognosis ______________________

PERITONEUM	**ENDOMETRIOSIS**	<1cm	1-3cm	>3cm
	Superficial	1	2	4
	Deep	2	4	6
OVARY	R Superficial	1	2	4
	Deep	4	16	20
	L Superficial	1	2	4
	Deep	4	16	20
	POSTERIOR CULDESAC OBLITERATION	Partial		Complete
		4		40
	ADHESIONS	<1/3 Enclosure	1/3-2/3 Enclosure	>2/3 Enclosure
OVARY	R Filmy	1	2	4
	Dense	4	8	16
	L Filmy	1	2	4
	Dense	4	8	16
TUBE	R Filmy	1	2	4
	Dense	4*	8*	16
	L Filmy	1	2	4
	Dense	4*	8*	16

*If the fimbriated end of the fallopian tube is completely enclosed, change the point assignment to 16.

Figure 29-8
American Fertility Society classification of endometriosis.

Reproduced with permission of the publisher, The American Fertility Society.

Treatment of pelvic endometriosis

Various therapeutic approaches have been used to treat pelvic endometriosis. Primary medical or surgical therapy, for all stages of the disease, has had variable results. The choice of treatment should be based on the extent of the disease and the reproductive desires of the patient. In severe cases, medical therapy should be followed by surgical correction.

Medical therapy

In the past 30 to 40 years, various hormonal preparations have been used for the treatment of pelvic endometriosis. Early medical treatment consisted of high-dose estrogen therapy, primarily diethylstilbestrol. Continuous estrogen therapy was given to suppress ovulation, in an effort to cause endometriosis to regress. This treatment regimen was soon abandoned, because the increasing dose of continuous estrogen therapy necessary to maintain amenorrhea was accompanied by severe side effects. Moreover, hyperstimulation of the endometrial cavity frequently resulted in irregular heavy bleeding and/or hyperplastic changes in the endometrium. In addition, with estrogen therapy alone, there was a low incidence of regression of the disease.

Current medical therapy for endometriosis consists of three different regimens: (1) combination of estrogens and progestins, that is, oral contraceptive (OC) suppression; (2) continuous progestins; and (3) danazol.[7] OCs have been used since 1958, when Kistner[8] first described their use in the so-called "pseudopregnancy" regimen. Combination OC tablets are ingested in a continuous fashion to make the patient amenorrheic for 6 to 9 months. Most often, combination formulations containing norgestrel are used, because this progestin has the most potent progestational activity. When breakthrough bleeding occurs during the OC regimen, the dosage is increased. The patient is started on 1 tablet daily; if spotting or breakthrough bleeding occurs, 2 tablets daily are administered until bleeding has ceased for 3 days. Then the dosage is decreased to 1 tablet daily. If bleeding starts again, the dosage is again increased to 2 tablets daily. The dosage is maintained at 2 unless breakthrough bleeding again occurs. In such cases, 3 tablets daily are administered until bleeding stops; then dosage is decreased to 2 tablets once again.

This type of stair-step pattern is followed until at least a 6-month interval of amenorrhea has been maintained. The mechanism of action of this form of therapy is thought to be a suppressant effect on the hypothalamic-pituitary axis, which blocks ovarian endogenous estrogen production. The result is decreased unopposed estrogen stimulation of aberrant endometrial implants. This suppressing action, as well as the direct antimitotic action of synthetic progestins on endometrial implants, is thought to help the implants regress. Side effects of the therapy are minimal, and are mainly the usual ones associated with OC use. A woman who has contraindications to OCs should obviously not be treated with this regimen.

A newer form of medical therapy that has replaced the OC regimen uses danazol, an ethinyltestosterone derivative that is a mild androgenic compound. Danazol began being specifically used for the therapy of endometriosis after initial studies in the 1970s found it useful. Danazol's mechanism of action is multiple. It affects hypothalamic-pituitary-ovarian function, blocks cyclic ovulatory function, and has a direct action on the endometrium.[9] It works mainly by interfering with ovarian steroidogenesis.[10] The result is disruption of ovulatory function, with a decrease in estrogen production. Unlike OC suppression therapy, no exogenous estrogen source is administered. Therefore, danazol therapy is considered a pseudomenopause regimen, because it induces low circulatory levels of estradiol and, often, estrogen-withdrawal symptoms.

Danazol's mechanisms of action, whether direct or indirect, primarily produce atrophic changes in the endometrium. The side effects, which have been reported extensively, are primarily dose- and time-dependent. Table 29-2 lists the major adverse effects. In 15% to 20% of patients, these become severe enough to necessi-

Table 29-2
Side effects associated with danazol therapy

Acne	Depression
Oily skin	Hair growth
Weight gain	Decrease in breast size
Hot flushes	Vaginal dryness
Mood swings	Deepening of the voice

Infertility

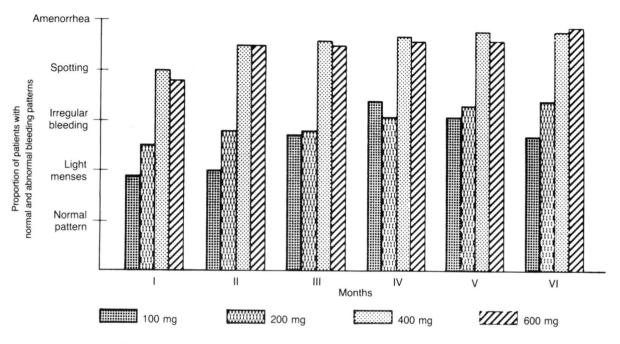

Figure 29-9
Effect of various dosages of danazol on bleeding patterns over time.

Reproduced, with permission, from Biberoglu KO, Behrman SJ: Dosage aspects of danazol therapy in endometriosis: Short-term and long-term effectiveness. Am J Obstet Gynecol 139:645, 1981

tate discontinuation of therapy. When danazol was first used to treat endometriosis, high doses were given—800 mg/day for 6 to 9 months. Several investigators found that lower doses can be effective yet cause fewer side effects.[11-14] A recent investigation reported irregular bleeding in a high percentage of patients receiving 100, 200, or 400 mg daily, but a minimal incidence in those receiving 600 mg (Figure 29-9).[12] Moreover, relief of symptoms occurred in most patients in all dosage groups (Figure 29-10).

At our institution, danazol is started at a 600-mg daily dose administered in 3 divided doses. If the patient remains amenorrheic for 8 weeks on 600 mg daily, then the dosage is decreased to 400 mg/day for the duration of the 6-month course of therapy. If irregular bleeding occurs, the dosage is increased to 600 mg/day or, in some cases, to 800 mg/day if bleeding persists. In our experience, a dosage of more than 600 mg/day is unnecessary for the vast majority of patients. Patients do not ovulate on the lower-dose treatment regimens, even though they may have irregular bleeding episodes.

The side effects observed with this type of regimen include symptoms of estrogen withdrawal; that is, hot flushes, moodiness, decrease in breast size, and sometimes vaginal dryness. Androgenic side effects such as acne, hair growth, or voice changes usually do not occur. Most patients will experience a 5- to 10-pound weight gain during a 6-month course of therapy.

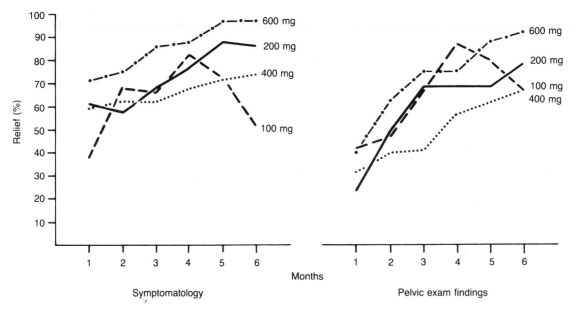

Figure 29-10
Symptomatic relief with various dosages of danazol.

This can be controlled by a good exercise schedule and careful control of dietary intake.

For patients who do not desire fertility following medical therapy for endometriosis, depo-medroxyprogesterone acetate (Depo-Provera) has been utilized with good success. This long-acting progestin is not an ideal choice for a young woman who desires to become pregnant soon after suppressive therapy of her disease process, because there is a prolonged period of anovulation after the drug is discontinued. The woman who has completed childbearing or has no desire for childbearing in the near future can have her disease treated successfully with depo-medroxyprogesterone acetate, 150 mg IM once a week for 4 weeks, then every 2 weeks for 1 month, and then once every 2 to 3 months for as long as necessary. Patients may have total amenorrhea with this treatment, or they may have very irregular bleeding and spotting. This regimen is useful for patients who have chronic pelvic pain, but who do not wish to undergo such

definitive surgical therapy as abdominal hysterectomy and bilateral salpingo-oophorectomy. In these women, long-term maintenance on the drug can be accomplished with a minimum of side effects. The regimen is also useful for patients who have recurrence of the disease after previous conservative surgical therapy.

One of the newest medical forms of therapy is a gonadotropin-releasing hormone (GnRH) agonist. A daily subcutaneous injection of GnRH agonist is given to create a "reversible medical oophorectomy" by down-regulating the GnRH receptors in the pituitary and decreasing gonadotropin production.[15] Patients receiving this agent have a cessation of hypothalamic-pituitary-ovarian cyclicity and enter a menopausal-like state, because ovarian steroidogenesis ceases and estrogen production is very low (Figure 29-11). There are menopausal side effects with this therapy, but no androgen-like side effects occur, such as those occasionally experienced with danazol. More research needs to be done with

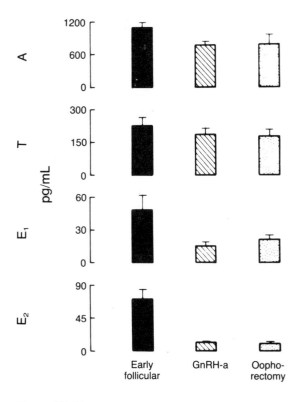

Figure 29-11
Hormone production with GnRH agonist therapy.

GnRH agonists, because only short-term studies (6 months) have been performed. The long-term therapeutic benefits of this treatment of pelvic endometriosis are unknown. It does appear, however, that an alternative method of administration with longer-acting agonists can be accomplished. This regimen of ovarian suppression for treatment of endometriosis may be optimal, because the side effects are few.

Surgical therapy

Patients with mild disease are treated primarily by medical therapy. Surgical therapy of pelvic endometriosis is reserved for those with moderate to severe disease, i.e., adhesions and/or endometriomas. Principles of surgical correction of endometriosis include removal of endometrial implants, removal of adhesions that have been caused by the inflammatory insult to the peritoneal surfaces, and normalization of the pelvic anatomy. For patients who desire childbearing after treatment, the surgical procedure is conservative. The principles of conservative surgery include the excision of endometrial implants (Figure 29-12), uterine suspension to elevate the adnexa from the pelvic floor (a common area of involvement) (Figure 29-13), and possibly a presacral neurectomy for patients with severe dysmenorrhea (Figure 29-14).[16]

A controversial aspect of conservative surgical management is the extent of excision of visible implants. In a small series, it appears that a conservative approach, instead of complete removal of all implants, yields better pregnancy rates (Table 29-3).[2] Specifically, when lesions involve the bowel or bladder, they should be left, rather than performing bowel resection or partial cystectomy. If there is no danger to the patient, as far as function of these organ systems, removal does not appear to be necessary to enhance fertility. Presacral neurectomy is used only when patients have midline pelvic pain or dysmenorrhea. In these patients, relief is prompt and satisfying after the presacral nerve plexus is divided.

Another area of controversy is conservation or removal of involved adnexa. The decision to remove adnexa should be made only when the organs are visualized during the surgical procedure. For patients with a large endometrioma involving one ovary—if the other ovary appears healthy, normal, and not involved—it is best to remove the involved ovary rather than to resect the large endometrioma and reconstruct the ovary. Most often, this ovary will not be functional, or it will become densely adherent to the side wall and remain nonfunctional. If both ovaries are equally involved, careful dissection and removal of the endometriomas and reconstruction of the ovaries should be performed.

The ovarian capsule should be closed care-

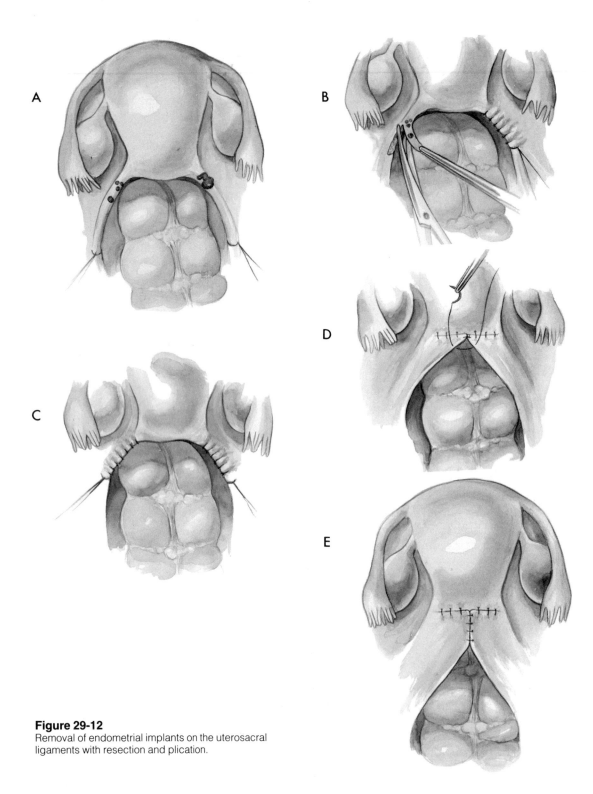

A

B

C

D

E

Figure 29-12
Removal of endometrial implants on the uterosacral
ligaments with resection and plication.

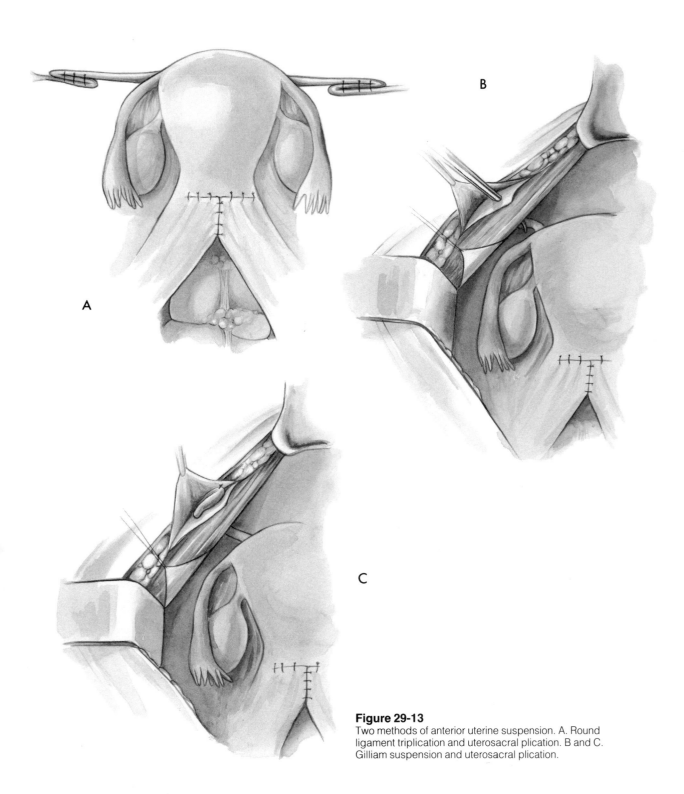

Figure 29-13
Two methods of anterior uterine suspension. A. Round ligament triplication and uterosacral plication. B and C. Gilliam suspension and uterosacral plication.

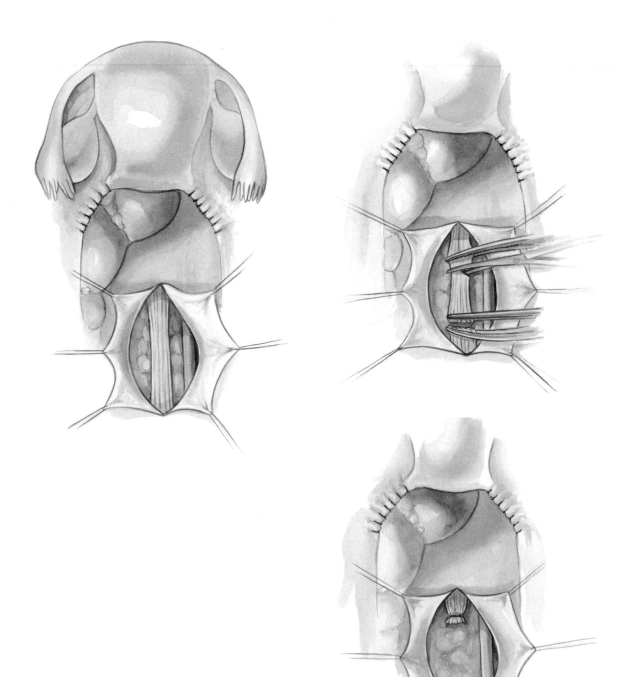

Figure 29-14
Presacral neurectomy. The retroperitoneal space is opened
over the sacral promontory. The presacral plexus is isolated
by blunt dissection and a portion is removed. The lateral
boundaries for dissection are the right ureter and the vena
caval fat pad.

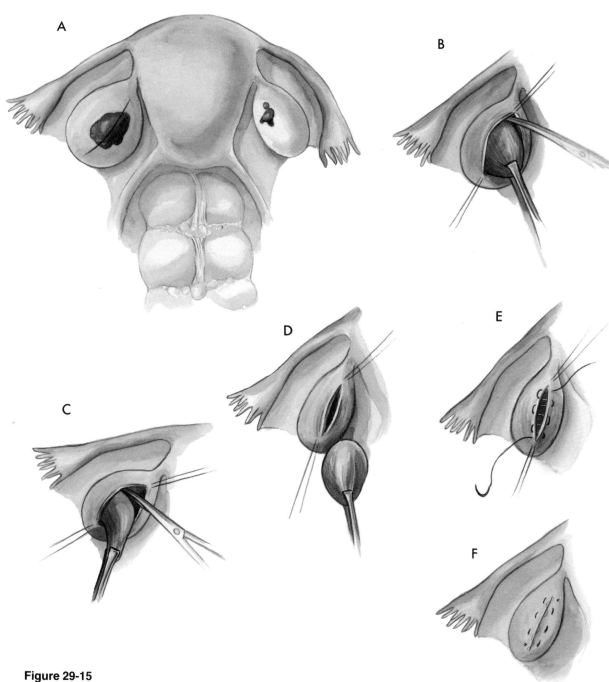

Figure 29-15
Removal of ovarian endometrioma. A. Incision of ovarian capsule. B. Identification of cyst wall. C. Sharp dissection of cyst wall from normal ovarian tissue. D. Removal of cyst wall. E. Running mattress suture to close dead space. F. Running subcapsular suture to close capsule.

Pelvic endometriosis

Table 29-3

Comparison of pregnancy rates in patients with complete removal (group I) versus incomplete removal (group II) of visible endometriosis

	Group	No. of patients	Pregnancy rate
Mild	I	8	6/8 (75%)
	II	61	51/61 (84%)
Moderate	I	60	30/60 (50%)
	II	32	24/32 (75%)
Severe	I	39	13/39 (33%)
	II	45	25/45 (56%)

Modified from Buttram VC Jr, Betts JW: Endometriosis. Curr Prob Obstet Gynecol 2:3, 1979.

fully with an imbricating stitch, so as not to expose raw surface areas. This overlapping helps prevent postoperative adhesions (Figure 29-15). Following the conservative operation, in order to lessen adhesion formation, it is best to place 200 mL of dextran-70 intraperitoneally. To further reduce adhesion formation, all patients should be given 4 mg of dexamethasone IV every 4 hours for 48 hours and 25 mg of promethazine IV every 6 hours for 48 hours. Broad-spectrum antibiotic therapy such as ampicillin or doxycycline is administered postoperatively for the first 48 hours.

For patients who desire no further childbearing and have symptoms related to their endometriosis, a conservative approach is unwarranted. In these women, definitive therapy should be undertaken—a total abdominal hysterectomy with or without salpingo-oophorectomy. The decision on ovarian removal should be based on the age of the patient. If the patient is under the age of 40, and complete resection of visible endometrial implants can be performed by removing the uterus, the ovaries should be preserved. In cases such as this, the incidence of reoperation for ovarian involvement or recurrence of endometriosis was 8% to 12% in a series from Duke University (Table 29-4).[17] If the patient is under 40, has severe endometriosis, and all lesions cannot be removed, then ovarian removal should be performed at the time of hysterectomy. In a small series, patients who fell into this category had an 85% chance of requiring a second operation to remove the ovaries

Table 29-4

Incidence of recurrent symptoms after ovarian conservation at the time of hysterectomy for endometriosis

Authors	No. of patients	Recurrence rate
Hoffman	11	8.1%
Ranney	129	0.7%
Andrews and Larsen[19]	130	2.3%
Williams and Pratt	153	6.5%
Buttram	14	7.1%
Hammond	13	85%

Infertility

and remove more endometriosis.[17] In patients over the age of 40, ovarian removal should also be performed. If all disease has been removed, estrogen replacement therapy can be given without fear of reinstituting the endometriosis. For patients who have a significant amount of disease after bilateral salpingo-oophorectomy and hysterectomy, a course of suppressive progestin therapy, either depo-medroxyprogesterone acetate or combination OCs, should be undertaken for 6 to 12 months before instituting sequential estrogen-progestin replacement therapy. The progestins will relieve hot flushes, as well as cause regression in the remaining endometrial implants.

Fertility following therapy for pelvic endometriosis

Medical outcomes

Of the medical therapies currently in use, OC suppression has been used for the longest period. Reported pregnancy rates following this method are about 50% in patients who have primarily surface lesions (mild disease). Pregnancy rates in series reporting treatment with the pseudopregnancy regimen, with all stages of disease, are given in Table 29-5.

More recently, a corrected pregnancy rate of 72% has been reported following danazol therapy in patients desiring fertility.[14] In several series now, overall uncorrected pregnancy rates range between 40% and 50% in patients treated

Table 29-5
Pregnancy rates after various pseudopregnancy regimens

Authors	Oral contraceptive	Pregnancy
Williams	Enovid	72%
Komides and Kistner	Norestrin	63%
	Ovral	54%
Andrews and Larsen[19]	Enovid	43%

with danazol (Table 29-6). These are obviously studies where good selection was applied before treatment, so that the patients in the moderate to severe category had minimal adhesions or endometriomas. Medical therapy with danazol does not cause regression of pelvic adhesive disease or ovarian endometriomas. To date, there have been no pregnancy rates reported for GnRH agonist therapy.

Surgical outcomes

Pregnancy rates after conservative surgery for pelvic endometriosis range from 70% for mild disease to 50% to 60% for moderate disease and 30% to 40% for severe disease (Table 29-7). Recently, most physicians treating moderate to severe endometriosis have combined preoperative danazol therapy with the operative procedure—in hopes of enhancing surgical outcome. In our institution, after an initial laparoscopic procedure is performed to determine the extent of the disease, 600 mg/day of danazol is given for 6

Table 29-6
Uncorrected pregnancy rates after danazol therapy for endometriosis

Authors	Dose (mg/day)/duration	Pregnancy rate
Friedlander	800 mg/6 months	41%
Greenblatt and Tzingomix	800 mg/6 months	50%
Dmowski & Cohen[14]	800 mg/6 months	46%
Barbieri et al[9,13]	800 mg/4 months	46%

Table 29-7
Pregnancy rates after conservative surgery for endometriosis

Authors	Mild	Moderate	Severe
Acosta et al[6]	75%	50%	33%
Garcia and David	66%	36%	29%
Sadighe et al	—	74%	48%
Buttram[16]	73%	56%	40%

weeks to 3 months, depending on disease severity, before conservative surgery is undertaken. Following this course of danazol, before proceeding to laparotomy, a laparoscopy is first performed to determine if the disease has regressed such that resection can be done through the laparoscope. This can usually be accomplished if the disease is not extensive and endometriomas are not present. Patients with moderate to severe disease, with adhesions that can be resected laparoscopically, should be treated with danazol after the operative laparoscopy for an additional 6 months.

It remains controversial whether preoperative danazol has any advantage over postoperative use. There are no studies comparing these treatment modalities.[18] Our current approach is to diagnose and stage the endometriosis at laparoscopy. Patients found to have extensive disease at the time of initial laparoscopy are placed on danazol, 600 mg daily for about 3 months. Laparotomy is then performed without a preoperative laparoscopy. We do not give postoperative danazol after excision of endometriosis by laparotomy in order not to delay the possibility of conception, which has the greatest chance of success soon after treatment.

For patients who receive only danazol suppressive therapy, almost 60% will have recurrence of symptoms suggestive of endometriosis within 12 months after therapy is discontinued, if pregnancy has not occurred (Figure 29-16).[14] This rapid recurrence is not seen in patients who have surgical therapy. The average time for re-

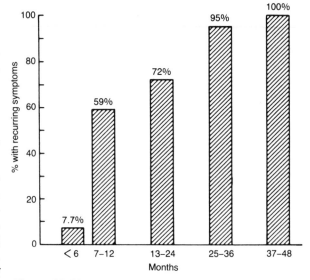

Figure 29-16
Time interval between end of treatment and recurrence of symptoms in 39 of 99 patients treated with danazol.

Modified from Dmowski WP, Cohen MR: Antigonadotropin (danazol) in the treatment of endometriosis: Evaluation of post-treatment fertility and 3-year follow-up data. Am J Obstet Gynecol 130:41, 1978.

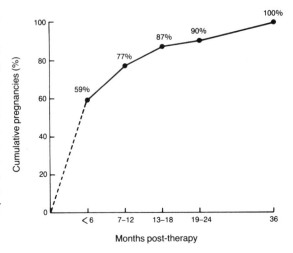

Figure 29-17
Cumulative monthly pregnancy rates following danazol therapy (39 patients).

Modified from Dmowski WP, Cohen MR: Antigonadotropin (danazol) in the treatment of endometriosis: Evaluation of post-treatment fertility and 3-year follow-up data. Am J Obstet Gynecol 130:41, 1978.

currence of symptoms is approximately 36 months following conservative surgery. Therefore, it appears that danazol therapy is a short-acting suppressive. More than half the pregnancies that occur after danazol will occur within 6 months after treatment is discontinued. Otherwise, the beneficial effect of the drug has been lost (Figure 29-17).[14] Surgery provides a more long-lasting symptom-free interval.[2,7,17,19] Pregnancies also occur most frequently within the first 12 to 18 months following surgical therapy (Figure 29-18).[20]

Therapeutic controversies

Recently, several major questions have been raised about the treatment of pelvic endometriosis and the effect of endometriosis on reproductive function. For many years, it was thought that mild endometriosis without adhesions was a cause of infertility. This concept has recently been challanged. Recent reports[21-23] have compared the use of danazol to expectant management for mild endometriosis. The pregnancy rate was higher in patients receiving no treatment at all when compared with patients who received danazol (Table 29-8). Other investigators compared pregnancy rates in patients with mild endometriosis after surgical resection of the disease to pregnancy rates in untreated patients. The results showed again that the surgical resection was no better than observation.[22,24] Therefore, whether mild disease should be treated at

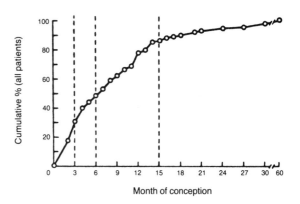

Figure 29-18
Cumulative monthly conception rate following surgery (121 patients).

From Buttram VC Jr: Conservative surgery for endometriosis in the infertile female: A study of 206 patients with implications for both medical and surgical therapy. Fertil Steril 31:117, 1979. Reproduced with permission of the publisher, The American Fertility Society.

all is debatable. If the patient desiring fertility has had long-standing mild endometriosis and no pregnancy has occurred for several years, then a course of danazol therapy is recommended for 6 months. If the patient has not been treated or evaluated for infertility previously and is found to have mild endometriosis at laparoscopy, then a waiting period of 6 to 12 months, with optimal timing of intercourse at the time of ovulation, should be tried before instituting medical or surgical therapy.[21-23]

Recently, the use of argon or CO_2 lasers has

Table 29-8
Comparison of pregnancy rates in mild endometriosis

Authors	No. of patients	Pregnancy rate (%)
Portnondo et al		
Donor male	10	9/10 (90%)
Fertile husband	21	10/21 (48%)
Schenken and Malinak	16	12/16 (75%)
Seibel et al		
Danazol	20	6/20 (30%)
No danazol	28	14/28 (50%)

been reported for treatment of patients with mild to moderate endometriosis. The laser systems can be used through endoscopic instruments, and visible surface lesions can be vaporized. Clinical trials judging improvement in pregnancy rates compared with other treatment modalities have not been reported. But in the near future, laser techniques may provide a therapeutic modality that is beneficial to the patient and requires a relatively minor surgical procedure.

Conclusion

In general, the infertile patient with endometriosis should be treated. The management plan should take into account the age of the patient, her pregnancy desires, and the stage of her disease. In patients with *mild disease*, as established by laparoscopy, who desire pregnancy, a period of observation is indicated before beginning medical therapy. If pregnancy does not occur within 6 to 12 months, with all other factors normal, then a 6-month course of danazol should be undertaken. In patients with *moderate disease* at the time of diagnostic laparoscopy, adhesions surrounding the tubes and ovaries should be removed if possible through the laparoscope and danazol therapy should be instituted for 6 months. Laparoscopy is then repeated. If disease that is unresectable through the laparoscope remains, surgical removal by laparotomy should be undertaken. For *moderate to severe disease* that cannot be corrected by laparoscopic surgery (severe adhesions and/or endometriomas of >1 cm), danazol is recommended for 6 weeks to 3 months preoperatively. Then conservative surgery should be performed by laparotomy. In patients finished with childbearing who have chronic recurrent symptoms from pelvic endometriosis, abdominal hysterectomy, with or without ovarian removal, is the treatment of choice. Patients who have symptomatic endometriosis, but who are not immediately desirous of childbearing, can be treated with any of the medical therapies that offer relief of symptoms. In young women, OCs are preferred, because the cost is low and side effects are few.

References

1. Sampson JA: Perforating hemorrhagic (chocolate) cysts of the ovary: Their importance and especially their relation to pelvic adenomas of endometrial type (adenomyoma) of the uterus, rectovaginal septum and sigmoid. *Arch Surg* 3:245, 1921

2. Buttram VC Jr, Betts JW: Endometriosis. *Curr Prob Obstet Gynecol* 2:3, 1979

3. Drake TS, O'Brien WF, Romwell PW: Elevated peritoneal fluid prostaglandins in unexplained infertility: A possible biochemical marker for microscopic endometriosis. *Abstr Fertil Steril* 37:302, 1982

4. Halme J, Becker S, Hammond MG, et al: Increased activation of pelvic macrophages in infertile women with mild endometriosis. *Am J Obstet Gynecol* 145:333, 1983

5. Muscato JJ, Haney AF, Weinberg JB: Sperm phagocytosis by human peritoneal macrophages: A possible cause of infertility in endometriosis. *Am J Obstet Gynecol* 144:503, 1982

6. Acosta AA, Buttram VC Jr, Besch PK, et al: A proposed classification of pelvic endometriosis. *Obstet Gynecol* 42:19, 1973

7. Hammond CB, Haney AF: Conservative treatment of endometriosis. In Wallach EE, Kempers RD (eds): *Modern Trends in Infertility and Conception Control.* Baltimore, Williams & Wilkins, 1979, p 41

8. Kistner RW: Endometriosis and infertility. In Berman SJ, Kistner RW (eds): *Progress in Infertility,* ed 2. Boston, Little, Brown, 1975, p 345

9. Barbieri RL, Canick JA, Makris A, et al: Danazol inhibits steroidogenesis. *Fertil Steril* 28:809, 1977

10. Barbieri RL, Ryan KJ: Danazol: Endocrine pharmacology and therapeutic applications. *Am J Obstet Gynecol* 141:453, 1981

11. Moore EE, Harger JA, Rock JA, et al: Management of pelvic endometriosis with low-dose danazol. *Fertil Steril* 36:15, 1981

12. Biberoglu KO, Behrman SJ: Dosage aspects of danazol therapy in endometriosis: Short-term and long-term effectiveness. *Am J Obstet Gynecol* 139:645, 1981

13. Barbieri RL, Evans S, Kistner RW: Danazol in the treatment of endometriosis: Analysis of 100 cases with a 4-year follow-up. *Fertil Steril* 37:737, 1982

14. Dmowski WP, Cohen MR: Antigonadotropin (danazol) in the treatment of endometriosis: Evaluation of post-treatment fertility and 3-year follow-up data. *Am J Obstet Gynecol* 130:41, 1978

15. Meldrum DR, Chang RJ, Lu J: "Medical oophorectomy" using a long-acting GnRH agonist—a possible new approach to the treatment of endometriosis. *J Clin Endocrinol Metab* 54:1081, 1982

16. Buttram VC Jr: Surgical treatment of endometriosis in the infertile female: A modified approach. *Fertil Steril* 32:635, 1979

17. Hammond OB, Rock JA, Parker RT: Conservative treatment of endometriosis: The effects of limited surgery and hormonal pseudopregnancy. *Fertil Steril* 27:756, 1976

18. Wheeler JM, Malinak LR: Postoperative danazol therapy in infertility patients with severe endometriosis. *Fertil Steril* 36:460, 1981

19. Andrews WC, Larsen GD: Endometriosis: Treatment with hormonal pseudopregnancy and/or operation. *Am J Obstet Gynecol* 118:643, 1974

20. Buttram VC Jr: Conservative surgery for endometriosis in the infertile female: A study of 206 patients with implications for both medical and surgical therapy. *Fertil Steril* 31:117, 1979

21. Seibel MM, Berger MJ, Weinstein FG, et al: The effectiveness of danazol on subsequent fertility in minimal endometriosis. *Fertil Steril* 38:534, 1982

22. Schenken RS, Malinak LR: Conservative surgery versus expectant management for the infertile patient with mild endometriosis. *Fertil Steril* 37:183, 1982

23. Muse KN, Wilson EA: How does mild endometriosis cause infertility? *Fertil Steril* 38:145, 1982

24. Garcia LR, David SS: Pelvic endometriosis: Infertility and pelvic pain. *Am J Obstet Gynecol* 129:740, 1977

Chapter 30

Role of Immunology in Infertility

Val Davajan, M.D.
Robert M. Nakamura, Ph.D.
Gerald S. Bernstein, Ph.D., M.D.

Immunologic incompatibility may be the cause of infertility in some patients who have previously been referred to as having unexplained infertility. Another infertility etiology, abnormal sperm-cervical mucus interaction, may also be due to an immune reaction, and can occur even when the cervical mucus and semen analysis are normal. An allergy to sperm is, at best, a misnomer, because true allergy causes a release of histamine and other vasoactive substances from plasma cells. This is an extremely rare sequela of intercourse.

The literature in this area deals with three major etiologic categories: (1) ABO blood-group incompatibility,[1] (2) autoimmunity in the male,[2] and (3) circulating sperm-agglutinating or immobilizing antibodies in the female.[3,4] Whether all of these immunologic reactions cause human infertility is unclear.

Antigens of the male reproductive tract

The antigenic system of the male reproductive tract has been subdivided into two unrelated categories: (1) spermatozoan and testicular antigens, and (2) antigens of the accessory glands of reproduction.[5,6]

Spermatozoan and testicular antigens

Many studies have been performed in an effort to establish the organ specificity and species specificity of the spermatozoan antigens and the testicular tissue antigens. It has been found that autoantibodies can be produced by injecting experimental animals with spermatozoa.

In 1957, using the mixed agglutination method, the ejaculate from a male with an AB blood group was found to contain a mixture of both A and B spermatozoa.[7] Serum with anti-A agglutinating antibodies, obtained by immunization of rabbits with A-group human spermatozoa, has been shown to cause agglutination of spermatozoa from the ejaculates of AB-group males.[8] Furthermore, using an immunofluorescent technique, ejaculated spermatozoa, unlike somatic cells, were found to bear only one ABO antigen on their surfaces.[9] These findings were challenged by researchers who found that A and B blood-group isoantigens were present on the membranes of seminal spermatozoa of secretors, but not on the spermatozoa of nonsecretors.[10] On the basis of these findings and those reported by other investigators,[11] it was assumed that the blood-group antigens on human spermatozoa did not originate in the sperm cells but were absorbed into the spermatozoa during their contact with seminal plasma in secretors. This concept was further substantiated when it was reported that washed spermatozoa from an O nonsecretor developed the ability to inhibit anti-A serum.[12] It is still unclear whether the seminal spermatozoa (1) contain only antigens of their own, (2) acquire antigens only from seminal plasma, or (3) contain their own as well as acquired antigens.

Antigens of male accessory reproductive glands

The immunologic properties of spermatozoa aspirated from the testes or the epididymis differ from those of spermatozoa obtained from semen. A study published in 1960 found immunologic evidence that the spermatocele spermatozoa lack the antigens that characterize seminal plasma or spermatozoa found in seminal plasma.[13] Spermatozoa and seminal fluid were immunologically indistinguishable when tested with immune sera against seminal spermatozoa or against sperm-free seminal plasma. This was observed for both humans and experimental animals. The antigens responsible for these immunologic reactions appeared to be very potent and stimulated antibody response in high titers. In another study, seminal plasma was found to be complement-fixing in high titers, and the ejaculates of azoospermic men were found to contain the full complement of the antigen.[14] Therefore, it was concluded that this was an antigen produced by the accessory glands and not a spermatozoan antigen being released into the seminal plasma by the sperm cell. Further work suggested that this antigen was excreted by the seminal vesicle. The antigen appeared to be coating the spermatozoa when they came into contact with the seminal vesicle secretions; therefore, it was called sperm-coating antigen

(SCA).[15] SCA was found to be quite stable under ordinary conditions. It was destroyed by boiling and was insoluble in common organic solvents.

Following this work, several authors studied the antigenic composition of human seminal plasma (HSP) by means of immunoelectrophoresis, using antiserum or HSP-specific proteins. Because of numerous and different techniques used and the different antisera chosen, the results have been difficult to compare. The number of HSP-specific proteins varies from three to eight in the different reports, but in all cases the most prominent antigens possessed β_1 and β_2 electrophoretic motility. There appear to be at least three HSP-specific antigens that originate in the prostate and two that appear to have their origin in the seminal vesicle. Antigens originating in the testes or epididymis have not yet been proven to exist. One of the seminal vesicle antigens appears to be lactoferrin, the iron-containing protein occurring in various other body secretions but not in blood plasma. It is lactoferrin that is thought to be the sperm-coating antigen found in the study mentioned above.[15]

A 1970 study used three different antisera produced by injecting rabbits with contents of spermatocele spermatozoa, whole semen, and seminal plasma obtained from vasectomized men.[16] These antisera were absorbed with extracts of normal serum, kidney, liver, and brain. On immunoelectrophoresis, the unabsorbed antiserum to vasectomized HSP formed 14 precipitation lines with whole semen, 12 with seminal plasma from vasectomized men, 4 with ejaculated spermatozoa extract, 8 with serum, 5 with kidney extract, and 3 each with liver and brain extracts—a pattern similar to that reported by other investigators.[6] It was concluded that there were at least four specific antigens in the seminal plasma and three HSP-specific antigens in the ejaculated spermatozoan extract.[16] Four specific antigens of human seminal plasma had previously been reported.[17] No specific antigens in the spermatozoa could be identified by any of these authors. At present, therefore, it can be stated that no sperm-specific antigen has yet been identified and that there appear to be at least four HSP-specific antigens that have their direct source in the prostatic fluid and the seminal vesicle.

Antibodies of the female reproductive tract

The immunoglobulins IgA, IgG, and IgM are the major types of antibodies in the human female genital tract. Each has distinct immunophysiologic properties. A fourth one that must be included in studies of antibodies against spermatozoa is a lytic complement-fixing antibody that has been found in animals as well as humans. Characterized as a slow IgG, it appears to be a naturally occurring antibody of obscure etiology. It has been shown to have the capacity to lyse spermatozoa and germinal cells in the testes.

Site of antibody production in the human female genital tract

In the human female, antibodies can be produced locally in the genital tract (IgA) as well as "leak in" from the systemic circulation (IgM). Locally produced antibodies appear to be responsible for the anaphylaxis-like uterine contractions reported to occur after intercourse in one subject. Locally produced antibodies that are cytotoxic to spermatozoa have also been found in a few infertile men and therefore could be present in some infertile women.[18] It has been reported that both circulating antibodies and locally produced antibodies can be induced by intravaginal immunization.[19]

The different fractions of immunoglobulins in cervical mucus have been quantitatively determined by an immunodiffusion technique. Immunoglobulin concentrations in whole cervical mucus have been reported to be 0.090 mg/mL

for IgA, 0.035 mg/mL for IgM, and 0.45 mg/mL for IgG.[20] The IgA:IgG ratio is 1:5, which is approximately equal to the ratio in serum. A 1970 study investigated the distribution of the secretory piece (described below), IgA, IgG, IgM, and lactoferrin in the human genital tract. IgA and IgG were found in all samples taken from the endometrium, tubes, cervix, and vagina.[21]

Whether antibodies in the human female genital tract are circulating or produced locally has been the subject of recent reports. Investigations of human external secretory glands (for example, salivary glands) have revealed that some immunoglobulins are secreted locally. Although the presence of antibodies in the secretions may be due to passive diffusion of circulating plasma components, more recent evidence suggests that an antibody may arise locally by a mechanism independent of circulating antibodies. IgA is thought to be locally produced. It is found in the lamina propria of mucosal epithelium and has been shown to combine with a glycoprotein synthesized by epithelial cells, called the secretory piece or T component. This combination of IgA and T component is known as secretory IgA and is considered the body's first line of defense against invading microorganisms.

The uterine cervix is biologically similar to other mucus-secreting glands, such as salivary, nasal, and lacrimal, in that it serves as a barrier preventing bacteria in the vagina from entering the sterile uterine cavity. The vagina can produce local antibodies against sperm. Using a fluorescein-tagged antibody technique, it has been shown that the human T component is localized in the endocervical epithelium and that IgA can be produced locally by the epithelium of the human cervix. These observations indicate that the ingredients necessary for local production of antibody in the endocervix, as well as in the vagina and, possibly, the endometrium and the fallopian tubes, are all present. Immunologic incompatibility thus is a very possible cause of certain cases of infertility.

Localization of antibody in the spermatozoa

Immunofluorescent techniques have disclosed these four different spermatozoa staining patterns: (1) staining of the acrosome, including the equatorial segment; (2) staining of the equatorial segment, a well-demarcated fluorescent band across the head at the equator; (3) staining of the postnuclear area; and (4) staining of the tail. A combination of these staining patterns has been reported. Staining of the postnuclear area was least frequent; only about 1% of sera tested exhibited this pattern.[22] Immunofluorescent staining in low titers (<4) was found in all groups of sera, whereas higher titers (>16) were found significantly more often in sera obtained from infertile women than in the control groups. The antibody levels also appeared to be significantly higher among women with unexplained infertility than among those in whom the infertility could be explained.

Immune reactions in unexplained infertility

When all diagnostic and therapeutic modalities available to the clinician dealing with infertility are exhausted, there still remains a large group of patients in whom the cause of infertility remains unsolved. Since 1952, numerous studies have implicated immunologic incompatibility in these patients. A discussion of the three major categories of possibly etiologic immune phenomena (ABO incompatibility, autoimmunity in men, and circulating sperm antibodies in women) follows.

ABO blood-group incompatibility

The incidence of ABO incompatibility was reported to be much higher in a group of couples with unexplained infertility than in a normal group.[1] This report stimulated further investigations into ABO incompatibility as a possible cause of human infertility. However, other investigators found no difference in incidence of ABO incompatibility between couples with known and couples with unknown causes of infertility.[23] In fact, it has been reported that spermatozoa from a type A donor seemed to survive better in anti-A immune sera than in the donor's own seminal plasma.

Nonspecific effects of anti-A and anti-B antisera on respiration and aerobic glycolysis of spermatozoa have also been reported. Exposure of spermatozoa to specific A or B antisera apparently does not adversely affect sperm motility, although adsorption of specific antibodies to the surface of spermatozoa has been noted. Because no effect on sperm motility or morphology has been noted, these agglutinins apparently are noncytotoxic and unrelated to infertility.

Autoimmunity in the human male

Autoimmunity as a cause of infertility in the human male was first reported in 1954.[24] Three infertile men were reported to have sperm agglutinins in both their seminal plasma and serum. The wives of two of these men later conceived following artificial donor insemination. About 3% of 2,000 husbands of infertile marriages were found to have serum sperm agglutinin titers in excess of 1:32.[25] This titer appeared to be critical for consideration of autoagglutination of spermatozoa as a causative factor in infertility. Of these men, 17 showed spontaneous agglutination of spermatozoa in their own seminal plasma. The control group of fertile men had sperm agglutination titers no greater than 1:16. Approximately 33% of the infertile men with titers above 1:32 had known occlusions of one or both vasa deferentia or, at least, blockage of one epididymal duct. Other authors have found similar results, all showing a higher incidence of sperm autoagglutinins in men with a history of infection or surgery involving the efferent reproductive ductal system.[26,27] In one study,[26] the presence of sperm-autoagglutinating antibodies in serum did not seem to interfere with fertility in every case.

Although autoagglutination does not always impair fertility, there appears to be a higher incidence of infertility in couples when the man has a history of trauma or infection of the genital tract. Therefore, it has been postulated that the resulting extravasation of spermatozoa into the interstitium or lymph vessels of the epididymis may provide the sperm access to the circulation and induce the production of antisperm agglutinating antibodies. In support of this hypothesis is a study that found sperm agglutinins in the blood of men from infertile marriages.[2] By in vitro testing methods, the ability of these men's sperm to penetrate cervical mucus was found to be markedly decreased. Both the sperm-agglutinating and sperm-immobilizing factors found in men seem to be antibodies mainly of the 7 S type. It is now generally accepted that male autoimmunity is a cause of infertility.

Sperm-agglutinating antibodies in the human female

Agglutination of the husband's sperm by the wife's serum has been reported by numerous authors. In 1964, it was reported that circulating sperm agglutinins were found in 72% of women with infertility of unknown etiology.[3] The control group had a 5.7% incidence of sperm agglutinins. The authors recommended sexual abstinence or the use of condoms by the husband for a period of 2 to 6 months to lower the antibody titer. Ten out of 13 women in the series showed a decline in titer, and 9 out of 10 became pregnant. However, by 1968, the same authors reported that the incidence of sperm-agglutinating antibodies in infertile women was only 48% compared with a control incidence of 13%.[28] In this report, some 57% of the patients became pregnant after using the recommended condom therapy. Of the 20 couples who refused condom therapy, only two (10%) achieved pregnancy.

Other authors have not found the incidence of sperm-agglutinating antibodies in infertile women as high as that published in the 1964 report. For example, rates of 37.5%[27] and 20%[29] have been reported in women with primary unexplained infertility. These authors found no correlation between positive sperm-agglutination tests and abnormal postcoital tests, or between the presence of sperm agglutinins and ABO incompatibility. In a large study published in 1969, the incidence of positive Kibrick tests was reported to be 23% and positive Franklin-Dukes tests to be 10% in couples with infertility of unexplained cause.[5] The controls were in the 2% to 3% range.

It now appears that the percentage of couples with infertility in which sperm agglutination is present may be much lower than suggested originally. At this time, the only statements that can be made on the subject are that sperm-agglutinating antibodies appear to exist in the serum of a small percentage of women in infertile couples and that if the phenomenon is a cause of infertility, it is most likely titer-dependent.

Sperm-immobilizing antibodies in the human female

Antibodies that immobilize spermatozoa have been found in the serum of some infertile women. These complement-dependent, sperm-immobilizing antibodies seem to have a greater specificity than those detected by agglutination tests; however, there appears to be an unacceptable level of false-negative results.[30] There are conflicting data about the incidence of these antibodies in fertile and infertile women, because different methods have been used to detect the antibodies. Some investigators have combined those patients with sperm-agglutinating antibodies and those with sperm-immobilizing antibodies into a common group with "positive tests," without differentiating between the two types of reactions.

It has been reported that 19.4% of women

with unexplained infertility had sperm-immobilizing antibodies in their serum,[4] compared with incidences of 26.5% and 60% for sperm-agglutinating antibodies as determined by the slide (Franklin-Dukes) and gelatin (Kibrick) agglutination tests. The proportion of pregnant women with positive results was 0%, 26.3%, and 53.8%, respectively, for the three types of tests.

Sperm-immobilizing antibodies have also been found in the cervical mucus of some infertile women. Cervical mucus studies must be interpreted with caution, however. For example, while sperm-agglutinating antibodies have been found in extracts of dissolved cervical mucus, in unaltered mucus the same antibodies may only immobilize sperm or cause them to lose their progressive motility rather than induce sperm agglutination. In some cases, there is impaired sperm migration through cervical mucus that contains antibodies. Considerably more work is required, however, to clarify the relationship between circulating sperm antibodies and the presence of antibodies in the cervical mucus. At present, it would be inaccurate to attribute an abnormality in the postcoital test to the presence of cervical mucus antibodies.

Test methods

At this institution, we recommend that the standardized immunologic tests be done to identify sperm antibodies. We use either the husband's own serum (autoimmunity) or the wife's serum if there is a suspicion of an immunologic factor in either partner or if infertility is unexplained. Numerous immunologic tests currently are being used in various research centers. These include the Kibrick and Franklin-Dukes tests for sperm-agglutinating antibodies, the Isojima test for sperm-immobilizing antibodies,[4] Shulman's modification of the Franklin-Dukes test, the Friberg microsyringe agglutination test,[31,32] various immunofluorescence techniques,[33] and the radiolabeled antiglobulin test.[33] The assays that are used in our laboratory are modifications of the gelatin agglutination (Kibrick) test and the sperm-immobilization (Isojima) test. They are performed as outlined below. The semen used in these assays is obtained both from donors with normal semen analyses and no sperm antibodies in their serum and from the husbands in infertile couples.

Test for sperm macroagglutinating antibodies in serum (Kibrick test)
This test is performed as follows:
1. Allow ejaculate to stand 30 to 60 minutes for complete liquefaction.
2. Count sperm and adjust sperm density to 60×10^6/mL with modified Baker's solution (MBS).
3. Allow diluted semen to stand 1 hour to let debris and dead sperm settle.
4. Remove supernatant, repeat sperm count, and adjust to 40×10^6 sperm/mL.
5. Dilute sperm suspension with an equal volume of 10% Difco gelatin prepared in MBS. The gelatin should be kept at 37°C to facilitate pipetting.
6. Heat-inactivate the test and control sera at 56°C for 30 minutes. This is to remove complement and prevent immobilization from complement-dependent immobilizing antibodies. The sera are then diluted in MBS as described below.
7. Place 0.2 mL of serum in a 65×5 mm test tube.
8. Add 0.2 mL of sperm-gelatin mixture to each test tube (final sperm concentration 10×10^6/mL).
9. Mix ingredients well and incubate for 1 hour. The agglutinated sperm are visible as flecks suspended in the gelatin.

Two controls are run with each test: (1) antigen plus known positive serum and (2) antigen plus known negative serum.

Sera are screened at dilutions of 1:4 and 1:16. If there is a positive reaction at either one, the serum is serially diluted. The titer is the highest dilution that gives a detectable reaction.

Modified Baker's solution consists of NaCl, 0.2 mg; Na_2HPO_4, 1.4 g; KH_2PO_4, 0.023 g; and glucose, 3 g; diluted to a final volume of 100 mL with distilled water. The pH is adjusted to 7.8.

Microagglutination tests

These two tests—the Franklin-Dukes and Friberg tests—identify microagglutinating antibodies. One test uses the tube-slide test described by Franklin and Dukes in 1964.[3] The tray-slide agglutination test is that of Friberg.[31,32] A positive Franklin-Dukes titer in patients with unexplained infertility has varied from 5.5% to 67.2%.[33] This variation has been attributed to factors other than antibodies that are known to agglutinate sperm (for example, bacteria, protein, chemicals, medication). With the Friberg test, the incidence of positive titers has been reported to be between 9% and 33%. Both tests have a high incidence of false positives reported among pregnant women and women using oral steroid contraceptives (10% to 45%).[31,32]

Test for sperm-immobilizing antibodies in serum

The Isojima test is a complement-dependent method that identifies circulating IgG or IgM antibodies. This test has been accepted as highly reproducible and reliable. The amount of complement used can apparently influence the results. Therefore, the test must be performed by skilled technicians. Beer has stated that he considers the Isojima test a more sensitive test than the spermatocytotoxic assays currently being used.[33] The Isojima test has been reported to be positive in 2% to 29% of an infertile population. This test does not appear to have false-positive results. The method is outlined below:

1. Take 0.250 mL of the patient's serum (heat-inactivated for 30 minutes at 56°C).

2. Add 0.025 mL of fresh semen adjusted to 60 × 10^6 sperm/mL with MBS.
3. Mix 0.050 mL of guinea pig complement made up in a solution of: 8.5 g NaCl; 0.04 g/L $MgCl_2 \cdot 6H_2O$ in distilled water.

Controls consist of known positive and negative sera. The tubes are incubated at 37°C for 1 hour, and the motility of the sperm in the test sera is compared with the control. The following formula is applied:

$$\frac{\% \text{ motility in negative control}}{\% \text{ motility in test serum}} = x$$

The test is considered positive if $x > 2$.

It is difficult to titer the sperm-immobilizing antibodies because, as the sera are diluted, the sperm sometimes lose their motility due to the decrease in protein concentration. To overcome this effect, negative serum has to be added to the diluent.

Test for antibodies in cervical mucus

The concentration of immunoglobulins found in mucus is approximately 1% of the amount found in the circulation. The cervical mucus antibody is most likely produced locally and is of the IgA type. The method is difficult, because the amount of the mucus sample is limited and extraction of the low-viscosity component (containing the antibody) from the high-viscosity component is troublesome. Different methods of separation have been reported using buffers (Baker's solution, human serum), ultracentrifugation, and the proteolytic enzyme bromelin. Bromelin does dissolve mucus; however, it should be kept in mind that it may be harmful to sperm.[30] Following extraction, both the microagglutination test and the immobilization test can be used to detect the antibodies.[34,35] For spermatozoa to be immobilized by antibody and lysed by complement in cervical mucus, at least 4 hours is required with at least 50% of the full complement cascade component available in the mucus.[36] The sperm-immobilizing antibody may be the etiologic factor in some cases of abnormal PCT due to sperm immobilization.

In examining thousands of postcoital tests during the past 18 years, we have not seen sperm agglutination in postcoital cervical mucus. The percentage of infertile patients with positive cervical mucus tests has been reported to be 8%.[37] More data are needed to correlate the results of these tests with those done for agglutinating and immobilizing antibodies in serum. If the assay is available as a clinical test and its cost is not prohibitive, it should be used in cases of an abnormal PCT with sperm immobilization and in unexplained infertility.

Recommended therapy

At present, we recommend condom therapy (occlusive therapy) for women with sperm-agglutinating or sperm-immobilizing antibodies. Immunologic tests should be repeated every 3 months until the results become negative or the titer drops to 1:4 or less. (Some authors accept a titer of 1:32 or less as normal.) Some authors report a pregnancy rate of approximately 50% in couples whose positive test reverts to normal.[28] The exact incidence of pregnancy among couples whose tests remain positive has not been established, but it should be made clear to such patients that pregnancies do occur even when the tests remain positive. At our institution, if a titer of 1:4 or less is not achieved within 6 months, condom therapy is discontinued.

Therapy for men who have autoantibodies to sperm is still debatable. Testosterone therapy to suppress spermatogenesis and thereby reduce the antigenic source has not been proven to be successful. Artificial insemination using the new washed sperm technique has just begun to be used at this institution, and it is too early to know whether bypassing the cervix will have any success. It has been reported that artificial insemination (husband) with washed sperm resuspended in 4% human albumin has been used in couples with male autoimmunity, but the success rate of this method has not been published. Finally, immunosuppression using corticosteroids is also being attempted, but again no conclusive results are available.

One recommended schedule of corticosteroid therapy is as follows:[30] 32 mg methylprednisolone, 3 times a day, for the last week of the wife's menstrual cycle; decreased to 16 mg methylprednisolone, 3 times a day, for the first week of the menstrual cycle; then 8 mg 3 times a day for the second week of the menstrual cycle.

Conclusion

There is undeniable experimental evidence that antibody production can be induced in female animals following immunization with antigen obtained from male reproductive organs. There is evidence that some infertile couples may have an immune phenomenon as the causative factor. But it is still debatable whether these observations can definitely be implicated as causative factors in human infertility. Most of the observations on human subjects were done in vitro, and the same phenomena have not been shown to occur in vivo. ABO incompatibility as a cause of human infertility is an example. This observation, which appeared both theoretically and by initial screening tests to be a factor in human infertility, proved to be totally unrelated to infertility when examined closely.

Although numerous authors have reported the presence of sperm isoagglutinins in the serum of infertile women, agglutination of sperm by serum has not yet been proven to be an absolute cause of infertility. Even with identification of circulating sperm-agglutinating antibody, it has yet to be demonstrated that agglutination of sperm occurs in the female lower genital tract. Failure to demonstrate this may be due to a flaw in methodology, not in the initial hypothesis. Nevertheless, at present, except in relatively few centers, the incidence of detection of isoagglutinins in infertile women has approached the incidence found in normal controls.

The observation that sperm-agglutinating antibodies, which may be the cause of infertility, exist in some infertile males is well established. This phenomenon is demonstrable in a very small percentage of infertile men, many of whom have had a previous vasectomy and a reversal procedure.

With all these contradictions, a clinician dealing with the problems of infertility must question whether antibody-antigen reactions are, in fact, a causative factor in any infertile patients. The techniques available for detection of antigen-antibody reactions in couples with unexplained infertility are very simple. Essentially, these methods rely on either sperm agglutination or immobilization as the endpoint of the test method when motile sperm are allowed to come into contact with either serum or cervical mucus.

Until more research is done in this field, and better tests are developed, we suggest that the immunologic factor of infertility be investigated only after all established diagnostic steps are undertaken. If a persistent positive test is found in an infertile couple, it is advisable to inform the couple that a pregnancy may occur and that a positive immunologic test is not reliable for contraceptive purposes.

References

1. Behrman SJ, Buettner-Janusch J, Hegler R, et al: ABO (H) blood incompatibility as a cause of infertility: A new concept. *Am J Obstet Gynecol* 79:847, 1960

2. Fjallbrant B, Obrant O: Clinical and seminal findings in men with sperm antibodies. *Acta Obstet Gynecol Scand* 47:451, 1968

3. Franklin RR, Dukes CD: Antispermatozoal antibody and unexplained infertility. *Am J Obstet Gynecol* 89:6, 1964

4. Isojima S, Li TS, Ashitaka Y: Immunologic analysis of sperm-immobilizing factor found in sera of women with unexplained sterility. *Am J Obstet Gynecol* 101:677, 1968

5. Shulman S: Antigenic analysis of the male tract. In Edwards RG (ed): *Immunology and Reproduction: Proceedings.* New York, International Publishing Service, 1969

6. Shulman S, Bronson P: Immunochemical studies on human seminal plasma. II. The major antigens and their fractionation. *J Reprod Fertil* 18:481, 1969

7. Gullbring B: Investigations on the occurrence of blood group antigens in spermatozoa from man and serological demonstration of the segregation of characters. *Acta Med Scand* 159:169, 1957

8. Popivanov R, Volchanov VH: Segregation of men's AB-group spermatozoa in A- and B-spermatozoa through agglutination with immuno rabbit and anti-A serum. *Z Immunitaetsforsch Exp Ther* 124:206, 1964

9. Shahani S, Southam AL: Immunofluorescent study of the ABO blood group antigens in human spermatozoa. *Am J Obstet Gynecol* 84:660, 1962

10. Edwards RG, Ferguson LC, Coombs RRA: Blood group antigens on human spermatozoa. *J Reprod Fert* 7:153, 1964

11. Holborow EJ, Brown PC, Glynn LE, et al: The distribution of the blood group A antigen in human tissues. *Br J Exp Pathol* 41:430, 1960

12. Boettcher B: Human ABO blood group antigens on spermatozoa from secretors and nonsecretors. *J Reprod Fert* 9:267, 1960

13. Weil AJ, Rodenburg JM: Immunological differentiation of human testicular (spermatocele) and seminal spermatozoa. *Proc Soc Exp Biol Med* 105:43, 1960

14. Weil AJ: Antigens of adnexal glands of the male genital tract. *Fertil Steril* 12:538, 1961

15. Weil AJ: The spermatozoa-coating antigen (SCA) of the seminal vesicle. *Ann NY Acad Sci* 124:267, 1965

16. Li TS, Behrman SJ: The sperm and seminal plasma-specific antigens of human semen. *Fertil Steril* 21:565, 1970

17. Quinlivan WLG: The specific antigens of human seminal plasma. *Fertil Steril* 20:58, 1969

18. Hamerlynck J, Rumke P: A test for detection of cytotoxic antibodies to spermatozoa in man. *J Reprod Fertil* 17:191, 1968

19. Behrman SJ, Nakayama MD: Antitestis antibody, its inhibition of pregnancy. *Fertil Steril* 16:37, 1965

20. Mancini G, Carbonara AO, Heremans JF: Immunochemical quantitation of antigens by single radial immunodiffusion. *Immunochemistry* 2:235, 1965

21. Lippes J, Ogra S, Tomasi TB, et al: Immunohistological localization of γG, γA, γM, secretory piece and lactoferrin in human female genital tract. *Contraception* 1:163, 1970

22. Hjort T, Hansen KB: Immunofluorescent studies on human spermatozoa. *Clin Exp Immunol* 8:9, 1971

23. Solish GI, Gershowitz H, Behrman SJ: Occurrence of titer of isohemagglutinins in secretions of the human uterine cervix. *Proc Soc Exp Biol Med* 108:645, 1961

24. Wilson L: Sperm agglutinins in human semen and blood. *Proc Soc Exp Biol Med* 85:652, 1954

25. Rumke P, Hellinga G: Autoantibodies against spermatozoa in sterile men. *Am J Clin Pathol* 32:357, 1959

26. Phadke AM, Padukone K: Presence and significance of autoantibodies against spermatozoa in the blood of men with obstructed vas deferens. *J Reprod Fertil* 7:163, 1964

27. Schwimmer WB, Ustay KA, Behrman SJ: An evaluation of immunologic factors of fertility. *Fertil Steril* 18:167, 1967

28. Dukes CD, Franklin RR: Sperm agglutinins and human infertility. *Fertil Steril* 19:263, 1968

29. Glass RH, Vaidya RA: Sperm-agglutinating antibodies in infertile women. *Fertil Steril* 21:657, 1970

30. Haas GG Jr: Female immunologic factor. In Garcia C-R, Mastroianni L Jr, Amelar RD, Dubin L (eds): *Current Therapy of Infertility, 1982-1983.* Trenton, NJ, B.C. Decker, 1982, p 179

31. Friberg J: Relation between sperm-agglutinating antibodies in serum and seminal fluid. *Acta Obstet Gynecol Scand (Suppl)* 36:73, 1974

32. Friberg J: Clinical and immunological studies on sperm-agglutinating antibodies in serum and seminal fluid. *Acta Obstet Gynecol Scand (Suppl)* 36:1, 1975

33. Beer AE: Immunology of reproduction. In *Handbook of Sixteenth Annual Postgraduate Course, Course No. 1.* Am Fert Soc, San Francisco Hilton, April 1983, p 84

34. Jones WR: Immunologic infertility: Fact or Fiction? *Fertil Steril* 33:577, 1980

35. Menge AC, Medley NE, Mangione CM, et al: The incidence and influence of antisperm antibodies in infertile human couples on sperm-cervical mucus interactions and subsequent fertility. *Fertil Steril* 38:439, 1982

36. Beer AE, Neaves WB: Antigenic states of semen from viewpoints of female and male. *Fertil Steril* 29:3, 1978

37. Moghissi KS, Sacco AG, Borin K: Immunologic infertility. I. Cervical mucus antibodies and postcoital tests. *Am J Obstet Gynecol* 136:941, 1980

Chapter 31

Occult Genital Infection and Infertility

Gerald S. Bernstein, Ph.D., M.D.

Infertile men and women who have had a symptomatic genital infection are likely candidates to have some damage to their reproductive tracts. Thus, evaluation for tubal damage should be performed early in the infertility workup of a woman with a history of hospitalization for salpingitis. There should also be concern about an obstructed epididymis in a man who has had a previous attack of epididymitis. In the past decade, besides the investigation of overt infection, there has been increased interest in the relationship between subclinical infection and reproductive impairment.

Concern has been expressed about infections that could cause obstruction of, or functional damage to, the male or female reproductive tract without producing symptoms. Other infections could interfere with sperm transport in the lower female tract or impair the functional properties of spermatozoa. Interest has centered on the mycoplasmas and *Chlamydia trachomatis*, but other organisms may also be involved.

Mycoplasmas

The mycoplasmas are named from their taxonomic order, Mycoplasmatales. They are unique microorganisms with some characteristics of both bacteria and viruses. They are the size of large viruses, but can survive and reproduce in cell-free media as bacteria do. They are surrounded by a triple-layered lipoprotein membrane, like animal cells, rather than having the cell wall of bacteria.

The mycoplasmas were once called pleuropneumonia-like organisms (PPLO), because the type originally isolated in 1898 caused pleuropneumonia in cattle. The mycoplasmas have been placed into the class Mollicutes, order Mycoplasmatales, family Mycoplasmataceae, and have been divided into three genera, two of which, *Mycoplasma* and *Ureaplasma*, are represented in the human. Five species of *Mycoplasma* have been isolated from the respiratory tract. Four of these exist as commensals in the human oropharynx, and a fifth, *Mycoplasma pneumoniae*, causes cold-agglutinin-positive primary atypical pneumonia. The organisms also colonize the genital tract and were first identified in the human in 1937 from material obtained from an abscess of Bartholin's gland. Three species of genital *Mycoplasma* have been identified: *M. hominis;* a relatively rare type, *M. fermentans;* and *Ureaplasma urealyticum.* The *Ureaplasma* species are differentiated from the *Mycoplasma* species by their ability to hydrolyze urea. They form very small colonies in culture and their original descriptive name was tiny, or T-strain, mycoplasma. Organisms that were earlier called T-mycoplasma are now correctly called *U. urealyticum.*

Genital colonization by mycoplasmas is related to sexual activity. The organisms are seldom found in prepubertal girls or sexually mature women who have not had intercourse. But *U. urealyticum* has been isolated in approximately 37% of women who have had intercourse with a single partner and in 75% of women who have had three or more sexual partners. The organisms are found frequently in women with venereal disease and vaginitis, and have been isolated from tuboovarian abscesses. *M. hominis* has been associated with salpingitis. *U. urealyticum* can cause nongonococcal urethritis in men and women.

Role in infertility

The major interest in these organisms has centered on their possible role as a cause of unexplained infertility. The older literature in this field has been reviewed by Friberg[1] and by Taylor-Robinson and McCormack.[2] The work of Gnarpe and Friberg[3,4] attracted attention in 1972 and 1973, when these authors reported that in 33 (92%) of 36 couples with unexplained infertility either the male (2 couples), female (3 couples), or both partners (28 couples) had positive cultures for *U. urealyticum.* The cultures were taken from semen and the endocervical ca-

nal. In two control groups evaluated, 9 (22%) of 40 pregnant women had positive cultures and 6 (26%) of 23 men whose wives were in the third trimester of pregnancy also had positive cultures. When the 36 infertile couples were treated with doxycycline, 15 (42%) of the women became pregnant within 3 months and 29 (84%) were pregnant within 1 year.

Other investigators have suggested that treatment of couples with antibiotics (usually tetracycline or doxycycline) will improve pregnancy rates.[1] However, this has not been supported by controlled studies, which have demonstrated no differences between the rates of pregnancies in treated and untreated couples (Table 31-1).[5,6]

Comparing data from various studies is difficult because of differences in the selection of patients and the amount of effort made to rule out other factors or infections that might be contributing to the infertility. There are also conflicting data relating the efficacy of treatment in eradicating the organism and the subsequent occurrence of pregnancy. In the study of Friberg and Gnarpe, it is not known whether all of the couples achieving pregnancy were cured by antibiotic treatment.[4] In a more recent study, Toth and co-workers followed 161 infertile couples in which the male partner's semen contained *U. urealyticum.* Both partners were treated with doxycycline, 100 mg twice a day for 4 weeks. In the group in which the male's infection was

Table 31-1
Controlled studies of outcome of therapy of couples with unexplained infertility and *U. urealyticum* infections

Authors	Treatment	No. of couples	No. of pregnancies	Conceptions (%)
Harrison et al[5]	Doxycycline	30	5	17
	Placebo	28	4	14
	None	30	5	17
Matthews et al[6]	Treated	51	10	20
	None	18	4	22

Infertility

Table 31-2
Factors affecting pregnancy outcome in 161 couples treated with doxycycline

Variable	3-Year pregnancy rate (%)	P*
Mycoplasma culture (semen)		
Negative	60	<0.001
Positive	5	
Hysterosalpingogram performed		
Yes	37	<0.001
No	57	
Tuboplasty		
Yes	14	<0.001
No	55	
D&C performed		
Yes	32	<0.002
No	53	
Fertility drugs given		
Yes	25	<0.001
No	57	

*Log rank test results comparing distributions of time until pregnancy and not the pregnancy rate. The last two variables were not significant when considered independently of the first three.

Modified from Toth A, Lesser ML, Brooks C, et al: Subsequent pregnancies among 161 couples treated for T-mycoplasma genital-tract infection. N Engl J Med 308:505, 1983.

cured (cultures were not done on the women), 60% of the women had a pregnancy and live birth, whereas only 5% had a successful pregnancy in the group in which the semen culture was still positive after therapy.[7] The median time to achieve pregnancy in the group with negative cultures was 10.6 months. Not all of these couples had unexplained infertility. In some cases the semen was abnormal; in others a female factor was involved. The outcome was partly related to other factors affecting fertility (Table 31-2).[7]

At present, it is unclear whether *U. urealyticum* is a major cause of unexplained infertility. One confounder is that only some serotypes of *U. urealyticum* may be pathogenic, and there has

been no information about *U. urealyticum* serotypes in the infertility literature. There is a need for further, well-controlled studies to establish the significance of this factor.

In some cases, *U. urealyticum* may produce changes in the semen that suggest possible infection. Some infected men have reduced sperm motility, reduced sperm counts, an increase in abnormal forms, and other changes including coiled tails and fine granular deposits on the tails.[8-10] Other infected men appear to have normal semen. It is possible that changes in the semen may be related to the site of infection or the number or serotype of the organisms present, but there is currently little information about these possibilities. The organisms themselves become attached to spermatozoa (Figure 31-1),[11]

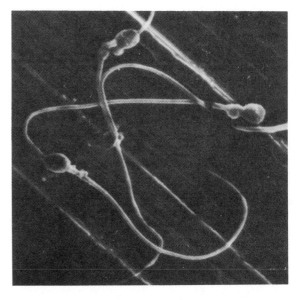

Figure 31-1
Scanning electron micrograph (× 1,860) of sperm from semen infected with *Ureaplasma urealyticum*. Note small outgrowths attached to spermatozoa, similar in appearance to *Ureaplasma* colonies grown in culture.

Reproduced, with permission, from Gnarpe H, Friberg J: T-mycoplasmas on spermatozoa and infertility. Nature 245:97, 1973.

but they can be observed only by means of scanning or transmission electron microscopy.

Infection with *U. urealyticum* may also be a cause of recurrent spontaneous abortion.[12-14]

There is no information about the mechanism by which *U. urealyticum* may affect fertility apart from its effect on semen quality. There is speculation that the organisms attached to spermatozoa may somehow impair fertilizing capacity or interfere with the early stages of development of the zygote. Berger et al did not find a difference in recovery rates of *U. urealyticum* from the semen of men with normal and abnormal hamster-egg penetration tests.[15] Mycoplasmas may also affect the oviducts. *M. hominis* has been shown to cause swelling of the cilia of the tubal endothelium in experimental infection of human oviducts grown in tissue culture.[16]

Diagnosis and management

We recommend that cultures for *M. hominis* and *U. urealyticum* be performed on both the male (semen) and female (cervix) members of couples with otherwise unexplained infertility, and in cases where the semen is abnormal or there is a history of nongonococcal urethritis. Cultures for these organisms are now readily available. Although it is controversial, we treat those individuals with positive cultures. *U. urealyticum* is usually sensitive to tetracycline and erythromycin. We follow the regimen recommended by Friberg and Gnarpe: doxycycline, 200 mg the first day, then 100 mg daily for another 9 days.[4] Both partners are treated from the 7th through the 16th day of the wife's menstrual cycle. If the cultures are still positive after the first treatment cycle, the couple should be treated the same way for 2 more cycles. An alternative method is to give doxycycline, 100 mg twice a day for 2 weeks. Doxycycline may give better cure rates and has to be taken less frequently than tetracycline HCl.[17] Some strains have become resistant to tetracycline. We do not advocate the use of antibiotics empirically, without cultures, because there is no assurance that one course of antibiotic treatment will cure the infection.

Chlamydia

The chlamydias are classified as prokaryotic cells (that is, not having a discrete nucleus) along with the mycoplasmas, rickettsias, and bacteria. They are obligate intracellular parasites that produce characteristic cytoplasmic inclusions in host cells and are susceptible to various antimicrobial agents. They have to be grown in cell cultures, or by other methods generally used to culture viruses.

The cytoplasmic inclusions consist of a group of small particles called elementary bodies and large particles called reticulate bodies. The elementary bodies can survive extracellularly and are the agents that invade new host cells. In order to multiply, the small particles have to reorganize within cells into large particles that replicate, and re-form into elementary bodies that can then leave the host cell.

The genus *Chlamydia* is divided into two species, *C. psittaci* and *C. trachomatis*. The organisms of the latter species form compact inclusion bodies that contain glycogen, and their growth is inhibited by sulfadiazine under standard conditions. Each species has a number of serotypes. The human diseases caused by *Chlamydia* include psittacosis, trachoma, inclusion conjunctivitis, lymphogranuloma venereum, nongonococcal urethritis in men, the urethral syndrome in women (symptoms of urethritis with negative bacterial cultures), and cervicitis and salpingitis (Table 31-3).

Chlamydia trachomatis accounts for at least 20% to 30% of the cases of salpingitis in Scandinavia and the US.[18,19] Studies in the US have generally shown lower rates than those in Scandinavia, but this is probably an artifact based on the populations studied and the techniques of sampling for culture.[20,21] Chlamydial salpingitis

Table 31-3
Chlamydia organisms that can cause disease in humans

Species	Disease	Immunotype
C. psittaci	Psittacosis	
C. trachomatis	Trachoma	A, B, Ba, C
	Inclusion conjunctivitis	D, E, F, G, H, I, J, K
	Genitourinary infections	D, E, F, H, I, J, K
	Lymphogranuloma venereum	L_1, L_2, L_3

tends to be more indolent than disease due to the gonococcus, and some women who develop chlamydial salpingitis may be asymptomatic.[22,23] Thus chlamydial infections are often treated later after the onset of infection than are gonococcal infections. Some infected women may not receive any treatment at all. Most gynecologists have had the experience of discovering tubal disease of varying degrees of severity in women with no clinical history of salpingitis. At least some of these infections have been associated with C. trachomatis.[23]

Women with cervical infections due to C. trachomatis generally have purulent cervicitis, but occasionally may have a normal-appearing cervix. They may have a vaginal discharge or no noticeable symptoms. Inflammation of this type might impair the migration of sperm through the cervix, but there is little information about this possibility.

In men, C. trachomatis can cause nongonococcal urethritis and epididymitis. The organisms can also be isolated from prostatic fluid in men with urethritis, but in these cases it is difficult to avoid contamination of the prostatic fluid sample with urethral organisms. A recent report, however, described the isolation of C. trachomatis from prostatic fluid in the absence of urethritis.[24] There is little information about asymptomatic chlamydial infection in the male and the effect of such infections on fertility. Chlamydia have been shown to adhere to human spermatozoa in vitro, but it is not known whether this occurs in vivo.[25]

Diagnosis and management

Women with suspected chlamydial cervicitis should have the infection documented. Facilities for culturing the organism are now generally available. There are also techniques for identifying organisms on direct smears by means of monoclonal antibodies and immunofluorescence. The female partners of men with nongonococcal urethritis should be treated empirically. The recommended therapy for men and women is a 7-day course of: tetracycline, 500 mg orally 4 times daily; doxycycline, 100 mg orally twice a day; or erythromycin, 500 mg orally 4 times a day.[26]

Other organisms

Other organisms inhabiting the male or female genital tract could also potentially interfere with fertility without causing significant symptoms.

In women, various organisms related to vaginitis can affect spermatozoa in vitro. For example, large numbers of Escherichia coli and Candida albicans can reduce sperm motility or cause clumping. This might have some effect on the delayed phase of sperm transport from the vagina into the cervical mucus. Leukocytes present in infected vaginal fluid may also have an effect on fertility, because these cells inhibit sperm motility and the ability of sperm to penetrate zona-free hamster eggs.[15] Cervical or vaginal infections may also alter cervical mucus to impair sperm entry. We have observed abnormal mucus and poor postcoital tests (PCTs) in women with subclinical vaginal infections due to a mixture of *Gardnerella vaginalis* and anaerobic bacteria, with return of the PCTs to normal after the infections have been treated. More information is needed about the effect of cervicovaginal infections on fertility.

The mechanism by which infection may affect male fertility, apart from causing permanent obstruction, is not clearly understood. It has been suggested that inflammation or other effects of infection may cause reversible obstruction of the epididymis or ejaculatory ducts, adversely alter the chemical composition of seminal plasma, interfere with sperm maturation in the epididymis, or affect spermatozoa through the influence of bacterial metabolites or products derived from leukocytes. There is little information about these possibilities. There have been some studies that relate abnormal semen to infections with *E. coli,* but most of these studies lack adequate controls.

The extent of the problem of subclinical genital infection as a factor in male fertility has not been defined.[27] Population studies have been inadequately controlled and there have been few attempts to determine whether organisms found in semen are derived from the urethra, prostate, or other sites in the male tract. Quantitative cultures and localizing tests have not always been done. However, it has been observed that some organisms are more likely to be present in the semen of some subgroups of infertile men. Toth and Lesser observed that *E. coli* was isolated more frequently from men with a history of prostatitis or urethritis (8% and 11%, respectively) than in infertile men without a history of genitourinary infections (2%) or fertile controls (0%).[17]

Treatment of asymptomatic men whose semen contains large numbers of coliforms sometimes results in a marked improvement in semen quality. Given the variation seen in semen quality over time, anecdotal cases do not prove cause

and effect. However, it is advisable to obtain a semen culture if there is some evidence that the semen may be infected.

The gram-negative enteric organisms, particularly *E. coli,* are usually the bacteria found in infected semen, although other organisms may be involved. Of particular interest are some of the agents commonly associated with vaginitis that can often be cultured from the semen of the infected woman's male partner. It is not clear whether these organisms (for example, *G. vaginalis* and anaerobes) are carried in the urethra or prostate, or whether they affect semen quality or sperm function. However, it is important to consider both partners in evaluating and treating infections in infertile couples. The infected male is a significant factor in perpetuating vaginal infections in his partner, and the combined effect may influence fertility. If either partner has evidence of infection by examination of the semen or vaginal fluid, both should be studied with appropriate cultures and both partners should be treated until cured.

References

1. Friberg J: Mycoplasmas and ureaplasmas in infertility and abortion. *Fertil Steril* 33:351, 1980

2. Taylor-Robinson D, McCormack WM: The genital mycoplasmas. *N Engl J Med* 302:1003, 1063, 1980 (Parts I & II)

3. Gnarpe H, Friberg J: Mycoplasma and human reproductive failure. I. The occurrence of different mycoplasmas in couples with reproductive failure. *Am J Obstet Gynecol* 114:727, 1972

4. Friberg J, Gnarpe H: Mycoplasma and human reproductive failure. III. Pregnancies in "infertile" couples treated with doxycycline for T-mycoplasmas. *Am J Obstet Gynecol* 116:23, 1973

5. Harrison RF, DeLouvois J, Blades M, et al: Doxycycline treatment and human infertility. *Lancet* 1:605, 1975

6. Matthews CD, Clapp KH, Tansing JA, et al: T-mycoplasma genital infection: The effect of doxycycline therapy on human unexplained infertility. *Fertil Steril* 30:98, 1978

7. Toth A, Lesser ML, Brooks C, et al: Subsequent pregnancies among 161 couples treated for T-mycoplasma genital-tract infection. *N Engl J Med* 308:505, 1983

8. Cassell GH, Younger JB, Brown MB, et al: Microbiological study of infertile women at the time of diagnostic laparoscopy. Association of *Ureaplasma urealyticum* with a defined subpopulation. *N Engl J Med* 308:502, 1983

9. Fowlkes DM, MacLeod J, O'Leary WM: T-mycoplasmas and human infertility: Correlation of infection with alterations in seminal parameters. *Fertil Steril* 26:1212, 1975

10. Toth A, Swenson CE, O'Leary WM: Light microscopy as an aid in predicting ureaplasma infection in human semen. *Fertil Steril* 30:586, 1978

11. Gnarpe H, Friberg J: T-mycoplasmas on spermatozoa and infertility. *Nature* 245:97, 1973

12. Horne HW Jr, Hertig AB, Kundsin RB, et al: Sub-clinical endometrial inflammation and T-mycoplasma: A possible cause of human reproductive failure. *Int J Fertil* 18:226, 1973

13. Stray-Pedersen B, Eng J, Reikvam TM: Uterine T-mycoplasma colonization in reproductive failure. *Am J Obstet Gynecol* 130:307, 1978

14. Sompolinsky D, Solomon F, Elkina L, et al: Infections with mycoplasma and bacteria in induced midtrimester abortion and fetal loss. *Am J Obstet Gynecol* 121:610, 1975

15. Berger RE, Karp LE, Williamson RA, et al: The relationship of pyospermia and seminal fluid bacteriology to sperm function as reflected in the sperm penetration assay. *Fertil Steril* 37:557, 1982

16. Mårdh PA, Westrom L, Von Mecklenburg C, et al: Studies in ciliated epithelia of the human genital tract. I. Swelling of the cilia of fallopian tube epithelium in organ cultures infected with *Mycoplasma hominis*. *Br J Vener Dis* 52:52, 1976

17. Toth A, Lesser ML: *Ureaplasma urealyticum* and infertility: The effect of different antibiotic regimens on the semen quality. *J Urol* 128:705, 1982

18. Mårdh PA, Ripa T, Svensson L, et al: *Chlamydia trachomatis* infection in patients with acute salpingitis. *N Engl J Med* 296:1377, 1977

19. Eschenbach DA, Buchanan TM, Pollock HM, et al: Polymicrobial etiology of acute pelvic inflammatory disease. *N Engl J Med* 293:166, 1975

20. Holmes KK, Eschenbach DA, Knapp JS: Salpingitis: Overview of etiology and epidemiology. *Am J Obstet Gynecol* 138:893, 1980

21. Mårdh PA: An overview of infectious agents of salpingitis, their biology and recent advances in methods of detection. *Am J Obstet Gynecol* 138:933, 1980

22. Svensson L, Westrom L, Ripa KT: Differences in some clinical and laboratory parameters in acute salpingitis related to culture and serologic findings. *Am J Obstet Gynecol* 138:1017, 1980

23. Henry-Suchet J, Catalan F, Loffredo V, et al: Microbiology of specimens obtained by laparoscopy from controls and from patients with pelvic inflammatory disease or infertility with tubal obstruction: *Chlamydia trachomatis* and *Ureaplasma urealyticum*. *Am J Obstet Gynecol* 138:1022, 1980

24. Goh BT, Morgan-Capner P, Lim KS: Isolation of *Chlamydia trachomatis* from prostatic fluid in association with inflammatory joint or eye disease. *Br J Vener Dis* 59:373, 1983

25. Wølner-Hanssen P, Mårdh PA: *In vitro* tests of the adherence of *Chlamydia trachomatis* to human spermatozoa. *Fertil Steril* 42:102, 1984

26. Centers for Disease Control: Sexually transmitted diseases treatment guidelines 1982. *MMWR* 31(2S):suppl, 1982

27. Berger RE, Holmes KK: Infection and male infertility. In Santeen RJ, Swerdoff RS (eds): *Male Sexual Dysfunction*, New York, Marcel Dekker, 1985

Chapter 32

Recurrent Abortion

Charles M. March, M.D.

Human reproduction is markedly inefficient. Overall, approximately 15% of ova exposed to sperm do not divide, and an equal number are fertilized but fail to implant. Data suggest that the postimplantation loss is 41% (Table 32-1).[1] Thus, only about 30% of possible fertilizations result in a viable fetus. Usually the losses are random events, and recurrent abortion is infrequent, affecting one in 200 couples and one in 500 pregnancies.

Recurrent abortion is defined as the spontaneous termination of three consecutive pregnancies before the 20th week of gestation. In one published report,[2] the rate of spontaneous abortion in women who had lost two preceding pregnancies was 26.2%. After three or more consecutive abortions, the spontaneous abortion rate was between 26% and 32%. In another report, the risk of spontaneous abortion was 28.6% after two spontaneous abortions in women with no prior term pregnancies and 26.9% in those with one or more prior term pregnancies (Table 32-2).[3] These rates are higher than the estimated 15% to 20% overall incidence of spontaneous abortion among all clinically diagnosed pregnancies.

The 26% to 32% observed rate of abortion after three consecutive abortions is much lower than the 73% to 83% rate computed from theoretical models.[4] These latter figures have been used incorrectly as controls to test the efficacy of a variety of treatment regimens for recurrent abortion. Because these models markedly exaggerate the actual recurrent abortion rate from 30% to 75%, the 70% rate of successful outcome of subsequent pregnancies following various treatment regimens is more correctly attributable to chance than to the therapy.

Table 32-1
Early conceptual loss among 148 women

Biochemical evidence of pregnancy only	47 (31.8%)
Clinically pregnant, spontaneous abortion	14 (9.5%)
Doing well after 20 weeks	87 (58.8%)

Adapted from Williamson EM, Miller JF: A prospective study into early conceptual loss. Clin Genet 17:93, 1980.

Table 32-2
Risk of spontaneous abortion relative to prior gestational outcome

Prior pregnancies		
Term	Abortions	Abortion rate (%)
0	0	12.7
0	1	22.8
0	2	28.6
0	3	33.3
≥1	0	14.0
≥1	1	24.9
≥1	2	26.9
≥1	3	48.7

From Naylor AF, Warburton D: Sequential analysis of spontaneous abortion. II. Collaborative study data show that gravidity determines a very substantial rise in risk. Fertil Steril 31:282, 1979.

Table 32-3
Etiology of recurrent abortion in 195 couples

Etiologic factor	First trimester		Second trimester		Primary abortion		Secondary abortion		Total	
	No.	%	No.	%	No.	%	No.	%	No.	%
Uterine defects	15	12.1	15	12.1	27	20.0	3	5.5	30	15.4
Cervical incompetence	4	3.2	21	29.6	17	12.6	8	13.3	25	12.8
Endocrine	9	7.3	1	1.4	9	6.7	1	1.7	10	5.1
Endometrial infection	20	16.1	9	12.7	21	15.6	8	13.3	29	14.9
Chromosomal	5	4.0	0	0	4	3.0	1	1.7	5	2.6
Systemic disorder	0	0	2	2.8	2	1.5	0	0	2	1.0
Oligospermia	7	5.6	1	1.4	8	5.9	0	0	8	4.1
Excessive smoking	1	0.8	0	0	1	0.7	0	0	1	0.5
Total known	61	49.2	49	69.0	89	65.9	21	35.0	110	56.4
Total unknown	63	50.8	22	31.0	46	34.1	39	65.0	85	43.6

Modified from Stray-Pedersen B, Stray-Pedersen S: Etiologic factors and subsequent reproductive performance in 195 couples with a prior history of habitual abortion. Am J Obstet Gynecol 148:140, 1984.

Recurrent abortion may occur in women who have never carried pregnancies to term (primary recurrent abortion) or who have had one or more successful gestations (secondary). This chapter discusses etiologies of recurrent abortion and offers an outline for management of women with recurrent abortion. In a report of 195 couples with a history of three or more consecutive abortions, it was possible to establish a diagnosis in 110, or 56.4%. (Table 32-3).[5]

Etiology

Chromosomal abnormalities

Abnormal chromosome distribution may occur during the first or second meiotic divisions of either oogenesis or spermatogenesis or during mitosis. Between 40% and 60% of first-trimester abortuses have chromosomal anomalies, whereas such anomalies are found in only 5% to 10% of second-trimester abortuses (Figure 32-1).[6] These data suggest that the pathophysiology of first- and second-trimester abortions differs.

Chromosomal abnormalities are present most frequently in very early abortions, and

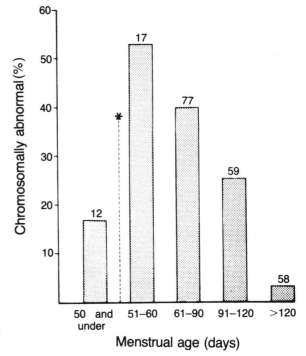

Figure 32-1
The frequency of chromosomal anomalies among abortuses, classified by menstrual age. The dotted line indicates the mean incidence of anomalies in abortuses of 60 days or less.

Reproduced, with permission, from Carr DH: Cytogenetic aspects of induced and spontaneous abortions. Clin Obstet Gynecol 15:203, 1972.

then decline in incidence with increasing gestational age. Autosomal trisomy is the most common type of chromosomal defect (50% to 60%) found in abortuses. These defects usually have a lethal effect upon the conceptus, thereby causing very early abortion. Trisomies 13, 18, and 21, however, are usually detected in late abortuses and in infants who survive.

Deletion of one sex chromosome with the resultant 45,X karyotype is the second most common type of anomaly, accounting for 15% to 25% of chromosomal defects in abortuses. Most fetuses with this karyotype are aborted. In the few who survive, the karyotype is manifested clinically with the stigmata of Turner's syndrome. Polyploidy is the least common major type of chromosomal defect, with an incidence of 15% to 20%. Triploidy (three times the germ cell number of chromosomes) is the most frequent defect in this group. Other uncommon abnormalities include autosomal monosomy and mosaicism. These defects follow errors in gametogenesis, chromosomal accidents at the time of fertilization, or during the first division of the fertilized ovum. In a study of 1,500 abortions, translocations that might have been present in one parent were found in only 3.8% of abortuses.[7] If the products of conception from the first abortion were normal, it was reported that the second abortus was chromosomally normal in 55 of 68 cases.[8] However, the second abortus was aneuploid in 40 of 57 cases in which the first abortus was aneuploid. A high rate of correlation has been found between the karyotype of the first abortus and that of the second abortus (Table 32-4).[9]

Most chromosomal defects occur as random errors in meiosis or mitosis or following exposure to toxic agents. Both advanced maternal (>35 years) and paternal (>55 years) age have been associated with an increase in chromosomal defects.[10] Maternal age of less than 17 years is also associated with a higher rate of chromosomal anomalies in abortuses.[6] Fetal karyotypic errors may also arise because of a chromosomal defect in an apparently normal parent. The most common defect of this type is a balanced translocation. Such persons are at high risk for transferring unbalanced genetic material to their offspring.

Translocations have been reported to occur in one in every 700 phenotypically normal persons.[6] However, the frequency of a translocation in one parent or the other is tenfold higher among couples with a history of recurrent spontaneous abortion (Table 32-5).[9] Translocations were noted most commonly among couples who had experienced a perinatal death of an infant in addition to one or more abortions. By using newer chromosomal banding techniques, minor chromosomal anomalies have been identified and reported in about 8% of couples with recur-

Table 32-4
Correlation between karyotype of first and second abortuses in four studies

First abortion	Second abortion					
	Normal	Monosomy	Trisomy	Polyploidy	Translocation	Total
Normal	34	2	6	5	0	47
Monosomy	4	1	2	1	0	8
Trisomy	4	1	20	1	0	26
Polyploidy	1	1	3	1	0	6
Translocation	0	0	0	0	4	4
Total	43	5	31	8	4	91

Reproduced with permission from Kajii T, Ferrier A: Cytogenetics of aborters and abortuses. Am J Obstet Gynecol 131:33, 1978.

**Table 32-5
Frequency of translocation in those who
abort in the general adult population**

General population	30/9,616	(0.3%)
All aborters	6/783	(0.8%)
Nonrecurrent aborters	4/710	(0.6%)
Recurrent aborters	2/73	(2.7%)
Aborters without perinatal death	4/727	(0.6%)
Aborters with perinatal death	2/56	(3.6%)

*Reproduced with permission from Kajii T, Ferrier A: Cytogenetics
of aborters and abortuses.* Am J Obstet Gynecol *131:33, 1978.*

rent abortion. The incidence is less than 3% in the general population.[11] Among couples with a history of both abortion and fetal anomalies, the frequency of a chromosomal abnormality in one parent is 23%.[12]

X-chromosome mosaicism has also been reported to cause recurrent abortion. Although an increased frequency of chromosomal defects has not been found in the abortuses of women treated with either oral contraceptives (OCs) or ovulatory drugs in the month before conception,[13] exposure to these drugs, and either maternal or paternal exposure to radiation, have been associated with a higher frequency of karyotypic abnormalities.[7] It has been suggested that most of the first-trimester abortions that are not due to chromosomal abnormalities are due to genetic disorders in the embryo, with normal chromosomes, that cannot as yet be diagnosed by genetic techniques.[12]

Uterine defects

Congenital anomalies
Anomalies of müllerian duct fusion have been found in 10% to 15% of women with recurrent abortion.[5,14] Most of these abortions occur in the second trimester. Although any of the various types of anomalies may be detected in a patient who has aborted, the anomalies related to in utero diethylstilbestrol (DES) exposure and septate uterus are the only ones that have been shown to be of etiologic importance in the pa-

tient with recurrent abortion. Abortion rates as high as 90% and 30% have been reported in women with septate uterus and DES-affected uterus, respectively.[15,16]

Patients with three or more first-trimester abortions and a septate uterus should have a complete investigation, including karyotype of both parents, to rule out other causes of reproductive wastage before surgical correction is attempted. Couples with multiple causes of recurrent abortion have been reported, and a comprehensive evaluation is needed. Those who have had one second-trimester abortion or only one or two first-trimester losses and who have a septate uterus need not have chromosomal studies before hysteroscopic incision of the septum.

Submucous leiomyomas
Infertility, premature labor, and an increased incidence of first- and second-trimester abortion have been reported in women with submucous leiomyomas.[5,17] The mechanism of recurrent first-trimester abortion is most likely to be a poor implantation site, secondary to impaired endometrial nutrition. In recurrent second-trimester abortion, the myoma(s) may impair uterine enlargement, and thereby cause premature expulsion of the fetus. To establish the diagnosis, it is best to use hysteroscopy. The size and location of the myoma(s), as well as the relation to the tubal ostia and the internal os, should be delineated. If this technique is not available, it is mandatory to obtain a hysterosalpingogram (HSG) before performing a myomectomy. The HSG not only provides preliminary information about the status of the fallopian tubes, but also documents the site of the defect, thus facilitating the surgical resection.

Intrauterine adhesions (IUA)
The significance of adhesions in the woman who has had recurrent abortions is uncertain. Extensive adhesions are associated with infertility and menstrual disturbances, whereas minimal or moderate adhesions are found often in patients

with recurrent abortion. Whether these adhesions have been an etiologic factor in the recurrent abortions or are merely the sequelae of multiple curettages is uncertain. Recent data, however, suggest that IUA do play a role in recurrent abortion. Hysteroscopic diagnosis and lysis of adhesions are the best management.[18]

Incompetent cervical os

Not every woman who has an incompetent cervical os reports the classic history of spontaneous late second-trimester rupture of membranes, followed by the painless delivery of a living fetus who immediately dies. However, most patients with cervical incompetence have some of these findings. Although a luteal phase HSG demonstrating a wide internal os, or the finding of a patulous internal os, may be used to suggest the presence of an incompetent cervix, the diagnosis is best made by careful review of the obstetric history rather than by laboratory studies or other diagnostic tests. Some patients have a prior history of trauma to the cervix. The risk of second-trimester abortion is markedly increased among nulliparous women who have had a prior elective abortion.[19]

Patients with an incompetent cervical os should be allowed to conceive again and should be examined biweekly during the first trimester. A real-time ultrasound examination should be performed at 12 to 14 weeks of gestation to document the presence of an intrauterine pregnancy of the expected duration and to detect fetal and cardiac activity. The optimum time to perform a cerclage is at 14 weeks' gestation.

The procedure of choice is the McDonald operation, because it is easier, faster, and associated with less morbidity than the Shirodkar procedure. A 5-mm double-armed Mersilene suture is placed in a purse-string manner into the cervical stroma, just distal to the level of the internal cervical os (Figure 32-2). This suture should be cut at 38 to 39 weeks of gestation to allow a vaginal delivery. The Lash procedure may cause infertility or permanent cervical scarring that might prevent dilatation, and it has no place in the management of cervical incompetence. Contraindications to cerclage include persistent

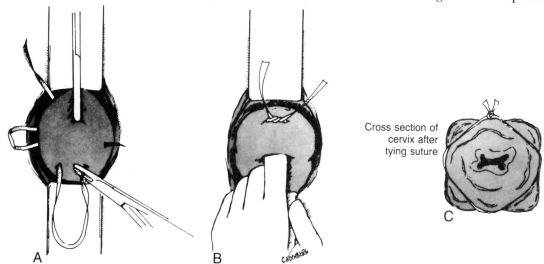

Cross section of cervix after tying suture

Figure 32-2
Steps in performing a McDonald cerclage using a Mersilene suture. The index finger is used to ensure closure of the internal os.

uterine contractions, rupture of membranes, cervical dilatation greater than 4 cm, or presence of a fetal anomaly. A 78% success rate has been reported for McDonald cerclage if performed electively, compared with 53% if performed after cervical dilatation occurs.[20]

Inadequate corpus luteum

This uncommon defect may be associated with very early abortion. Many of these abortions are subclinical and may be detected only with the use of the most sensitive assays for human chorionic gonadotropin (hCG). The β-subunit radioimmunoassay for hCG may be used to detect occult pregnancies in patients who have luteal phase defects.

The underlying abnormality in luteal phase defects is inadequate progesterone production. This may be manifested either by a luteal phase of normal length (as defined by an elevated basal body temperature, or BBT) but low serum progesterone levels and/or out-of-phase endometrial histology, by a short luteal phase (less than 10 days), or by combinations of these. The evaluation of patients with recurrent abortion should include both a midluteal phase serum progesterone level and a late (day 26) luteal phase endometrial biopsy. The former should be greater than 10 ng/mL[21] and the latter, using the criteria of Noyes and co-workers, should be within 2 days of the expected date.[22] Both studies are best performed in a cycle in which the BBT is

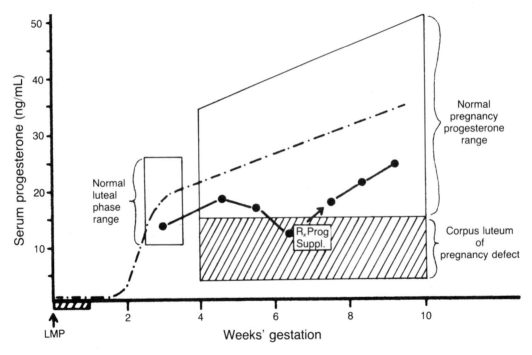

Figure 32-3
Serum progesterone levels in a patient with corpus luteum of pregnancy dysfunction (solid circles). Treatment with progesterone suppositories (25 mg twice daily) was instituted when the serum progesterone level fell below 15 ng/mL.

From Hensleigh PA, Fainstat T: Corpus luteum dysfunction: Serum progesterone levels in diagnosis and assessment of therapy for recurrent and threatened abortion. Fertil Steril 32:396, 1979. Reproduced with permission of the publisher, The American Fertility Society.

recorded, and the results should be correlated with both the day of the thermogenic shift and the onset of the next menstrual period.

In a study of eight patients with recurrent abortion and poor luteal function as determined by both progesterone levels and endometrial biopsies,[23] five were found to have luteal phase corpus luteum dysfunction and seven had low progesterone levels (<15 ng/mL) in early pregnancy. The former defect was treated with clomiphene citrate and the latter with progesterone vaginal suppositories, 25 mg twice daily. All eight women treated this way carried their pregnancies to term.

The same authors also treated 11 of 12 patients who had vaginal bleeding and/or cramping within the first 10 weeks after the last menstrual period by means of progesterone vaginal suppositories. All 12 patients had serum progesterone levels in pregnancy below 15 ng/mL. The patient who was not treated aborted. All of the nine patients whose progesterone levels rose above 15 ng/mL delivered at term, except for one patient who had an anencephalic infant. Figure 32-3[23] depicts the progesterone levels of one patient who was treated successfully.

Further support for the relation of luteal insufficiency and recurrent abortion was provided by measurement of serum progesterone during early pregnancy in 15 women with a prior histo-

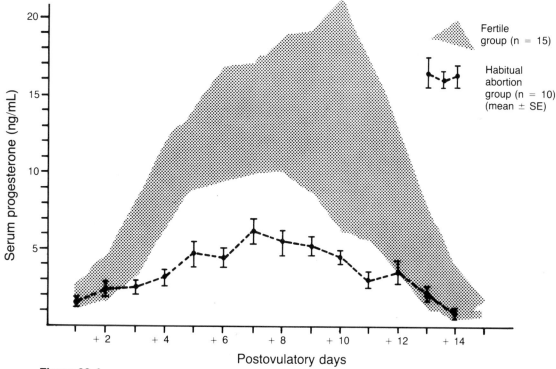

Figure 32-4
Serum progesterone levels (means ± SE) during the luteal phase of the menstrual cycle. Shaded area shows range in 15 women with normal menses and proven fertility (group 2); broken line shows range in 10 women who habitually aborted (group 1).

From Hernandez-Horta JL, Gordillo Fernandez J, Soto de Leon B, et al: Direct evidence of luteal insufficiency in women with habitual abortion. Obstet Gynecol 49:705, 1977. Reprinted with permission from The American College of Obstetricians and Gynecologists.

ry of three to seven spontaneous abortions.[24] In 10 of these women, serum progesterone levels were also measured during the luteal phase and were found to be significantly lower than in controls (Figure 32-4).[24] Among those who aborted again, serum progesterone levels were between 4.0 and 5.0 ng/mL in early pregnancy, compared with normal levels of 14 to 35 ng/mL.

Infections

Toxoplasma, Ureaplasma urealyticum (T-mycoplasma), *Listeria, Brucella, Chlamydia,* cytomegalovirus, and herpes simplex have all been associated with abortion. Intrauterine infection may prevent implantation or interfere with organogenesis. Infection may be primarily intrauterine or may result from transplacental transmission from the mother. However, cause and effect relationships between these organisms and recurrent abortion have not been well documented.

In developing countries, some women with recurrent abortion have been shown to have positive titers for *Toxoplasma*. One study in the US reported the isolation of *U. urealyticum* from the endometrium in 28% of recurrent aborters compared with 7% of a control group.[25] Unfortunately, no investigators have found bacteria to be present before pregnancy loss. The ideal study—isolating *U. urealyticum* from the endometrium and randomly assigning patients to a treatment or a placebo group—is not ethical. Perhaps randomly assigning patients with repeated abortion of unknown etiology to antibiotic treatment or a placebo group without detection of these pathogens and assessing the results may provide some answers.

Other etiologies

In a carefully performed case control study, it was shown that the incidence of spontaneous abortion and of repetitive abortion was not increased among diabetics.[26] Most maternal diseases, even if severe, may be associated with an increased risk of fetal demise or intrauterine growth retardation, but do not cause abortion. Severe congenital heart disease, especially when accompanied by cyanosis, has been associated with high rates of fetal wastage. Hypothyroidism and renal disease with hypertension have been incriminated as etiologic agents in abortion.[27,28]

Endometriosis has also been reported in association with abortions. In a study of women with endometriosis, 46% of all pregnancies and 63% of pregnancies occurring less than 2 years before treatment of endometriosis were reported to have terminated in abortion.[29] Some authors have reported an increased frequency of luteal phase defects in women with endometriosis.[30] Systemic lupus erythematosus (SLE) is associated with a significant increase in the rate of abortion, and recurrent reproductive failure may occur before other clinical manifestations of SLE are present.

The lupus anticoagulant, an immunoglobulin directed against the phospholipid portion of the prothrombin activator complex, has been identified in the plasma of a group of women with recurrent abortion. This globulin has been found in the plasma of women with and without SLE. This anticoagulant prolongs the activated partial thromboplastin time and tissue thromboplastin test, which are uncorrected by dilution with normal plasma. However, rather than having an increased bleeding tendency, these women often have thromboembolic phenomena. Treatment with prednisone, 40 to 60 mg/day, and aspirin, 40 to 80 mg/day, has resulted in term pregnancies.[31]

If nephrosis and hypertension are present in a patient with SLE, the prognosis for pregnancy is worse than it is for all pregnancies that occur during "active" stages of the disease. Increasing gravidity, independent of advancing maternal age, has also been associated with an increased risk of spontaneous abortion.[3]

Immunologic factors

More recently, a role for immunologic factors in recurrent abortion has been postulated. Protection from rejection by the maternal immune system is conferred on the fetus by a number of mechanisms. These include the elaboration of serum blocking antibodies that prevent the recognition of paternal antigens and the incompatibility of histocompatibility locus antigens (HLA) between a woman and her partner. These mechanisms might be related, as homozygosity of major HLA antigens between the mother and the fetus might prevent the maternal formation of blocking antibodies that probably coat fetal antigens—thus preventing rejection. A marked increase in abortion rate has been demonstrated among one population that was heavily inbred and thus presumably was homozygous for many genes.[32] Antisperm antibodies, as measured by the Franklin-Dukes test, have also been shown to be associated with an increased abortion rate.[33] This observation has been confirmed by many investigators.

In one study, a significantly increased rate of HLA antigen sharing at the A and B loci was found among couples with recurrent unexplained abortion compared with those whose abortions were due to a known etiology.[34] In another study, three women who had previously lost three pregnancies each, and who shared HLA antigens with their partners, were treated with multiple leukocyte transfusion during pregnancy; all delivered at term.[35] However, a study of 12 recurrent aborters found that only half shared one or more HLA antigens with their partners.[36] Without treatment, three of six pregnancies went to term, including a conception in one couple who shared two antigens and another couple who had three antigens in common. Thus more data are necessary to place the role of immunology in proper perspective for those with recurrent abortion. Leukocyte transfusions must still be regarded as experimental.

Management

The investigation and therapy of the patient with recurrent abortion depend on the history and examination (Table 32-6). Investigation should begin after only one second-trimester abortion. Of all abortions, 90% occur in the first trimester; the occurrence of a single second-trimester abortion should alert the clinician to suspect a uterine etiology. At the time of the ini-

Table 32-6
Indications and diagnostic procedures for recurrent aborters

Indication	Test or procedure
Recurrent abortion (all)	TSH
	Cervical/endometrial culture for *Ureaplasma urealyticum*
First-trimester abortions	Karyotype
	Late-luteal-phase endometrial biopsy
	Mid-luteal-phase serum progesterone level
	Hysteroscopy or hysterosalpingography
	LE prep, AN antibodies, HLA typing
Second-trimester abortions (one or more)	Hysteroscopy or hysterosalpingography
Abortion with hypomenorrhea	Hysteroscopy or hysterosalpingography
Abortion with family history of thyroid disease	TSH
Abortion with abnormal fetus or child	Karyotype

Table 32-7
Frequency of diagnostic evaluation with all results normal

Live births	Pregnancy losses			
	≥4 (%)	3 (%)	2 (%)	Total (%)
0	10/26 (38)	10/41 (24)	8/37 (22)	28/104 (27)
≥1	6/17 (35)	9/22 (41)	6/12 (50)	21/51 (41)
Total	16/43 (37)	19/63 (30)	14/49 (29)	49/155 (32)

From Harger JH, Archer DF, Marchese SG, et al: Etiology of recurrent pregnancy losses and outcome of subsequent pregnancies. Obstet Gynecol 62:574, 1983. Reprinted with permission from The American College of Obstetricians and Gynecologists.

tial consultation, a barrier method of contraception should be prescribed so that the evaluation may be completed with no risk of conception and so that endometrial histology may be assessed. The entire workup should be explained, and the couple advised that an etiology cannot be detected in as many as 40% of cases (Table 32-7).[37] Normal diagnostic evaluations are more common in couples with at least one live birth in addition to recurrent abortion.

Empirical treatment of women who have had repeated abortions is not indicated. The use of progestins has been associated with the prolonged retention of nonviable pregnancies resulting in missed abortion, a complication that is more difficult to treat than incomplete abortion and one that frequently leads to IUA. The use of

estrogens, particularly DES, has been associated with the later development of vaginal adenosis, clear-cell carcinoma, and uterine anomalies in female offspring and with urethral abnormalities in male offspring. The use of these regimens and other medications is based on little or no scientific data. Inaccurate theoretic estimates that placed the risk of recurrent abortion in excess of 70%[4] were used to support the efficacy of various treatment regimens.

The occurrence of a single second-trimester abortion, especially if a living infant was delivered or if the fetus was alive before the onset of labor, suggests that there is an abnormality of the uterine cavity. The uterine cavity should be carefully explored at the time of abortion or subsequent curettage. If this is not done, the diag-

Table 32-8
Abnormal laboratory tests associated with recurrent pregnancy losses

Test	Pregnancy losses			
	≥4 (%)	3 (%)	2 (%)	Total (%)
Karyotype	5/88 (5.7)	12/112 (10.7)	4/72 (5.6)	21/272 (7.7)
Hysterosalpingogram	8/30 (27)	11/45 (24)	11/37 (30)	30/112 (27)
Thyroid function	0/30	2/52 (3.9)	0/37	2/119 (1.7)
Antinuclear antibody	1/32 (3.1)	5/51 (10)	3/37 (8.1)	9/120 (7.5)
Cervical culture				
M. hominis	7/40 (18)	8/61 (13)	7/46 (15)	22/147 (15)
U. urealyticum	22/40 (55)	27/61 (44)	22/46 (48)	71/147 (48)

From Harger JH, Archer DF, Marchese SG, et al: Etiology of recurrent pregnancy losses and outcome of subsequent pregnancies. Obstet Gynecol 62:574, 1983. Reprinted with permission from The American College of Obstetricians and Gynecologists.

nostic evaluation should be initiated following the first spontaneous menstrual period. Investigation should be started after the first second-trimester loss, and any intrauterine defects that are detected should be corrected. There is no benefit in delaying the diagnostic evaluation or treatment until the patient has had recurrent second-trimester losses. Such patients should have hysteroscopy; or an HSG should be performed. It has been reported that among all studies performed for 155 couples with two or more abortions, the HSG was abnormal in 27% (Table 32-8).[37]

If submucous myomas are detected in a woman who has had one or more second-trimester abortions, myomectomy should be performed. In a recent review, a reduction in the abortion rate from 41% preoperatively to 19% after myomectomy was reported.[17] If a uterine septum is detected in a patient who has had one or more first- or second-trimester abortions, the septum should be incised under hysteroscopic control. If the history is consistent with cervical incompetence, a McDonald cerclage is the treatment of choice. Following metroplasty, myomectomy, or cerclage, term gestation rates of about 75% have been reported.[15,17,37]

Because most first-trimester abortions are due to chromosomal defects, a patient with early pregnancy wastage who has a submucous leiomyoma or a uterine septum should not undergo surgery, unless more than one loss has occurred and all other studies (Table 32-6) are normal. A karyotype with trypsin Giemsa banding should be obtained on both partners in all couples with two or more primary first-trimester abortions or with one or more abortions and the delivery of an abnormal fetus or child. Counseling by a geneticist should be provided for couples with a discovered chromosomal defect. A 32% term delivery rate of normal infants has been reported among couples with a genetic etiology for recurrent abortion (Table 32-9).[14] If the abnormality is present in the man, donor insemination may be considered.

If the patient has recurrent first-trimester abortion with no karyotype abnormality, a midluteal (day 20 to 22) serum progesterone level should be obtained, and an endometrial biopsy should be performed late in the luteal phase (day 26 to 27). The serum progesterone level should be at least 10 ng/mL. The endometrial tissue should be dated, and this must be correlated with the date of the BBT rise and the onset of the next menstrual period. If the endometrial histology is more than 2 days behind what is expected, the biopsy should be repeated during the next menstrual cycle. If the histologic dating

Table 32-9
Reproductive outcome in couples with recurrent abortion due to different etiologies

Etiology	Total couples	Successful couples	Success rate (%)
Genetic	25	8	32
Müllerian	15	9	60
Endocrine	23	21	91
Unknown	37	23	62
Combined endocrine and unknown	60	44	73

From Tho PT, Byrd JR, McDonough PG: Etiologies and subsequent reproductive performance of 100 couples with recurrent abortion. Fertil Steril 32:389, 1979. Reproduced with permission of the publisher, The American Fertility Society.

is still out of phase by more than 2 days, progesterone substitution therapy should be started and continued until 10 weeks of gestation. If only a low serum progesterone level is found, treatment with clomiphene citrate should be started. Following these regimens, term gestation rates of about 75% have been reported.[38]

In patients with hypomenorrhea and either first- or second-trimester recurrent abortion, IUA should be suspected. Even if the menstrual history is normal, adhesions may be present and should be considered as a possible etiology in the patient who has had prior intrauterine instrumentation. Hysteroscopy should be performed for both diagnosis and therapy. The outcome of pregnancies following hysteroscopic lysis of adhesions is excellent.[18]

In the absence of factors that suggest a specific etiology for recurrent spontaneous abortion, the cervix and the endometrium should be cultured for *U. urealyticum* (T-mycoplasma). If positive, treatment with doxycycline should be instituted. Both partners should receive 200 mg on the seventh day of the menstrual cycle and 100 mg daily for the next 9 days. Doxycycline therapy should be continued for three successive cycles, then cultures should be repeated to document a cure. In addition, SLE and antinuclear antibody testing should be performed and, if available, HLA typing. The significance of these studies is unclear today. Furthermore, a partial thromboplastin time should be performed, and if prolonged, attempts should be made to identify the lupus anticoagulant antibody. If present, treatment with aspirin and prednisone as outlined above is indicated.

Finally, serum thyroid-stimulating hormone should be measured to rule out subclinical hypothyroidism in all women with recurrent abortion. It is also appropriate for those who have had one or more abortions and have a family history of thyroid disease. Although glucose tolerance tests are commonly advised as part of the evaluation of recurrent aborters, neither gestational nor frank diabetics have an increased rate of repetitive early pregnancy loss.[26]

References

1. Williamson EM, Miller JF: A prospective study into early conceptual loss. *Clin Genet* 17:93, 1980

2. Warburton D, Fraser FC: Spontaneous abortion risks in man: Data from reproductive histories collected in a medical genetics unit. *Am J Hum Genet* 16:1, 1964

3. Naylor AF, Warburton D: Sequential analysis of spontaneous abortion. II. Collaborative study data show that gravidity determines a very substantial rise in risk. *Fertil Steril* 31:282, 1979

4. Malpas P: A study of abortion sequences. *J Obstet Gynaecol Brit Emp* 45:932, 1938

5. Stray-Pedersen B, Stray-Pedersen S: Etiologic factors and subsequent reproductive performance in 195 couples with a prior history of habitual abortion. *Am J Obstet Gynecol* 148:140, 1984

6. Carr DH: Cytogenetic aspects of induced and spontaneous abortions. *Clin Obstet Gynecol* 15:203, 1972

7. Boué J, Boué A, Lazar P: Retrospective and prospective epidemiological studies of 1500 karyotyped spontaneous abortions. *Teratology* 12:11, 1975

8. Hassold TJ: A cytogenetic study of repeated spontaneous abortions. *Am J Hum Genet* 32:723, 1980

9. Kajii T, Ferrier A: Cytogenetics of aborters and abortuses. *Am J Obstet Gynecol* 131:33, 1978

10. Rodrigo Guerrero V, Rojas OI: Spontaneous abortion and aging of human ova and spermatozoa. *N Engl J Med* 293:573, 1975

11. Buckton KE, O'Riordan ML, Ratcliff S, et al: A G-band study of chromosomes in live born infants. *Ann Hum Genet* 43:227, 1980

12. Tho SPT, Reindollar RH, McDonough PG: Recurrent abortion. In Sciarra JJ (ed): *Gynecology and Obstetrics*. Philadelphia, Harper & Row, 1984, pp 259-281

13. Heinonen OP, Slone D, Shapiro S: Hormones, hormone antagonists, and contraceptives. In *Birth Defects and Drugs in Pregnancy*. Littleton, Mass, Publishing Sciences Group, 1977, p 388

14. Tho PT, Byrd JR, McDonough PG: Etiologies and subsequent reproductive performance of 100 couples with recurrent abortion. *Fertil Steril* 32:389, 1979

15. Rock JA, Jones HW Jr: The clinical management of the double uterus. *Fertil Steril* 28:798, 1977

16. Kaufman RH, Adam E, Binder GL, et al: Upper genital tract changes and pregnancy outcome in offspring exposed in utero to diethylstilbestrol. *Am J Obstet Gynecol* 137:299, 1980

17. Buttram VC, Jr, Reiter RC: Uterine leiomyomata: etiology, symptomatology and management. *Fertil Steril* 36:433, 1981

18. March CM, Israel R: Gestational outcome following hysteroscopic lysis of adhesions. *Fertil Steril* 36:455, 1981

19. Harlap S, Shiono PH, Ramcharan S, et al: A prospective study of spontaneous fetal losses after induced abortions. *N Engl J Med* 301:677,1979

20. Harger JH: Comparison of success and morbidity in cervical cerclage procedures. *Obstet Gynecol* 56:543, 1980

21. Hull MGR, Savage PE, Bromham DR, et al: The value of a single serum progesterone measurement in the midluteal phase as a criterion of a potentially fertile cycle ("ovulation") derived from treated and untreated conception cycles. *Fertil Steril* 37:355, 1982

22. Noyes RW, Hertig AT, Rock J: Dating the endometrial biopsy. *Fertil Steril* 1:3, 1950

23. Hensleigh PA, Fainstat T: Corpus luteum dysfunction: Serum progesterone levels in diagnosis and assessment of therapy for recurrent and threatened abortion. *Fertil Steril* 32:396, 1979

24. Hernandez Horta JL, Gordillo Fernandez J, Soto de Leon B, et al: Direct evidence of luteal insufficiency in women with habitual abortion. *Obstet Gynecol* 49:705, 1977

25. Stray-Pedersen B, Eng J, Reikvam TM: Uterine T-mycoplasma colonization in reproductive failure. *Am J Obstet Gynecol* 130:307, 1978

26. Crane JP, Whal N: The role of maternal diabetes in repetitive spontaneous abortion. *Fertil Steril* 36:477, 1981

27. Winikoff D, Malinek M: The predictive value of thyroid "Test Profile" in habitual abortion. *Br J Obstet Gynaecol* 82:760, 1975

28. Felding C: Pregnancy following renal diseases. *Clin Obstet Gynecol* 11:579, 1968

29. Naples JD, Batt RE, Sadigh H: Spontaneous abortion rate in patients with endometriosis. *Obstet Gynecol* 57:509, 1981

30. Radawanska E, Dmowski WP: Luteal function in infertile women with endometriosis. *Infertility* 4:269, 1981

31. Lubbe WF, Graham C, Liggins MB: Lupus anticoagulant and pregnancy. *Am J Obstet Gynecol* 153:322, 1985

32. Ober C, Martin AO, Elias S, et al: Adverse effect of HLA compatibility on reproductive outcome. Presented at the 29th Annual Meeting of the Society for Gynecologic Investigation, Dallas, Texas, March 24-27, 1982

33. Jones WR: Immunological aspects of infertility. In Scott JS and Jones WR (eds): *Immunology of Reproduction.* New York, Academic Press, 1976, p 375

34. Beer AE, Quebbeman JF, Ayers JWT, et al: Major histocompatibility complex antigens, maternal and paternal immune responses, and chronic habitual abortions in humans. *Am J Obstet Gynecol* 141:987, 1981

35. Taylor C, Faulk WP: Prevention of recurrent abortion with leucocyte transfusions. *Lancet* 2:68, 1981

36. Caudle MR, Rote NS, Scott JR, et al: Histocompatibility in couples with recurrent spontaneous abortion and normal fertility. *Fertil Steril* 39:793, 1983

37. Harger JH, Archer DF, Marchese SG, et al: Etiology of recurrent pregnancy losses and outcome of subsequent pregnancies. *Obstet Gynecol* 62:574, 1983

38. Downs KA, Gibson M: Clomiphene citrate therapy for luteal phase defect. *Fertil Steril* 39:34, 1983

Suggested reading

Carr DH: Chromosomes and abortion. In Harris H, Hirschhorn K (eds): *Advances in Human Genetics,* vol 2. New York, Plenum Press, 1971, pp 201-257

Daling JR, Emanuel I: Induced abortion and subsequent outcome of pregnancy in a series of American women. *N Engl J Med* 297:1241, 1977

Gill TJ: Immunogenetics of spontaneous abortions in humans. An overview, *Transplantation* 35:1, 1983

Hertig AT, Rock J. Adams EC, et al: Thirty-four fertilized human ova, good, bad and indifferent, recovered from 210 women of known fertility. A study of biologic wastage in early human pregnancy. *Pediatrics* 23:202 (suppl), 1959

Jones HW, Jones GES: Double uterus as an etiological factor in repeated abortion: Indications for surgical repair. *Am J Obstet Gynecol* 65:325, 1953

McDonald IA: Incompetent cervix as a cause of recurrent abortion. *J Obstet Gynaecol Br Commonw* 70:105, 1963

Richardson JA, Dixon G: Effects of legal termination on subsequent pregnancy. *Br Med J* 1:1303, 1976

Tsenghi C, Metaxotou-Stavridaki C, Strataki-Benetou M, et al: Chromosome studies in couples with repeated spontaneous abortions. *Obstet Gynecol* 47:463, 1976

Upadhyaya M, Hibbard BM, Walker SM; The role of mycoplasmas in reproduction. *Fertil Steril* 39:814, 1983

Warburton D, Fraser FC: Genetic aspects of abortion. *Clin Obstet Gynecol* 2:22, 1959

Warburton D, Fraser FC: On the probability that a woman who has a spontaneous abortion will abort in subsequent pregnancies. *J Obstet Gynaecol Br Commonw* 68:784, 1961

Chapter 33

Luteal Phase Defects

Charles M. March, M.D.

Luteal phase defects are defined as abnormalities of corpus luteum function with insufficient progesterone production. The incidence, pathophysiology, and effects of certain abnormalities classified as luteal phase defects are impossible to document accurately. The defects are found in 1% to 3% of infertile couples, but are seen much more commonly in those with recurrent abortion. In one study, one-third of women with recurrent abortion had luteal phase defects.[1] Inadequate production of progesterone results in prevention of pregnancy or lack of adequate support to maintain the early embryo. Although abnormalities of uterine contractility, defects in the tubal transport of gametes or fertilized ova, and deficient secretions to nourish the conceptus are possible sequelae of reduced progesterone secretion, the most likely effect is an endometrium that is inadequately prepared to permit implantation or to maintain the recently implanted blastocyst.

In patients with luteal phase defects, either the amount and/or the duration of progesterone secretion may be deficient, while the production of estrogen usually remains normal. Normal corpus luteum function depends upon an intact hypothalamic-pituitary-ovarian axis. The ovulatory process begins with recruitment of the cohort of follicles that will develop during the subsequent menstrual cycle. The selection and emergence of the dominant follicle is followed by the preovulatory rise in estradiol that is needed to induce a luteinizing hormone (LH) surge. This surge results in ovulation and changes in ovarian steroidogenesis that produce formation and, finally, maintenance of the corpus luteum until either menses onset or placental steroidogenesis becomes adequate. Derangements at any point in this process may cause luteal phase abnormalities due to insufficient progesterone production.

A second etiology may be an inadequate effect of progesterone action on the endometrium, despite normal production. Classically, the diagnosis of luteal phase defects has depended on interpretation of a properly timed endometrial biopsy. The risk of interrupting a pregnancy by taking a single anterior fundal sample of endometrium in the late luteal phase is minimal. Serum progesterone levels alone cannot be used to establish the diagnosis, even if they are obtained daily throughout the luteal phase, unless the peak value is below 10 ng/mL. Many patients with histologically proven luteal phase defects have serum progesterone levels that overlap the values obtained in normal fertile women. Basal body temperature (BBT) graphs cannot be used for the diagnosis of these defects, because such abnormalities as a slow or irregular rise in BBT reported by some to reflect this diagnosis, are frequently found in normal fertile women.

Classification

Short luteal phase
The length of an ovulatory cycle is reduced in the patient with a short luteal phase. This de-

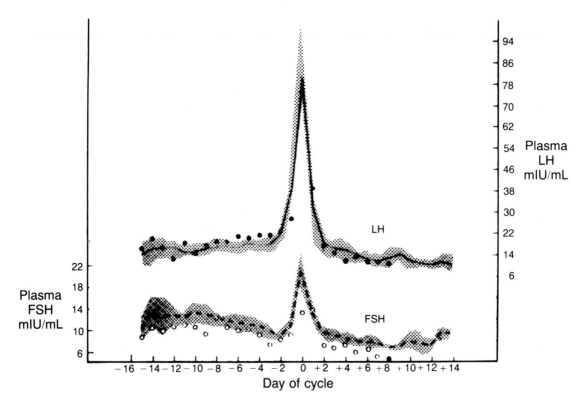

Figure 33-1
Plasma FSH and LH in normal and short luteal phase cycles. The normal means ± SE are shown as the solid lines and shaded areas, respectively. The means of plasma gonadotropin levels in short luteal phases are shown as superimposed circles.

Reproduced, with permission, from Strott CA, Cargille CM, Ross GT, et al: The short luteal phase. J Clin Endocrinol Metab 30:246, 1970. © 1970, The Endocrine Society.

crease is due entirely to shortening of the interval between the LH peak and the onset of menses to 10 days or less (Figure 33-1).[2] The defect can also be detected by a review of the BBT that shows a luteal phase temperature rise of 10 days or less. When the timing of the endometrial biopsy is correlated with the day of the LH peak or the BBT shift, the endometrial response is usually in phase. The pattern of follicle-stimulating hormone (FSH) and LH secretion throughout the cycle is normal; however, the mean FSH levels are below normal. The FSH/LH ratios in short luteal phase cycles are significantly re-

duced. The peak serum progesterone concentration is lower and occurs sooner after the LH surge than in a normal cycle. Some women who have a short luteal phase have a menstrual cycle of normal length, because the follicular phase is prolonged. This defect appears to occur most frequently in young women before complete maturation of the hypothalamic-pituitary-ovarian axis.

Because the corpus luteum can be maintained by endogenous human chorionic gonadotropin (hCG) produced by the recently implanted blastocyst, some have suggested that the short luteal phase has little or no effect upon fertility. However, recent ultrasound studies have demonstrated delayed follicular development together with irregular shape and reduced maximal diameter of the dominant follicle in women with short luteal phases.[3] These women also had no sonographic evidence of corpus luteum formation despite normal LH surges, biphasic BBTs, and adequate progesterone production. These data suggest that the inadequate FSH stimulation leads to poor folliculogenesis in women with short luteal phases.

Inadequate luteal phase

The inadequate luteal phase defect may be diagnosed in an ovulatory cycle of normal length in which the endometrial histologic pattern (using the criteria of Noyes and associates[4]) is more than 2 days behind the expected pattern for that day of the cycle. *This defect must be demonstrated in at least 2 cycles.* Dating of the endometrium must be correlated with both the apparent date of ovulation and the first day of the next menstrual period. The importance of documenting this defect in at least 2 cycles cannot be overemphasized. An out-of-phase endometrium has been reported to occur in a single cycle in as many as 20% of fertile women, but the incidence is only 3% or less if 2 cycles are examined.[1]

Another endometrial defect noted in women with luteal phase insufficiency is a discrepancy between the pattern of stroma and glands. Or the stroma may maintain an estrogenic pattern with persistent mitoses, abundant nuclear chromatin, and loose organization. In some studies, reduced levels of nuclear and cytosol estradiol (E_2) and progesterone receptors have been reported in women with luteal phase defects.[5] Many of those patients also have lower E_2 and progesterone levels, suggesting a central etiology. Recently, reduced follicular phase FSH levels and FSH/LH ratios have been reported in women with histologically proven luteal phase defects.[6] These data add further support to the concept of a central etiology.

Table 33-1
Number of cycles with normal and inadequate progesterone levels and endometrial histologic features

Progesterone	Adequate histologic features	Inadequate histologic features	Total
Adequate	10	9	19
Inadequate	12	11	23
Total	22	20	42

$X^2 = 0.079$; $P \doteq 0.779$.

From Shangold M, Berkeley A, Gray J: Both midluteal serum progesterone levels and late luteal endometrial histology should be assessed in all infertile women. Fertil Steril 40:627, 1983. Reproduced with permission of the publisher, The American Fertility Society.

Diagnosis

In some patients with luteal phase inadequacy, peak serum progesterone levels remain below 10 ng/mL. It has been shown in several reports that in conception cycles, maximum luteal phase progesterone levels are consistently above 10 ng/mL.[7] If the peak level is below 10 ng/mL repeatedly, the diagnosis of luteal insufficiency may be made with certainty and treatment instituted without performing an endometrial biopsy. Thus, as a screening test for luteal phase function, a serum progesterone level should be obtained before other studies.

The patient should record her BBT daily, and the serum progesterone level should be measured 1 week after the temperature rise. Many investigators have found a lack of correlation between endometrial histology and peak serum progesterone levels (Table 33-1).[8] Thus, an endometrial biopsy should also be performed and appropriate therapy should be based upon the results of both studies (Figure 33-2). The biopsy is obtained 12 days after the thermogenic shift (5 days after the progesterone level is measured), that is, 2 days before the expected onset of menses, on day 26 of a 28-day cycle. On this date, the endometrium reflects the estradiol and progesterone stimulation from almost the entire life span of the corpus luteum.

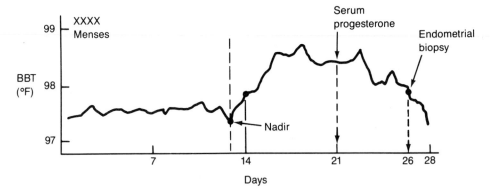

Figure 33-2
Method of evaluating luteal phase function in patients with biphasic BBT. Serum progesterone (P) level is measured 7 days after temperature shift, and an endometrial biopsy is obtained 5 days after the progesterone level.

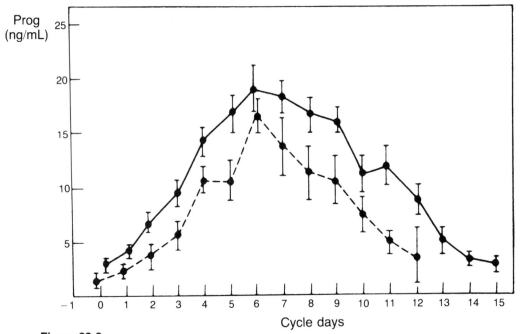

Figure 33-3
Mean progesterone levels in 28 cycles with normal corpus luteum function (solid line) and in 10 patients with luteal defects (broken line). Progesterone decline starts on the sixth luteal day in the defective cycles, whereas it is observed on the ninth luteal day in the normal cycles. The difference between the areas under the two curves is significant ($P < 0.001$).

From Jones GS, Aksel S, Wentz AC: Serum progesterone values in the luteal phase defects. Effect of chorionic gonadotropin. Obstet Gynecol 44:26, 1974. Reprinted with permission from The American College of Obstetricians and Gynecologists.

Abnormal BBT charts cannot be used to establish the diagnosis of luteal phase inadequacy, because the BBT does not reflect a specific serum progesterone level. A maximal increase in BBT may occur with as little as 3 ng/mL of progesterone in serum.[9] However, neither random nor multiple luteal phase progesterone assays can be used to establish the diagnosis, unless, as mentioned above, the peak concentration is consistently less than 10 ng/mL. Mean daily progesterone values in 10 patients with histologically proven luteal phase defects and 28 patients with normal luteal function are shown in Figure 33-3.[10] Although the areas under the curves are significantly different, it is not always possible to establish the diagnosis by measurement of individual or multiple progesterone levels in a given patient.

Etiology

Hypothalamic-pituitary defects

Four types of hypothalamic-pituitary defects may lead to luteal insufficiency:

1. Inadequate or asynchronous FSH stimulation during the preceding luteal phase and/or the subsequent follicular phase. diZerega and co-workers treated normally menstruating monkeys with charcoal-extracted porcine follicular fluid (pFF) on days 1 through 5 of the cycle.[11] This substance selectively suppresses FSH levels and maintains LH levels. The midcycle LH/FSH surge was delayed significantly when pFF was also administered on days 9 to 11. FSH and estradiol levels also fell significantly, as did luteal phase progesterone levels (Figure 33-4).[11]
2. Asynchronous or inadequate FSH and/or LH surges. Aksel has demonstrated an absent FSH surge at midcycle in women with short luteal phases (Figure 33-5).[1]
3. Inadequate tonic luteal phase LH stimulation. This is probably a theoretical etiology

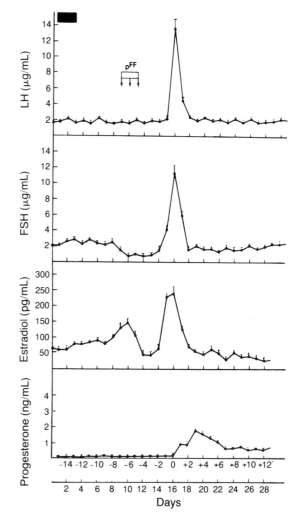

Figure 33-4

Composite patterns of LH, FSH, estradiol, and progesterone from the sera of three monkeys treated with charcoal-extracted pFF (5 to 10 mL, IV, for 3 days) beginning on the day after serum estradiol levels first exceeded 100 pg/mL. The decreases in serum FSH and estradiol levels concomitant with pFF therapy were significant. Although ovulation apparently occurred, as manifested by the subsequent elevation in serum levels, luteal phase progesterone levels were clearly below those of normal ovulatory cycles. The bar indicates menses.

Reproduced, with permission, from diZerega GS, Turner CK, Stouffer RL, et al: Suppression of follicle-stimulating hormone-dependent folliculogenesis during the primate ovarian cycle. J Clin Endocrinol Metab 52:451, 1981. © 1981, The Endocrine Society.

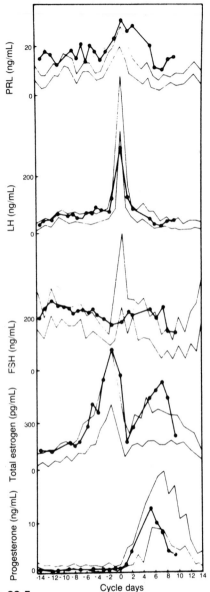

Figure 33-5
PRL, LH, FSH, total estrogen, and progesterone
concentrations in a cycle of a woman studied by Aksel,
plotted against normal range in the background
(mean ± 1 SD).

*From Aksel S: Sporadic and recurrent luteal phase defects in cyclic
women: Comparison with normal cycles. Fertil Steril 33:372, 1980.
Reproduced with permission of the publisher, The American Fertility
Society.*

only. Many patients without functioning pituitary glands will have normal luteal phases
following ovulation induction with human
menopausal gonadotropins (hMG) and hCG,
even if additional hCG is not given to support
the luteal phase.

4. Hyperprolactinemia. Elevated prolactin concentrations may interfere with the release of
gonadotropins and gonadotropin-releasing
hormone. In vitro studies have shown that
progesterone synthesis by the corpus luteum
is reduced by high levels of prolactin.[12] This
latter mechanism is not clinically significant
in all hyperprolactinemic women, because
many conceive after treatment with either
clomiphene or hMG/hCG while serum prolactin levels remain elevated.

Ovarian defects

Two ovarian defects may result in luteal insufficiency. The first is deficient response to gonadotropins with inadequate follicular development
or premature atresia of follicles. Elevated local
levels of androgens have been shown to retard
follicular development.[13] Poor corpus luteum
function with inadequate progesterone production may be a second cause. This etiology may be
the result of defective or inadequate numbers of
ovarian LH receptors. The failure to develop
sufficient numbers of LH receptors may be secondary to inadequate FSH stimulation of the
granulosa cells. This stimulation is necessary to
induce functional LH receptors.

Endometrial defects

Although luteal insufficiency is of central or
ovarian origin, a similar histologic pattern may
be seen in the patient whose endometrium responds inadequately to a normal hormonal milieu. The inadequate response may not occur
uniformly throughout the endometrium or may
be manifested by asynchronous development of
the endometrial glands and stroma. The cause is
probably a defect in endometrial receptors. One

Infertility

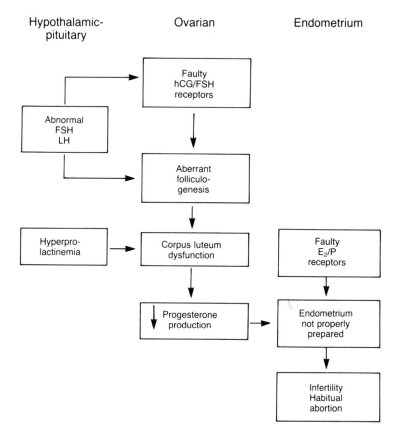

Figure 33-6
Pathophysiology of luteal phase defects.

such patient has been reported by Keller and co-workers.[14] The pathophysiology of these different defects is shown in Figure 33-6.

Therapy

Five types of treatment have been recommended for patients with an inadequate luteal phase: progesterone, hCG, clomiphene citrate, hMG, and bromocriptine. The ideal approach to therapy depends on identifying the specific etiology and planning specific treatment.

Progesterone

One 25-mg suppository* is inserted into the vagina or rectum twice a day, or 12.5 mg progesterone in oil is given IM daily beginning with the day of the BBT rise and continuing until menses onset (Figure 33-7). Accurate BBT recording is essential if this treatment is to be effective. Treatment cannot be started before the tem-

---

*Progesterone suppositories are not commercially available and must be made by a pharmacist. Suppositories with a concentration of 25 mg each are made using this formula: progesterone powder, 25 mg per suppository, in a water-soluble base of polyethylene glycol 400, USP, 60%, and polyethylene glycol 6000, USP, 40%. A rectal suppository mold is used.

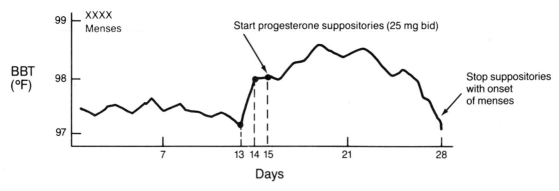

Figure 33-7
Use of BBT record to initiate progesterone replacement therapy.

perature rise, because premature therapy may block ovulation or inhibit cervical mucus production. Treatment begun after a missed menses is inadequate, because the nidation site has not been prepared properly. Therapy must be given with progesterone, not synthetic progestins, because the synthetic drugs may be luteolytic and do not produce normal endometrial histology. If conception occurs, as documented by a sensitive hCG assay, treatment should be continued for 8 weeks—that is, 10 weeks from the last menstrual period. Approximately 2 weeks before this time, the luteoplacental shift in steroidogenesis has occurred, and placental production of progesterone is sufficient to maintain the pregnancy.

Figure 33-8[10] represents the BBT and levels of estrone (E_1), estradiol (E_2), and progesterone in a control and a treatment cycle in a patient with an inadequate luteal phase. One disadvantage of progesterone therapy is that it maintains an elevated BBT and delays menses. Thus, both patient and physician may believe that a conception has occurred. If menses are delayed more than 6 days (20 days of elevated BBT), a sensitive serum pregnancy test should be obtained (Figure 33-9). It is mandatory to document that the defect has been corrected by repeating the endometrial biopsy. If the lag in the

histologic pattern persists and if suppository therapy has been used, the daily dose of progesterone should be doubled or treatment with IM progesterone in oil prescribed. Of patients with luteal insufficiency treated with progesterone suppositories, 70% will conceive and three-fourths of those pregnancies will be delivered at term.[15]

Human chorionic gonadotropin
A dose of 2,500 to 5,000 IU is given IM every other day, beginning the day after the BBT rise and continuing until menses begin, or, if conception has occurred, until the beginning of the second trimester. Figure 33-10[10] diagrams progesterone levels in a control and treatment cycle. This method has been reported to be less successful than progesterone substitution in reversing the defect.[10] Although hCG may prolong corpus luteum function and increase steroidogenesis, it will not correct the defect in patients with inadequate ovarian LH receptors or those with poor follicular development. If this method of treatment is used, qualitative serum pregnancy tests cannot be used to document pregnancy. Quantitative tests that demonstrate serial increases consistent with a normal intrauterine gestation must be used instead. Because of these factors, hCG therapy is not recommended.

Clomiphene citrate

Some authors have recommended this drug be used as therapy for the inadequate luteal phase; others have incriminated it as inducing ovulatory cycles with luteal phase defects. Those who support the latter position may merely be observing a partial correction of the anovulatory state that, in turn, may be rectified by increasing the dose of clomiphene. Clomiphene citrate is the treatment of choice for patients with a short luteal phase. These patients have reduced levels of FSH in the early follicular phase and, thus, inadequate follicular development. Clomiphene citrate, 50 or 100 mg per day on days 2 through 6 of the cycle, is usually sufficient to cause augmented FSH release. (Usually clomiphene is administered on days 5 through 9.) Adequate early follicular phase FSH, together with E_2, is necessary to achieve maximal granulosa cell biosynthesis. Without the latter, folliculogenesis is abnormal and abnormal corpus luteum function is guaranteed. An overall pregnancy rate of 41% has been reported with the use of clomiphene in 41 patients with long-standing infertility and luteal phase defects.[16] Similar results were reported among 69 infertile women whose midluteal serum progesterone levels were below 15 ng/mL before clomiphene therapy.[17]

Human menopausal gonadotropins

Small doses of gonadotropins have been reported to correct luteal phase inadequacy in some patients. The mechanism is presumably the induction of better follicular recruitment and early development. Treatment should be begun with 1 or 2 ampules per day, starting on day 2 of the cycle. These patients should be monitored as are anovulatory patients treated with hMG/hCG. Too few data are available to know the true value of hMG in the therapy of luteal phase defects. This modality should be reserved for patients who fail to respond to other drugs or who develop drug-related complications.

Bromocriptine

Administration of bromocriptine (Parlodel) results in the return of serum prolactin levels to normal in most patients who have hyperprolactinemia. Elevated serum prolactin levels have been reported in some patients with luteal phase defects. Preliminary studies have indicated that bromocriptine therapy results in normalization of the menstrual cycles of patients with luteal phase defects. In one published study, 18 wom-

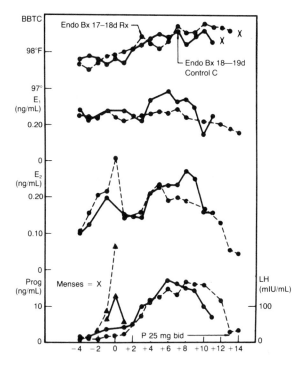

Figure 33-8
Basal body temperature chart (BBTC), estrone (E_1), estradiol (E_2), and progesterone (Prog) levels of a patient during a control cycle (solid line) and treatment cycle (broken line). Endometrial biopsy (Endo Bx) in the control cycle was 5 days out of phase. This defect was adequately corrected with progesterone suppositories (25 mg twice a day) used from the third postovulatory day.

From Jones GS, Aksel S, Wentz AC: Serum progesterone values in the luteal phase defects. Effect of chorionic gonadotropin. Obstet Gynecol 44:26, 1974. Reprinted with permission from The American College of Obstetricians and Gynecologists.

en with hyperprolactinemia and short luteal phases were treated with bromocriptine.[18] Suppression of prolactin values to normal resulted in a slight increase in follicular phase FSH levels and a significant increase in midcycle FSH and LH levels. Luteal phase estradiol, 17-hydroxyprogesterone, and progesterone levels also rose significantly compared with pretreatment levels. Only those women with hyperprolactinemia should receive bromocriptine.

Adequate correction of the defect can be proven only by histologic examination of the endometrium during the treatment cycle. Successful pregnancies may be achieved in up to 75% of

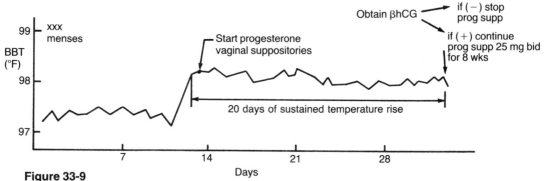

Figure 33-9
Method of treating luteal phase defects with progesterone replacement. The β-hCG level is obtained if temperature remains elevated for 20 days.

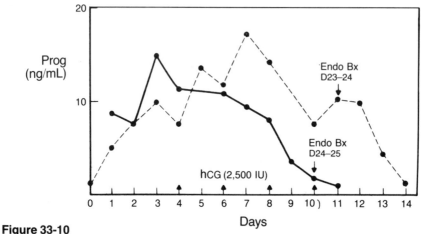

Figure 33-10
Progesterone levels in control (solid line) and treatment (broken line) cycles of a patient. hCG (2,500 IU) was given on the 4th, 6th, 8th, and 10th postovulatory days. There is a 47% increase in the area covered by the progesterone curve in the treatment cycle compared with the control. The luteal phase is prolonged 2 days and the endometrial biopsy (Endo Bx), which had been 2 days behind, has come into phase.

From Jones GS, Aksel S, Wentz AC: Serum progesterone values in the luteal phase defects. Effect of chorionic gonadotropin. Obstet Gynecol 44:26, 1974. Reprinted with permission from The American College of Obstetricians and Gynecologists.

women who have only this cause for their reproductive failure.[19]

Treatment selection

Luteal phase defects may be caused by hypothalamic, pituitary, ovarian, or endometrial abnormalities. Before treatment can be planned, a complete investigation, including measurement of serum progesterone and prolactin levels and endometrial biopsy, is needed. Moreover, after beginning therapy, the response can be considered adequate only if all chemical or histologic abnormalities have been corrected. Methods of selecting the proper drug and monitoring the response are outlined in Table 33-2. For those with peak serum progesterone levels below 10 ng/mL, the initial treatment should be with clomiphene citrate, irrespective of endometrial histology. Hyperprolactinemic patients should be given bromocriptine (those with minimal elevations could also receive clomiphene). Progesterone supplementation is reserved for those who have normal serum prolactin and progesterone levels but an out-of-phase endometrium. Follow-up must include documenting that the defect(s) is (are) corrected. Combination therapy may be necessary in some patients. Treatment with hMG should be reserved for those whose defect is not corrected by clomiphene, whether or not other drugs are also used. This approach is most likely to result in a term pregnancy.

References

1. Aksel S: Sporadic and recurrent luteal phase defects in cyclic women: Comparison with normal cycles. *Fertil Steril* 33:372, 1980
2. Strott CA, Cargille CM, Ross GT, et al: The short luteal phase. *J Clin Endocrinol Metab* 30:246, 1970

Table 33-2
Selection of treatment for a patient with a luteal phase defect

Abnormality	Treatment	Follow-up
Low Prog Normal PRL Endometrium in phase	Clomiphene citrate	Prog
Low Prog Normal PRL Retarded endometrium	Clomiphene citrate	Prog EMB
Low Prog ↑PRL Endometrium in phase	Bromocriptine	PRL Prog
Low Prog ↑PRL Retarded endometrium	Bromocriptine	PRL Prog EMB
Retarded endometrium ↑PRL Normal Prog	Bromocriptine	PRL EMB
Retarded endometrium Normal Prog Normal PRL	Progesterone	EMB

Low Prog, peak serum progesterone level below 10 ng/mL; "retarded," more than 2 days out of phase; EMB, endometrial biopsy. Follow-up peak serum progesterone levels should be ≥15 ng/mL. Combination therapy may be necessary in some patients.

3. Geisthovel F, Skubsch U, Zabel G, et al: Ultrasonographic and hormonal studies in physiologic and insufficient menstrual cycles. *Fertil Steril* 39:277, 1983

4. Noyes RW, Hertig AT, Rock J: Dating the endometrial biopsy. *Fertil Steril* 1:3, 1950

5. Gautray JP, de Brux J, Tajchner G, et al: Clinical investigation of the menstrual cycle. III. Clinical, endometrial, and endocrine aspects of luteal defect. *Fertil Steril* 35:296, 1981

6. Cook CL, Rao CV, Yussman MA: Plasma gonadotropin and sex steroid hormone levels during early, midfollicular, and midluteal phases of women with luteal phase defects. *Fertil Steril* 40:45, 1983

7. Hull MGR, Savage PE, Bromham DR, et al: The value of a single serum progesterone measurement in the mid-luteal phase as a criterion of a potentially fertile cycle ("ovulation") derived from treated and untreated conception cycles. *Fertil Steril* 37:355, 1982

8. Shangold M, Berkeley A, Gray J: Both midluteal serum progesterone levels and late luteal endometrial histology should be assessed in all infertile women. *Fertil Steril* 40:627, 1983

9. Israel R, Mishell DR Jr, Stone SC, et al: Single luteal phase progesterone assay as an indicator of ovulation. *Am J Obstet Gynecol* 112:1043, 1972

10. Jones GS, Aksel S, Wentz AC: Serum progesterone values in the luteal phase defects. Effect of chorionic gonadotropin. *Obstet Gynecol* 44:26, 1974

11. diZerega GS, Turner CK, Stouffer RL, et al: Suppression of follicle-stimulating hormone-dependent folliculogenesis during the primate ovarian cycle. *J Clin Endocrinol Metab* 52:451, 1981

12. McNatty KP, Sawyers RS, McNeilly AS: A possible role for prolactin in control of steroid secretion by the human Graafian follicles. *Nature* 250:653, 1974

13. Lobo RA, Wellington LP, Goebelsmann U: Serum levels of DHEA-S in gynecologic-endocrinopathy and infertility. *Obstet Gynecol* 57:607, 1981

14. Keller D, Wiest W, Askin F, et al: Pseudocorpus luteum insufficiency: A local defect of progesterone action on endometrial stroma. *J Clin Endocrinol Metab* 48:127, 1979

15. Rosenberg SM, Luciano AA, Riddick DH: The luteal phase defect: The relative frequency of, and encouraging response to, treatment with vaginal progesterone. *Fertil Steril* 34:17, 1980

16. Downs KA, Gibson M: Clomiphene citrate therapy for luteal phase defect. *Fertil Steril* 39:34, 1983

17. Hammond MG, Talbert LM: Clomiphene citrate in the management of infertile women with low luteal phase progesterone levels. *Am J Obstet Gynecol* 59:275, 1982

18. Muhlenstedt D, Bohnet HG, Hanker JP, et al: Short luteal phase and prolactin. *Int J Fertil* 23:213, 1978

19. Andersen AN, Larsen JF, Eskildsen PC, et al: Treatment of hyperprolactinemic luteal insufficiency with bromocriptine. *Acta Obstet Gynecol Scand* 58:379, 1979

Suggested reading

Niswender GD, Menon RMJ, Jaffe RB: Regulation of the corpus luteum during the menstrual cycle and early pregnancy. *Fertil Steril* 23:432, 1972

Rosenfeld DL, Chudow S, Bronson RA: Diagnosis of luteal phase inadequacy. *Obstet Gynecol* 56:193, 1980

Rosenfeld DL, Garcia ER: Comparison of endometrial histology with simultaneous plasma progesterone determination in infertile women. *Fertil Steril* 28:443, 1977

Tredway DR, Mishell DR, Jr, Moyer DL: Correlation of endometrial dating with the luteinizing hormone peak. *Am J Obstet Gynecol* 117:1030, 1973

Chapter 34

Human In Vitro Fertilization

State of the Art

Richard P. Marrs, M.D.
Joyce M. Vargyas, M.D.

In vitro techniques of mammalian reproduction have been studied for many years in various animal species. Many attempts have been undertaken to extrapolate these techniques to the human. However, because of species differences, full, detailed knowledge of human reproduction is still lacking. Direct visualization of extracorporeal gamete fertilization, embryo development, and early gestation in animals ultimately led to application of in vitro fertilization (IVF) techniques to human reproduction. After many years of trials with IVF procedures, Edwards and Steptoe, in 1978, reported the first human birth resulting from IVF.[1] Since then, the human IVF and embryo replacement (ER) process has been modified, refined, and improved. Today, IVF-ER not only provides the infertile couple with the hope of producing a child of their own but also provides the investigator with a "physiologic window" through which a dynamic view of human reproduction can be studied and understood.

Initially, IVF-ER was designed to provide a reproductive mechanism for women who had no fallopian tube function. It was merely a way to bypass the tube. However, with increased success and knowledge, other forms of infertility are now treated by this process.

Currently, the indications for IVF-ER include not only tubal disease but also male factor infertility as well as idiopathic or unexplained infertility. Although IVF-ER has not replaced conventional forms of therapy for infertility, this procedure should be used when conventional methods have not resulted in a successful outcome. It is expected that in the future, as pregnancy success increases, IVF-ER will replace many of the conventional surgical therapies that attempt to treat female reproductive failure.

Technical aspects of IVF-ER

The evolution of human extracorporeal fertilization has been rapid. Initially, Edwards and Steptoe used stimulated ovarian cycles, but this method was discontinued when no pregnancies resulted.[2] As the use of oocyte recovery during a spontaneous ovulatory cycle resulted in the first human IVF pregnancy in 1978, investigators in the field used the spontaneously cycling female. Oocyte recovery was timed by ultrasound and measurement of estradiol (E_2) and luteinizing hormone (LH). Daily measurements of E_2 were performed to determine the time of the preovulatory E_2 peak. As the dominant follicle approached 18 mm in diameter, urinary LH measurements were performed every 3 to 4 hours to identify the beginning of the preovulatory LH increase. Laparoscopy for oocyte collection was performed 26 to 28 hours from the start of the LH increase. In 1981, Trounson and associates reported the use of clomiphene citrate, 150 mg on cycle days 5 through 9, in an effort to recover more than one ovum. They established pregnancies from multiple embryo transfer in nine of 103 treatment cycles.[3] Thereafter, IVF teams worldwide began using some form of ovarian stimulation before oocyte recovery.

Ovarian stimulation methods

Various regimens of ovarian stimulation have been used to induce multiple follicle development for the purpose of IVF. In primates, exogenous ovarian stimulation needs to occur early in the cycle if multiple dominant follicles are to be generated.[4]

In the past 2 years, we have studied various regimens of ovarian stimulation. Initially clomiphene citrate, 150 mg daily for 5 days, was the primary method. Since studies in the primate indicated that dominant follicle selection occurred early in the cycle, an initial study was performed giving clomiphene citrate at various times in the cycle to determine if multiple follicle development could be more successful if initiated early.[5]

Clomiphene, 150 mg/day, was given beginning on day 3, 4, 5, or 7 of the menstrual cycle. In this group of patients, the number of follicles generated, oocytes collected and fertilized, and embryos transferred per cycle were found to be optimal when clomiphene was begun on day 5. Significant decreases in the number of eggs collected and fertilized and the number of embryos transferred occurred when clomiphene was begun on days 3, 4, and 7 (Figures 34-1 and 34-2). These data diverged somewhat from what was expected from studies in the primate model.

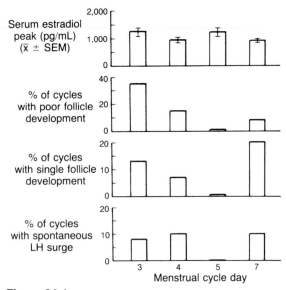

Figure 34-1
Effect of time of initiation of clomiphene citrate on multiple follicle development.

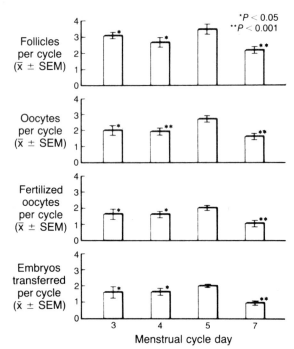

Figure 34-2
Laparoscopic outcome after clomiphene citrate.

When the day 3 clomiphene group was looked at more closely, however, it appeared—using ultrasound scanning—that early in the treatment cycle multiple follicles developed. But the majority of these follicles did not continue to develop.

Therefore, we performed a second study using combinations of clomiphene citrate and human menopausal gonadotropin (hMG) to determine whether a prolonged stimulation cycle would result in larger numbers of multiple follicles.[6] In this study, the patients received either clomiphene citrate, 150 mg on days 3 through 7 (group 1), or clomiphene citrate, 150 mg on days 3 through 7, followed by 2 ampules of hMG dai-

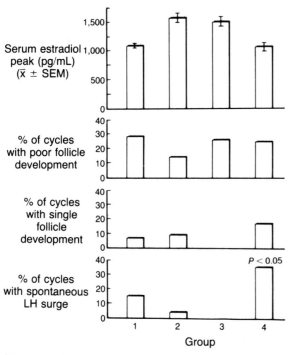

Figure 34-3
Follicle and oocyte production after clomiphene citrate and hMG stimulation.

From Vargyas JM, Morente C, Shangold G, et al: The effect of different methods of ovarian stimulation for human in vitro fertilization and embryo transfer. Fertil Steril 42:745, 1984. Reproduced with permission of the publisher, The American Fertility Society.

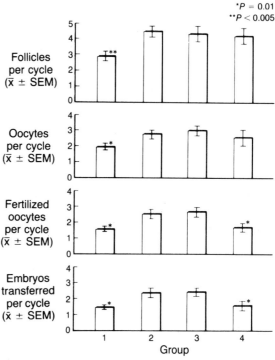

Figure 34-4
Laparoscopic outcome of clomiphene citrate and hMG stimulation.

From Vargyas JM, Morente C, Shangold G, et al: The effect of different methods of ovarian stimulation for human in vitro fertilization and embryo transfer. Fertil Steril 42:745, 1984. Reproduced with permission of the publisher, The American Fertility Society.

ly thereafter until two follicles 18 mm or larger were visualized by ultrasound, at which time hMG was discontinued (group 2). Patients in group 3 received clomiphene citrate, 150 mg on days 3 through 7, combined with hMG, 2 ampules/day administered on days 3, 5, and 7 and daily thereafter until two follicles reached 18 mm. Group 4 patients received hMG alone, 2 ampules daily beginning on day 3 of the cycle, and continuing until two follicles 18 mm or larger were visualized.

In all groups, E_2 concentrations were measured daily until a plateau occurred, at which time human chorionic gonadotropin (hCG),

4,000 IU, was administered. The E_2 plateau was defined as a failure of the E_2 to increase at the same increment as the previous day. Results of this study revealed that the patients receiving clomiphene citrate followed by hMG or clomiphene citrate combined with hMG had optimal numbers of mature follicles, oocyte recovery rates, fertilization rates, and embryo transfer rates (Figures 34-3 and 34-4). The group receiving hMG stimulation alone had a lower oocyte recovery rate and lower embryo transfer rate. This was thought to be due to overstimulation of the follicles, which caused difficulty in retrieving eggs because of the thick, luteinized follicular contents. Moreover, the immature oocytes recovered with this stimulation technique were difficult to fertilize in vitro. Interestingly, there was a significant increase in spontaneous endogenous LH release before administration of hCG in this group of hMG-stimulated patients.

Since 1983, we have used primarily two regimens of ovarian stimulation. Clomiphene citrate, 150 mg on days 3 through 7, followed by hMG, 2 ampules per day, was the regimen used in approximately half the patients treated. The hMG was administered daily until two follicles 18 mm or larger were visualized. Beginning on day 8 of the cycle, E_2 measurements were performed daily until a plateau occurred; then hCG was administered. The rest of the patients received a modified hMG treatment: Three ampules of hMG were given daily, beginning on day 3 of the cycle and continuing until two follicles 15 mm or larger were visualized. Thereafter, when the E_2 plateau occurred, hCG was administered. In both groups, laparoscopy was performed 36 hours after the E_2 plateau.

In the group receiving only hMG stimulation, an average of 5.5 ± 0.4 oocytes were recovered per laparoscopy, of which 3.6 ± 0.4 were fertilized and ultimately 2.8 ± 0.2 embryos were transferred per cycle. In the group receiving clomiphene followed by hMG, an average of 3.3 ± 0.2 oocytes were retrieved per follicle aspiration cycle, 2.5 ± 0.2 were fertilized, and 2.3 ± 0.2 embryos were transferred. There was no significant difference between these results. In comparison with these types of stimulation, patients receiving only clomiphene, 150 mg, had fewer oocytes recovered and fertilized and embryos transferred (2.7 ± 0.3, 2.0 ± 0.1, and 2.0 ± 0.1, respectively), which was significantly less than resulted from the combination treatment or from hMG alone (Table 34-1).

Currently, a modification of the combination therapy is being utilized. Clomiphene citrate, 100 mg/day, is given on days 3 through 7 concurrently with 1 ampule/day of hMG. The hMG is continued at that dosage until two follicles 18 mm or larger are visualized on ultrasound. hCG is administered when the E_2 plateau occurs. Thus far, with this regimen, an average of 4.3 ± 0.3 oocytes have been collected per cycle by laparoscopy, of which 3.7 ± 0.3 have been fertilized and 3.1 ± 0.3 embryos transferred per cycle. Pregnancy rates with the various stimula-

Table 34-1
Comparison of stimulation regimens

Type	No. of oocytes	No. of fertilizations	No. of transfers
Clomiphene citrate, 150 mg	2.7 ± 0.3	2.0 ± 0.1	2.0 ± 0.1
Clomiphene citrate, 150 mg, + hMG	3.3 ± 0.2	2.5 ± 0.2	2.3 ± 0.2
hMG	5.5 ± 0.4	3.6 ± 0.4	2.8 ± 0.2
Clomiphene citrate, 100 mg, + hMG	4.3 ± 0.3	3.7 ± 0.3	3.1 ± 0.3

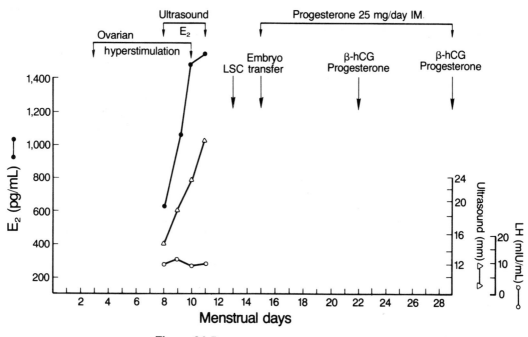

Figure 34-5
Diagram of IVF protocol. LSC = laparoscopy.

tion methods have shown an increasing trend. With clomiphene citrate alone, pregnancy occurred in 12% of laparoscopy cycles. The combination of clomiphene citrate followed by hMG resulted in a 21% rate of pregnancy initiation per laparoscopy, whereas 20% of hMG-stimulated cycles that went to laparoscopy resulted in pregnancy. The combination of clomiphene citrate and menotropins has, to date, produced a pregnancy rate of 26% per laparoscopy.

Monitoring ovarian response

When using the stimulated ovarian cycle, judgment of optimal response is of prime importance. Measurement of follicle size by real-time ultrasound correlates well with hormonal determinations of follicular growth in spontaneous and stimulated ovarian cycles.[7,8] To determine precise timing of oocyte/follicle maturation for

IVF-ER, it is best to use a combination of ovarian ultrasound scanning and daily measurement of LH and peripheral E_2 (Figure 34-5).

Initially, ultrasound is used to determine the number and size of follicles developing after stimulation (Figure 34-6). This is correlated with secretion of E_2. In clomiphene citrate/hMG combination regimens, hMG is continued after the initial 5 days of clomiphene administration until two or more follicles are at least 18 mm in diameter. After the discontinuation of hMG, an ovulatory dose of hCG, 4,000 IU, is given when the levels of E_2 plateau. Laparoscopic aspiration is performed precisely 36 hours later. The same basic approach is followed for hMG-induced follicular growth, except that the agent is discontinued when two or more follicles reach or exceed a diameter of 15 mm. This method has produced an improvement in oocyte quality and collection,

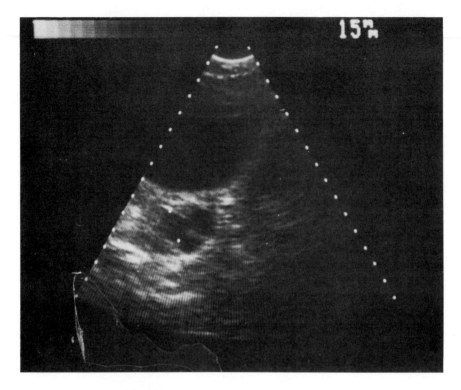

Figure 34-6
Ultrasound scan of ovarian response after stimulation.

since luteinization is not present, as was the case when hMG was administered until follicle size was ≥18 mm. With both regimens, LH levels are measured daily to ensure that endogenous LH release has not occurred before hCG administration, necessitating earlier oocyte recovery.

Oocyte recovery

From the initiation of human IVF procedures, the laparoscope has been the primary instrument for oocyte collection. In our program, we use an offset or operating laparoscope, because this allows the surgeon an extra operating channel when severe adhesions are encountered. A secondary puncture site is used suprapubically in the midline for placement of a grasping instrument, which stabilizes the ovaries during follicle aspiration. A third puncture site is placed midline for the small sleeve through which the needle aspirator is placed. We use the Cook Teflon-lined needle aspiration system (Figure 34-7). This needle system is connected to a constant suction source adjusted to 100 to 140 mm Hg of negative pressure. Under direct visualization, the aspirating needle is inserted into the follicle and, as the needle enters the follicle wall, suction is begun. The needle is removed after follicle collapse is visualized, then the needle is flushed with 0.5 mL of Hepes medium. With the use of this system and no follicle washing or flushing, oocytes are collected from approximately 80%

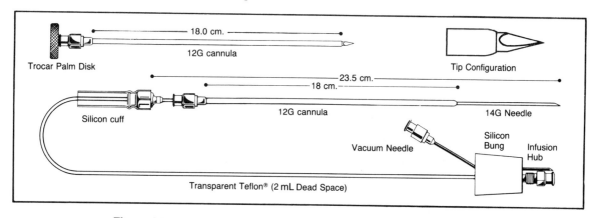

Figure 34-7
Diagram of Cook Teflon-lined aspiration system (Cook, Inc., Melbourne, Australia).

of follicles aspirated (Table 34-2).[9]

If an oocyte is not obtained in the follicle aspirate, a heparinized Hepes solution can be instilled through the aspiration needle after reintroduction into the follicle, and the follicle can be rinsed. This may allow oocyte recovery from those follicles that did not yield an oocyte in the original aspirate.

Recently, a number of European centers have reported the use of ultrasound-directed aspiration. Utilizing an 18-gauge thin-walled needle and a real-time ultrasound transducer, the needle is placed transcutaneously through the bladder into the visualized follicles. The advantage of this technique is that it does not require general anesthesia. Moreover, it is best for patients with severe pelvic-abdominal adhesions, because the follicle is entered from the interface between the follicle wall and the bladder wall, making abdominal access unnecessary. So far, the rate of oocyte recovery per follicle is reported to range from 50% to 75%.[10,11] Complications such as hematuria or intraabdominal bleeding have been negligible. Even with multiple puncture sites through the bladder, no urinary tract damage or complications have been reported. If this oocyte recovery rate is confirmed by other centers, ultrasound-directed aspiration may replace laparoscopy for oocyte collection. This would reduce costs and allow the entire procedure to be performed in an outpatient setting.

Table 34-2
Results of laparoscopy (constant suction)

Patient group (No.)	No. of follicles	No. of oocytes	Mean follicle volume (mL)
Tubal disease (26)	78	62 (79%)	6.5 ± 0.04
Idiopathic infertility (8)	21	18 (86%)	6.7 ± 0.1
Male factor (2)	5	3 (60%)	7.0 ± 0.5

From Marrs RP, Vargyas JM, Gibbons WE et al: A modified technique of human in vitro fertilization and embryo transfer. Am J Obstet Gynecol 147:318, 1983.

Table 34-3
Preparation of culture medium

1. Stock solution
   a. Dissolve one package of powdered Ham's F-10 with glutamine in 250 mL of twice-distilled water
   b. Add penicillin G, 75 mg/L, and streptomycin, 50 mg/L
2. Culture medium
   a. Add 62.5 mL of stock solution to 187.5 mL of twice-distilled water (250-mL volume)
   b. Add calcium lactate, 61.3 mg; sodium bicarbonate, 420.1 mg; and potassium bicarbonate, 126.9 mg
   c. Adjust osmolarity to 280 mOsm
   d. Adjust pH to 7.3–7.4
   e. Filter medium through 0.22 μm filters and store refrigerated in sterile 17 × 100 snap-top tubes

Oocyte-embryo culture system

A rigidly controlled, strictly defined laboratory environment must be maintained for successful IVF and embryo growth. Over the years, various tissue culture media have been used for oocyte culture, but the most commonly used medium is Ham's F-10. Fresh Ham's medium is prepared every week as detailed in Table 34-3. Before use for culturing of human gametes, the medium is tested with mouse embryos to determine normal growth-promoting properties. Only medium that demonstrates a hatching rate of greater than 70% of mouse blastocysts after 96 hours of culture is used in the human culture system.

Ham's medium is supplemented with heat-inactivated (56°C for 30 minutes), Millipore-filtered patient serum that is collected immediately before hCG administration. The serum is added in 10% concentration to the insemination plates. After the first 18 to 24 hours of culture, the embryos are transferred to media containing 20% heat-inactivated, Millipore-filtered human serum for further growth.

Culture conditions are extremely important, and the culture environment must be rigidly controlled. Different centers use various containers for the culturing of oocytes. In a study done at our institution, oocyte fertilization rates were significantly increased when the culturing was carried out in organ culture plates rather than in tissue culture tubes[12] (Figure 34-8). The egg is placed in an atmosphere consisting of 90% nitrogen, 5% oxygen, and 5% carbon dioxide at 37°C and 100% humidity. Some centers use an

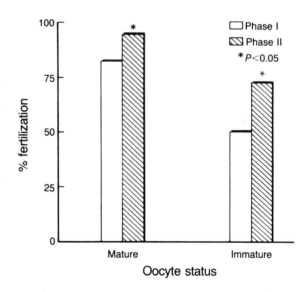

Figure 34-8
Fertilization rates in tube cultures (phase I, unfilled bars) and dish cultures (phase II, hatched bars) in mature and immature oocytes.

atmosphere of 5% carbon dioxide in air with good success.[13]

The determination of oocyte maturity at the time of recovery is as important as the culture environment. Fertilization rates have increased from 40% to as much as 80% to 90% since 1982, partly because of increased knowledge in identifying oocyte maturation. Immature oocytes are often recovered during stimulated cycles and must mature in culture medium before fertilization attempts. Immature oocytes either fail to be fertilized or undergo polyspermic fertilization. A morphologic grading system has been established.[12] With preincubation of immature oocytes (for as long as 36 hours) a higher fertilization rate is obtained.

The oocytes are identified in the follicular aspirate by viewing aliquots of the follicular fluid with a dissecting microscope set at 6× magnifi-

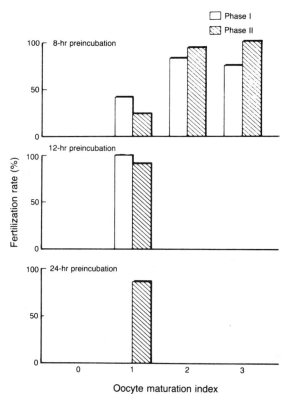

Figure 34-10
Fertilization success with variable preincubation times.

From Marrs RP, Saito H, Yee B, et al: Effect of variation of in vitro *culture techniques upon oocyte fertilization-embryo development in human* in vitro *procedures. Fertil Steril 41:519, 1984. Reproduced with permission of the publisher, The American Fertility Society.*

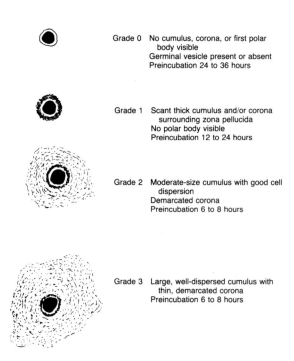

Figure 34-9
Oocyte grading system to judge morphologic maturation.

cation. Once identified, the oocyte can be inspected under higher magnification (40× to 400×) with an inverted-head, phase-contrast microscope to try to stage the maturity morphologically (Figure 34-9). Once the stage of maturity is determined, the oocyte is placed in an organ culture plate and incubated with Ham's F-10 medium containing 10% human serum for variable time periods before the sperm is added. With this variable preincubation schedule, an increased fertilization rate has been obtained with immature oocytes (Figure 34-10).[12]

Sperm preparation and insemination

In cases where the man has a normal semen analysis, a routine semen culture is done before initiating a treatment cycle. If bacterial growth is present in the sperm, antibiotic treatment with doxycycline, 100 mg twice a day, is instituted for 4 to 6 weeks before performing IVF.

If the semen profile is normal, a standard two-step washing procedure is performed. A 0.5-mL aliquot of fresh semen, obtained by masturbation, is mixed with 3 mL of Ham's F-10 medium and centrifuged at $300 \times g$ for 10 minutes. Then the supernatant is removed, and the sperm pellet is resuspended in 2 mL of Ham's F-10 medium and centrifuged at $300 \times g$ for 10 minutes. The supernatant is again removed, and the sperm pellet is resuspended in 1 mL of Ham's F-10 medium and incubated for 2 to 6 hours. Before spermatozoa are added to the oocyte culture dish, the supernatant is removed and a precise determination of sperm count and motility is performed on a 0.1-mL ali-quot of the sample. Thereafter, 25 million motile cells are added to each oocyte culture dish (Figure 34-11).

If IVF is being performed because of an abnormality in the semen analysis, screening is done with the hamster-egg penetration assay. Penetration of the hamster egg correlates fairly well with the IVF system. If penetration rates are below the normal fertile range (<15%), the ejaculate is treated in an attempt to improve spermatozoa quality.[14] The three primary methods for improving penetration ability are albumin gradient separation, "swim-up" separation, and Percoll gradient separation. These washing techniques are described in Figures 34-12, 34-13, and 34-14. The improvement in sperm penetrating ability seems to be greatest with Percoll separation (Table 34-4). If the rate of sperm penetration of zona-free hamster eggs improves with one of these methods, that method is used during the IVF treatment cycle. If the penetration rate on two separate hamster-egg penetration tests is zero, IVF should be performed only if donor semen is acceptable to the couple. However, because so few spermatozoa are necessary

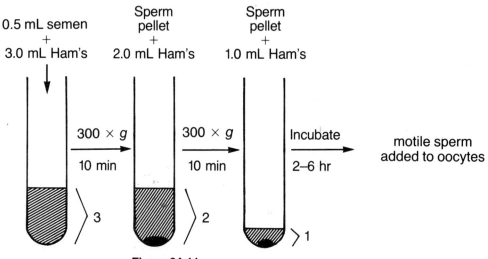

Figure 34-11
Sperm-washing technique (two-step wash).

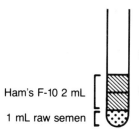

1. Incubate ×.30 min and remove 0.5-mL layer

2. Incubate × 60 min and remove 7% albumin

3. Dilute with Ham's F-10 and recover motile cells

0.5 mL washed sperm

1.0 mL 7% albumin

1.0 mL 17% albumin

Figure 34-12
Albumin gradient sperm separation.

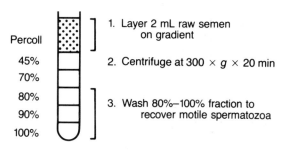

1. Place 1 mL raw semen beneath 2 mL Ham's

2. Remove upper 1 mL Ham's after 60 min

3. Remove 1 mL Ham's after 60 min more and recover motile sperm

Ham's F-10 2 mL

1 mL raw semen

Figure 34-13
Swim-up sperm separation technique.

Percoll

45%
70%
80%
90%
100%

1. Layer 2 mL raw semen on gradient

2. Centrifuge at 300 × g × 20 min

3. Wash 80%–100% fraction to recover motile spermatozoa

Figure 34-14
Percoll sperm separation technique.

Table 34-4
Comparison of separation techniques

Technique	Sperm recovery (%)	Motility enhancement (%)	Hamster-egg penetration
Two-step wash	66*	46*	Unchanged
Swim-up	28	79	Unchanged
Albumin	40	92	Unchanged
Percoll	35	88	Improved†

*$P < 0.01$.
†$P < 0.05$.

for successful IVF, severely oligozoospermic men can now produce pregnancies. Fertilization rates in our program range from 63%, in men producing fewer than 10 million total spermatozoa, to 86%, in men producing more than 10 million total spermatozoa.

Embryo culturing

Once spermatozoa are placed in the oocyte culture dish, the coincubation time is 18 hours. At that time, the corona cells are gently removed from the egg by dissection with 28-gauge needles under a dissecting microscope. Visualization with the dissecting microscope of male and female pronuclear formation signifies fertilization (Figure 34-15). Multiple pronuclei signify polyspermic (Figure 34-16) fertilization. Since these oocytes may begin normal cleavage, an abnormal fertilization process may not be detected unless they are inspected 18 hours after fertilization. If the fertilization process is completed normally, oocytes are transferred to Ham's F-10 medium with 20% human serum, cultured for another 24 hours, inspected, and replaced in the uterine cavity at a two-cell to eight-cell stage of development (Figure 34-17). Embryos showing evidence of fragmentation (Figure 34-18) or polyspermic fertilization are not replaced in the uterus.

Embryo replacement

Cleaving embryos are placed in the uterine cavity by a transcervical approach. The patient is brought into the operating room, adjacent to the embryo culture laboratory, and placed in the lithotomy position. The replacement of the embryo(s) is performed with a side-hole Teflon catheter (Figure 34-19). The embryo(s) is loaded into the catheter in 30 µL of the patient's serum

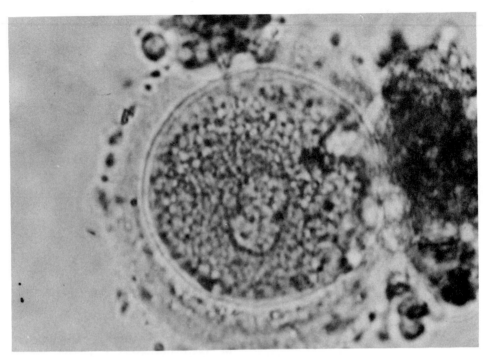

Figure 34-15
Normal fertilization after pronucleus formation.

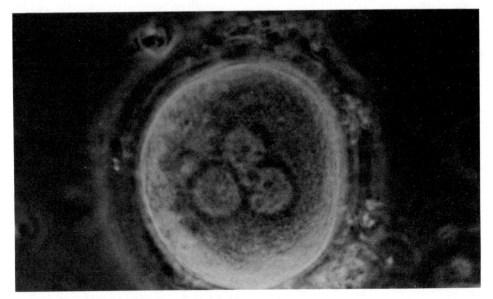

Figure 34-16
Polyspermic fertilization.

Infertility

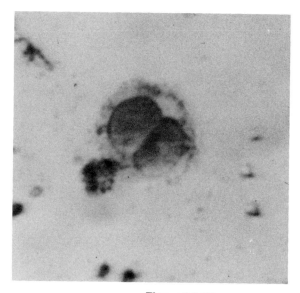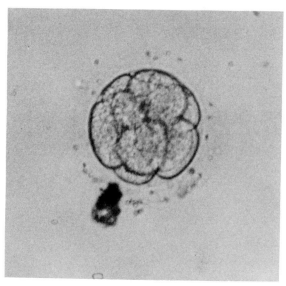

Figure 34-17
Normal cleavage development of human embryo (2- and 8-cell).

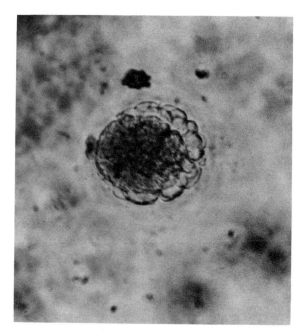

Figure 34-18
Fragmented human embryos.

and then expelled after the catheter is placed in the region of the uterine fundus. No anesthetic is required for this part of the procedure, but the patient is given diazepam, 10 mg orally, 45 minutes prior to replacement. Following the procedure, the patient is kept in a slight Trendelenburg position for 4 to 6 hours in the recovery room before returning home.

Pregnancy success

A steady increase in rates of successful outcome with IVF-ER has been observed in this decade. Before the use of stimulated cycles, pregnancy success was approximately 3% to 12% per laparoscopy.[1,15] With use of ovarian stimulation techniques, pregnancy rates in 1983 ranged between 15% and 25% per laparoscopy.[13,16] One factor that appears to affect pregnancy occurrence is the number of embryos replaced (Table 34-5). There is a substantial improvement in

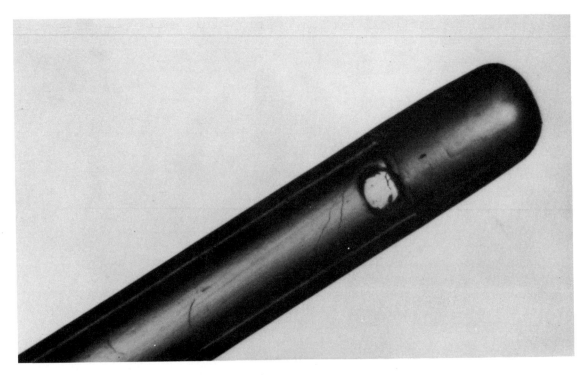

Figure 34-19
Transfer catheter.

outcome when the number of embryos replaced is two or more. Spontaneous abortions appear to occur somewhat more frequently after IVF-ER than after normal fertilization, with an abortion rate ranging from 20% to 40% after evidence of pregnancy establishment. "Biochemical" pregnancies have been reported from all centers. These are defined by a detectable low-level increase of β-hCG 14 days after embryo replacement and a delay of menses. Menstrual bleeding ensues, however, and hCG disappears. Approximately 10% to 30% of all conceptions occurring following IVF are characterized as biochemical pregnancies.

There appears to be an increasing incidence of survival of multiple gestations (twins, triplets, and quadruplets) with improving laboratory conditions. This finding necessitates a reevalua-

tion of the optimal number of embryos to be replaced during an IVF-ER cycle. Currently, we replace a maximum of three or four embryos to minimize the risk of multiple gestation. If patients produce more than four embryos during the treatment cycle, they are frozen and stored for future use.[17]

Some IVF centers use exogenous progesterone to support the luteal phase; however, preg-

Table 34-5
Pregnancy rates correlated with number of embryos per replacement

Embryos replaced	Pregnancy per replacement (%)
1	12
2	18
3	33

Infertility

nancy outcome does not appear to be affected by the use of progesterone.

Future considerations

Factors that possibly affect the incidence of pregnancy with IVF include the number of embryos replaced, maturity of the embryo(s) at the time of replacement, the overall quality of the embryos, and the receptivity of the endometrium at the time of replacement. Moreover, the quality of the luteal phase during a stimulated cycle may be less likely to promote pregnancy initiation or maintenance than a natural cycle.

One method that may avoid many problem areas is embryo cryopreservation and storage. Animal data support the successful use of embryo cryopreservation for breeding purposes. From this experience, freezing techniques have been adapted to the human. If embryos produced by IVF are frozen for later use, several theoretical advantages become evident. Because ovarian hyperstimulation is generally utilized for IVF-ER, the hormonal or endocrine milieu may not be conducive to implantation in many patients. However, if embryos are frozen and then transferred when the patient is in a spontaneous ovulatory cycle, implantation may occur more readily. Moreover, if embryo replacement is not done during the recovery cycle, the embryo can be allowed to develop to an advanced stage, either before or after cryopreservation. Therefore, it will be easier to recognize viable preimplantation embryos. More important, the incidence of implantation may be greater when the embryo has reached a preimplantation stage of development than with replacement at the two- to eight-cell stage.

Other advantages of freezing include a decrease in the number of treatment cycles necessary for pregnancy occurrence. Therefore, the financial cost per pregnancy is less. Even though embryo cryopreservation has theoretical advantages, clinical trials are necessary to demonstrate its real clinical benefit in the human IVF-ER process.

In summary, the technique of IVF-ER is in its infancy. The knowledge that is being compiled will allow even greater advances in the future. The use of gene splicing and DNA probes to eradicate various types of hereditary diseases will become a reality.

Even though ethical and moral controversies regarding IVF-ER have been raised in the past, and most certainly will be raised in the future, the underlying factor that will continue to interest investigators in this area of research is the eradication of human infertility and inherited disease. The advancement of knowledge in human reproductive function continues as we experiment more with IVF-ER.

References

1. Edwards RG: Test-tube babies. *Nature* 293:253, 1981
2. Steptoe PC, Edwards RG: Laparoscopic recovery of preovulatory human oocytes after priming of ovaries with gonadotropins. *Lancet* 1:683, 1970
3. Trounson AD, Leeton JF, Wood C, et al: Pregnancies in humans by fertilization *in vitro* and embryo transfer in the controlled ovulatory cycle. *Science* 212:681, 1981
4. Goodman AL, Nixon WE, Johnson DK, et al: Regulation of folliculogenesis in the cycling rhesus monkey: Selection of the dominant follicle. *Endocrinology* 100:175, 1977
5. Marrs RP, Vargyas JM, Shangold GM, et al: The effect of the time of initiation of clomiphene citrate on multiple follicle development for human *in vitro* fertilization and embryo replacement procedures. *Fertil Steril* 41:682, 1984
6. Vargyas JM, Morente C, Shangold G, et al: The effect of different methods of ovarian stimulation for human *in vitro* fertilization and embryo transfer. *Fertil Steril* 42:745, 1984
7. Hackelöer BJ, Fleming R, Robinson HP, et al: Correlation of ultrasonic and endocrinologic assessment of human follicular development. *Am J Obstet Gynecol* 135:122, 1979
8. Vargyas JM, Marrs RP, Kletzky OA, et al: Correlation of ultrasonic measurement of ovarian follicle size and serum estradiol levels in ovulatory patients using clomiphene citrate for *in vitro* fertilization. *Am J Obstet Gynecol* 144:569, 1982
9. Marrs RP, Vargyas JM, Gibbons WE, et al: A modified technique of human *in vitro* fertilization and embryo transfer. *Am J Obstet Gynecol* 147:318, 1983

10. Lenz S, Lauritsen JG: Ultrasonically guided percutaneous aspiration of human follicles under local anesthesia: A new method of collecting oocytes for in vitro fertilization. *Fertil Steril* 38:673, 1982

11. Wikland M, Nilsson L, Hansson R, et al: Collection of human oocytes by the use of sonography. *Fertil Steril* 39:603, 1983

12. Marrs RP, Saito H, Yee B, et al: Effect of variation of *in vitro* culture techniques upon oocyte fertilization-embryo development in human *in vitro* procedures. *Fertil Steril* 41:519, 1984

13. Jones HW Jr, Jones GS, Andres MC, et al: The program for *in vitro* fertilization at Norfolk. *Fertil Steril* 38:14, 1982

14. Berger T, Marrs RP, Moyer DL: Comparison of techniques for selection of motile spermatozoa. *Fertil Steril* 43:268, 1984

15. Lopata A, Johnston IW, Hoult IJ, et al: Pregnancy following intrauterine implantation of an embryo obtained by *in vitro* fertilization of preovulatory egg. *Fertil Steril* 33:117, 1980

16. Lopata A: Concepts in human *in vitro* fertilization and embryo transfer. *Fertil Steril* 40:289, 1983

17. Sato F, Brown J, Marrs RP: Effect of freezing on embryo viability and sister chromatid exchange (SCE). *Fertil Steril* 41:23, 1984 (Supplement abstracts of the March 1984 American Fertility Society Annual Meeting, New Orleans)

Part IV

Contraception

Chapter 35

Contraceptive Use and Effectiveness

Daniel R. Mishell Jr., M.D.

Reversible contraception is defined as the temporary prevention of fertility. Sterilization should be considered the permanent prevention of fertility. A perfect method of contraception has not yet been developed. All techniques have advantages and disadvantages. Therefore, when giving advice on contraception, the clinician should explain to the couple the advantages and disadvantages of each method, so that they will be fully informed and can rationally choose the method most suitable for them. Because no contraceptive method other than the condom has as yet been developed for use by the male, the physician usually discusses various contraceptive techniques with the woman. In this discussion, the physician should inform the patient if there are medical reasons that contraindicate the use of certain methods and offer her alternatives.

Contraceptive use in the US

The use of contraceptives has increased steadily in the US since 1960. According to the 1982 National Survey of Family Growth, the latest pub-

lished survey conducted by the National Center for Health Statistics, the proportion of married women in the US between the ages of 15 and 44 who practice contraception increased from 50.4% in 1960 to 67.7% in 1976. But it then stabilized, rising to no more than 68% by 1982.[1,2] The survey also showed that by 1982 about one-third (20 million) of the 54 million women in that age group were not exposed to unwanted pregnancy (they either were not having sexual intercourse, had a hysterectomy for reasons other than sterility, or were infertile, pregnant, or attempting to conceive). Of the remaining 34 million women who were exposed to the risk of pregnancy, all but 4 million (7.4%) used a method of contraception (Table 35-1).[1,2]

Sterilization was the method of preventing conception most frequently used by these 30 million women, accounting for 32.7% (10.8% male, 21.9% female). Of the nonsurgical methods of contraception, oral contraceptives (OCs) were most popular, being used by 16% of all women in this age group. OCs were followed in frequency of use by the condom, diaphragm, intrauterine device (IUD), spermicides, and withdrawal (Table 35-1).[1,2] Overall, 28.6% of women

Table 35-1

Percentage distribution of US women aged 15 to 44, by contraceptive status and method, 1982

Contraceptive status*	Percentage	Contraceptive method†	Percentage
Contraceptive users	54.5	Sterilization:	
Pregnant, postpartum, or		Male	10.8
seeking pregnancy	9.2	Female	21.9
Noncontraceptively sterile	9.4	OCs	28.6
Other nonusers:		IUD	7.3
Never had intercourse	13.6	Barrier:	
No intercourse in last 3 months	5.9	Diaphragm	8.3
Had intercourse in last 3 months	7.4	Condom	12.2
		Spermicides	2.4
		Periodic abstinence	4.0
		Withdrawal	2.0
		Douche	0.2
		Other	2.3

*All women (n = 54,099,000)

†Contraceptive users only (n = 29,498,000)

From Bachrach CA: Contraceptive practice among American women, 1973-1982. Fam Plan Perspect 16:253, 1984.

Data from Mosher WD: Vital and health statistics, Series 23, Data from the National Survey of Family Growth, No. 7, DHHS Publication PHS 81-1983.

practicing contraception used OCs. This method was most popular among women 15 to 24 years of age. Among married women younger than 25 practicing contraception in 1982, more than half (54%) used OCs. For women over 35, the condom was the most popular method of nonsurgical contraception; OCs were used by fewer than 10% of women in this age group who were exposed to pregnancy. Sterilization was used by 62% of married women over 35 who were exposed to the risk of pregnancy.

Sterilization use increased dramatically among married US women 15 to 44 years of age—from 7.8% in 1965 to 27.5% by 1982 (Table 35-2).[1,2] In 1982, female sterilization was nearly twice as frequent as male sterilization. OC use among the same group of women increased from 15.3% in 1965 to a high of 25.1% in 1973. Pharmacy purchases of OCs began declining in the US in 1975. By 1982, OCs were used by only 13.4% of all married US women in this age group. IUD use by these women increased from 0.7% in 1965 to 6.7% in 1973 and then declined to 6.3% in 1976 and 4.8% in 1982. Thus, since

1976, although sterilization has become more frequent, use of the two most effective nonsurgical methods of contraception, OCs and the IUD, has declined. There has been a concomitant increase in use of the less effective barrier methods, the diaphragm, condom, and foam.[2]

Contraceptive effectiveness

It is difficult to determine the actual effectiveness of a contraceptive method, because of the many factors that affect contraceptive failure. The terms "method effectiveness" and "use effectiveness" (or "method failure" and "patient failure") have been used to describe conception occurring while the contraceptive method was being used correctly vs. incorrectly. In general, methods used at the time of coitus, such as the diaphragm, condom, foam, rhythm, and withdrawal, have much greater method effectiveness than use effectiveness. There is less difference between method and use effectiveness with methods not related to the time of coitus, such as

OCs and the IUD. Because less motivation is required, their overall effectiveness is greater than that of coitus-related methods.

The overall value of a contraceptive method as used by a couple (correctly or incorrectly) is determined by calculating the actual effectiveness and the continuation rate. Actuarial methods should be used to determine these rates. The most useful of the life-table methods currently used in contraceptive studies is the log-rank method described by Azen and associates.[3] This method is suitable for a rigorous statistical comparison of various contraceptive methods, different types of the same method, or various parameters, such as age and parity, affecting the use of a single method.

Even with use of these excellent statistical techniques, it is difficult to determine the effectiveness of a contraceptive method in actual practice. Most studies undertaken for this purpose are performed under carefully controlled clinical trials. During these studies, frequent contact with supportive clinic personnel results in lower failure rates and higher continuation rates than actually occur in field use. Furthermore, these clinical trials are infrequently performed in a comparative randomized manner. Therefore, clinicians cannot accurately compare results of a trial of one type of contraceptive method with those of another.

Several other factors also influence contraceptive failure rates. One of the most important is motivation. Contraceptive failure is more likely to occur in couples seeking to delay a wanted birth, compared with those seeking to prevent any more births, especially for coitus-related methods. The woman's age has a strong negative correlation with failure of a contraceptive method, as does socioeconomic status and level of education. Thus, many variables must be considered when evaluating the effectiveness of any method of contraception for an individual patient. Failure rates reported in prospective studies are also consistently lower than those of retrospective interview studies.

For example, Vessey and colleagues reported failure rates of various contraceptive methods among the more than 17,000 women who were enrolled in the Oxford/Family Planning Association Contraceptive Study.[4] This study included married women, 25 to 39 years of age, who had been using the diaphragm, IUD, or

Table 35-2
Distribution of US married women aged 15 to 44, categorized by contraceptive status and method

Contraceptive status and method	Distribution (%)			
	1965*	1973*	1976*	1982†
All women	100.0	100.0	100.0	100.0
Contraceptors	63.9	69.6	67.7	68.0
Surgical (sterilization)	7.8	16.4	18.6	27.5
Nonsurgical	56.1	53.2	49.2	40.5
OCs	15.3	25.1	22.5	13.4
IUD	0.7	6.7	6.3	4.8
Other methods	40.1	21.4	20.3	22.3
Noncontraceptors	36.1	30.4	32.3	32.0

*From Mosher WD: Vital and health statistics, Series 23, Data from the National Survey of Family Growth, No. 7, DHHS Publication PHS 81-1983.
†From Bachrach CA: Contraceptive practice among American women, 1973-1982. Fam Plan Perspect 16:253, 1984.

Contraceptive use and effectiveness

OCs for at least 5 months before enrollment. Most of the women were well educated and of high socioeconomic status. This select population was comprised of women who were motivated to attend family-planning clinics and who had been under observation for an average of $9\frac{1}{2}$ years. Failure rates per 100 woman-years were very low for several contraceptive methods. They were approximately 0.3 for OCs, 1.3 for the IUD, 1.9 for the diaphragm, 3.6 for the condom, 11.9 for spermicides, and 15.5 for the rhythm method (Table 35-3).[4] Failure rates declined with increasing age and increasing dura-

Table 35-3
Contraceptive failures
with various methods

Method	Failure rate (per 100 woman-years)
Sterilization	
Male	0.02
Female	0.13
OCs	
< 50 μg estrogen	0.27
50 μg estrogen	0.16
> 50 μg estrogen	0.32
Progestogen only	1.2
IUD	
Copper T	1.2
Copper 7	1.5
Dalkon Shield	2.4
Loop A	6.8
Loop B	1.8
Loop C	1.4
Loop D	1.3
Saf-T-Coil	1.3
Not known	1.8
Diaphragm	1.9
Condom	3.6
Withdrawal	6.7
Spermicides	11.9
Rhythm	15.5

Data from Oxford/Family Planning Association Contraceptive Study. Vessey M, Lawless M, Yeates D: Efficacy of different contraceptive methods. Lancet 1:841, 1982.

tion of use, especially for barrier methods and the IUD. However, with the exception of the diaphragm, there was no substantial difference in failure rates among women wishing to delay or prevent a pregnancy.

In contrast, data obtained from questionnaires used in the 1973 and 1976 National Surveys of Family Growth indicated that first-year failure rates of each of these methods of contraception were higher than those reported in the Oxford Study.

When Grady and associates analyzed data obtained from married women, aged 15 to 44, they found failure rates lowest for OCs, 2.5%, and highest for the rhythm method, 18.8% (Table 35-4).[5,6]

Grady and co-workers also found a marked difference in failure rates among women of various age groups wishing to prevent, but not delay, a pregnancy. For all methods, the failure rate was 10.7% among women 15 to 24 years of age, compared with 1.4% among women 35 to 44 (Table 35-5).[5] This age-related difference was most marked among preventers using methods other than OCs and the IUD. First-year failure rates were also inversely related to the level of education (Table 35-6).[5]

Schirm and associates analyzed the same data in a somewhat different manner and arrived at similar conclusions.[6] They found that age, motivation, and income (socioeconomic level) influenced failure rates for all methods, with the least variation being for OCs and the greatest for rhythm. OC failure rates exceeded 5% only for women younger than 22 whose annual income was less than $15,000. Failure rates were very high for diaphragm users under age 22, ranging from 18% to 52%, depending on such factors as annual income and desire for more children. Failure rates for the condom declined sharply with age. According to this study, failure rates for the condom were lower than those for the IUD for couples in which the woman was over 30.

Contraception

Table 35-4
Percentage of US married women aged 15 to 44
experiencing a first-year contraceptive failure,
by contraceptive method (1970 to 1975)

Contraceptive method	All women*	Women over 30 (annual income > $15,000) wishing to prevent pregnancy†
Sterilization	0.0	0.0
OCs	2.5	0.8
IUD	4.8	1.5
Condom	9.6	0.9
Diaphragm	14.4	6.4
Foam, cream, jelly, suppository	17.7	6.1
Rhythm	18.8	8.3
Other	11.5	4.0

*From Grady WR, Hirsch MB, Keen N, et al: Contraceptive failure and continuation among married women in the United States, 1970-75. Stud Fam Plan 14:9, 1983.

†From Schirm AL, Trussell J, Menken J, et al: Contraceptive failure in the United States: The impact of social, economic and demographic factors. Fam Plan Perspect 14:68, 1982.

Failure rates from these studies are use failure rates. Theoretically, method failure rates could be estimated by the lowest failure rate found in any of the subgroups of women. The lowest failure rate was found in women who wished to prevent a pregnancy, had the highest income, and were over age 30. In this group, first-year failure rates were: OCs, 0.8%; condom, 0.9%; IUD, 1.5%; spermicide, 6.1%; diaphragm, 6.4%; and rhythm, 8.3% (Table 35-

Table 35-5
Percentage of US married women aged 15 to 44
experiencing a first-year contraceptive failure,
by contraceptive method, intention, and age (1970 to 1975)

Age	Modern methods (OCs and IUD)	Barrier methods	All methods
Prevent conception			
15–44	2.4	10.3	4.0
15–24	4.1	36.5	10.7
25–34	1.1	6.8	2.7
35–44	0.0	3.6	1.4
Delay conception			
15–44	3.3	17.3	8.3
15–24	3.2	17.8	7.4
25–34	3.8	16.8	10.5
35–44			

From Grady WR, Hirsch MB, Keen N, et al: Contraceptive failure and continuation among married women in the United States, 1970-75. Stud Fam Plan 14:9, 1983.

Table 35-6
Percentage of US married women aged 15 to 44 experiencing a first-year contraceptive failure, by education, contraceptive intention, and method (1970 to 1975)

Education	OCs and IUD	Barrier methods
Prevent conception		
All educational levels	2.4	10.3
<12 years	4.4	11.6
12 years	1.9	10.8
>12 years	1.7	8.4
Delay conception		
All educational levels	3.3	17.3
<12 years	3.9	19.0
12 years	3.4	20.9
>12 years	2.6	12.7

From Grady WR, Hirsch MB, Keen N, et al: Contraceptive failure and continuation among married women in the United States, 1970-75. Stud Fam Plan 14:9, 1983.

4).[5,6] The lowest first-year failure rates in women under 30 were somewhat higher: OCs, 1.2%; IUD, 2.3%; condom, 5.7%; spermicide, 9.4%; diaphragm, 9.7%; and rhythm, 12.6%. When first-year failure rates were standardized for desire to have more children, income, and age, the rates were similar to those found by Grady and co-workers.[5,6]

Further data from these surveys indicate that 1-year continuation rates for the various contraceptive methods were highest for the IUD and lowest for the diaphragm, condom, and spermicide (Table 35-7).[5]

Spermicides: vaginal foams, creams, and suppositories

All these agents contain a spermicidal ingredient, usually nonoxyl 9, which immobilizes or kills sperm on contact. They also provide a mechanical barrier and need to be placed into the vagina before each coital act. There are no data comparing the efficiency of the various types of vaginal spermicides; however, as noted above, their effectiveness increases with increasing age of the woman and is similar to that of the diaphragm in all age and income groups. The increased effectiveness of vaginal spermicides in older women is probably due to increased motivation. Also, coitus is more likely to be less spontaneous and to occur less frequently than in younger women.

A spermicide incorporated into a vaginal sponge that can be left in place for 24 hours avoids the need of insertion before each coital act. However, this device had slightly higher 1-year pregnancy rates than the diaphragm in clinical trials (Table 35-8).[7] Although it has been reported that contraceptive failures with spermicides may be associated with an increased incidence of congenital malformations, this finding has not been confirmed in several large studies and is not believed to be valid.[8-10]

Diaphragm

A diaphragm must be carefully fitted by the physician or nursing personnel. The largest size that does not cause discomfort or undue pressure on the vaginal mucosa should be used. After the fitting, the patient should remove the diaphragm and reinsert it herself. She should then

Table 35-7
Percentage of US married women aged 15 to 44 continuing same method for 1 year,* by contraceptive method (1970 to 1975)

Contraceptive method	All women
All methods except sterilization	69.3
Pill	74.1
IUD	78.6
Condom	61.9
Diaphragm	64.3
Foam, cream, jelly, suppository	53.8
Rhythm	71.4
Other (excluding sterilization)	66.5

From Grady WR, Hirsch MB, Keen N, et al: Contraceptive failure and continuation among married women in the United States, 1970-75. Stud Fam Plan 14:9, 1983.
*Only method-related reasons for stopping (excluding unintended pregnancy) are considered.

Contraception

Table 35-8
12-month cumulative life-table discontinuation rates (per 100 women)

	Contraceptive method mainly used			
	Used vaginal contraceptive before		Did not use vaginal contraceptive before	
Event	Contraceptive sponge (n=264)	Diaphragm (n=249)	Contraceptive sponge (n=452)	Diaphragm (n=470)
Pregnancy	13.2*	5.9	16.1	12.0
Medical reasons	7.0*	2.4	7.5	3.9
Discomfort	1.8	2.2	7.0*	3.5
Planned pregnancy	3.1	3.8	5.5	8.8
Other personal reasons	18.3	22.7	24.1	28.5
Continuation rate	62.7	66.9	51.7	53.2

*P < 0.05.

From Edelman DA, Smith SC, McIntyre S: Comparative trial of the contraceptive sponge and diaphragm: A preliminary report. J Reprod Med 28:781, 1983.

be examined to make sure the diaphragm is covering the cervix. The diaphragm should be used with contraceptive cream or jelly and be left in place for at least 8 hours after coitus. If repeated intercourse takes place or coitus occurs more than 8 hours after insertion of the diaphragm, additional contraceptive cream or jelly must be used. Diaphragm users should also be cautioned not to leave the device in place for more than 24 hours.

Data from the Oxford/Family Planning Association Contraceptive Study indicate that the diaphragm is an effective method of contraception.[11] Women who have been using it successfully should be encouraged not to switch to another method. Prospective new users should be informed that it is an effective method after the first few months of use.

Cervical cap

The cervical cap, a cup-shaped plastic or rubber device that fits around the cervix, has been used as a barrier contraceptive for decades, mainly in Britain and other parts of Europe. Each type of device is manufactured in different sizes and should be fitted to the cervix by a clinician. The cervical cap should not be left in place for more than 72 hours because of the possibility of ulceration, unpleasant odor, and infection. Although this device is not currently approved for general use in the US, it is a popular method of contraception among a segment of the population. Clinical trials with the cervical cap among motivated women report first-year failure rates of about 9%.[12]

Condom

Use of the condom by individuals with multiple sex partners should be encouraged. It is the contraceptive method most effective in preventing transmission of sexually transmitted diseases. The condom should not be applied tightly. The tip should extend beyond the end of the penis by about $\frac{1}{2}$ inch to collect the ejaculate. Care must be taken upon withdrawal not to spill the ejaculate. In the Oxford/Family Planning Association Contraceptive Study, all condom users had previously used another method, mainly OCs.[13] During 12,497 woman-years of exposure, 449 unplanned pregnancies occurred, for a use-pregnancy rate of 3.6/100 woman-years. The pregnancy rate increased linearly over time: from 0.7/100 woman-years at 3 months to 8.4/100 woman-years at 24 months. Accidental pregnancy rates were slightly lower among women over 35 years of age and among women who had completed their families, even when these factors were standardized for the other characteristics. This study is one of the largest for which findings have been published. The results are consistent with those of several older studies, which show a similar high level of effectiveness for the condom when used by couples with enough motivation for the woman to attend a family-planning clinic.

Rhythm method

The Roman Catholic church officially proscribes all methods of contraception other than rhythm, or periodic abstinence. The rationale for the rhythm method is based on three assumptions: (1) the human ovum is capable of being fertilized for only about 24 hours after ovulation; (2) spermatozoa retain their fertilizing ability for only about 48 hours after coitus; and (3) ovulation usually occurs 12 to 16 days (14 ± 2 days) before the onset of the subsequent menses. According to these assumptions, after the woman records the length of her cycles for several months, she establishes her fertile period by subtracting 18 days from the length of her previous shortest cycle and 11 days from her previous longest cycle. Then, in each subsequent cycle, the couple abstains from coitus during this calculated fertile period.

The use effectiveness of this calendar method of periodic abstinence is poor. According to the US Survey of Family Growth, the failure rate was 18.8%.[5] The reasons for this lack of success, as summarized by Mastroianni, are numerous, despite advances in knowledge of human reproductive physiology.[14] Significantly, there is no evidence to indicate that the three assumptions stated above, upon which the rhythm method is based, have scientific validity. Furthermore, women have great irregularity in menstrual cycle length. Even women with previously regular

cycles have occasional marked variations. Cycle irregularity is common in perimenarcheal and perimenopausal women, for whom most pregnancies are unwanted. In addition, because a woman is menstruating during several of the nonfertile days and most couples do not have coitus during this time, the period of abstinence is frequently greater than the time during which sexual relations may be practiced.

To increase the effectiveness of the rhythm method, instead of relying solely on the calendar method described above, it is advisable to also measure the basal body temperature (BBT) daily. Because progesterone causes an increase in BBT, if the couple abstains from intercourse from the start of menses until at least 48 hours after the rise in BBT (2 days after ovulation), sexual relations will take place only after the ovum is no longer capable of being fertilized. Data from several sources indicate that the use of daily BBTs for determining the days of periodic abstinence increases the effectiveness of the rhythm method. One British study reported a failure rate of only 6.6 per 100 woman-years in women practicing the temperature method for determining the time of periodic abstinence.[15]

There have been reports that women could detect changes in the quality and quantity of their cervical mucus and consequently could be taught to predict the time when ovulation was going to occur.[16] Although some enthusiasts report extraordinary success with this method, careful analysis of their results suggests that its actual effectiveness is substantially less than claimed.

Thus, periodic abstinence, or the rhythm method, requires a high degree of motivation, communication, and sophistication. Even with these qualities, the rhythm method of family planning is associated with a very high failure rate, and this fact should be made known to all couples choosing to use this method of family planning.

References

1. Bachrach CA: Contraceptive practice among American women, 1973-1982. *Fam Plan Perspect* 16:253, 1984

2. Mosher WD: *Vital and health statistics,* Series 23, Data from the National Survey of Family Growth, No. 7, DHHS Publication PHS 81-1983

3. Azen SP, Roy S, Pike MC, et al: A new procedure for the statistical evaluation of intrauterine contraception. *Am J Obstet Gynecol* 128:329, 1977

4. Vessey M, Lawless M, Yeates D: Efficacy of different contraceptive methods. *Lancet* 1:841, 1982

5. Grady WR, Hirsch MB, Keen N, et al: Contraceptive failure and continuation among married women in the United States, 1970–75. *Stud Fam Plan* 14:9, 1983

6. Schirm AL, Trussell J, Menken J, et al: Contraceptive failure in the United States: The impact of social, economic and demographic factors. *Fam Plan Perspect* 14:68, 1982

7. Edelman DA, Smith SC, McIntyre S: Comparative trial of the contraceptive sponge and diaphragm: A preliminary report. *J Reprod Med* 28:781, 1983

8. Linn S, Schoenbaum SC, Monson RR, et al: Lack of association between contraceptive usage and congenital malformations in offspring. *Am J Obstet Gynecol* 147:923, 1983

9. Mills JL, Harley EE, Reed GF, et al: Are spermicides teratogenic? *JAMA* 248:2148, 1982

10. Shapiro S, Sloane D, Heinonen OP, et al: Birth defects and vaginal spermicides. *JAMA* 247:2381, 1982

11. Vessey MP, Wiggins P: Use-effectiveness of the diaphragm in a selected family planning clinic population in the United Kingdom. *Contraception* 9:15, 1974

12. Koch JP: The Prentif contraceptive cervical cap: A contemporary study of its clinical safety and effectiveness. *Contraception* 25:135, 1982

13. Glass R, Vessey M, Wiggins P: Use-effectiveness of the condom in a selected family planning clinic population in the United Kingdom. *Contraception* 10:591, 1974

14. Mastroianni L Jr: Rhythm: Systematized chance-taking. *Fam Plan Perspect* 6:209, 1974

15. Marshall J: A field trial of the basal-body-temperature method of regulating births. *Lancet* 2:8, 1968

16. Ovulation method of family planning. *Lancet* 2:1027, 1972

Chapter 36

Oral Steroid Contraceptives

Daniel R. Mishell Jr., M.D.

The oral steroid contraceptives (OCs) first became available for use by women in 1960. Shortly thereafter, they became the most widely used method of contraception in developed countries among both married and unmarried women. The main reasons for the popularity of this method were ease of administration and an extremely high rate of effectiveness. Although accompanying side effects that did not endanger health, such as nausea, breakthrough bleeding, and breast tenderness, were not uncommon, serious side effects, such as thromboembolism, were relatively rare. Thus, by 1965, OCs were used by about 24% of married women in the US practicing contraception. This incidence had risen to 36% by 1970 and remained there until 1976. In that year, it was estimated that OCs were used by about 33% of married women in the US using contraception.[1]

However, in 1975, articles linking use of OCs with an increased risk of fatal myocardial infarction (MI) and stroke appeared in the medical literature. During the same year, the use of exogenous estrogens was reported to be causally related to development of endometrial carcinoma when given in large dosages for prolonged periods to postmenopausal women. Since women were aware that OCs also contained estrogen, they were concerned that OCs might also be car-

cinogenic. Furthermore, the results of the scientific articles were frequently misinterpreted by lay writers, who then wrote articles exaggerating the hazards of OCs. As a result of the exaggeration of the risks of OCs, retail sales declined in the US after 1975. By 1982, OCs were being used by only 19.7% of married women in the US practicing contraception.[2]

Pharmacology

There are three major types of oral steroid contraceptive formulations: fixed-dose combination, combination phasic, and daily gestagen. The combination formulations are the most widely used and most effective. They consist of tablets containing both an estrogen and a gestagen (progestin) given continuously for 3 weeks. The original sequential type, which is no longer marketed, provided a regimen of estrogen alone given for about 2 weeks, followed by 1 week of combination estrogen/gestagen tablets. Recently, combination formulations have been marketed that contain two or three different amounts of the same estrogen and gestagen. Each of the tablets containing one of these various dosages is given for intervals varying from 5 to 11 days during the 21-day medication period. These

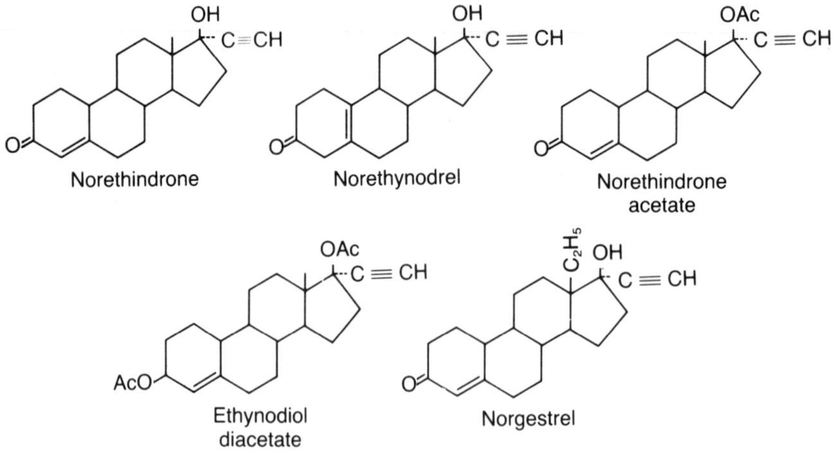

Figure 36-1
Structures of the five gestagens used in US combination OCs.

formulations have been described as biphasic or triphasic and are generally referred to as multiphasic. The rationale for this type of formulation is that a lower total dose of steroid is administered without increasing the incidence of breakthrough bleeding. In the usual regimen for combination OCs, no medication is given for 1 week out of 4 to allow withdrawal bleeding to occur. The third type of contraceptive formulation, consisting of tablets containing a gestagen without any estrogen, is designed to be taken daily without a steroid-free interval.

OCs currently being used are formulated from synthetic steroids and contain no natural estrogens or gestagens. There are two major types of synthetic gestagens: (1) derivatives of 19-nortestosterone and (2) derivatives of 17α-acetoxyprogesterone. The latter group are C_{21} gestagens, consisting of such steroids as medroxyprogesterone acetate and megestrol acetate. They are not used in current contraceptive formulations. In contrast to the 19-nortestosterone derivatives, when high dosages of the C_{21} gestagens were given to female beagle dogs, the animals developed an increased incidence of mammary cancer. Because of this carcinogenic effect, contraceptives containing these gestagens are not marketed.

All OC formulations now available in the US consist of varying dosages of one of the following five 19-nortestosterone gestagens: norethynodrel, norethindrone, norethindrone acetate, ethynodiol diacetate, or norgestrel (Figure 36-1). With the exception of two daily gestagen-only formulations, the gestagens are combined with varying dosages of two estrogens, ethinylestradiol and ethinylestradiol 3-methyl ether, also known as mestranol (Figure 36-2). All the synthetic estrogens and gestagens in OCs have an ethinyl group at position 17. The presence of this ethinyl group enhances the oral activity of these agents, because their essential functional groups are not as rapidly hydroxylated and then conjugated as they initially pass through the liver via the portal system, in contrast with what occurs when natural sex steroids are ingested orally. The synthetic steroids thus have greater oral potency per unit of weight than the natural steroids.

The various modifications in chemical

Contraception

structure of the different synthetic gestagens and estrogens also affect their biologic activity. Thus, one cannot judge the pharmacologic activity of the gestagen or estrogen in a particular contraceptive steroid formulation only by the amount of steroid present. The biologic activity of each steroid also has to be considered. Using established tests for progestational activity in animals, it has been found that a given weight of norgestrel is several times more potent than the same weight of norethindrone. Studies in humans, using delay of menses[3] or endometrial histologic alterations such as subnuclear vacuolization[4,5] as endpoints, also conclude that norgestrel is several times more potent than the same weight of norethindrone. Norethindrone acetate and ethynodiol diacetate are metabolized in the body to norethindrone. The human studies, measuring progestational activity as described above, as well as other studies comparing the effects on serum lipids in humans, indicate that each of these three gestagens have approximately equal potency per unit of weight, while levonorgestrel is 10 to 20 times as potent.[6]

The two estrogenic compounds used in OCs, ethinylestradiol and its 3-methyl ether, mestranol, also have different biologic activity in women. To become biologically effective, mestranol must be demethylated to ethinylestradiol, because mestranol does not bind to the estrogen cytosol receptors. The degree of conversion of mestranol to ethinylestradiol varies among individuals; some are able to convert it completely, while others convert only a portion of it. Thus, in some women, a given weight of mestranol is as potent as the same weight of ethinylestradiol, while in other women it is only about half as potent. Overall, it has been estimated that ethinylestradiol is about 1.7 times as potent as the same weight of mestranol. This factor was determined using human endometrial response and effect on liver corticosteroid-binding globulin (CBG) production as endpoints. Thus, it is important to evaluate the biologic activity as well as the quan-

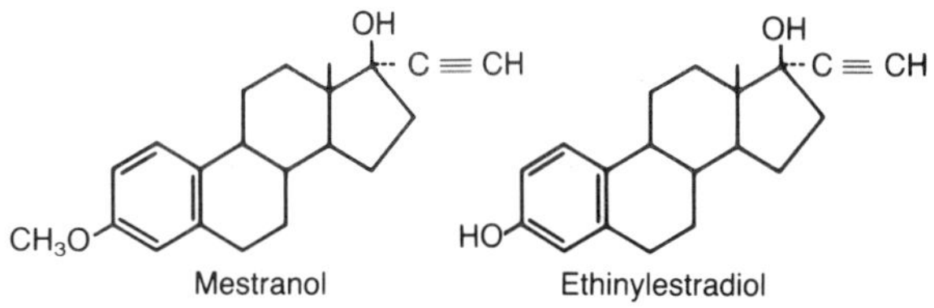

Figure 36-2
Structures of the two estrogens used in US combination OCs.

tity of both steroid components when comparing potency of the various formulations.

Radioimmunoassay methods have been developed to measure blood levels of these synthetic estrogens and gestagens. Peak plasma levels of ethinylestradiol occur about 1 hour after ingestion, then rapidly decline.[7] However, measurable amounts of ethinylestradiol are still found in plasma 24 hours after ingestion. With mestranol, peak levels of ethinylestradiol are lower than with ethinylestradiol, and occur from 2 to 4 hours after ingestion. This delay is due to the time necessary for mestranol to be demethylated to ethinylestradiol in the liver.

When different doses of norgestrel were administered to women, we found that the serum levels of levonorgestrel were related to the dosage.[7] Peak serum levels were found $\frac{1}{2}$ to 3 hours after oral administration, followed by a rapid, sharp decline (Figure 36-3).[8] However, 24 hours after ingestion, 20% to 25% of the peak level of levonorgestrel was still present in the serum. After 5 days of norgestrel administration, measurable amounts of levonorgestrel were present for at least the following 5 days.

We measured serum levels of levonorgestrel, follicle-stimulating hormone (FSH), luteinizing hormone (LH), estradiol, and progesterone 3 hours after ingestion of a combination OC containing 0.5 mg of dl-norgestrel and 50 μg of ethinylestradiol in three women during two consecutive cycles, as well as during the intervening pill-free interval. Daily levels of levonorgestrel

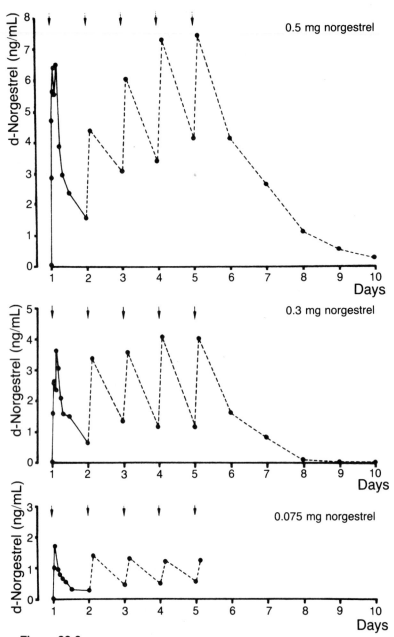

Figure 36-3
Serum *d*-norgestrel levels in three women at various times after ingestion of 0.5, 0.3, and 0.075 mg of *dl*-norgestrel once a day for 5 days. Arrows indicate days drug was ingested.

From Mishell DR Jr, Stanczyk F, Hiroi M, et al: Steroid contraception. In Crosignani PG, Mishell DR Jr (eds): Ovulation in the Human. London, Academic Press, 1976.

rose during the first few days of medication, plateaued thereafter, and declined after ingestion of the last pill (Figure 36-4).[7] Nevertheless, substantial amounts of levonorgestrel remained in the serum for at least the first 3 to 4 days after the last pill was ingested. These steroid levels were sufficient to suppress gonadotropin release; thus follicle maturation, as evidenced by rising estradiol levels, does not occur during the pill-free interval.

From these data, it seems reasonable to conclude that accidental pregnancies during OC use probably do not occur because of a failure to ingest 1 to 2 pills more than a few days after a treatment cycle is initiated, but rather because initiation of the next cycle of medication is delayed for a few days. Therefore, it is very important that the pill-free interval be limited to no more than 7 days. This is best accomplished by administering either a placebo or iron pill daily during the steroid-free interval (the so-called 28-day package). Alternatively, treatment may be started on the first Sunday after menses begins instead of the first or fifth day of the cycle.

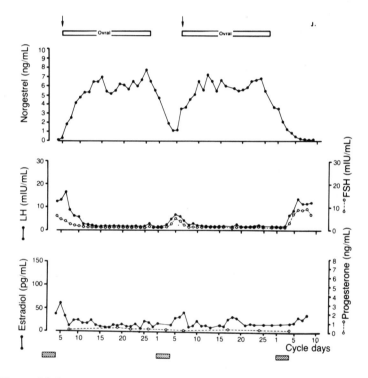

Figure 36-4

Serum *d*-norgestrel, FSH, LH, estradiol, and progesterone levels in a subject during and following oral administration of 500 µg of *dl*-norgestrel and 50 µg of ethinylestradiol (Ovral) for two subsequent 21-day periods interrupted by a pill-free interval of 6 days.

From Brenner PF, Mishell DR Jr, Stanczyk FZ, et al: Serum levels of d-norgestrel, luteinizing hormone, follicle-stimulating hormone, estradiol, and progesterone in women during and following ingestion of combination oral contraceptives containing dl-norgestrel. *Am J Obstet Gynecol 129:133, 1977.*

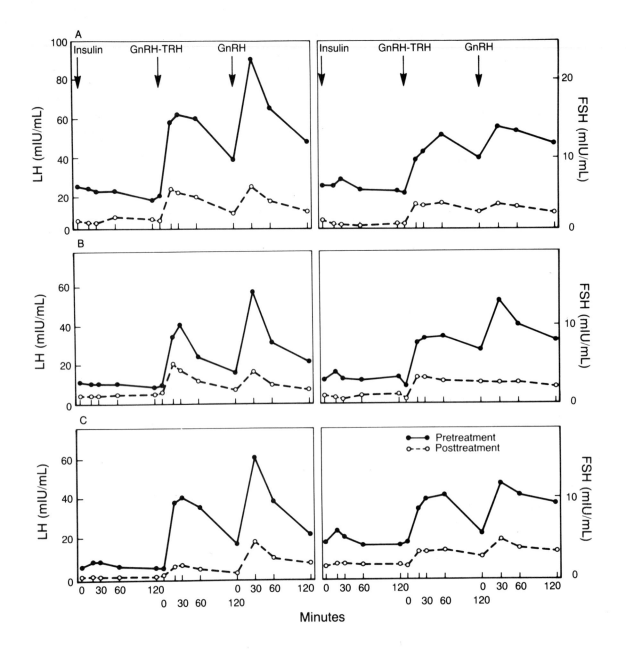

Figure 36-5
LH and FSH basal levels and following stimulation with two boluses of GnRH in three subjects before (filled circles) and three weeks after (open circles) receiving a combination oral contraceptive.

From Mishell DR Jr, Kletzky OA, Brenner PF, et al: The effect of contraceptive steroids on hypothalamic-pituitary function. Am J Obstet Gynecol 128:60, 1977.

It is easier to remember to start the new package on a Sunday. Patients should be warned that the most important pill to remember to take is the first one of each cycle.

Physiology

Mechanism of action

The estrogen/gestagen combination is the most effective type of OC formulation, because it consistently inhibits the midcycle gonadotropin surge, and thus prevents ovulation. Such formulations also act on other aspects of the reproductive process. They alter the cervical mucus, making it thick, viscid, and scanty, thus preventing sperm penetration. They also alter motility of the uterus and oviduct, thus impairing transport of both ova and sperm. Furthermore, they alter the endometrium, so that its glandular production of glycogen is diminished and less energy is available for the blastocyst to survive in the uterine cavity. Finally, they may alter ovarian responsiveness to gonadotropin stimulation. Nevertheless, neither gonadotropin production nor ovarian steroidogenesis is completely abolished. Levels of endogenous estradiol in the peripheral blood during ingestion of combination OCs are similar to those found in the early follicular phase of the normal cycle.[9]

Contraceptive steroids prevent ovulation mainly by interfering with release of gonadotropin-releasing hormone (GnRH) from the hypothalamus. In rats, and in a few studies in humans, this inhibitory action of the contraceptive steroids could be overcome by the administration of GnRH. However, in most other human studies, including ours, most women who had been ingesting combination OCs had suppression of the release of LH and FSH following infusion of GnRH (Figure 36-5).[10] This suggests that the steroids had a direct inhibitory effect on the pituitary as well as on the hypothalamus.

It is possible that when hypothalamic inhibition is prolonged, the mechanism for synthesis and release of gonadotropins may become refractory to the normal amount of GnRH stimulation. However, in a few OC users studied, after serial daily administration of GnRH, there was still a refractory response to a GnRH infusion. Thus, the combination contraceptive steroids probably do have a direct inhibitory effect on the gonadotropin-producing cells of the pituitary, in addition to affecting the hypothalamus. This effect occurs in about 80% of women ingesting combination OC steroids. It is unrelated to the age of the patient or the duration of steroid use, but is related to the potency of the preparations. The effect is more pronounced with formulations containing a more potent gestagen (Figure 36-6)[11] and with those containing 50 μg or more of estrogen than with 30 to 35 μg formulations (Figure 36-7).[12] It is unknown whether the amount of pituitary suppression is related to the occurrence of postpill amenorrhea, but if there is a relationship, lower-dose formulations should be associated with a lower frequency of this entity.

The daily gestagen-only preparations do not consistently inhibit ovulation. They exert their contraceptive action via the other mechanisms listed above, but because of the inconsistent ovulation inhibition, their effectiveness is significantly less than that of the combined type, with failure rates of 2% to 8% per year.[13] Because a lower dose of gestagen is used, it is important that they be consistently taken at the same time of day to ensure that blood levels do not fall below the effective contraceptive level.

Although no significant difference in clinical effectiveness has been demonstrated among the various combination formulations currently available in the US (Table 36-1), the one containing only 20 μg of ethinylestradiol may be slightly less effective. Provided no tablets are omitted, the pregnancy rate is less than 0.2% at the end of 1 year with all combination formulations.

Metabolic effects

It is important to realize that the OCs do produce certain adverse effects (Table 36-2), although the incidence of these effects has been exaggerated. Fortunately, in most cases the more common adverse effects are relatively mild. The majority are produced by the estrogenic component; the rest are produced by the gestagenic component alone or by a combination of the two. The most frequent symptoms produced by the estrogenic component include nausea, breast tenderness, and fluid retention, which usually does not exceed 3 to 4 pounds of body weight.

The synthetic estrogens in OCs cause an increase in the hepatic production of several globulins. The amount of increase is related to the

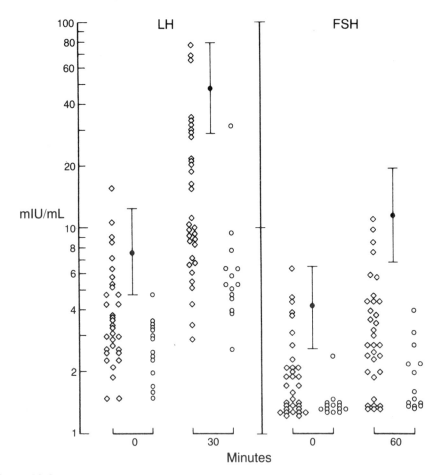

Figure 36-6
Serum LH and FSH levels in 33 subjects using mestranol and norethindrone (diamonds) and 14 subjects using ethinylestradiol and norgestrel (circles) before and 30 and 60 minutes after stimulation with GnRH. Bars represent means and 95% confidence limits for control subjects.

From Scott JA, Brenner PF, Kletzky OA, et al: Factors affecting pituitary gonadotropin function in users of oral contraceptive steroids. Am J Obstet Gynecol 130:817, 1978.

amount of the estrogenic component in the formulation (Table 36-3).[14] Increased levels of one of the globulins, angiotensinogen, may cause an increase in angiotensin II, which may result in the development of elevated blood pressure. Although a small percentage of OC users will develop increased blood pressure, the effect is temporary and will disappear when the medication is discontinued. Other globulins are involved in the blood clotting process, and their increase may cause a hypercoagulable state and the development of thrombosis in certain OC users.

The estrogenic component can also produce changes in mood, including mental depression, as a result of diversion of tryptophan metabolism from its minor pathway in the brain to its major pathway in the liver. The end product of tryptophan metabolism, serotonin, is thus

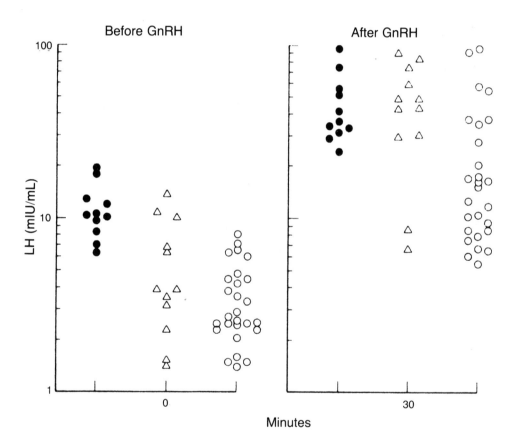

Figure 36-7
Serum LH levels before and after GnRH stimulation in control subjects (filled circles) and in subjects using formulations with less than 50 μg of estrogen (triangles) and 50 μg of estrogen or more (open circles).

From Scott JA, Kletzky OA, Brenner PF: Comparison of the effects of contraceptive steroid formulations containing two doses of estrogen on pituitary function. Fertil Steril 30:141, 1978. Reproduced with permission of the publisher, The American Fertility Society.

Table 36-1
Composition of OCs currently marketed in the US

Product	Type	Progestin	Estrogens	Manufacturer
Brevicon	Comb	0.5 mg norethindrone	35 μg ethinylestradiol	Syntex
Norinyl 1+ 35	Comb	1.0 mg norethindrone	35 μg ethinylestradiol	Syntex
Norinyl 1+ 50	Comb	1.0 mg norethindrone	50 μg mestranol	Syntex
Norinyl 1+ 80	Comb	1.0 mg norethindrone	80 μg mestranol	Syntex
Norinyl 2	Comb	2.0 mg norethindrone	100 μg mestranol	Syntex
Nor-QD	Prog	0.35 mg norethindrone		Syntex
Tri-Norinyl 7/	Comb-triphasic	0.5 mg norethindrone	35 μg ethinylestradiol	Syntex
9/		1.0 mg norethindrone	35 μg ethinylestradiol	
5		0.5 mg norethindrone	35 μg ethinylestradiol	
Demulen 1+ 35	Comb	1.0 mg ethynodiol diacetate	35 μg ethinylestradiol	Searle
Demulen 1+ 50	Comb	1.0 mg ethynodiol diacetate	50 μg ethinylestradiol	Searle
Ovulen	Comb	1.0 mg ethynodiol diacetate	100 μg mestranol	Searle
Enovid-E	Comb	2.5 mg norethynodrel	100 μg mestranol	Searle
Enovid 5	Comb	5.0 mg norethynodrel	75 μg mestranol	Searle
Enovid 10	Comb	9.85 mg norethynodrel	150 μg mestranol	Searle
Loestrin 1+ 20	Comb	1.0 mg norethindrone acetate	20 μg ethinylestradiol	Parke-Davis
Loestrin 1.5+ 30	Comb	1.5 mg norethindrone acetate	30 μg ethinylestradiol	Parke-Davis
Norlestrin 1+ 50	Comb	1.0 mg norethindrone acetate	50 μg ethinylestradiol	Parke-Davis
Norlestrin 2.5+ 50	Comb	2.5 mg norethindrone acetate	50 μg ethinylestradiol	Parke-Davis
Lo/Ovral	Comb	0.3 mg norgestrel	30 μg ethinylestradiol	Wyeth
Nordette	Comb	0.15 mg levonorgestrel	30 μg ethinylestradiol	Wyeth
Ovral	Comb	0.5 mg norgestrel	50 μg ethinylestradiol	Wyeth
Ovrette	Prog	75 μg norgestrel		Wyeth
Triphasil 6/	Comb-triphasic	50 μg levonorgestrel	30 μg ethinylestradiol	Wyeth
5/		75 μg levonorgestrel	40 μg ethinylestradiol	Wyeth
10		125 μg levonorgestrel	30 μg ethinylestradiol	Wyeth
Ovcon-35	Comb	0.4 mg norethindrone	35 μg ethinylestradiol	Mead Johnson
Ovcon-50	Comb	1.0 mg norethindrone	50 μg ethinylestradiol	Mead Johnson
Modicon	Comb	0.5 mg norethindrone	35 μg ethinylestradiol	Ortho
Ortho-Novum 1+ 35	Comb	1.0 mg norethindrone	35 μg ethinylestradiol	Ortho
Ortho-Novum 1+ 50	Comb	1.0 mg norethindrone	50 μg mestranol	Ortho
Ortho-Novum 1+ 80	Comb	1.0 mg norethindrone	80 μg mestranol	Ortho
Ortho-Novum 2	Comb	2.0 mg norethindrone	100 μg mestranol	Ortho
Ortho-Novum 10/	Comb-biphasic	0.5 mg norethindrone	35 μg ethinylestradiol	Ortho
11		1.0 mg norethindrone	35 μg ethinylestradiol	
Micronor	Prog	0.35 mg norethindrone		Ortho
Ortho-Novum 7/	Comb-triphasic	0.5 mg norethindrone	35 μg ethinylestradiol	Ortho
7/		0.75 mg norethindrone	35 μg ethinylestradiol	
7		1.0 mg norethindrone	35 μg ethinylestradiol	

Table 36-2
Metabolic effects of contraceptive steroids

	Effects	
	Chemical	Clinical
ESTROGEN—ETHINYLESTRADIOL		
Proteins		
Albumin	↓	None
Amino acids	↓	None
Globulins	↑	
1. Angiotensinogen		↑ Blood pressure
2. Factors VII & X		Hypercoagulability
3. Carrier proteins (CBG, TBG, transferrin, ceruloplasmin)		None
Carbohydrate		
Plasma insulin	None	None
Glucose tolerance	None	None
Lipids		
Cholesterol	None	None
Triglyceride	↑	None
HDL-Cholesterol	↑	None
LDL-Cholesterol	↓	None
Electrolytes		
Na excretion	↓	Fluid retention Edema
Tryptophan metabolism	↓	Depression Mood changes Sleep disturbance
Vitamins		
B complex	↓	None
Ascorbic acid	↓	None
Vitamin A	↑	None
Skin		
Sebum production	↓	Less acne
Pigmentation	↑	Chloasma
Target tissues		
Breast	↑	Breast tenderness
Endometrial receptors	↑	Hyperplasia
GESTAGENS—19-NORTESTOSTERONE DERIVATIVES		
Proteins	None	?
Carbohydrate		
Plasma insulin	↑	None
Glucose tolerance	↓	None
Lipids		
Cholesterol	↓	None
Triglyceride	↓	None
HDL-Cholesterol	↓ ⎫	? ↑ Cardiovascular disease
LDL-Cholesterol	↑ ⎭	
Nitrogen retention	↑	↑ Body weight
Skin—Sebum production	↑	↑ Acne
Androgenic effect	↑	Nervousness
Endometrial receptors	↓	↓ Endometrial cancer

decreased in the central nervous system. This decrease in serotonin levels can produce depression in some women and sleepiness and other mood changes in others. This is a reversible symptom that, fortunately, is not too common and disappears when the OCs are stopped. All these estrogenic side effects occur much less frequently now than they did a decade ago, because the OC formulations in use today contain only one-fifth as much estrogen as those used in the 1960s and 1970s.

Because they are structurally related to testosterone, the gestagens produce certain adverse androgenic effects. These include weight gain, acne, and a symptom perceived by some women as nervousness. Some women gain a considerable amount of weight when they take OCs. This is caused by the anabolic effect of the gestagenic component. Although estrogens decrease sebum production, gestagens increase it and can cause acne to develop and/or worsen. Thus, patients with acne should be given a formulation with a low gestagen/estrogen ratio. Temporary alterations in glucose metabolism may also be produced by certain gestagens, but these changes disappear when OC use is discontinued. There is no evidence that the use of OCs produces either diabetes mellitus or permanent hypertension. The gestagenic component can produce failure of withdrawal bleeding or amenorrhea, because it decreases the endometrial estrogen receptors and, thus, endometrial growth. This symptom is not important medically, but because bleeding serves as a signal that the patient is not pregnant, it is desirable to have some amount of periodic withdrawal bleeding during the days the steroid formulation is not being taken. Finally, both the estrogenic and gestagenic portions of the formulation can act together to produce irregular bleeding and/or chloasma. Breakthrough bleeding, which is usually the result of insufficient estrogen or too much gestagen or a combination of both, as well as failure of withdrawal bleeding, can be alleviated by switch-

ing to a formulation containing more estrogen. Chloasma (pigmentation of the malar eminences) is accentuated by sunlight and usually takes many years to disappear after OCs are stopped.

In addition to these more common adverse effects, there is an increased risk of more serious problems that can lead to death or severe morbidity. Although the incidence of cholelithiasis is increased about twofold in the first few years of OC use compared with its incidence in controls, data from a study by the Royal College of General Practitioners (RCGP) in the UK indicate that, after 4 years of OC use, the incidence of cholelithiasis is decreased in OC users compared with controls.[15] Thus, OCs appear to accelerate the process of cholelithiasis, but do not increase its overall incidence. The risk of deep vein thrombophlebitis is also increased about three to four times, as is the risk of thromboembolism. However, the absolute incidence of these disorders, which are not necessarily related (that is, patients with thromboembolism do not necessarily have clinical symptoms of thrombophlebitis), is on the order of about 1/10,000 users annually for thrombophlebitis and about 1/30,000 users annually for thromboembolism. OCs probably increase the incidence of thrombotic and possibly hemorrhagic stroke. The epidemiologic data relating OC use to stroke are conflicting, however, and indicate that the increased risk of stroke,

Table 36-3
Mean Factor VII and fibrinogen levels*
by OC usage and estrogen dose

	Not on OCs	OC estrogen dose	
		30 μg	50 μg
No. of patients	243	15	65
Factor VII (%)	83.0	96.6	121.1
Fibrinogen (g/L)	2.52	2.84	2.89

*Age-adjusted values
From Meade TW: Oral contraceptives, clotting factors, and thrombosis. Am J Obstet Gynecol 142:758, 1982.

like MI, is limited mainly to women who have underlying vascular disorders such as hypertension or who are older and smoke. Although the relative risk of stroke is possibly increased about three times in OC users, the actual incidence remains quite low, about 1/20,000 to 1/30,000 users per year.

Benign liver adenomas occur very rarely in OC users, with an estimated frequency of about 1/30,000 to 1/50,000 users per year. The incidence is increased in women who have used OCs for more than 5 years. Also, although there is epidemiologic evidence that women over 35 who smoke or have other associated risk factors, such as hypertension or hypercholesterolemia, have an increased risk of MI with OC use, the actual incidence of MI in this group is also low, about 1/5,000 users annually.

Major concerns

Women have three major concerns about OCs: the possibilities of (1) an increased risk of cancer, (2) problems with future childbearing, and (3) an increased risk of heart attack and stroke. These concerns are mostly unwarranted.

Neoplastic effects

A thorough review of the literature reveals only scant evidence in the 25 years since OCs were introduced that their use increases the risk of any type of cancer, including breast, uterine, cervical, and liver cancer. Three large prospective studies of OC users were started in 1968: two in the UK, the RCGP study[15] and the Oxford Family Planning Association study,[16] and one in the US, the Walnut Creek study.[17] The last was sponsored by the National Institutes of Health. Each of these studies was set up to compare large groups of women using OCs with a similar number of control women using other methods of contraception. To date, none of these studies has found an increased risk of any type of can-

cer, except for two possible exceptions: An increased risk of cervical cancer has been found in the Oxford study, but it may be due to confounding factors. And although data from the Walnut Creek study indicate that women using OCs and exposed to large amounts of sunlight may have an increased risk of melanoma, this association has not been found in other studies.

Breast cancer

At present, the women using OCs in these and other studies do not have a higher incidence of cancer of the breast than a control group of women of similar age who are using other methods of contraception. Concern that OCs may increase the risk of breast cancer has arisen because estrogens are known to stimulate normal breast tissue. In women who already have cancer of the breast, estrogens can stimulate growth of the malignant tissue. There is no evidence in humans, however, that estrogens can initiate the development of cancer from normal breast tissue. Furthermore, OCs contain a gestagen in addition to the estrogen. The gestagen counteracts the stimulatory action of the estrogen on target tissues. For this reason, women ingesting OCs have a lower incidence of nonmalignant cystic disease of the breast than do controls.

A recent multicenter epidemiologic study conducted by the US Centers for Disease Control (CDC), the Cancer and Steroid Hormone (CASH) study, has shown no increased risk of breast cancer in OC users overall, as well as in various subgroups of OC users, such as those with a family history of breast cancer, those with and without benign breast disease, and those starting OCs before their first pregnancy.[18] Furthermore, there was no change in the risk of breast cancer with increasing duration of OC use or time since first OC use (Table 36-4).

Another recent epidemiologic study indicated that women under 25 ingesting OCs for more than 5 years with a high dose of certain gestagens, such as those used in the 1960s, may

Table 36-4
Relative risk* of breast cancer† with OC use

Time since first OC use (years)	Duration of OC use (years)					All ever-users
	<2	2–5	6–7	8–10	≥11	
<10	0.7	2.0	2.8	0.8		1.4
10–12	1.2	2.0	0.3	0.9	1.2	1.2
13–15	0.9	1.0	1.2	0.8	1.1	1.0
≥16	0.9	1.0	0.8	0.7	0.8	0.9
All	0.9	1.2	1.0	0.7	0.9	0.9

*Relative to never-users of OCs.

†By time since first OC use and duration of OC use. Excludes women with unknown duration of OC use.

Adapted from Centers for Disease Control Cancer and Steroid Hormone Study: Long-term oral contraceptive use and the risk of breast cancer. JAMA 249:1591, 1983.

have an increased risk of developing breast cancer.[19] In the same study, no increased risk was found in a similar group of young women ingesting formulations without high gestagenic potency.

Following the publication of that study, data from both the CDC study and the Boston Collaborative Drug Surveillance Program were analyzed thoroughly and were unable to confirm the results.[20] Both these studies, with much larger numbers of women, revealed no increased relative risk of breast cancer in women under the age of 25 taking any type of OC for more than 5 years. After careful analysis of all available data, the Advisory Committee to the US Food and Drug Administration recently concluded that a significant risk of breast cancer has not been demonstrated in any subgroup of OC users, or with any particular type of OC. The FDA agreed with these recommendations and has not advised a change in product labeling.

Endometrial cancer

There is no evidence of an increased incidence of carcinoma of the endometrium in OC users. In fact, data from several recently published epidemiologic studies, including the CASH study, indicate that women using OCs are less likely to develop cancer of the endometrium than are a

control group of women who do not use OCs.[21] The mistaken belief that OCs may increase the incidence of uterine cancer resulted from findings suggesting that postmenopausal women taking large doses of estrogen without gestagens for more than 5 years had an increased incidence of endometrial cancer when compared with postmenopausal women not taking estrogen. OCs contain estrogen, but they also contain a gestagen, and the gestagen counteracts the stimulatory effect of the estrogen on the endometrium. For estrogen to cause growth of the endometrium, it has to react with a receptor protein in the endometrial cell. Gestagens inhibit the synthesis of these estrogen receptors and thus, when given with an estrogen, prevent the estrogen's growth-promoting action. Several investigators have reported that when gestagens are given with estrogen to postmenopausal women, the combination is not associated with an increased incidence of endometrial cancer.

Cervical cancer

There is evidence from only one epidemiologic study (the Oxford study) that users of OCs have an increased incidence of cancer of the cervix.[16] In this and other epidemiologic studies, OC users have been found to have a higher incidence of cervical dysplasia (including carcinoma in

Contraception

situ), than women using other methods of contraception. Dysplasia, as well as epidermoid cancer of the cervix, has been linked with onset of sexual intercourse at a young age and with multiple sexual partners. Thus, women who began having sexual intercourse while young teenagers, and who have had a large number of sexual partners, have a greater chance of developing cervical dysplasia than women with fewer sexual partners and later onset of sexual activity.

In the studies showing a higher incidence of dysplasia in OC users than in controls using other contraceptive methods, it was also found that the OC users had more sexual partners and earlier onset of sexual activity. Thus, the studies determined not that the increased incidence of dysplasia was due to OC use, but that it most likely was due to other factors, including more sexual partners and more frequent cytologic screening among OC users, as well as increased protection provided by diaphragms or condoms used by some controls. A similar problem may have occurred in the Oxford study, which recently reported a significantly higher incidence of cervical cancer in OC users than in IUD users. The OC users may have had earlier onset of sexual activity than the IUD-using controls.

Liver tumors
Cancer of the liver is very uncommon in young women, and OC users do not have a greater chance of developing it. Women using OCs for

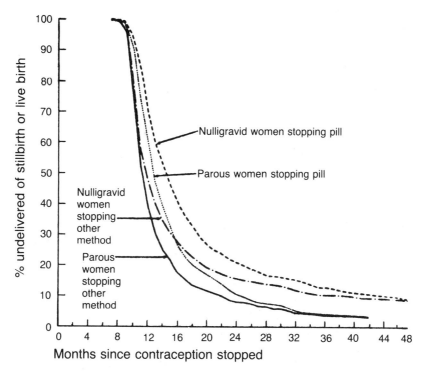

Figure 36-8
Fertility after stopping different methods of contraception in order to conceive.

From Vessey MP, Wright NH, McPherson K, et al: Fertility after stopping different methods of contraception. Br Med J 1:265, 1978.

more than 5 years appear to have a greater chance of developing benign liver adenomas. These tumors usually decrease in size and eventually disappear after OCs are discontinued. Thus, these adenomas, which occur in only about 1/30,000 to 1/50,000 OC users per year, are temporary and do not become malignant. In rare cases, however, they may rupture and cause life-threatening bleeding.

Effects on future reproduction

Although the rate of return of fertility in both nulligravid and parous women after stopping OCs is delayed when compared with women who stop using other contraceptive methods, such as the diaphragm or IUD, eventually the percentage of women who conceive after stopping all methods is the same. Thus, although OCs produce a period of temporary infertility in some women after discontinuation, this infertility usually is not permanent. As reported by the Oxford Family Planning Association study,[22] after a 2- to 3-year interval, fertility rates were the same among groups of former OC users and former users of other contraceptive methods (Figure 36-8).

In an attempt to determine whether the reproductive endocrine system recovers normally after cessation of OC therapy, we measured serum levels of FSH, LH, estradiol, progesterone, and prolactin in six women every day for 2 months after they discontinued use of OCs.[23] Except for a variable prolongation of the follicular phase of the first postcontraceptive cycle, the patterns and levels of all of these hormones were indistinguishable from those found in normal ovulating subjects (Figure 36-9). In these six women, the initial LH peak occurred from 21 to 28 days after ingestion of the last tablet. These results indicate that after a variable, but usually short, interval following the cessation of oral steroids, their suppressive effect on the hypothalamic-pituitary-ovarian axis disappears. Following the initial recovery, completely normal endocrine function occurs.

Since the resumption of ovulation is delayed for variable periods after OCs are stopped, it is difficult to estimate the expected date of delivery if conception takes place before spontaneous menses return. For this reason, when women stop OCs in order to conceive, it is probably best that they use barrier methods for about 1 to 2 months until regular cycles resume. If conception occurs before resumption of spontaneous menses, gestational age should be estimated by serial sonography.

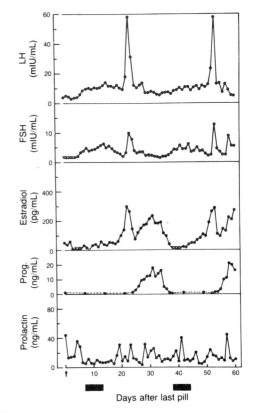

Figure 36-9
Serum levels of LH, FSH, estradiol, progesterone, and prolactin after discontinuation of OCs. Day of discontinuation is indicated by arrow. Shaded bars indicate menstruation.

From Klein TA, Mishell DR Jr: Gonadotropin, prolactin and steroid hormone levels after discontinuation of oral contraceptives. Am J Obstet Gynecol 127:585, 1977.

Contraception

The spontaneous abortion rate in women who conceive in the first or subsequent months after stopping OCs is the same as the rate in the general population or in women who stop using other contraceptive methods. An early study reported a high incidence of lethal chromosomal abnormalities in abortuses of women who conceived within a few months after stopping OCs. However, more recent studies have shown that the abortuses of women who did not use OCs had the same incidence of these chromosomal abnormalities.[24-25]

In several large studies of infants born to women who stopped using OCs, the infants had no increased risk of any type of birth defect.[26-30] The incidence of congenital anomalies was the same in infants born to former OC users as in infants born to women who had previously used other contraceptive methods or no method.

Cardiovascular disease

One problem with the retrospective case-control epidemiologic studies performed to determine drug risks is that they provide a figure called a relative risk or "times" rate. For example, in studies of OCs it has been stated that MI occurs three times more often in OC users than nonusers. Nevertheless, because young women rarely experience MI, in terms of absolute risk, the chance of MI occurring in any one woman is extremely low. Although the relative risk figure may seem frightening, the absolute risk figure is more important.

As another example, the relative risk of dying in an automobile accident is much higher if one drives frequently. Nevertheless, most people drive frequently because the absolute risk is so low. The three prospective studies of OC users mentioned above, which have been ongoing for more than 10 years, indicate that the absolute risk of any OC user developing cardiovascular disease is very low. In the US and UK, death rates for heart attacks have decreased in women aged 20 to 45 during the past 15 years—years in which OC use increased dramatically.[31] Furthermore, the decrease in heart attack death rates in these countries has been similar for men and women. If OCs, which are used by about 35% of women of this age group, were responsible for a great increase in the number of fatal heart attacks, one would expect that the decline in mortality rates would be different for men and women during this period.

Analysis of the latest results from the three prospective OC studies indicates that a significantly increased risk of developing cardiovascular disease occurs only in current OC users over 35 who smoke or in those of any age who have some type of preexisting vascular disease, such as hypertension, diabetes, or hypercholesterolemia (Tables 36-5 and 36-6).[16-17,32] There is no definitive evidence that nonsmokers under 45 and smokers under 35 who use OCs have a significantly increased chance of dying from a heart attack, provided they have no other vascular diseases. Thus, if a woman is under 35 and is a smoker, she can still use OCs, but she should be advised to discontinue smoking. Likewise, a woman between 35 and 45 can continue to use OCs, provided she does not smoke or have any other type of vascular disease such as hypertension, diabetes, or hypercholesterolemia.

Data from a recent study conducted in the state of Washington provide confirmation for these recommendations.[33] The morbidity of more than 10,000 healthy OC users and 30,000 healthy controls, ages 15 to 44, was analyzed for the periods 1977 to 1979 and 1980 to 1982. During the time of study, there were no heart attacks among OC users and one in controls. Only one of these healthy OC users and 14 controls suffered strokes. Although this study showed an increased risk of venous thromboembolism in OC users, there was no positive association between current OC use and stroke or MI.

A few years ago, there was some concern that duration of OC use should possibly be limited to 5 years, because analysis of mortality data

Table 36-5
Circulatory disease mortality rates (per 100,000 woman-years) by age, smoking status, and OC use

Age	Mortality rate (No. of deaths) Ever-users	Mortality rate (No. of deaths) Controls	Ever-users vs. controls (95% confidence limits) Relative risk
15–25			
Nonsmokers	0.0 (0)	0.0 (0)	
Smokers	10.5 (1)	0.0 (0)	
25–34			
Nonsmokers	4.4 (2)	2.7 (1)	1.6
Smokers	14.2 (6)	4.2 (1)	3.4
35–44			
Nonsmokers	21.5 (7)	6.4 (2)	3.3
Smokers	63.4 (18)	15.2 (3)	4.2*
45+			
Nonsmokers	52.4 (4)	11.4 (1)	4.6
Smokers	206.7 (17)	27.9 (2)	7.4*

*Significantly different.

Adapted from Royal College of General Practitioners' Oral Contraceptive Study: Further analysis of mortality in oral contraceptive users. Lancet 1:541, 1981.

Table 36-6
Walnut Creek Study: Effect of OC use on risk of diseases of the circulatory system

Disease	Standard rates Never used OCs	Standard rates Current OC users	Standard rates Past OC users	Relative risk Current OC users	Relative risk Past OC users
Acute MI	0.23	0.27	0.20	1.1	0.8
Ischemic heart disease	0.79	1.09	0.90	1.4	1.1
Subarachnoid hemorrhage	0.04	0.43	0.10	10.1*	2.3*
Cerebral thrombosis	0.24	0.53	0.29	2.2*	1.2
Arterial thrombosis	0.24	0.76	0.24	3.2*	1.0
Pulmonary embolism	0.38	0.22	0.29	0.6	0.0
Thrombophlebitis	0.51	0.42	0.48	0.8	1.8

*Not significantly different overall. Significantly different only in smokers over 40 years of age.

Adapted from Ramcharan S, Pellegrin FA, Ray RM, et al: The Walnut Creek Contraceptive Drug Study: A prospective study of the side effects of oral contraceptives, vol 3. NIH Pub. #81-564. Washington, DC, US Govt Printing Office, 1981.

from the RCGP study suggested an increased risk of dying from cardiovascular disease with longer durations. Recent data from the same study indicate that this concern was not valid, as the incidence of cardiovascular deaths did not increase with duration of use (Table 36-7).[32] This information, together with data from many other epidemiologic studies that show no increase in deaths from MI in former OC users, indicates that MI or stroke in OC users is due to arterial thrombosis, not atherosclerosis.

These thromboses occur mainly in women with narrowing of the arteries from cigarette smoking or other arterial disease such as that caused by hypertension, diabetes, or hypercholesterolemia. Despite data indicating that certain OC formulations decrease high-density lipoprotein (HDL) cholesterol and raise low-density lipoprotein (LDL) cholesterol (theoretically atherogenic changes), there is no evidence that long-term use of OCs produces an atherosclerotic or other permanent harmful effect on the blood vessels. Furthermore, the adverse lipid alterations produced by some formulations, especially those with high gestagen potency, are small and within the normal range. Although of theoretical concern, there are no data indicating that these small alterations increase the incidence of atherosclerosis in humans. Thus, women can take OCs for an unlimited period, no matter how old they are when they start. There also is no evidence that a rest period is needed after a few years of OC use. A rest period does not serve any purpose.

Other concerns

Another concern about OCs that has proven untrue is that vitamin supplements are necessary to compensate for OC-induced deficiencies. Although OCs slightly lower blood levels of the B-complex vitamins and vitamin C, these lower levels are not accompanied by any clinical evidence of deficiency. Supplementation is not necessary.

There has also been some concern that OCs

Table 36-7
Circulatory disease* mortality rates with OC use

Duration of OC use (months)	Rate (per 100,000 woman-years)	Relative risk
0	7.0 (10)	1.0
1–24	32.5 (5)	4.6
25–48	23.5 (4)	3.4
49–72	28.4 (5)	4.1
73–96	32.3 (5)	4.6
97+	20.4 (4)	2.9

*ICD 390–458.
From Royal College of General Practitioners' Oral Contraceptive Study: Further analysis of mortality in oral contraceptive users. Lancet 1:541, 1981.

should not be prescribed to young teenagers, because their use might produce permanent changes in the hypothalamic-pituitary-ovarian axis as well as premature epiphyseal closure, causing cessation of growth. Both these concerns have proven to be unfounded, and OCs can be used by women of any age who have started to have regular menstrual cycles.

Finally, there has been concern that OCs should not be taken by women with morphologic alterations of the vagina or uterus due to diethylstilbestrol (DES) exposure during fetal life. There is no evidence of an increase in cancer or other harmful alterations when OCs are ingested by women with adenosis or other genital tract changes due to antenatal DES exposure. Therefore, OCs can be used safely by these women.

Contraindications to OC use

OCs can be prescribed for the majority of women of reproductive age, because these women are young and generally healthy; however, there are certain absolute contraindications. These include a present or past history of vascular disease, including thromboembolism, thrombophlebitis, atherosclerosis, and stroke; or systemic disease that may affect the vascular system, such as lupus erythematosus or hemoglobin SS disease. Hypertension, diabetes mellitus with vascular disease, and hyperlipidemia are also contraindications, because OC use in women with these disorders can increase the risk of stroke or MI. One of the contraindications listed by the FDA is cancer of the breast or endometrium, although there are no data indicating OCs are harmful to women with these diseases.

Pregnant women should not ingest OCs because of the masculinizing effect of gestagens on the external genitalia of female fetuses. Concerns that OCs might produce other deleterious fetal effects, such as limb reduction and heart defects, have not proven valid. These concerns were raised by articles linking ingestion of any progestational agent in pregnancy to an increased incidence of congenital abnormalities. However, the major use of progestins in pregnancy has been for treatment of threatened abortion.[34] Bleeding in pregnancy is itself associated with an increased incidence of anomalies. The incidence of birth defects has not decreased since the use of progestins for threatened abortion has been discontinued. There is no definitive evidence that OC use per se during pregnancy increases the incidence of any fetal anomalies other than masculinization of the female external genitalia. This effect will not occur before 8 weeks of gestation.

Patients with functional heart disease should not use OCs, because the fluid retention they produce could result in congestive heart failure. There is no evidence, however, that individuals with a prolapsed mitral valve should not use OCs. Patients with active liver disease should not take OCs, because the steroids are metabolized in the liver. However, women who have recovered from liver disease, such as viral hepatitis, and whose liver function tests have returned to normal, can safely take OCs.

Relative contraindications to OC use include heavy cigarette smoking, migraine headaches, amenorrhea, and depression. Migraine headaches can be worsened by OC use, and patients who develop strokes while taking OCs frequently have an increased incidence of headaches of the migraine type, fainting, temporary loss of vision or speech, or paresthesias prior to the stroke. If any of these symptoms develop in an OC user, the use of OCs should be stopped.

Patients who are amenorrheic for a cause other than polycystic ovary syndrome should probably not take OCs, because a pituitary microadenoma may be present. OC use usually masks both amenorrhea and galactorrhea, the symptoms produced by enlargement of the adenoma. Thus, amenorrheic patients should not receive OCs until the diagnosis is established. OCs should be stopped if galactorrhea develops, and after 2 weeks, a serum prolactin level should be measured. If prolactin is elevated, further diagnostic evaluation, such as x-rays of the sella turcica, are indicated. A recent NIH study reported by the Pituitary Adenoma Study Group confirmed other findings that OCs do not produce prolactin secretory pituitary adenomas; the incidence of these tumors was the same in OC users and controls.[35] Patients with gestational diabetes can take low-dose OC formulations, because these low-dose gestagens do not affect glucose tolerance.

Starting OCs

Adolescents

In deciding whether a sexually active pubertal girl should use OCs for contraception, the clinician should be more concerned about compliance with the regimen than about possible physiologic harm. Provided she has demonstrated maturity of the hypothalamic-pituitary-ovarian axis with at least three regular, presumably ovulatory, menstrual cycles, it is safe to prescribe OCs without concern that permanent damage to the reproductive process will result. It is probably best not to prescribe OCs for women of any age with oligomenorrhea, except those with polycystic ovary syndrome, because of their increased likelihood of developing postpill amenorrhea. Oligomenorrhea is more frequent in adolescence than in later life. Postpill amenorrhea that lasts more than 6 months is not produced by OCs but becomes manifest after discontinuing OCs, because OCs will mask the development of the symptoms of amenorrhea. It is not necessary to be concerned about accelerating epiphyseal closure in the postmenarcheal female. Endogenous estrogens have already initiated the process a few years before menarche, and the contraceptive steroids will not hasten it.

Following pregnancy

The first episode of menstrual bleeding in the postabortal woman is usually preceded by ovulation. Following a term delivery, the first episode of bleeding is usually, but not always, anovulatory. Ovulation occurs sooner after an abortion, usually between 2 and 4 weeks, than after a term delivery, in which case ovulation is usually delayed beyond 6 weeks. But it may occur as early as 4 weeks after delivery in a woman who is not breast-feeding.

Thus, after spontaneous or induced abortion of a fetus of less than 12 weeks' gestation, OCs should be started immediately to prevent conception following the first ovulation. For patients who deliver after 28 weeks' gestation and are not nursing, the combination pills should be initiated 2 weeks after delivery. If pregnancy ends at between 21 and 28 weeks' gestation, OCs should be started 1 week later. The reason for delay in the latter two instances is that the normally increased risk of thromboembolism occurring in the postpartum period may be further enhanced by the hypercoagulable state associated with contraceptive steroid ingestion. As the first ovulation is delayed at least 4 weeks after a term delivery, there is no need to expose the patient to this enhanced risk.

It is probably best for nursing women to avoid combination OCs, because they appear to diminish the amount of breast milk produced.[36] Estrogen inhibits prolactin's action on the breast. Women who are breast-feeding every 4 hours, including at night, will not ovulate until at least 10 weeks after delivery and thus do not need contraception before then.[37] Since only a small percentage of breast-feeding women will ovulate as long as they continue full nursing, either a barrier method or the progestin-only OC can be used. The latter does not diminish the amount of breast milk and is effective in this group of women.

All patients

At the initial visit, after a history and physical examination have determined that there are no medical contraindications to OCs, the patient should be informed about the benefits and risks. For medicolegal reasons, it is best to use a written informed consent signed by the patient and to note on the patient's medical record that benefits and risks have been explained to her.

Choice of formulation

It is best initially to prescribe a formulation containing 30 or 35 μg of ethinylestradiol. Data from Sweden demonstrate that as the dosage of estrogen in the formulation has decreased, there has been a concomitant decrease in the incidence of thromboembolism.[38] A study from the UK showed that the increase in levels of serum globulins, including angiotensinogen and those involved with coagulation, is also directly related to the dose of estrogen administered.[14] In the same study, the incidence of total deaths, as well as deaths due to arterial causes alone, was significantly decreased in patients using formulations with 30 μg of ethinylestradiol, as compared with 50 μg. Furthermore, the incidence of ischemic heart disease and stroke was significantly decreased in women using the lower-dose estrogen formulations (Table 36-8)[39].

There is some indication from the RCGP study that the incidence of total arterial disease in OC users is related to the dose of gestagen when the estrogen dosage is unchanged. For this reason, it would appear reasonable to use formulations with the lowest dosage of a particular gestagen, as well as low estrogen dosage. The new multiphasic formulations have less total steroid per cycle with the same incidence of breakthrough bleeding as the fixed-dose formulations. Theoretically, they should be safer.

Evidence that some highly gestagenic formulations lower HDL cholesterol levels more than others has caused concern that they may also increase the risk of MI more than other formulations. However, there is no evidence that artificially lowering or raising HDL cholesterol levels in humans affects the incidence of MI, and the alterations in HDL cholesterol produced by OCs are minimal. Furthermore, as noted above, the cause of OC-related MI appears to be thrombotic, not atherosclerotic, as the risk is not increased in ex-users and is not related to duration of use. The FDA has stated that the product prescribed should be one containing the least amount of estrogen and gestagen compatible with a low failure rate and the needs of the individual patient. Use of the new multiphasic products, with lower total steroid dosage per cycle than the fixed-dose OCs, should help achieve this goal.

The contraceptive formulations containing gestagens without estrogen are associated with a lower incidence of adverse metabolic effects. Since the factors that predispose to thromboembolism are caused by the estrogenic component, the incidence of thromboembolism is not increased in women taking gestagen-only agents. Furthermore, blood pressure is not affected, nausea and breast tenderness are eliminated, and, in lactating women, milk production and quality are unchanged. Despite these advantages, the gestagen-only agents are associated with a high frequency of intermenstrual and other abnormal bleeding patterns, including amenorrhea, and a lower rate of effectiveness, all of which limit their use. The actual use-failure rate of these agents has been reported to vary between 2% and 8% per year, and a relatively high percentage of the resulting pregnancies are ectopic.[13]

As mentioned above, one indication for prescribing gestagen-only OCs is concomitant breast-feeding by a mother who desires oral contraception. Since these women have reduced fertility and are amenorrheic, the major disadvantages are minimized. Furthermore, the production and quality of the breast milk are unaffected, in contrast with the changes produced by combination pills. However, a small portion of the synthetic steroid has been detected in the breast milk of women taking gestagens. The long-term effects, if any, on the infant are not known, but appear to be nonexistent. Although theoretically one must be concerned about prescribing any synthetic steroids to a nursing mother, the use of gestagen-only OCs does not appear to be harmful to the infant.

Follow-up

If the patient has no contraindications to OC use, the only routine laboratory tests indicated at the initial visit are a complete blood count, urinalysis, and Pap smear. At the end of 3 months, the patient should be seen again; at this time, a nondirected history should be obtained and the blood pressure measured. After this visit, the patient should be seen annually; a nondirected history should again be taken; blood pressure and body weight measured; a physical examination, including a breast, abdominal, and pelvic examination done; and a Pap smear performed.

It is important to perform annual Pap smears on OC users, because they constitute a

Table 36-8
Ratio of observed to expected events by estrogen dose, in UK (1974 to 1977)

Event	Ethinylestradiol 50 μg	Ethinylestradiol 30 μg
Venous deaths	1.40	0.65
Nonvenous deaths	1.52	0.53*
Ischemic heart disease	1.48	0.54*
Stroke	1.20	0.80
Pregnancy	0.62	1.33*

*$P < 0.05$

Adapted from Meade TW, Greenberg G, Thompson SG: Progestogens and cardiovascular reactions associated with oral contraceptives and a comparison of the safety of 50- and 30-μg estrogen preparations. Br Med J 280:1157, 1980.

relatively high-risk group for development of cervical neoplasia. The routine use of other laboratory tests is not indicated, unless the patient is over 35 or has a family history of diabetes or vascular disease. For patients over 35 who wish to continue taking OCs, it is advisable to obtain a lipid panel, including HDL and LDL cholesterol, total cholesterol, and triglycerides. If the lipid levels are abnormal, another method of contraception may be safer. Because of the increased incidence of diabetes after age 35, a 2-hour postprandial blood glucose should also be obtained; if this is elevated, a full glucose tolerance test should be performed. If results of this test are abnormal, the OCs should probably be stopped.

Routine use of these tests in women under 35 is not indicated, because the incidence of positive results is extremely low. However, if the patient has a family history of vascular disease, such as MI in a family member under the age of 50, it would be advisable to obtain a lipid panel before and after starting OCs. A patient of any age with a family history of diabetes, or evidence of diabetes during pregnancy, should be tested with a 2-hour postprandial blood glucose measurement both before and after starting OCs. In patients with a past history of liver disease, a liver panel should be obtained to make certain that liver function is normal before starting OCs.

Drug interactions

Although synthetic sex steroids can retard the biotransformation of certain drugs, such as antipyrine and meperidine, through substrate competition, such interference is not important clinically. Otherwise, OC use has not been shown to inhibit drug action. However, some drugs can clinically interfere with the action of the OCs by inducing liver enzymes that convert the steroids to more polar and less biologically active metabolites. Certain drugs have been shown to accelerate the biotransformation of steroids in the human. These include barbiturates, sulfonamides, cyclophosphamide, and rifampicin. Several investigators have reported a relatively high incidence of OC failure in women ingesting rifampicin, and OCs and rifampicin should not be given concurrently.[40]

The clinical data concerning OC failure in users of antibiotics other than rifampicin (such as penicillin, ampicillin, and sulfonamides), and in users of analgesics and barbiturates, are less clear. A few anecdotal studies have appeared in the literature, but reliable evidence for a clinical inhibitory effect, such as occurs with rifampicin, is not available. Until controlled studies are performed, it would appear prudent to suggest use of a barrier method in addition to the OCs when antibiotics are given simultaneously. Women with epilepsy requiring medication are best treated with 50-μg estrogen formulations, because a high incidence of bleeding irregularities has been reported in these women with the use of lower-dose estrogen formulations.[41]

Noncontraceptive health benefits

In addition to being the most effective nonsurgical contraceptive method, and thus preventing the medical problems associated with pregnancies, OCs provide several other health benefits.[42] Some are due to the fact that the combination OCs contain a potent, orally active gestagen, as well as an orally active estrogen. Since the same two steroids are ingested throughout the cycle, and since endogenous estradiol secretion is markedly suppressed, there is no time when the estrogenic target tissues are stimulated by estrogen without gestagen (unopposed estrogen).

Antiestrogenic effect of progestins

It has been known for many years that both natural progesterone and the synthetic progestins inhibit the proliferative effect of estrogen, the so-called antiestrogenic effect. Recent studies have elucidated the mechanism of this effect. Estrogens increase the synthesis of both estrogen and progesterone receptors, whereas progesterone decreases their synthesis. Thus, one mechanism of progesterone's antiestrogenic effect is decreased estrogen receptor synthesis. Relatively little progestin is needed to do this, and the amount present in OCs is sufficient. Another way progesterone produces its antiestrogenic effect is by stimulating the activity of the enzyme 17β-estradiol dehydrogenase within the endometrial cell. This enzyme converts the more potent estrogen, estradiol, to the less potent estrone, reducing intracellular estrogenic action.

As a result of the antiestrogenic action of the progestins in OCs, the height of the endometrium is less than in an ovulatory cycle, and there is less proliferation of the glandular epithelium. These changes produce several substantial benefits for the OC user. One is a reduction in blood loss at the time of endometrial shedding. In an ovulatory cycle the mean blood loss during menstruation is about 35 mL, compared with 20 mL for women ingesting OCs. This decreased blood loss makes iron-deficiency anemia less likely. Data from the RCGP study showed that users of OCs were about half as likely to develop iron-deficiency anemia as were controls.[15] Moreover, the beneficial effect persisted to a similar degree in women who had previously used OCs, proba-

Table 36-9
Relationship between OC use and incidence of iron-deficiency anemia

OC use	Rate (per 1,000 woman-years)	Relative risk
Current	5.67	0.58*
Ever	5.44	0.56*
Never	9.77	1.0

*P < 0.01.

From Royal College of General Practitioners: Oral Contraceptives and Health. An Interim Report from the Oral Contraceptive Study of the Royal College of General Practitioners. New York, Pitman Medical Publishing, 1974.

bly because of an increase in the iron stores that remained for several years after the drug was discontinued (Table 36-9).

Since the OCs produce regular withdrawal bleeding, it would be expected that OC users would have fewer menstrual disorders than nonusers. The results of the RCGP study confirmed the fact that OC users were significantly less likely to develop menorrhagia, irregular menstruation, or intermenstrual bleeding (Table 36-10).[15] Because these disorders are frequently treated by curettage, OC users require this procedure less frequently.

Since progestins inhibit the proliferative effect of estrogens on the endometrium, their constant ingestion should reduce the incidence of endometrial hyperplasia. This condition occurs mainly in anovulatory women as a result of the unopposed action of estrogen. Because women with unopposed endogenous or exogenous estrogen also have an increased incidence of endometrial adenocarcinoma, it is not surprising that OC users have been found significantly less likely to develop this estrogen-stimulated cancer. Data from several retrospective case-control studies, including the CASH study, indicate that the relative risk of endometrial cancer among OC users was only half that of controls (Table 36-11).[21] The protective effect of OCs increased the longer these agents were used, and the reduced risk of endometrial cancer persisted for at

Contraception

Table 36-10
Relationship between OC use and incidence of menstrual disorders

Menstrual disorder	Rate (per 1,000 woman-years)		
	OC users	Controls (No.)	Relative risk
Menorrhagia	12.48	23.82 (1,004)	0.52*
Irregular menses	5.19	13.08 (326)	0.65*
Intermenstrual bleeding	3.04	5.26 (178)	0.72*

*$P < 0.01$.

From Royal College of General Practitioners: Oral Contraceptives and Health. An Interim Report from the Oral Contraceptive Study of the Royal College of General Practitioners. New York, Pitman Medical Publishing, 1974.

Table 36-11
Risk of endometrial cancer by duration of OC use

Duration of OC use (years)	Cases*	Controls*	Relative risk (95% confidence interval)†
Never	99	540	1.0 (referent)
<1	33	175	1.1 (0.7–1.8)
1–5	16	266	0.4 (0.2–0.7)
>5	21	251	0.6 (0.4–0.9)
Total	169	1,232	

Excludes 14 cases and 60 controls with history of sequential OC use and 4 cases and 28 controls with unknown duration of OC use.

†*Standardized for age. Test for trend with referent category equals less than 1 year of OC use; $X^2 = -3.055$; P (two-tailed) = 0.002. Less than 1 year of OC use means 1 to 11 months of use.*

From Centers for Disease Control Cancer and Steroid Hormone Study: Oral contraceptive use and the risk of endometrial cancer. JAMA 249:1600, 1983.

least 5 years after treatment was discontinued.

Estrogen exerts a proliferative effect on breast tissue, which also contains estrogen receptors. Progestins probably inhibit the synthesis of estrogen receptors in this tissue as well, producing an antiestrogenic action on the breast. At least 10 published studies have shown that OCs reduce the incidence of benign breast disease, and two prospective studies have indicated that this reduction is directly related to the amount of progestin in the formulations.

Data from the 1974 RCGP study revealed a significantly decreased incidence of chronic cystic breast disease, but not of fibroadenomas, among users of OCs. This reduced incidence became apparent after 2 years of OC use, and a further reduction was reported with increasing use.[15] A prospective study beginning in 1970 in Boston also found a significant reduction in fibrocystic disease, but not fibroadenomas, among OC users compared with controls. The reduced risk developed after 1 to 2 years of OC use. Women taking OCs for more than 2 years had a 65% reduction in the incidence of fibrocystic disease and a nonsignificant 50% reduction in the incidence of fibroadenomas.[43]

Data from the Oxford study indicate that three types of benign breast disease were found

Table 36-12
Relative risk of benign breast disease

OC use	Fibroadenoma	Cystic disease	Breast lumps	Other
Never	1.00 (49)	1.00 (113)	1.00 (169)	1.00 (34)
Ever	0.35 (25)*	0.66 (101)*	0.58 (162)*	0.63 (36)
Current	0.16 (7)*	0.47 (41)*	0.52 (77)*	0.60 (21)

*$P < 0.01$.

From Brinton LA, Vessey MP, Flavel R, et al: Risk factors for benign breast disease. Am J Epidemiol 113:203, 1981 (Oxford Family Planning Study).

significantly more frequently among controls than among OC users.[44] The largest reduction in risk occurred for fibroadenomas, where the relative risk was 0.35, or 65% reduction. Low risks were also discovered for chronic cystic breast disease, 0.66, a 34% reduction, and nonbiopsied breast lumps, 0.58, a 42% reduction (Table 36-12). Current users of OCs were at lowest risk of developing benign breast disease, with a significant reduction of 84% for fibroadenomas, 53% for chronic cystic disease, 48% for nonbiopsied breast lumps, and a nonsignificant reduction of 40% for other breast diseases. The first three categories showed decreased risk with increasing duration of OC use. After 6 or more years of use, there was a 50% reduction in these three categories of benign breast disease. This reduced risk persisted for about 1 year following discontinuation of OCs, after which no reduction was observed.

Inhibition of ovulation

Other noncontraceptive health benefits of OCs result from their main action, inhibition of ovulation. The occurrence of ovulatory menstrual cycles throughout most of a woman's reproductive years is a relatively recent phenomenon. A few generations ago, most of a woman's reproductive years were anovulatory because she was either pregnant or lactating. Thus, what has been termed "incessant ovulation" is really a result of modern civilization. Some disorders, such as dysmenorrhea and premenstrual tension, oc-

cur much more frequently in ovulatory than anovulatory cycles. In fact, inhibition of ovulation by exogenous steroids has been used as therapy for severe dysmenorrhea for decades. The 1974 report of the RCGP study showed that OC users had 63% less dysmenorrhea and 29% less premenstrual tension than controls.[15]

Another serious adverse effect that can result from ovulatory menstrual cycles is the development of functional ovarian cysts, specifically, follicular and luteal cysts, which frequently require laparotomy because of enlargement, rupture, or hemorrhage. When ovulation is inhibited, functional cysts do not usually develop. The RCGP study found the incidence of benign ovarian neoplasms to be reduced by 64%.[15] In a survey performed by the Boston Collaborative Drug Surveillance Program, fewer than 2% of women with a discharge diagnosis of functional ovarian cysts were taking OCs, in contrast with 20% of a control group of women of similar age hospitalized without ovarian cysts.[45] In contrast, 20% of women with nonfunctional cysts were taking OCs, an incidence similar to that observed in the controls (Table 36-13).

Another disorder linked with incessant ovulation is ovarian cancer. Several case-control studies have shown that the risk of ovarian cancer decreases as the number of pregnancies increases; one study reported that the incidence of ovarian cancer correlated inversely with the number of children born.[46] Trauma to the ovarian surface epithelium produced by incessant

Table 36-13
Surgically removed ovarian cysts in OC users

	Controls (n = 842)	Functional cysts (n = 60)	Nonfunctional cysts (n = 70)
OC users	170 (20%)	1 (1.7%)	14 (20%)
Relative risk	1.0	0.07*	1.0

*P < 0.02.

Data from the Boston Collaborative Drug Surveillance Program (24 hospitals).

From Ory HW: Functional ovarian cysts and oral contraceptives. JAMA 228:68, 1974.

Table 36-14
Duration of OC use and risk of ovarian cancer

Duration of OC use	Cases	Controls	Relative risk (95% confidence interval)*
None	86	683	1.0 (referent)
Ever-use†	90	921	0.6 (0.4–0.9)
<3 mo	16	106	1.0 (0.5–1.9)
3–11 mo	13	133	0.7 (0.4–1.4)
1–2 yr	32	213	0.8 (0.5–1.4)
3–4 yr	12	137	0.5 (0.2–1.0)
≥5	17	332	0.4 (0.2–0.6)

*Standardized by age. Test for trend, never-users excluded, $X^2 = 3.20$ and $P = 0.002$, two-tailed.

†Excludes three cases and 38 controls with unknown duration of OC use.

From Centers for Disease Control Cancer and Steroid Hormone Study: Oral contraceptive use and the risk of ovarian cancer. JAMA 249:1596, 1983.

ovulation may, in some way, contribute to the development of ovarian cancer. Data from another case-control study indicated that the relative risk of ovarian cancer decreased as the number of live births and incomplete pregnancies as well as OC use increased.[46] When the anovulatory years from all three factors were added, the decreased relative risk was statistically significant. The protective effect of OCs was about the same as pregnancy with 12 months of OC use; i.e., a year of OC use was about equivalent to one live birth in degree of protection. Several recent case-control studies, including the CASH study, reported that the risk of ovarian cancer in OC users was only about half as great as in nonusers. This protection persisted for at least 10 years after OCs were stopped (Table 36-14).[47]

Other benefits

The RCGP study showed that the risk of rheumatoid arthritis in OC users was only about half the risk in controls. Additional evidence of this protective effect was obtained from the Rochester (Minnesota) Epidemiologic Program Project, which showed that the incidence of rheumatoid arthritis increased from 1950 to 1964 in men and women but declined in women after that date with no decline in men.[48] This decline occurred during the time when OC use increased in the US. However, some recent reports have failed to confirm OCs' protective effect against rheumatoid arthritis.

Another benefit of OC use is protection against salpingitis, commonly referred to as pelvic inflammatory disease (PID). There have

Table 36-15
Hospitalizations prevented annually by OC use

Disease	Rate (per 100,000 pill users)	No. of hospitalizations*
Benign breast disease	235	20,000
Ovarian retention cysts	35	3,000
Iron-deficiency anemia†	320	27,200
Pelvic inflammatory disease (first episodes)		
Total episodes†	600	51,000
Hospitalizations	156	13,300
Ectopic pregnancy	117	9,900
Rheumatoid arthritis†	32	2,700
Endometrial cancer‡	5	2,000
Ovarian cancer‡	4	1,700

*Except where noted, figures refer to hospitalizations prevented among the estimated 8.5 million current OC users in the US.

†Episodes prevented regardless of whether hospitalizations occurred.

‡Based on an estimated 39 million US women who have ever used OCs.

From Ory HW: The noncontraceptive health benefits from oral contraceptive use. Fam Plan Perspect 14:182, 1982.

been at least 11 published epidemiologic studies estimating the relative risk among OC users of developing PID. Seven of these studies compared OC use with nonuse of any other contraception. The relative risk of PID among OC users in most of these studies was about 0.5. The largest study analyzing PID in OC users was the RCGP study, which reported that the rate of PID in OC users was reduced about 50%.[15] A recent CDC study also reported that the relative risk of PID among all OC users was 0.5, decreasing to 0.3 after 1 year of OC use.[49]

It has been estimated that about 15% of women with cervical gonorrheal infection will develop salpingitis. In a Swedish study of women with cervical gonorrhea, investigators were able to confirm all cases of suspected salpingitis by laparoscopic visualization 1 day after admission.[50] Of those who used contraception other than the IUD and oral steroids, 15% developed salpingitis; only about half as many (8.8%) of those who used OCs developed salpingitis. The results of this study indicate that OCs reduce the clinical development of salpingitis in women in-

fected with gonorrhea. This protection may be related to the decreased duration of menstrual flow, which permits a smaller number of gonococcal organisms to ascend to the upper genital tract and allows the body's defenses to eliminate them more easily.

Data were compared on the use of contraceptives and the incidence of PID among 20- to 29-year-old women in Lund, Sweden, between 1970 and 1974.[51] Among sexually active women using no contraception, the rate of PID was 3.42/100 woman-years, whereas in OC users the rate of PID was only 0.91/100 woman-years. Increased use of OCs by the population at greatest risk—sexually active women between 15 and 24 years of age—would greatly reduce the incidence of this disease with its high cost of treatment and resultant infertility. One of the sequelae of PID is ectopic pregnancy, an entity that has tripled in incidence in the past decade. OCs reduce the risk of ectopic pregnancy by more than 90% among current users and may reduce the incidence in former users by decreasing their chance of developing salpingitis.

To summarize these benefits, it was recently estimated that OC use will prevent 320 cases of iron-deficiency anemia, 32 cases of rheumatoid arthritis, and 600 cases of PID per 100,000 OC users in the US each year.[52] There will be an estimated 156 fewer women hospitalized for PID, 235 fewer hospitalized for breast disease, 35 fewer hospitalized for ovarian tumors, and 117 fewer hospitalized for ectopic pregnancies (Table 36-15). It is also estimated that about 1/750 OC users per year will not develop a serious disease that would otherwise have developed and that OC use prevents 50,000 women from being hospitalized in the US each year. It is unfortunate that the infrequent adverse effects of OCs receive widespread publicity, while information about their more common noncontraceptive health benefits attracts little attention.

References

1. Mosher WD: Vital and health statistics, Series 23. Data from the National Survey of Family Growth, No 7. DHHS Pub PHS 81-1983

2. Bachrach CA: Contraceptive practice among American women, 1973-1982. *Fam Plan Perspect* 16:253, 1984

3. Swyer GIM: Potency of progestogens in oral contraceptives—further delay of menses data. *Contraception* 26:23, 1982

4. Ferin J: Orally active progestational compounds. Human studies: Effects on the utero-vaginal tract. In *International Encyclopedia of Pharmacology and Therapeutics*, vol 2, ch 30. Oxford, Pergamon Press, 1972

5. Grant ECG: Hormone balance of oral contraceptives. *J Obstet Gynaecol Br Commonw* 74:908, 1967

6. Dorflinger L: Relative potency of progestins used in oral contraceptives. *Contraception* 31:557, 1985

7. Brenner PF, Mishell DR Jr, Stanczyk FZ, et al: Serum levels of d-norgestrel, luteinizing hormone, follicle-stimulating hormone, estradiol, and progesterone in women during and following ingestion of combination oral contraceptives containing dl-norgestrel. *Am J Obstet Gynecol* 129:133, 1977

8. Mishell DR Jr, Stanczyk F, Hiroi M, et al: Steroid contraception. In Crosignani PG, Mishell DR Jr (eds): *Ovulation in the Human*. London, Academic Press, 1976

9. Mishell DR Jr, Thorneycroft IH, Nakamura RM, et al: Serum estradiol in women ingesting combination oral contraceptive steroids. *Am J Obstet Gynecol* 114:923, 1972

10. Mishell DR Jr, Kletzky OA, Brenner PF, et al: The effect of contraceptive steroids on hypothalamic-pituitary function. *Am J Obstet Gynecol* 128:60, 1977

11. Scott JA, Brenner PF, Kletzky OA, et al: Factors affecting pituitary gonadotropin function in users of oral contraceptive steroids. *Am J Obstet Gynecol* 130:817, 1978

12. Scott JZ, Kletzky OA, Brenner PF, et al: Comparison of the effects of contraceptive steroid formulations containing two doses of estrogen on pituitary function. *Fertil Steril* 30:141, 1978

13. World Health Organization Task Force on Oral Contraceptives: A randomized, double-blind study of two combined and two progestogen-only oral contraceptives. *Contraception* 25:243, 1982

14. Meade TW: Oral contraceptives, clotting factors, and thrombosis. *Am J Obstet Gynecol* 142:758, 1982

15. Royal College of General Practitioners: *Oral Contraceptives and Health. An Interim Report from the Oral Contraceptive Study of the Royal College of General Practitioners.* New York, Pitman Medical Publishing, 1974

16. Vessey M, Doll R, Peto R, et al: A long-term follow-up study of women using different methods of contraception—an interim report. *J Biosoc Sci* 8:373, 1976

17. Ramcharan S, Pellegrin FA, Ray RM, et al: The Walnut Creek Contraceptive Drug Study: A prospective study of the side effects of oral contraceptives, vol 3. NIH Pub #81-564. Washington, DC, US Govt Printing Office, 1981, p 349

18. Centers for Disease Control Cancer and Steroid Hormone Study: Long-term oral contraceptive use and the risk of breast cancer. *JAMA* 249:1591, 1983

19. Pike MC, Henderson BE, Krailo MD, et al: Breast cancer in young women and use of oral contraceptives: Possible modifying effect of formulation and age at use. *Lancet* 2:926, 1983

20. Centers for Disease Control: OC use and the risk of breast cancer in young women. *MMWR* 33:353, 1984

21. Centers for Disease Control Cancer and Steroid Hormone Study: Oral contraceptive use and the risk of endometrial cancer. *JAMA* 249:1600, 1983

22. Vessey MP, Wright NH, McPherson K, et al: Fertility after stopping different methods of contraception. *Br Med J* 1:265, 1978

23. Klein TA, Mishell DR Jr: Gonadotropin, prolactin and steroid hormone levels after discontinuation of oral contraceptives. *Am J Obstet Gynecol* 127:585, 1977

24. Jacobsen C: Cytogenic study of immediate post contraceptive abortion. Report of a study under Food and Drug Administration contract, 1974

25. Vosbeck E: Cytogenic, morphological and clinical aspects of 453 cases of human spontaneous abortions. PhD dissertation, George Washington University School of Graduate Studies, 1975

26. Harlap S, Davies AM: The pill and births: The

Jerusalem Study. 2. Tables. Final Report. Rockville, Md, National Institute of Child Health and Development, January 1978, p 119

27. Rothman KJ, Louik C: Oral contraceptives and birth defects. *N Engl J Med* 299:522, 1978

28. Royal College of General Practitioners' Oral Contraceptive Study: The outcome of pregnancy in former oral contraceptive users. *Br J Obstet Gynaecol* 83:608, 1976

29. Vessey M, Meisler L, Flavel R, et al: Outcome of pregnancy in women using different methods of contraception. *Br J Obstet Gynaecol* 86:548, 1979

30. Janerich DT, Piper JM, Glebatis DM: Oral contraceptives and birth defects. *Am J Epidemiol* 112:73, 1980

31. Beral V: Cardiovascular-disease mortality trends and oral-contraceptive use in young women. *Lancet* 2:1047, 1976

32. Royal College of General Practitioners' Oral Contraceptive Study: Further analysis of mortality in oral contraceptive users. *Lancet* 1:541, 1981

33. Porter JB, Hunter JR, Danielson DA, et al: Oral contraceptives and nonfatal vascular disease—recent experience. *Obstet Gynecol* 59:299, 1982

34. Wilson JG, Brent RL: Are female sex hormones teratogenic? *Am J Obstet Gynecol* 141:567, 1981

35. Pituitary Adenoma Study Group: Pituitary adenomas and oral contraceptives: A multi-center case-control study. *Fertil Steril* 39:753, 1983

36. World Health Organization Task Force on Oral Contraceptives: Effects of hormonal contraceptives on milk volume and infant growth. *Contraception* 30:505, 1984

37. Perez A, Vela P, Masnick GS, et al: First ovulation after childbirth: The effect of breast-feeding. *Am J Obstet Gynecol* 114:1041, 1972

38. Böttiger LE, Boman G, Eklund G, et al: Oral contraceptives and thromboembolic disease: Effects of lowering oestrogen content. *Lancet* 1:1097, 1980

39. Meade TW, Greenberg G, Thompson SG: Progestogens and cardiovascular reactions associated with oral contraceptives and a comparison of the safety of 50- and 30-μg estrogen preparations. *Br Med J* 280:1157, 1980

40. Back DJ, Breckenridge AM, Crawford FE, et al: The effects of rifampicin on the pharmacokinetics of ethinylestradiol in women. *Contraception* 21:135, 1980

41. Diamond MP, Greene JW, Thompson JM, et al: Interaction of anticonvulsants and oral contraceptives in epileptic adolescents. *Contraception* 31:623, 1985

42. Mishell DR Jr: Noncontraceptive health benefits of oral steroidal contraceptives. *Am J Obstet Gynecol* 142:809, 1982

43. Ory H, Cole P, Mac Mahon B, et al: Oral contraceptives and reduced incidence of benign breast disease. *N Engl J Med* 294:419, 1976

44. Brinton LA, Vessey MP, Flavel R, et al: Risk factors for benign breast disease. *Am J Epidemiol* 113:203, 1981

45. Ory HW: Functional ovarian cysts and oral contraceptives. *JAMA* 228:68, 1974

46. Casagrande JT, Louie EW, Pike MC, et al: "Incessant ovulation" and ovarian cancer. *Lancet* 2:170, 1979

47. Centers for Disease Control Cancer and Steroid Hormone Study: Oral contraceptive use and the risk of ovarian cancer. *JAMA* 249:1596, 1983

48. Linos A, Worthington JW, O'Fallon WM, et al: The epidemiology of rheumatoid arthritis in Rochester, Minnesota: A study of incidence, prevalence, and mortality. *Am J Epidemiol* 111:87, 1980

49. Rubin GL, Ory HW, Layde PM: Oral contraceptives and pelvic inflammatory disease. *Am J Obstet Gynecol* 144:630, 1982

50. Rydén G, Fahraeus L, Molin L, et al: Do contraceptives influence the incidence of acute pelvic inflammatory disease in women with gonorrhoea? *Contraception* 20:149, 1979

51. Weström L: Incidence, prevalence, and trends of acute pelvic inflammatory disease and its consequences in industrialized countries. *Am J Obstet Gynecol* 138:880, 1980

52. Ory HW: The noncontraceptive health benefits from oral contraceptive use. *Fam Plan Perspect* 14:182, 1982

Chapter 37

Long-Acting Contraceptive Steroids and Interception

Daniel R. Mishell Jr., M.D.

Oral contraceptives in current use need to be ingested daily. In many countries, as well as in the US, it would be advantageous to provide methods of administering contraceptive steroid formulations at infrequent intervals. To be acceptable, these long-acting formulations should be as effective as the daily orally administered steroids and have a lower incidence of undesirable side effects. Thus far, three types of long-acting steroid formulations have been developed and undergone clinical testing. This chapter reviews the current status of the three methods—injectable suspensions, subdermal polysiloxane capsules, and vaginal polysiloxane rings—and also discusses postcoital contraception (interception).

Injectable suspensions

Depo-medroxyprogesterone acetate

Several injectable steroid formulations are currently in use for contraception throughout the world. Of these, depo-medroxyprogesterone acetate (DMPA) is the most widely used and the most studied. More than 500 scientific articles have been written about it since it was first made available for contraceptive use 20 years ago. More than 11 million women have used DMPA, and currently there are more than 2 million users in the world. It is approved for use as a contraceptive in more than 50 countries, including Sweden and the United Kingdom, but not the US. Currently, in the US, the drug is approved only for the treatment of endometrial cancer; however, with physician and patient consent it can be used for contraception.

DMPA is extremely effective. The failure rates in various studies range from 0.0 to 1.2 per 100 woman-years. In a recent World Health Organization (WHO) multiclinic study of 1,587 users of DMPA, the failure rate at the end of 1 year was only 0.1%, and at the end of 2 years, 0.4%.[1]

DMPA is formulated as a crystalline suspension. It should be given by injection in the upper outer quadrant of the gluteal region. The area should not be massaged, so that the drug is released slowly into the circulation. Administering the drug by this method should result in a very low failure rate.

We measured serum levels of MPA as well as estradiol and progesterone in three women at frequent intervals for 7 to 9 months after injec-

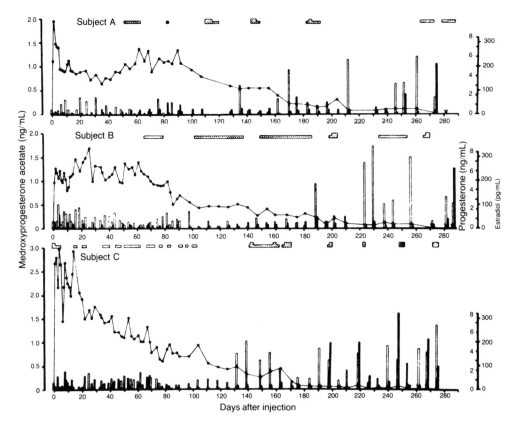

Figure 37-1
Serum medroxyprogesterone acetate (MPA, dots), estradiol (open bars), and progesterone (solid bars) concentrations in three women (subjects A, B, and C) following IM injection of 150 mg of DMPA. Uterine bleeding and spotting are indicated by hatched horizontal bars of full and half thickness, respectively. Undetectable levels of MPA are indicated by V.

From Ortiz A, Hiroi M, Stanczyk FZ, et al: Serum medroxyprogesterone acetate (MPA) concentrations and ovarian function following intramuscular injection of depo-MPA. J Clin Endocrinol Metab 44:32, 1977.

tion of 150 mg of DMPA.[2] For a few days after the injection, MPA levels in the serum ranged from 1.5 to 3 ng/mL. Thereafter, MPA levels gradually declined, but remained relatively constant at about 1 ng/mL for 2 to 3 months. They declined gradually thereafter, reaching 0.2 ng/mL during the sixth month, and they became undetectable about 7½ to 9 months following administration (Figure 37-1).[2]

Serum estradiol levels remained at early fol-licular phase levels for 4 to 6 months after the DMPA injection. When serum levels of MPA fell below 0.5 ng/mL, estradiol rose to preovulatory levels. Ovulation, however, as evidenced by elevated serum progesterone levels, did not occur, apparently because the luteinizing hormone (LH) peak was suppressed by positive feedback inhibition. When serum MPA levels fell below 0.1 ng/mL, about 7 to 9 months after the injection, cyclic ovulatory ovarian function resumed.

Thus, the delay in ovulation after receiving injections of DMPA is due to prolonged MPA release and persists until serum levels of MPA become very low. The time required for the drug to disappear from serum after the last of several injections should be approximately the same as that following a single injection, because MPA is rapidly cleared from the bloodstream. The prolonged presence in serum is related to the slow release from the injection site.

MPA acts by inhibiting the midcycle gonadotropin surge. Levels of LH and follicle-stimulating hormone (FSH) remain in the follicular-phase range and are not completely suppressed. Mean estradiol levels remain relatively constant, about 40 pg/mL, for up to 5 years of treatment (Figure 37-2).[3] These estradiol levels are higher than menopausal levels, and patients receiving DMPA do not develop signs or symptoms of estrogen deficiency.

We examined a group of patients 1 to 5 years after initiation of DMPA therapy and none of them had evidence of vaginal atrophy or objective or subjective changes in breast size. Patients do not develop hot flushes or have increased urinary excretion of calcium while receiving DMPA. On the contrary, it has been shown that DMPA is effective therapy for amelioration of hot flushes, as well as for decreasing urinary calcium excretion in postmenopausal women.[4] As a result of the high progestin and low estrogen levels, the endometrium becomes low-lying and atrophic. The glands are narrow and widely spaced with deciduoid stroma. With this atrophic type of endometrium, many patients develop amenorrhea.

The major side effect of DMPA is complete disruption of the menstrual cycle. In the first 3 months after the first injection, about 30% of the patients are amenorrheic and another 30% have irregular bleeding and spotting occurring more than 11 days per month.[5] As duration of therapy increases, the incidence of frequent bleeding steadily declines and the incidence of amenor-

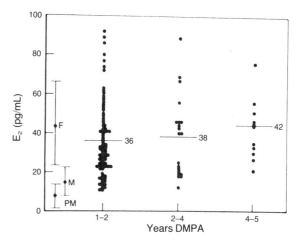

Figure 37-2

Serum estradiol levels in 121 women who had used DMPA for contraception for more than 1 year. The horizontal bar in each time period represents the mean value. Vertical bars represent means (circles) ± SD of serum estradiol levels in cycling women in the early follicular phase (F), normal males (M), and postmenopausal women (PM).

From Mishell DR Jr, Kharma KM, Thorneycroft IH, et al: Estrogenic activity in women receiving an injectable progestogen for contraception. Am J Obstet Gynecol 113:372, 1972.

rhea steadily increases, so that at the end of 2 years about 70% of the patients are amenorrheic (Figure 37-3).[5]

After treatment with DMPA is discontinued, about half of the patients resume a regular cyclic menstrual pattern within 6 months and about three-quarters have regular menses within 1 year.[6] When bleeding does resume after the effect of the last injection is dissipated, it is initially regular in about half the patients and irregular in the remainder.

Additional side effects include slight weight gain and a slight deterioration of glucose tolerance that is not clinically significant. Because of the long duration of action of the drug, there is a delay in return of fertility.

Fertility rates have been calculated for couples discontinuing barrier methods and the IUD in order to conceive. At the end of 3 months, about 50% of these women are pregnant; at the end of a year, about 90% are pregnant. For DMPA users, the curve is shifted to the right, so the 50% pregnancy rate does not occur until about a year, a delay of about 9 months compared with women discontinuing barrier methods (Figure 37-4).[7] The 90% pregnancy rate is also delayed about 9 months. Fertility rates are about the same 21 months after discontinuing a barrier method or IUD and discontinuing DMPA. Therefore, DMPA does not cause sterility, but causes a temporary period of infertility. A major benefit of the prolonged effect of the drug is that when patients do not return for their scheduled injection on time, but delay for a month or two, pregnancy rates remain very low.

Because DMPA does not increase liver globulin production as does the estrogen component of oral contraceptives (ethinylestradiol), no alteration in blood clotting factors or angiotensinogen levels is associated with its use. Thus, unlike OCs, DMPA has not been associated with increases in hypertension or thromboembolism. A recent WHO study reported that blood pressure measurements were unchanged in DMPA users after 2 years of injections.[1]

Concern has also been raised that DMPA may be associated with an increased incidence of abnormal cervical cytology. However, there is no evidence that the drug causes an increase in cervical dysplasia or carcinoma. An increased incidence of abnormal cervical cytology among contraceptive steroid users appears to be related to confounding factors, such as failure to use a diaphragm or many sexual partners.

DMPA has been associated with an increased incidence of two types of carcinoma in animals but not in humans. When given in high

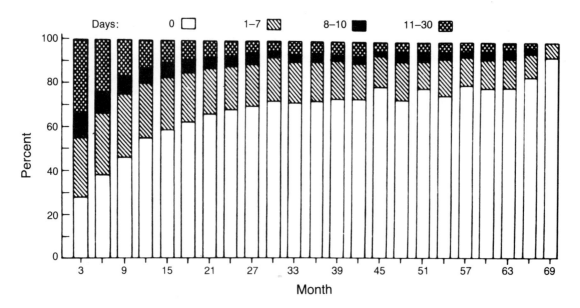

Figure 37-3
Percentage of women with bleeding and/or spotting 0, 1 to 7, 8 to 10, and 11 to 30 days per 30-day cycle while receiving injectable DMPA, 150 mg every 3 months.

From Schwallie PC, Assenzo JR: Contraceptive use—Efficacy study utilizing medroxyprogesterone acetate administered as an intramuscular injection once every 90 days. Fertil Steril 24:331, 1973.

Contraception

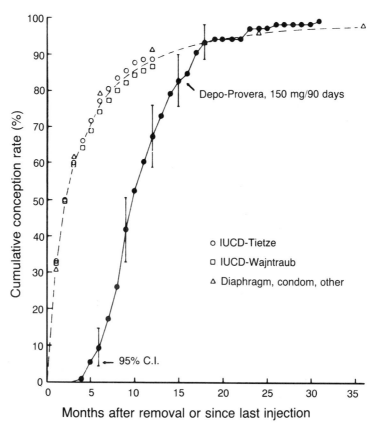

Figure 37-4
Cumulative conception rates of women who discontinued a method to become pregnant.

From Schwallie PC, Assenzo JR: The effect of depo-medroxyprogesterone acetate on pituitary and ovarian function, and the return of fertility following its discontinuation: A review. Contraception 10:181, 1974.

doses to beagle dogs, it is associated with an increase in mammary cancer; however, the beagle is a poor model for study of steroid action in the human, because progestins are metabolized differently in the two species. Beagles develop a high incidence of breast carcinoma after receiving various types of progestins.

After 20 years of study with this agent in humans, there is no evidence of an increased incidence of breast carcinoma. In long-term monkey studies, two monkeys developed adenocarcinoma of the endometrium when treated with high doses of DMPA for 10 years; however, there is no evidence that DMPA produces endometrial cancer in humans, because it produces an atrophic endometrium and actually is used to treat metastatic endometrial carcinoma. Nevertheless, concern about carcinogenicity has prevented approval of this drug for use as a contraceptive in the US.

Norethindrone enanthate

Norethindrone enanthate (NET-EN) is another injectable progestogen that is being used in Europe but not in the US. It is administered in an oily suspension, and thus has different pharmacodynamics from DMPA.

Using radioimmunoassay, we measured levels of norethindrone, FSH, LH, estradiol, and progesterone in a group of women for 6 months after a single injection of 200 mg of NET-EN.[8] About 1 week after the injection, peak serum levels of norethindrone of 12 to 17 ng/mL were reached. These high serum levels lasted for about 3 weeks and decreased thereafter, first precipitously and then gradually (Figure 37-5). Serum levels of norethindrone of 4 ng/mL or more suppressed gonadotropin levels and follicular development. Norethindrone levels in this range persisted only for approximately 1 to 2 months after the injection. With a further fall in norethindrone levels, follicular maturation, as determined by estradiol peaks, occurred. Nevertheless, these peaks were not followed by ovulation, because of positive feedback inhibition as long as the serum norethindrone levels stayed above 1.8 ng/mL. Ovulation occurred at variable intervals in the subjects, when their norethindrone concentrations ranged from 0.1 to 1.8 ng/mL. Thus, a variability of positive feedback inhibition was observed among different patients. These findings indicate why some patients conceive in the last few weeks of NET-EN therapy with an injection interval of 12 weeks.

Furthermore, if the patient does not return exactly when scheduled for a subsequent injection, the possibility of pregnancy increases greatly. In a comparative study done by the WHO in 10 centers around the world in 1977, at the end of 1 year the pregnancy rate with DMPA treatment was 0.7%, whereas with NET-EN given every 12 weeks it was 3.6%, significantly higher.[9] Because the rate of discontinuation for amenorrhea was higher with DMPA than with NET-EN, it was decided to administer the latter drug at more frequent intervals, in an attempt to lower the pregnancy rate.

In a subsequent comparative study using DMPA and NET-EN, NET-EN was given every 60 days to one group of subjects; a second group received NET-EN every 60 days for the first 6 months, followed by every 84 days thereafter. With both these regimens, at the end of 1 year, the pregnancy rates with NET-EN were more comparable to the 0.1% rate found with DMPA: 0.4% for the 60-day regimen and 0.6% for the 60/84-day regimen.[1] At the end of 2 years, the pregnancy rate for the 60-day regimen was still 0.4%, the same as with DMPA, whereas with the 60/84-day regimen it was 1.4%. For this reason, it is now recommended that NET-EN be given every 60 days for at least the first 6 months and no less often than every 12 weeks thereafter.

NET-EN is also associated with irregular menstrual bleeding and few systemic effects other than weight gain. In the WHO study, mean weight gain with both DMPA and NET-EN was approximately 1.8 kg at the end of 1 year and 3.3 kg at the end of 2 years. Fewer NET-EN users than DMPA users became amenorrheic and, at the end of 1 year, more women discontinued the use of DMPA for this reason than NET-EN. About 55% of DMPA users were amenorrheic at 1 year and 62% at 2 years, in contrast with about 30% and 40% of NET-EN users after the same periods. Nevertheless, total discontinuation rates for the two methods were similar at the end of 1 and 2 years, about 50% and 75%, respectively (Table 37-1).

Progestin-estrogen injectable formulations

Various injectable combinations of estrogen and progestogens have been investigated.[10] The two formulations most widely studied have been dihydroxyprogesterone acetophenide, 150 mg, with estradiol enanthate, 10 mg (Deladroxate, Perlutal); and medroxyprogesterone acetate, 50 or 25 mg, with estradiol cypionate, 10 or 5 mg

Contraception

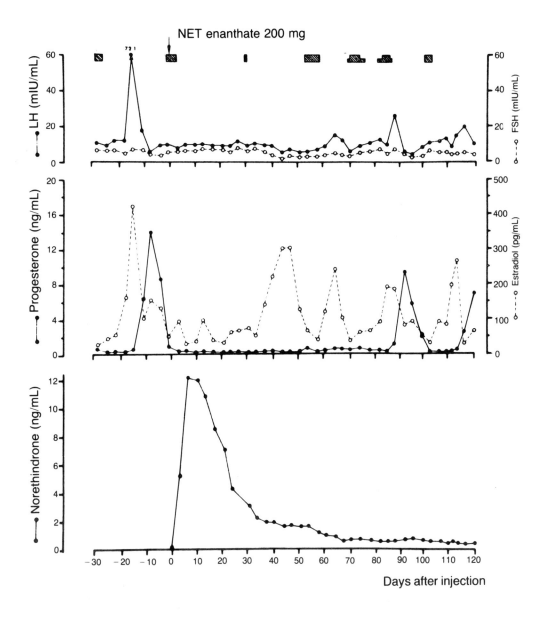

Figure 37-5
Serum levels of LH, FSH, progesterone, estradiol, and norethindrone before and 4 months after a single injection of norethindrone enanthate. The hatched bars represent uterine bleeding (full thickness) and spotting (half thickness).

From Goebelsmann U, Stanczyk FZ, Brenner PF, et al: Serum norethindrone (NET) concentrations following intramuscular NET enanthate injection. Effect upon serum LH, FSH, estradiol, and progesterone. Contraception 19:283, 1979.

Long-acting contraceptive steroids and interception

Table 37-1
Net termination rates per 100 women in WHO comparative study
of DMPA and norethindrone enanthate (NET-EN)

Reason	1-year net cumulative event rates			2-year net cumulative event rates		
	DMPA	NET-EN 60 days	NET-EN 60/84 days	DMPA	NET-EN 60 days	NET-EN 60/84 days
Pregnancy	0.1	0.4	0.6	0.4	0.4	1.4
Amenorrhea	11.9	6.8	8.4	24.2	14.7	14.6
Bleeding	15.0	13.6	13.7	18.8	18.4	21.8
Medical	11.8	13.7	12.7	15.0	16.0	16.7
Personal	20.7	24.5	22.8	38.8	42.6	40.2
Total	51.4	49.7	50.3	73.5	70.7	72.4

From World Health Organization Expanded Programme of Research, Development and Research Training in Human Reproduction Task Force on Long-Acting System Agents for the Regulation of Fertility: Multinational comparative clinical evaluation of two long-acting injectable contraceptive steroids: norethisterone enanthate and medroxyprogesterone acetate. Final report. Contraception 28:1, 1983.

(Cyclo-Provera). Because these estrogen esters are effective for only about 1 month, formulations containing them have to be given monthly. These formulations cause less abnormal bleeding than do the injectable contraceptives without estrogen; however, not all subjects have regular cycles, and irregular bleeding and amenorrhea do occur in some. Because of concerns about the toxicity of high doses of estrogen, as well as the need for monthly injections, these formulations are not available for use in most countries; however, they are widely used in Mexico and some other countries in Latin America. It is reported that other monthly injectable formulations are used in the People's Republic of China.

Subdermal implants

Subdermal implants of capsules made of polysiloxane (Silastic) and containing levonorgestrel have been developed and patented by the Population Council as Norplant®. As with all steroid-containing Silastic devices, the rate of steroid delivery is directly proportional to capsule surface area, while duration of action depends on the amount of steroid in the capsules. To pro-

duce effective blood levels of norgestrel, it was found necessary to use six capsules filled with crystalline levonorgestrel with the ends sealed with Silastic plugs. The cylindrical capsules are 3 cm long and 2.4 mm in outer diameter.

Insertion is performed in an outpatient area, and the entire procedure takes about 5 minutes. After infiltration of the skin with local anesthesia, a small (3-mm) incision is made, usually in the upper arm, although the lower arm and the inguinal and gluteal regions have also been used. The capsules are implanted into the subcutaneous tissue in a radial pattern through a large (11-gauge) trocar, and the incision is closed with adhesive. Stitches are not necessary. Because polysiloxane is not biodegradable, the capsules have to be removed through another incision when all the steroid has been released.

After insertion, blood levels of levonorgestrel are nearly uniform, with a mean of about 400 pg/mL, which is usually sufficient to inhibit ovulation (Figure 37-6).[11] From in vitro studies, it was estimated that the amount of norgestrel in the capsules would last for 6 to 7 years. When the amount of steroid was measured in capsules removed from patients after various times, it was found that the rate of release was fairly constant.

Mean blood levels of levonorgestrel are also constant, remaining at about 400 pg/mL for up to 6 years of use.

With this low level of levonorgestrel, gonadotropin levels are not completely suppressed, and follicular activity results in periodic peaks of estradiol. The irregular estradiol levels are accompanied by irregular bleeding episodes. The major side effect of this method, therefore, is a highly irregular menstrual pattern. Most of the bleeding is characterized as spotting, and total blood loss averages about 25 mL per month, a little less than the normal monthly blood loss of cycling women. Clinical studies with these implants revealed no significant change in hemo-globin or blood pressure, although there was a slight increase in total body weight.[12]

Studies of electrolytes, metabolites, and liver function tests have revealed no significant alterations; however, lipid levels are altered slightly. These implants produce a decrease in serum cholesterol, triglycerides, low-density lipoprotein (LDL) cholesterol, and high-density lipoprotein (HDL) cholesterol. However, the ratio of total cholesterol to HDL cholesterol is not changed significantly, and the slight decreases in the lipids are within the normal range and not believed to be clinically meaningful.[13]

With this preliminary clinical information, in 1975, the Population Council began a com-

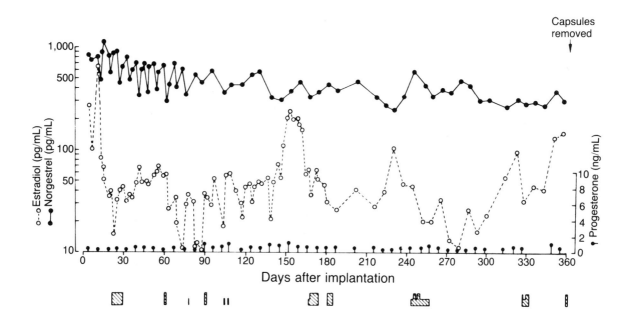

Figure 37-6
Serum levels of estradiol, progesterone, and *d*-norgestrel in a subject with six polysiloxane capsules, each containing 33.9 mg of *d*-norgestrel, implanted on day 0. Hatched bars represent uterine bleeding.

From Moore DE, Roy S, Stanczyk FZ, et al: Bleeding and serum d-norgestrel, estradiol, and progesterone patterns in women using d-norgestrel subdermal polysiloxane capsules for contraception. Contraception 17:315, 1978.

parative study of Norplant® subdermal implants and the IUD. Although there was a higher rate of removal due to bleeding problems with these implants than with the IUD, at the end of 1 year the continuation rates with the implants were about the same as with the IUD (Table 37-2).[14] In this study, the approximately 75% continuation rate was higher than the 50% continuation rate observed after 1 year with OCs and injectable agents.

Both subdermal implants and the IUD require a positive act on the part of the patient to discontinue use. Women cannot stop using these methods by themselves, but must visit a clinical facility. This is the main reason why Norplant® implants and the IUD have the highest continuation rates of any methods of contraception in use today.

Norplant® implants are very effective. After 5 years of use in clinical studies coordinated by the Population Council, the net cumulative pregnancy rate was only 1.5 per 100 women (Table 37-3). This method is now recommended for 5-year use. It has an annual use-pregnancy rate of less than 0.5%, significantly lower than OCs or the IUD. The main reasons for discontinuation of Norplant® use are bleeding problems and other medical problems. In the Population Council studies, more than 80% of women were still using the method at the end of the first year, and at the end of 3 years, 50% were still using it. At the end of 5 years, 40% of the women were still active users.[15]

If a woman wishes to become pregnant or have the device removed because of bleeding or other problems, the capsules can be removed with a hemostat through a small incision made under local anesthesia. Serum levels of levonorgestrel decline rapidly following removal, and ovulation resumes promptly. At the end of 12 months, 77% of the patients discontinuing the method in order to conceive have become pregnant,[16] comparable with rates after discontinuation of barrier methods of contraception. Be-

Table 37-2
One-year net termination rates
per 100 women in
Population Council comparative study

Reason	Norplant® (492)	IUD (402)
Pregnancy	0.6	1.2
Bleeding	12.3	3.8
Other medical	4.1	7.6
Other method	0.6	2.6
Personal	3.2	3.4
Technical	4.6	0.3
Total term	25.4	18.9
Continuation	74.6	81.9

From Population Council, International Committee for Contraception Research: Contraception with long-acting subdermal implants: I. An effective and acceptable modality in international clinical trials. Contraception 18:315, 1978.

cause of knowledge obtained from the nearly 2,000 women involved in the six-country phase III studies, this method has been approved for distribution in Finland and has been introduced into family-planning programs in Colombia, Ecuador, Egypt, Indonesia, and Thailand. Large-scale clinical studies of Norplant® are currently under way in the US, preparatory to obtaining FDA approval.

Manufacture of the capsules is complicated, and placing or removing six capsules creates some difficulties; therefore, norgestrel has been fabricated into solid rods that are a homologous mixture of Silastic and crystalline levonorgestrel covered with Silastic tubing. The rods are easier to manufacture, insert, and remove than the capsules. Because of different properties of diffusion, with the rods higher blood levels of norgestrel are achieved with a smaller total surface area. Thus, with two 4-cm covered rods with the same diameter as the capsules, the same release rate for norgestrel—about 50 μg/day—can be achieved as with placement of six 3-cm capsules. During a 2-year clinical study comparing rods and capsules, the serum norgestrel levels, bleeding patterns, and incidence of elevated progesterone levels were similar.[13] Thus, if large-scale clinical studies confirm these findings, the two covered rods will be used instead of six capsules.

Contraceptive vaginal rings (CVRs)

Another method of contraception that the Population Council has been studying for the past 12 years is the administration of contraceptive steroids through a donut-shaped Silastic vaginal ring. Originally, the ring was impregnated with a variety of gestagens alone; more recently, it has been impregnated with a combination of levonorgestrel and estradiol. Different fabrications of Silastic were studied, but the design used now, the so-called shell design, has three layers—an inert inner core, a middle layer in which the steroid is placed, and an outside Silastic tubing through which the steroid diffuses (Figure 37-7).[17] These CVRs have an outside diameter of 50 or 58 mm with a width of 7 to 9 mm and are placed in the vagina by the patient herself for a period of 3 weeks, beginning on the fifth day after menses begins, and then removed for 1 week to allow withdrawal bleeding to occur.

While the rings are in place, the steroids are released from the surface and absorbed through the vaginal epithelium into the circulation at a fairly constant rate. The serum level of steroids found in patients using the rings varies between 1 and 2 ng/mL, which is sufficient to inhibit ovulation, but several times less than the peak levels obtained with daily ingestion of OC steroids (Figure 37-8).[17] Ovulation continues to be inhibited during the week the rings are removed.

With the use of rings containing a combination of levonorgestrel and estradiol, breakthrough bleeding is infrequent and similar to that with the combination OCs. The daily release rate of levonorgestrel is about 300 μg/day, and of estradiol, 180 μg/day. Withdrawal bleeding after the ring is removed usually occurs within a day or two, lasts for 3 or 4 days, and is similar in amount to the normal flow.

The rings are very comfortable, and most women are not aware they are in place. They usually are not noticed by either partner during sexual intercourse, and they seldom cause dyspareunia. No local adverse changes have been observed in the vagina colposcopically or histologically, except for an occasional patient who has developed erosion of the vaginal epithelium. These erosions healed rapidly after removal of the CVR, without additional therapy. The incidence of vaginitis has not been found to be increased in CVR users.

We performed bacteriologic studies of the vaginal flora of CVR and OC users during a 6-month period. There were changes in the flora

Table 37-3
First-segment net termination rate per 100 women using Norplant® subdermal implants

	1 year	2 years	3 years	4 years	5 years
Pregnancy	0.3	0.4	0.7	1.3	1.5
Bleeding	8.6	12.9	14.4	15.2	16.6
Medical	4.7	8.2	10.2	12.0	12.8
Total term	20.6	41.7	51.0	56.8	60.7
No. at risk	787	331	174	92	51
Woman-months	10,601	16,334	18,785	20,147	20,823

From Sivin I (personal communication).

Long-acting contraceptive steroids and interception

of women using both types of contraception, but there were no significant differences between the changes observed with the two methods.[18] The amount of estrogen in the ring is not sufficient to raise the levels of serum globulins. We have measured levels of angiotensinogen, corticosteroid-binding globulin, and sex hormone-binding globulin in CVR and OC users. Levels of these globulins were not increased in CVR users, in contrast with the severalfold increase that occurs with ingestion of OCs.[19] Reasons for this lack of hepatic effect with the CVRs are: (1) the use of estradiol instead of ethinylestradiol, which is used in OCs and affects liver globulin production more than estradiol; (2) the small amount of estrogen that is absorbed from the CVR; and (3) the systemic absorption of the CVR estrogen, precluding the first-pass effect on the liver that occurs with OCs.

Liver function tests and measurements of glucose metabolism in CVR users have revealed no changes except for a slight but clinically insignificant decrease in alkaline phosphatase levels.[20] There is no change in glucose tolerance with CVR use. Decreases in lipid levels are associated with these rings; however, because LDL cholesterol decreases nearly as much as HDL cholesterol, there is little likelihood that use of the CVR will prove to be atherogenic.[21]

The Population Council performed a multicenter study in seven countries comparing the use of CVRs with OCs containing levonorgestrel and ethinylestradiol. Most of the women were young (70% were between 20 and 29) and of low parity. Use of the CVR was associated with relatively little change in body weight, hemoglobin,

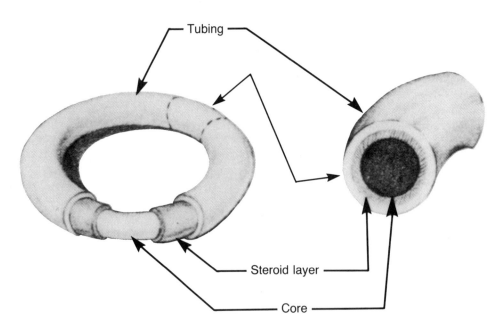

Figure 37-7
Schematic drawing of three-layered shell design of contraceptive vaginal ring.

From Mishell DR Jr, Moore DE, Roy S, et al: Clinical performance and endocrine profiles with contraceptive vaginal rings containing a combination of estradiol and d-norgestrel. Am J Obstet Gynecol 130:55, 1978.

Contraception

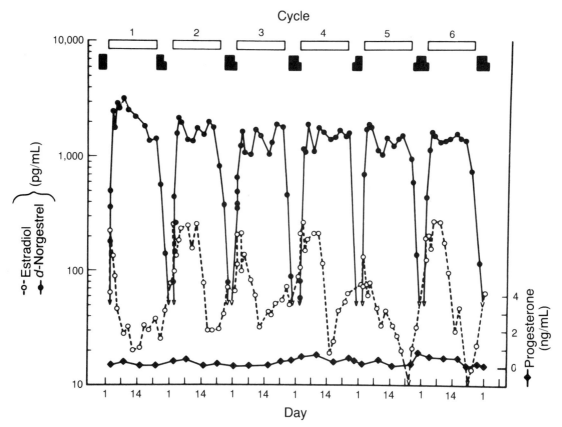

Figure 37-8
Serum estradiol and *d*-norgestrel levels on a log scale and progesterone levels during six treatment cycles with vaginal rings. Rings were inserted on day 1 and removed on day 21 during each cycle. Open bars represent 3-week treatment cycles with rings in place. Black bars represent bleeding days (full height for bleeding and half height for spotting).

From Mishell DR Jr, Moore DE, Roy S, et al: Clinical performance and endocrine profiles with contraceptive vaginal rings containing a combination of estradiol and d-norgestrel. Am J Obstet Gynecol 130:55, 1978.

or blood pressure. Pregnancy rates at the end of 1 year were similar for CVR and OC users, between 1% and 2% (Table 37-4).[22] There was a higher discontinuation rate for medical reasons and use-related reasons among the CVR users than the OC users, but at the end of 1 year the continuation rates were approximately the same with the two methods.

When the medical termination rates were analyzed for various causes, it was found that CVR users had a slightly higher discontinuation rate for menstrual and vaginal problems than did OC users; however, OC users had a significantly higher discontinuation rate for other medical reasons, such as headache, nausea, and depression. Use-related reasons for CVR discontinuation included expulsion, problems with coitus, odor, and storage difficulties. Patients using the CVR perceived that they had substantially less menstrual flow and fewer bleeding days, but they had more intermenstrual bleeding than did OC users.

The CVR, unlike the diaphragm, can be removed for intercourse as long as it is not left out for more than 3 hours; however, only about 20% of sexual partners complained about the presence of the CVR. In a study in Latin America, about 76% of CVR users never removed the ring for coitus, 13% removed it sometimes, and 10% always.[23] At the end of 2 years of the comparative Population Council study, pregnancy rates were still similar for the CVR and OCs, and continuation rates were slightly higher for the CVR. In summary, the CVR has convenient, once-a-month self-administration, an acceptable rate of breakthrough bleeding and spotting, a good level of effectiveness because of inhibition of ovulation, prompt withdrawal bleeding, and a prompt return of ovulation. Patient and consort acceptance is good. The metabolic effects and systemic side effects are minimal, and less than those of OCs because of the smaller amount of estrogen absorbed.

Pregnancy interception

Morris and Van Wagenen suggested in 1966 that high doses of estrogen administered in the early postovulatory period will prevent implantation in women. Morris has suggested that the term "interception" be used for what is commonly referred to as the "morning-after pill." The estrogen compounds that have been used by various investigators for interception include diethylstilbestrol, 25 to 50 mg/day; diethylstilbestrol diphosphate, 50 mg/day; ethinylestradiol, 1 to 5 mg/day; and conjugated estrogens, 20 to 30 mg/day. Treatment is continued for 5 days. If it is begun within 72 hours after an isolated midcycle act of coitus, its effectiveness is very good. If more than one episode of coitus has occurred, or if treatment is initiated later than 72 hours after coitus, the method is much less effective.

Morris and Van Wagenen summarized the literature in 1973 and found that in 9,000 cases of midcycle exposure treated with estrogen, a total of 29 pregnancies occurred, for a pregnancy rate of approximately 0.3%.[24] Only three pregnancies appeared to be due to method failure, yielding a Pearl Index of 0.4 per 100 woman-years. Of the 29 pregnancies, three were ectopic, an incidence of approximately 10%. A later review of 4,595 treatment cycles reported a failure rate of 0.7%.[25]

Side effects associated with this high-dose estrogen therapy are, as expected, nausea and vomiting, breast soreness, and menstrual irregularities. The US Centers for Disease Control performed a five-center study comparing use of ethinylestradiol, 5 mg/day, with conjugated estrogens, 30 mg/day, for 5 days. The pregnancy rate was slightly lower with ethinylestradiol (0.7%) than with conjugated estrogens (1.6%).[26] However, patients treated with ethinylestradiol had a greater incidence of nausea and vomiting, indicating that its potency may have been greater. If treatment was begun 2 days after coitus, the pregnancy rate was 1.7 times greater than if it was begun the day after coitus. Thus, it is best to start treatment within 24 hours of coitus.

Table 37-4
One-year net termination rates per 100 women in Population Council comparative study

	CVR 50	CVR 58	OC
Pregnancy	1.8	1.0	2.0
Medical	23.5	22.5	18.7
Use	6.6	4.4	2.0
Personal	8.8	9.7	11.2
Move	2.0	2.1	2.0
Lost-to-follow-up	8.5	9.9	25.9
Continuation with lost-to-follow-up	48.8	50.4	38.2
Continuation without lost-to-follow-up	54.0	56.8	55.4

From Sivin I, Mishell DR Jr, Victor A, et al: A multicenter study of levonorgestrel-estradiol contraceptive vaginal rings. I. Use effectiveness. Contraception 24:341, 1981.

Contraception

Because the side effects of high-dose estrogens cause some women to fail to complete the 5-day treatment course, a regimen of 4 tablets of an ethinylestradiol, 0.05 mg, and *dl*-norgestrel, 0.5 mg, combination (Ovral), given in doses of 2 tablets 12 hours apart, has been tested in Canada. Effectiveness is comparable to the high-dose estrogen regimen, with a shorter duration of adverse symptoms.

The experience with the use of this regimen among 692 women treated in 24 clinics was recently summarized.[27] There were 11 pregnancies (1.6%), but four of these subjects had unprotected intercourse more than 72 hours before treatment and, therefore, should not have been included in the study. Excluding those four, the pregnancy rate was 1.0%. About half of the subjects (42.4%) had no side effects, while nausea and/or vomiting occurred in 51.7%. Other side effects, such as mastalgia and menorrhagia, were infrequent, each occurring in fewer than 2% of the women.

Thus, the effectiveness of this method is similar to that of higher dosages of estrogen alone, and a lower incidence of abnormal and delayed menses results. Side effects appear to be less frequent and, because of the 1-day treatment regimen, patient compliance is greater with this technique. If the patient has a continuing need for contraception after the cycle in which interception is used, one of the conventional methods should be prescribed.

References

1. World Health Organization Expanded Programme of Research, Development and Research Training in Human Reproduction Task Force on Long-Acting Systemic Agents for the Regulation of Fertility: Multinational comparative clinical evaluation of two long-acting injectable contraceptive steroids: norethisterone enanthate and medroxyprogesterone acetate. Final report. *Contraception* 28:1, 1983

2. Ortiz, A, Hiroi M, Stanczyk FZ, et al: Serum medroxyprogesterone acetate (MPA) concentrations and ovarian function following intramuscular injection of depo-MPA. *J Clin Endocrinol Metab* 44:32, 1977

3. Mishell DR Jr, Kharma KM, Thorneycroft IH, et al: Estrogenic activity in women receiving an injectable progestogen for contraception. *Am J Obstet Gynecol* 113:372, 1972

4. Lobo RA, McCormick W, Singer F, et al: Depo-medroxyprogesterone acetate compared with conjugated estrogens for the treatment of postmenopausal women. *Obstet Gynecol* 63:1, 1984

5. Schwallie PC, Assenzo JR: Contraceptive use—efficacy study utilizing medroxyprogesterone acetate administered as an intramuscular injection once every 90 days. *Fertil Steril* 24:331, 1973

6. Gardner JM, Mishell DR Jr: Analysis of bleeding patterns and resumption of fertility following discontinuation of a long-acting injectable contraceptive. *Fertil Steril* 21:286, 1970

7. Schwallie PC, Assenzo JR: The effect of depo-medroxyprogesterone acetate on pituitary and ovarian function, and the return of fertility following its discontinuation: A review. *Contraception* 10:181, 1974

8. Goebelsmann U, Stanczyk FZ, Brenner PF, et al: Serum norethindrone (NET) concentrations following intramuscular NET enanthate injection. Effect upon serum LH, FSH, estradiol and progesterone. *Contraception* 19:283, 1979

9. World Health Organization Expanded Programme of Research, Development and Research Training in Human Reproduction Task Force on Long-Acting Systemic Agents for the Regulation of Fertility: Multinational comparative clinical evaluation of two long-acting injectable contraceptive steroids: norethisterone enanthate and medroxyprogesterone acetate. I. Use-effectiveness. *Contraception* 15:5, 1977

10. Hall P, Fraser I: Monthly injectable contraceptives. In Mishell DR Jr (ed): *Advances in Contraceptive Technology*, vol 2. New York, Raven Press. 1983

11. Moore DE, Roy S, Stanczyk FZ, et al: Bleeding and serum d-norgestrel, estradiol, and progesterone patterns in women using d-norgestrel subdermal polysiloxane capsules for contraception. *Contraception* 17:315, 1978

12. Population Council, International Committee for Contraception Research: Contraception with long-acting subdermal implants. II. Measured and perceived effects in international trials. *Contraception* 18:335, 1978

13. Roy S, Robertson D, Krauss RM, et al: Long-term reversible contraception with levonorgestrel-releasing Silastic rods. *Am J Obstet Gynecol* 148:1006, 1984

14. Population Council, International Committee for Contraception Research: Contraception with long-acting subdermal implants. I. An effective and acceptable modality in international clinical trials. *Contraception* 18:315, 1978

15. Sivin I: personal communication, 1985

16. Sivin I: Clinical effects of NORPLANT® subdermal implants for contraception. In Mishell DR Jr (ed): *Advances in Human Fertility and Reproductive Endocrinology*, vol 2: *Long-Acting Steroid Contraception*. New York, Raven Press, 1983, p 89

17. Mishell DR Jr, Moore DE, Roy S, et al: Clinical performance and endocrine profiles with contraceptive vaginal rings containing a combination of estradiol and d-norgestrel. *Am J Obstet Gynecol* 130:55, 1978

18. Roy S, Wilkins J, Mishell DR Jr: The effect of a contraceptive vaginal ring and oral contraceptives on the vaginal flora. *Contraception* 24:481, 1981

19. Roy S, Mishell DR Jr, Gray G, et al: Comparison of metabolic and clinical effects of four oral contraceptive formulations and a contraceptive vaginal ring. *Am J Obstet Gynecol* 136:920, 1980

20. Ahren T, Victor A, Lithell H, et al: Comparison of the metabolic effects of two hormonal contraceptive methods: An oral formulation and a vaginal ring. I. Carbohydrate metabolism and liver function. *Contraception* 24:415, 1981

21. Roy S, Kraus RM, Mishell DR Jr, et al: The effect on lipids and lipoproteins of a contraceptive vaginal ring containing levonorgestrel and estradiol. *Contraception* 14:429, 1981

22. Sivin I, Mishell DR Jr, Victor A, et al: A multicenter study of levonorgestrel-estradiol contraceptive vaginal rings. I. Use effectiveness. *Contraception* 24:341, 1981

23. Faundes A, Hardy E, Reyes C, et al: Acceptability of the contraceptive vaginal ring by rural and urban population in two Latin American countries. *Contraception* 24:393, 1981

24. Morris JM, Van Wagenen G: Interception: The use of postovulatory estrogens to prevent implantation. *Am J Obstet Gynecol* 115:101, 1973

25. Garcia C-R, Huggins GR, Rosenfeld DL, et al: Post-coital contraception: Medical and social factors of the morning after pill. *Contraception* 15:445, 1977

26. Dixon GW, Schlesselman JJ, Ory HW, et al: Ethinyl estradiol and conjugated estrogens as postcoital contraceptives. *JAMA* 244:1336, 1980

27. Yuzpe AA, Smith RP, Rademaker AW: A multicenter clinical investigation employing ethinyl estradiol combined with dl-norgestrel as a postcoital contraceptive agent. *Fertil Steril* 37:508, 1982

Chapter 38

Intrauterine Devices

Daniel R. Mishell Jr., M.D.

The main benefits of IUDs are: (1) a high level of effectiveness, (2) a lack of associated systemic metabolic effects, and (3) the need for only a single act of motivation for long-term use. In contrast to other types of contraception, there is no need for frequent motivation to ingest a pill daily or to use a coitus-related method consistently. These characteristics, as well as the necessity for a visit to a health-care facility to discontinue the method, account for the fact that IUDs have the highest continuation rate of all currently available reversible methods of contraception. Of course, it is desirable for all women to make at least annual visits to a health-care facility, but in some areas of the world this is not possible.

Unlike other contraceptives, such as the barrier methods, which rely on use by the individual for effectiveness and therefore have higher use-failure rates than method-failure rates, the IUD has similar method-effectiveness and use-effectiveness rates. First-year failure rates are generally reported to range from 2% to 3%; however, pregnancy rates are related to the skill of the clinician inserting the device. With experience, correct high-fundal insertion occurs more frequently, and there is a lower incidence of partial or complete expulsion, with resultant lower pregnancy rates. Furthermore, the annual incidence of accidental pregnancy decreases steadily after the first year of IUD use and after several years of use is similar to that of oral contraceptives. The incidence of all major adverse events with IUDs, including pregnancy as well as expulsion or removal for bleeding and/or pain, also steadily decreases with increasing age. Women over 35 have pregnancy rates of less than 2% in the first 2 years of use of the loop (Table 38-1).[1] Thus, the IUD is especially suited for older parous women who wish to prevent further pregnancies.

Mechanism of action

The IUD's main mechanism of contraceptive action in the human is spermicidal, produced by a local sterile inflammatory reaction caused by the presence of the foreign body in the uterus. We found a nearly 1,000% increase in the number of leukocytes in washings of the human endometrial cavity 18 weeks after the insertion of an IUD, compared with washings obtained before insertion.[2] Tissue breakdown products of these leukocytes are toxic to all cells, including sperm and the blastocyst. Small IUDs do not produce as great an inflammatory reaction as larger ones do. Therefore, smaller IUDs have higher pregnancy rates than larger devices of the same design. The addition of copper increases the inflammatory reaction. We found that the short phase of sperm transport from the cervix to the oviduct is markedly impaired in women wearing IUDs.[3] Thus, because of this spermicidal action, very few, if any, sperm reach the oviducts, and

Table 38-1
Two-year net cumulative event rates with the loop D (per 100 women)

Events	Age at insertion (years)			
	15–24	25–29	30–34	35–49
Pregnancies	5.8	4.7	2.8	1.5
Expulsions	17.4	9.8	7.1	5.4
Removals for bleeding/pain	18.0	17.7	16.8	16.2
Continuation rate	58.0	66.7	72.0	75.4
First insertions	2,753	2,082	1,397	1,187
Woman-months of use	41,758	34,574	23,874	19,912

From Tietze C, Lewit S: Evaluation of intrauterine devices: Ninth progress report of the Cooperative Statistical Program. Stud Fam Plan 1:55, 1970.

the ovum usually does not become fertilized.

Recently, further evidence was found for this spermicidal action of IUDs.[4] A group of Chilean investigators performed oviductal flushings in 54 women, with and without IUDs, who were sterilized by salpingectomy soon after ovulation and also had unprotected sexual intercourse shortly before ovulation. Normally cleaving ova were found in the tubal flushings of about half of the women not wearing IUDs, whereas none were found in the oviducts of the women wearing IUDs.

In rabbits, the sterile inflammatory reaction changes the receptiveness of the endometrium to the nidation of the blastocyst, preventing implantation. The same effect is believed to occur in humans if fertilization does take place. Copper ions, as well as the locally released prostaglandins, probably also act to prevent the normal process of implantation.

Upon removal of both copper-bearing and noncopper-bearing IUDs, the inflammatory reaction rapidly disappears. Resumption of fertility following IUD removal is not delayed and occurs at the same rate as resumption of fertility following discontinuation of mechanical methods of contraception, such as the condom and diaphragm. Of a reported group of 378 women who had IUDs removed in order to conceive, 59.4% had conceived at the end of 3 months and

88.2% at the end of 1 year.[1] These rates are similar to those found with women discontinuing barrier methods.

Another study reported that pregnancy rates of women who discontinued using IUDs were similar to those of women discontinuing barrier methods at 1 and 2 years.[5] The only exception was for women discontinuing IUDs for medical problems, including infection, who had a slightly lower pregnancy rate at these time intervals (Table 38-2).

Types of IUDs

In the past 25 years, many types of IUDs have been designed and used clinically. Although many of these devices are available for use in Europe, Canada, and elsewhere, at present only the progesterone-releasing IUD is being marketed in the US. While the barium-impregnated plastic loop and the copper-bearing copper 7, copper T 200B, and copper T 380A (Figure 38-1) are currently approved by the FDA for use in the US, they are no longer being sold because the costs of product liability litigation exceed the profits from their sale. Nevertheless, these devices need not be removed from women wearing them. Production and distribution of the shield device with a multifilament tail were discontin-

Contraception

Table 38-2

Fertility of parous women in various contraceptive groups

Results are percentages (±SE) of women remaining undelivered of live birth or stillbirth at given intervals after stopping contraception to plan pregnancy.

Groups of women studied	Mean age (years)	Women remaining undelivered (%)					
		12 months	18 months	24 months	30 months	36 months	42 months
Method of contraception stopped to plan pregnancy							
IUD	31.4	48.8 ± 2.4	18.1 ± 1.9	10.6 ± 1.6	9.3 ± 1.5	6.7 ± 1.4	6.3 ± 1.4
Oral contraceptive	30.6	60.7 ± 1.2	20.4 ± 1.0	10.8 ± 0.8	7.6 ± 0.7	5.4 ± 0.6	4.5 ± 0.6
Diaphragm	30.9	36.8 ± 1.5	13.8 ± 1.1	8.2 ± 0.9	6.2 ± 0.9	4.6 ± 0.8	4.2 ± 0.8
Other method	31.8	39.4 ± 1.5	16.2 ± 1.3	10.6 ± 1.1	7.8 ± 1.0	6.2 ± 0.9	5.0 ± 0.9
Any method of contraception stopped to plan pregnancy in							
Ever-users of IUD	31.9	48.7 ± 2.0	18.7 ± 1.6	11.6 ± 1.4	9.8 ± 1.3	7.4 ± 1.2	7.0 ± 1.2
Never-users of IUD	30.9	48.7 ± 0.8	17.4 ± 0.7	9.8 ± 0.6	7.1 ± 0.5	5.2 ± 0.4	4.3 ± 0.4
Ever-users of IUD never using OCs	31.6	45.7 ± 2.7	16.1 ± 2.1	10.0 ± 1.8	8.2 ± 1.6	5.9 ± 1.5	5.9 ± 1.5
Never-users of IUD never using OCs	30.8	37.2 ± 1.6	15.0 ± 1.2	9.5 ± 1.1	7.4 ± 1.0	5.6 ± 0.9	5.2 ± 0.9
IUD users in past, stopped for medical reasons	32.7	49.3 ± 4.7	19.1 ± 4.1	13.6 ± 3.8			

From Vessey MP, Lawless M, McPherson K, et al: Fertility after stopping use of intrauterine contraceptive device. Br Med J 286:106, 1983.

ued in 1974. Because of the increased risk of infection reported with shield IUDs, those still in place should be removed. All IUDs now approved for distribution have monofilament tails.

The T- and 7-shaped plastic devices are smaller than most noncopper-bearing types of IUDs. When T-shaped devices without copper underwent clinical trials, they were found to have a much higher pregnancy rate than the larger loops and coils. With the addition of copper wire, the effectiveness of these IUDs was increased and is now comparable with that of the other IUDs.

Because of the constant dissolution of copper, which amounts daily to less than that ingested in the normal diet, copper IUDs have to be replaced periodically. The necessary interval was originally estimated to be 2 to 3 years, but now is believed to be 4 to 5 years. There have been five published studies indicating that the annual pregnancy rates with the copper 7 and copper T 200 devices do not increase in the fourth and fifth years after insertion. The World Health Organization stated in 1982 that the copper 7 is safe and effective for at least 4 years of use,[6] and the copper T 200B is now approved in the US for 4 years of use. At the scheduled time of removal, the device can be removed and another inserted during the same office visit.

Adding a reservoir of progesterone to the vertical arm also increases the effectiveness of

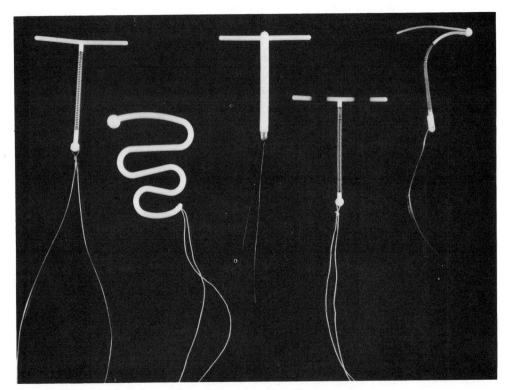

Figure 38-1
IUDs currently approved by the FDA for use in the US: Copper T 200B, loop, progesterone-releasing device, Copper T 380A, and Copper 7.

Contraception

the T-shaped devices. The currently marketed progesterone IUD releases 65 μg of progesterone daily. This amount is sufficient to prevent pregnancy by local action within the endometrial cavity, but it is not enough to cause a measurable increase in peripheral serum progesterone levels. The currently approved progesterone-releasing IUD needs to be replaced annually, because the reservoir of progesterone becomes depleted after about 18 months of use.

There is no need to change a nonmedicated plastic IUD unless the patient develops increased bleeding after it has been in place for more than a year. Calcium salts are deposited on the plastic over time, and their roughness can cause ulceration and bleeding of the endometrium. If increased bleeding develops after a loop or double coil has been in the uterus for a year or more, the old IUD should be removed and a new device inserted.

Time of insertion

Although it is widely believed that the optimal time for insertion of an IUD is during the men-

ses, there are data indicating that if a woman is not pregnant, the IUD can be safely inserted on any day of the cycle. An analysis was made of 2-month event rates of about 10,000 women who had copper T 200s inserted on various days of the cycle.[7] Rates of expulsion were lower when insertion occurred during the week after menses stopped, while rates of removal for bleeding and pain as well as pregnancy were higher with insertions after cycle day 18. However, the differences were small and of little clinical relevance (Table 38-3).

It has also been recommended that IUDs not be inserted until more than 2 to 3 months have elapsed after a pregnancy. However, in 1982 we analyzed event rates in our clinic among women who had copper T IUDs inserted between 4 and 8 weeks postpartum and more than 8 weeks postpartum.[8] The 1- and 2-year event rates for all causes were similar for the two groups, indicating that copper T IUDs can be safely inserted at the time of the routine postpartum visit (Table 38-4).[8] No perforations occurred in our series, in which the withdrawal technique of insertion was used. Although a recent report suggested that the perforation rate

Table 38-3
IUD termination rates* during the third and fourth postinsertion months, by menstrual cycle day of insertion

Reason for termination	Menstrual cycle day of insertion				
	1–5	6–10	11–17	≥18	All cycle days
Expulsion	12.1	9.5	12.2	12.2	11.3
Pregnancy	4.0	6.8	3.5	2.7	4.8
Pain and bleeding	19.0	14.8	8.7	20.3	17.0
Miscellaneous medical	4.0	3.8	3.5	4.1	3.9
Personal	17.8	14.8	13.9	12.2	16.0
Pelvic infection	1.4	1.1	0	0	1.1
Total	58.3	50.8	41.8	51.5	54.1
Women beginning ordinal month 3	4,220	2,633	575	740	8,168

*Rate per 1,000 insertions.
From White MK, Ory HW, Rooks JB, et al: Intrauterine device termination rates and the menstrual cycle day of insertion. Obstet Gynecol 55:220, 1980.

Table 38-4
IUD closure rates for various events
1 and 2 years after insertion
at 4 to 8 weeks and >8 weeks postpartum

Termination event	1 year			2 years		
	4–8 wks	8+ wks	P	4–8 wks	8+ wks	P
Pregnancy	2.0	2.9	NS	5.9	4.6	NS
Expulsion	7.1	5.6	NS	10.8	6.5	NS
Bleeding and pain	8.2	9.2	NS	17.3	16.9	NS
Other medical indications	0.6	1.3	NS	2.6	3.6	NS
Planning pregnancy	2.4	3.6	NS	10.8	10.1	NS
Personal indications	3.5	2.9	NS	5.8	7.0	NS
Cumulative relevant terminations*	16.8	16.7	NS	27.3	23.0	NS
Cumulative relevant continuations	83.2	83.3		72.7	77.0	
Cumulative total terminations†	30.2	30.3	NS	53.1	50.0	NS
Cumulative total continuations	69.8	69.7		46.9	50.0	
Lost to follow-up	10.6	9.4	NS	17.6	16.1	NS
Woman-months at risk‡	4,164	11,647		6,816	19,733	

*Includes pregnancy, expulsion, and bleeding and pain.

†Includes all termination events listed.

‡Calculated by dividing woman-days at risk by 30.44, the average number of days per month.

From Mishell DR Jr, Roy S: Copper intrauterine contraceptive device event rates following insertion 4 to 8 weeks postpartum. Am J Obstet Gynecol 143:29, 1982.

may be higher if the IUD is inserted when a woman is lactating, this finding has not been confirmed in other studies.

Adverse effects

Incidence

In general, in the first year of use, IUDs have about a 2% pregnancy rate, a 10% expulsion rate, and a 15% rate of removal for medical reasons, mainly bleeding and pain. The incidence of each of these events, especially expulsion, diminishes steadily in subsequent years.[1]

Since the most extensively studied type of IUD is the loop D, more information is available concerning event rates with this device than any other. A large enough population of women had this device inserted so that reliable data for 6 years of use are available (Table 38-5). At the end of the first year in a group of nearly 10,000 mainly multiparous women, 22.6% had discontinued use of the loop D, with a steadily declining rate of discontinuation thereafter.[1] At the end of 6 years, 42.6% of women originally inserted with a loop D were still wearing it. A total of 5.4% of the terminations during 6 years were due to pregnancy, a little less than 1% per year. Thus, although the pregnancy rate during the first year is greater with the IUD than with oral contraceptives (OCs), within the framework of longer time periods, the use-pregnancy rate with the IUD is similar to that of the combination OCs.

Although the incidence of expulsion is about 10% during the first year, in most cases, another loop D is inserted. Therefore, at the end of 6 years, only about 7% of women with a loop D will have discontinued using it because they have expelled the device one or more times.

Table 38-5

Net annual and cumulative rates of closures per 100 women during 6 years of using the loop D

Year	Pregnancy	Expulsion		Removals				Total closures	Active
		Initial	Later	Bleeding and pain	Medical	Planned pregnancy	Personal		
1	2.4	2.9	1.9	10.4	2.5	0.6	1.9	22.6	77.4
2	1.6	0.9	0.7	6.3	2.2	1.5	2.1	15.3	65.6
3	1.0	0.5	0.6	6.4	1.3	1.9	1.9	13.6	56.6
4	1.1	0.3	0.2	5.0	1.2	1.9	2.2	11.9	49.9
5	0.4	0.1	0.0	2.2	2.1	2.2	1.6	8.6	45.4
6	0.6	0.0	0.0	2.2	0.3	1.1	2.1	6.3	42.6
Total	5.4	7.1		31.3		13.6		57.4	42.6

Adapted from Tietze C, Lewit S: Evaluation of intrauterine devices: Ninth progress report of the Cooperative Statistical Program. Stud Fam Plan 1:55, 1970.

Table 38-6

Cumulative net event rates per 100 acceptors, by device and year

Events	1		2		3		4		5	
	Nova T	Copper T	Nova T	Copper T	Nova T	Copper T200	Nova T	Copper T	Nova T	Copper T
Pregnancies	0.7	1.9	1.4	3.8	1.9	4.9	2.0	5.1	2.2	5.8
Expulsion	5.5	4.2	6.9	5.2	8.1	5.7	8.7	6.8	9.3	7.2
Removals										
Bleeding and pain	11.1	11.4	17.0	14.9	21.1	19.7	24.1	22.8	26.7	23.7
Infection	2.3	1.8	2.9	2.3	3.7	3.6	4.2	4.2	4.8	4.3
Other medical	0.8	1.4	1.6	2.7	2.0	3.4	2.3	5.0	2.9	5.2
Planning pregnancy	2.5	1.9	6.1	5.3	10.5	8.7	12.9	10.8	14.5	12.3
Other personal	1.0	0.5	2.2	1.1	4.7	2.9	5.1	4.8	6.4	5.5
Continuation	76.1	77.0	62.0	64.7	48.2	51.1	39.8	40.5	33.2	36.0

From Luukkainen T, Allonen H, Nielsen NC, et al: Five years' experience of intrauterine contraception with the Nova-T and Copper-T-200. Am J Obstet Gynecol 147:885, 1983.

About half of all women discontinuing use of the loop D by the end of 6 years have done so because of bleeding, pain, and/or other medical reasons.

A randomized, multiclinic study compared the results of 5 years' experience of 947 women wearing the copper T 200 with data on the Nova T (a copper-bearing T-shaped IUD of modified design not yet available in the US).[9] In this study, 27% of the copper T users were nulliparous and 33% were less than 25 years of age. Nevertheless, despite this high proportion of young users, at the end of 5 years the net pregnancy rate was only 5.8% (about 1% per year), the discontinuation rate for expulsion was 7.2%, and the removal rate for bleeding and pain was 23.7%. The Nova T was associated with a 5-year pregnancy rate of only 2.2%, significantly less than the copper T 200. Other event rates were similar (Table 38-6).

The recently approved copper T 380A IUD, which has copper on the horizontal as well as the vertical arm, also has a very low pregnancy rate. The net cumulative pregnancy rate with this copper T device at the end of 4 years was reported to be only 1.9%.[10] Thus, the addition of copper on the horizontal arm appears to lower the pregnancy rate, as well as increase the estimated duration of action to 8 years or more.

Among IUDs currently available, there is little evidence to indicate any significant differences in the rates of the major adverse events associated with their use. This assumption was made after careful evaluation of reports of IUD performance in multiclinic as well as single-clinic studies. These revealed that there is likely to be at least as much variation in event rates among different clinics using the same type of IUD as among different types of IUDs used in the same clinic.[11]

There are several reasons for these marked variations among clinics. First is disparity among patient populations. Both age and parity have been shown to affect IUD performance. Physician skill is a second factor. As noted earlier, insertion of the device into its correct high-fundal position is extremely important. Incorrect placement will increase downward displacement and expulsion rates, resulting in an increased pregnancy rate. Third, patients, nurses, and physicians may vary greatly in their tolerance of side effects. Finally, there is variation in the use of additional methods of contraception, mainly vaginal foam. For all these reasons, the only valid method of comparison of different IUDs is randomized insertion of the devices in the same clinics, using the same paramedical and physician personnel, during the same period, with life-table analysis of the results. Published reports claiming superior performance for any particular IUD cannot be considered valid unless randomized studies of its performance are conducted using another type of IUD, which has previously undergone extensive clinical testing, for comparison. To determine whether the differences in the event rates are significant, statistical analysis must be performed.

Uterine bleeding

As mentioned above, the majority of women discontinuing this method of contraception do so for medical reasons. Nearly all medical reasons accounting for IUD removal involve one or more types of abnormal bleeding: heavy and/or prolonged menses or intermenstrual bleeding. We have shown that the IUD does not affect the pattern or level of gonadotropins and steroid hormones during the menstrual cycle.[12] The IUD therefore does not influence follicular maturation, the time or incidence of ovulation, or corpus luteum function. Nevertheless, the IUD does exert a local effect on the endometrium, causing menses to begin about 2 days earlier than normal, when steroid levels are higher than in control cycles. It is possible that this early onset of menses may be produced by a premature and increased rate of release of prostaglandins, brought about by the presence of the intrauter-

Contraception

ine foreign body. The stimulation of uterine contractions by excessive levels of prostaglandins may prolong the duration of the menstrual flow, which is significantly longer in women wearing IUDs.[13]

The amount of blood loss in each menstrual cycle is also significantly greater in women wearing inert as well as copper-bearing IUDs than in nonwearers. In a normal menstrual cycle, the mean amount of menstrual blood loss (MBL) is about 35 mL. After insertion of a loop IUD, the mean MBL increases to 70 to 80 mL.[14,15] The increase is less with copper-bearing devices. With the copper 7 IUD, the mean MBL has been found to vary from 50 to 55 mL,[14-16] while with the copper T 200, mean MBL varies from 50 to 60 mL.[15,17] In contrast, with the progesterone-releasing IUD, the amount of blood loss is actually reduced to about 25 mL/cycle.[18]

Some investigators report that the increase in MBL with copper-bearing IUDs is greatest in the first cycle after IUD insertion and that it declines steadily thereafter,[13,19] while others report that the increase in MBL is similar during each menses for 1 year after insertion of copper IUDs.[16,17] After insertion of copper as well as inert IUDs, a greater percentage of women have MBL in excess of 80 mL, an amount that has been shown to produce severe iron deficiency.[14] In a study of English women inserted with either the loop or copper 7,[14] there was a decrease in mean hemoglobin levels after 1 year, as well as a significant increase in the percentage of women with hemoglobin levels below 12 g/dL. As expected, because the mean MBL increase and the percentage of women losing more than 80 mL were greater with the loop than with the copper 7, the decrease in mean hemoglobin levels, as well as the incidence of anemia, was less with the copper 7 than with the loop. In a study of Swedish women inserted with the copper 7 or copper T 200, there was no significant change in mean values for hemoglobin concentration, serum iron, and total iron-binding capacity 6 and 12

months after IUD insertion when compared with mean values before insertion.[18]

A sensitive indicator of tissue iron stores is the serum ferritin level. Several studies have shown that both copper-bearing IUDs and nonmedicated plastic IUDs are associated with significant decreases in serum ferritin levels overall, as well as with an increase in the percentage of women with extremely low ferritin levels (less than 16 μg/L), indicative of an absence of iron in bone marrow.[20-22] Low serum ferritin levels are a good predictor of the development of anemia. Therefore, ideally both ferritin and hemoglobin levels should be measured annually in all women wearing nonsteroid-releasing IUDs. If either level decreases significantly, supplemental iron should be administered.

The exact mechanism whereby IUDs cause increased MBL is not completely understood, despite extensive investigative efforts. Histologic studies of endometrium obtained by biopsy and hysterectomy have demonstrated two types of lesions in association with IUDs. Vascular erosions have been seen in areas of direct contact with the IUD, and evidence of increased vascular permeability has been found in areas not in direct contact with the IUD. Both types of lesions could cause increased MBL as well as intermenstrual bleeding. An increased concentration of proteolytic enzymes and plasminogenic activators that may lead to increased fibrinolytic activity has been found in the endometrial tissue adjacent to the device. This increase in fibrinolytic activity adversely affects hemostasis and increases MBL.

Excessive bleeding in the first few months following IUD insertion should be treated with reassurance and supplemental oral iron. The bleeding may diminish with time, as the uterus adjusts to the presence of the foreign body. Excessive bleeding that continues or develops several months or more after IUD insertion may be treated by systemic administration of one of the prostaglandin synthetase inhibitors.

Mefenamic acid ingested in a dosage of 500 mg three times a day during the days of menstruation has been shown to reduce MBL significantly in IUD users.[23] If excessive bleeding continues despite this treatment, the device should be removed. After a 1-month interval, another kind of device may be inserted if the patient still wishes to use an IUD for contraception. The new device should be a copper or a progesterone-releasing IUD, because these smaller devices are associated with less blood loss than the larger ones.

Nulliparous women tolerate the smaller copper and progesterone-releasing IUDs better than the larger nonmedicated plastic ones. However, since event rates have not been shown to be significantly different with either type of IUD, in multiparous women the advantages of less blood loss with a medicated device should be weighed against the disadvantages of necessary periodic replacement. Until randomized, comparative studies demonstrate the superior performance of a particular device, the decision as to which type to use in a multiparous woman should be made by the physician and patient after considering the relative advantages and disadvantages of each.

Perforation

Although uncommon, one of the potentially serious complications associated with use of the IUD is perforation of the uterine fundus. Perforation initially occurs at insertion. It can best be prevented by straightening the uterine axis with a tenaculum and then probing the cavity with a uterine sound before IUD insertion. Sometimes only the distal portion of the IUD penetrates the uterine muscle at insertion. Then uterine contractions over the next few months force the IUD into the peritoneal cavity. IUDs correctly inserted entirely within the endometrial cavity do not wander through the uterine muscle into the peritoneal cavity. The incidence of perforation is generally related to the shape of the device and/or amount of force used during its insertion, as well as the experience of the clinician performing the insertion.

Perforation rates with the loop have been reported to be about 1/1,000 insertions.[1] In large multiclinic studies, perforation rates for the copper 7 and the copper T are in the same range as those for the loop. The clinician should always suspect perforation if a patient says she cannot feel the appendage but did not notice that the device was expelled. One should not assume that an unnoticed expulsion has occurred. Frequently, the device has rotated 180° and the appendage has been withdrawn into the cavity. In this situation, after pelvic examination has been performed and the possibility of pregnancy excluded, the uterine cavity should be probed.

In a study of 100 patients at this institution who had no IUD appendages visible at the time of a routine examination, it was found that 69 had the IUD in utero with the strings drawn up into the endometrial cavity, 17 had an unnoticed expulsion, 10 had a uterine perforation, and in 4 the cause was unknown.[24] If the device cannot be felt with a uterine sound or biopsy instrument, an x-ray or sonogram should be ordered. It is preferable to obtain both anteroposterior and lateral x-ray views with contrast medium or a uterine sound inside the uterine cavity. If the IUD is located in the cul-de-sac, the diagnosis may be missed with only an anteroposterior film.

Any type of IUD found to be outside the uterus should be electively removed, because such complications as adhesions and bowel obstruction have been reported. Both the copper IUDs and the shields have been found to produce severe peritoneal reactions. Therefore, it is best to remove these devices as soon as possible after the diagnosis of perforation is made. Unless severe adhesions have developed, most intraperitoneal IUDs can be removed by means of laparoscopy, avoiding the need for laparotomy.

Perforation of the cervix has also been reported with devices having a straight vertical arm such as the copper T or 7. The incidence of downward perforation into the cervix has been reported to range from about 1/600 to 1/1,000 insertions. When follow-up examinations are performed on patients with these devices, the cervix should be carefully inspected and palpated, because often perforations do not extend completely through the ectocervical epithelium. Cervical perforation is not a major problem, but devices that have perforated downward should be removed through the endocervical canal with uterine packing forceps. Their downward displacement is associated with reduced contraceptive effectiveness.

Complications related to pregnancy

Congenital anomalies

When pregnancy occurs with an IUD in place, implantation takes place away from the device itself, so the device is always extra-amniotic. Although there is a paucity of published data, so far there is no evidence of an increased incidence of congenital anomalies in infants born with an IUD in utero. In a study of spontaneously aborted tissue, 21% of the embryos conceived with an IUD in situ had evidence of abnormalities.[25] This was considerably less than the 44% incidence of abnormalities in abortuses of women using no contraception, and was similar to the incidence of embryonic abnormalities in abortuses of women having induced abortions. This suggests that the presence of an IUD has no influence on embryonic development and that the increased incidence of spontaneous abortion in IUD users is not due to a greater incidence of embryonic abnormalities.

In a study of 166 embryos conceived with an intrauterine copper T in place and large enough to permit adequate examination, only one had a congenital anomaly, a fibroma of the vocal cords.[26] In a series of 167 pregnancies that reached viability with the copper 7 in place, 159 normal babies were born.[27] No details were given regarding three infants, and the other five had a variety of anomalies. The incidence of congenital defects, 3%, was similar to the usually expected rate. Thus, there is no evidence from these studies to indicate that the presence of a copper IUD in the uterus exerts a deleterious effect on fetal development. Although relatively few infants have been born with a progesterone-releasing IUD in the uterus, careful examination of these infants has revealed no increased incidence of cardiac or other anomalies.

Spontaneous abortion

In all reported series of pregnancies with any type of IUD in situ, the incidence of fetal death was not significantly increased; however, a significant increase in spontaneous abortion has been consistently observed. In the first 7 years of the prospective Oxford Family Planning Association study, there were a total of 494 unplanned pregnancies among women using IUDs, OCs, or diaphragms.[28] After the electively terminated pregnancies were excluded, the rates of spontaneous abortion were 55.7% for women using IUDs, 13.6% for women using OCs, and 18.1% for women using diaphragms. This significantly greater incidence in the IUD-failure group is similar to the spontaneous abortion rate of 55.6% reported among 233 women who became pregnant with nonmedicated IUDs in place and did not have the devices removed.[29] In a study of 157 women who became pregnant with copper T devices in place that were not subsequently removed, the spontaneous abortion rate was 54.1%.[26] These three studies indicate that if a patient conceives while wearing an IUD that is not subsequently removed, the incidence of spontaneous abortion is about 55%, approximately three times greater than would occur without an IUD.

After conception, if the IUD is spontaneously expelled, or if the appendage is visible and the IUD is removed by traction, the incidence of spontaneous abortion is significantly reduced. Of 201 women conceiving with a loop in place, the abortion rate was 48.3% if the device was not removed and only 29.6% if it was removed.[30] In the study mentioned above of women who conceived with copper T devices in place,[26] the incidence of spontaneous abortion was only 20.3% if the device was removed or spontaneously expelled. This figure is similar to the normal incidence of spontaneous abortion and significantly less than the 54.1% incidence of abortion reported in the same study among women retaining the devices in utero. Thus, if a woman conceives with an IUD in place and wishes to continue the pregnancy, the IUD should be removed if the appendage is visible. This will significantly reduce the chance of spontaneous abortion. If the appendage is not visible, the uterine cavity should not be probed in an attempt to locate the IUD, because the probing may increase the chance of abortion as well as sepsis.

Septic abortion

If the IUD cannot be easily removed, or if the appendage is not visible, available evidence suggests that the risk of septic abortion may be increased if the IUD remains in place. Most of the evidence is based on data from women who conceived while wearing the shield type of IUD. This device, with its multifilament tail, was widely used from 1971 to 1974. It has been shown that the structure of the shield's appendage allowed bacteria to enter the spaces between the filaments of the tail underneath the sheath. This contrasts with the inability of bacteria to enter the monofilament tails of other devices.[31] During pregnancy, when the shield was drawn upward into the uterus as gestation advanced, the bacteria in the tail had the potential for causing a severe and sometimes fatal uterine infection, usually in the second trimester of pregnancy.

Although there is theoretical and actual evidence of an increased risk of septic abortion if a patient conceives with a shield IUD in place, there is no conclusive evidence of an increased risk if a patient conceives with a device other than the shield in place. In the Oxford study, there was no significant difference in the incidence of septic abortion between women who conceived with an IUD in place and those who conceived while using other methods.[32] Of 115 spontaneous abortions, 58 occurred in the IUD group and 57 in women using other methods. There was evidence of sepsis in six of these abortions—four in the IUD group and two in the others, an insignificant difference. None of the women with septic abortions were seriously ill, and all responded promptly to treatment. In a study of 918 women who conceived with the copper T in situ, there were only two cases of septic abortion, both occurring in the first trimester.[26] This evidence does not suggest an increase in sepsis in pregnancy due to the presence of an IUD, except that about 2% of all spontaneous abortions are septic, and IUDs increase the rate of spontaneous abortion.

Thus, if a patient with a shield IUD in place conceives and wishes to continue the pregnancy, and the device cannot be removed without entering the uterine cavity, she should be fully informed of the risks. Because of the increased incidence of fatal sepsis in pregnancy that has been reported with the shield IUD, it is advisable that the device be removed and the pregnancy terminated. However, while there is no conclusive evidence of an increased incidence of sepsis with other types of IUDs, the patient should be informed of the possibility of a greater chance of sepsis and, if she wishes to continue the pregnancy, of the need to report symptoms of infection promptly. If an intrauterine infection does occur during pregnancy with an IUD in place, treatment should proceed in the same manner as if the IUD were absent. In such a situation, the endometrial cavity should be evacuated following a short interval of appropriate antibiotic treatment.

Ectopic pregnancy

As stated above, the IUD's main mechanism of contraceptive action is the production of a continuous sterile inflammatory reaction in the uterine cavity due to foreign body presence. As the large numbers of leukocytes stimulated to enter the uterine cavity by the inflammatory reaction are catabolized, their breakdown products exert a toxic effect on sperm and the blastocyst. Less of this inflammatory reaction reaches the oviducts, so the IUD prevents intrauterine pregnancy more effectively than it prevents ectopic pregnancy.

It was estimated that if the 30,000 women enrolled in the Population Council IUD study did not have their rate of fertilization changed by use of the IUD, during the 45,000 woman-years of use, about 180,000 fertilized ova and 900 ectopic pregnancies would be expected.[33] Of the ectopic pregnancies, 845 would be tubal and approximately five ovarian.

Actually, during that time there were 1,046 pregnancies with IUDs in situ, 45 of which were ectopic: 40 tubal and five ovarian. From analysis of these data it was concluded that IUD use reduces uterine implantation by 99.5%, tubal implantation by about 95%, and ovarian pregnancy not at all. Thus, a pregnancy occurring with an IUD in place is more likely to be ectopic than one occurring in the absence of an IUD. Several additional studies have confirmed this finding.[28]

If a patient conceives with an IUD in place, her chances of having an ectopic pregnancy range from 3% to 9%. This incidence is about 10 times greater than the reported ectopic pregnancy frequency of 0.3% to 0.7% of total births in similar populations. In two large Population Council studies, the ectopic pregnancy rate in IUD wearers was about 1.0 to 1.2 per 1,000 woman-years.[1,34]

Thus, if a patient conceives with an IUD in place, ectopic pregnancy should be suspected. There appears to be a higher frequency of ectopic pregnancy with the progesterone-releasing IUD, and patients conceiving while wearing this device should have sonography performed early in gestation.[35] In addition, the possibility of ovarian pregnancy should always be considered. IUD users with a clinical diagnosis of ruptured corpus luteum may, in fact, have an unrecognized ovarian pregnancy. If any patient with an IUD has an elective termination of pregnancy, the evacuated tissue should be examined histologically to be certain that the gestation was intrauterine.

Despite the increased incidence of ectopic pregnancy in women conceiving with an IUD in place, overall the IUD reduces the incidence of ectopic pregnancy. A recent Centers for Disease Control (CDC) study indicates that women using IUDs have only about 40% as great a chance of developing ectopic pregnancy as women using no method of contraception.[36] This is similar to the protection against ectopic pregnancy provided by barrier methods, but not as effective as that provided by OCs.

Prematurity

In the previously cited study of conceptions occurring in the presence of copper T devices,[26] the rate of prematurity among live births was four times greater when the copper T was left in place than when it was removed. Although the sample size was small and the rate of prematurity in the IUD-removal group was only 4.3%, the higher incidence of prematurity when the device was left in situ was significant. In a study of pregnancies with the loop in situ,[30] the incidence of prematurity was also higher if the device was left in place, but the numbers were small and the differences were not significant. A higher incidence of prematurity with IUDs in utero was also noted in the Oxford study.[28] It was reported that 13.6% of infants conceived during IUD use weighed less than 2,800 g at birth, compared with 3% of infants conceived during the use of other contraceptive methods.

If a pregnant patient has an IUD in place

and the device cannot be removed but the patient wishes to continue gestation, she should be warned of the increased risk of prematurity as well as that of spontaneous abortion and ectopic pregnancy. She should also be informed of the possible increased risk of septic abortion and advised to report promptly the first signs of pelvic pain or fever. There is no evidence that pregnancies with IUDs in utero are associated with an increased incidence of other obstetric complications. There is also no evidence that earlier use of an IUD results in a greater incidence of complications in subsequent pregnancies.

Infection in the nonpregnant IUD user

In the 1960s, despite great concern among gynecologists that use of the IUD would markedly in-crease the incidence of salpingitis, or pelvic inflammatory disease (PID), there was little evidence that such an increase did occur. During that decade, the IUD was inserted mainly into parous women, and the incidence of sexually transmitted disease was not as high as it is currently. In 1966, we prepared aerobic and anaerobic cultures of homogenates of endometrial tissue obtained transfundally from uteri removed by vaginal hysterectomy at various intervals after loop insertion.[37] During the first 24 hours, the normally sterile endometrial cavity was consistently infected with bacteria. Nevertheless, in 80% of cases, the women's natural defenses destroyed these bacteria within 24 hours. In our study, the endometrial cavity, the IUD, and the portion of the thread within the cavity were con-

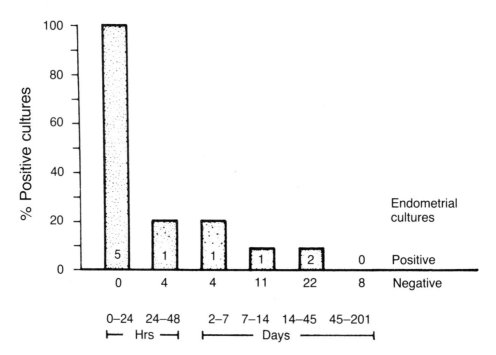

Figure 38-2
Relationship of incidence of positive endometrial cultures to duration of use of loop IUD.

From Mishell DR Jr, Bell JH, Good RG, et al: The intrauterine device: A bacteriologic study of the endometrial cavity. Am J Obstet Gynecol 96:119, 1966.

Contraception

sistently found to be sterile when transfundal cultures were obtained more than 30 days after insertion (Figure 38-2). These findings indicate that development of PID more than a month after insertion of the loop IUD is of venereal origin and unrelated to the presence of the device.

These findings agree with the incidence of clinically diagnosed PID found in a group of 23,977 mainly parous women wearing IUDs.[1] When PID rates were computed according to the duration of IUD use, the rates were highest in the first 2 weeks after insertion and then steadily diminished. Rates after the first month were in the range of 1 to 2.5 per 100 woman-years (Table 38-7).

The results of both of these studies indicate that an IUD should not be inserted into a patient who may have been recently infected with gonococci or *Chlamydia*. Insertion of the device will transport these pathogens into the upper genital tract. If there is clinical suspicion of infectious endocervicitis, cultures should be done and the IUD insertion delayed until negative results are obtained. It does not appear to be cost-effective to administer systemic antibiotics routinely with IUD insertion, but the insertion technique should be as aseptic as possible.

Following the introduction and widespread use of the shield device, particularly among nul-liparous women (in whom IUDs were previously inserted only occasionally), several published studies suggested that IUD use increased the relative risk of PID.

A prospective case-control study of patients at an emergency room in Atlanta demonstrated a relative risk of 5.1 for IUD-related febrile PID versus non-IUD-related febrile PID.[38] In the prospective Oxford Family Planning Association study based on inpatient illness, the incidence of PID was about three times greater in IUD users than in diaphragm or oral contraceptive users.[39] In a prospective case-control study from Sweden, the diagnosis of PID was made by laparoscopy, and the controls were chosen by questionnaire.[40] Analysis of these data showed that the relative risk for development of PID in IUD users versus nonusers was 2.9 for all women, 6.8 for nulliparous women, and only 1.7 for parous women.[41] The relative risk of PID decreased with age when parity was standardized, and it showed a marked drop in nulliparous women over age 25.

A retrospective case-control study found the relative risk of PID among IUD users versus nonusers to be 4.4 for all women, 2.8 for gonococcal PID, and 6.5 for nongonococcal PID.[42] This study also found an increased risk of PID in nulliparous compared with parous IUD users.

Table 38-7
Rate of pelvic inflammatory disease,
categorized by period of diagnosis

Period	Cases	Woman-years	Rate per 100 woman-years (95% confidence limits)
1–25 days	75	969	7.7 (6.0–9.5)
16–30 days	34	913	3.7 (2.5–5.0)
2–12 months	421	16,144	2.6 (2.4–2.9)
13–24 months	236	10,588	2.2 (1.9–2.5)
25–36 months	94	6,068	1.5 (1.2–1.9)
37–72 months	40	4,420	0.9 (0.6–1.2)

From Tietze C, Lewit S: Evaluation of intrauterine devices: Ninth progress report of the Cooperative Statistical Program. Stud Fam Plan 1:55, 1970.

An additional study also reported that IUD users had a greater relative risk of developing PID than nonusers.[43]

There are several problems with all these studies. One is that uniform guidelines were not used for the diagnosis of PID (or salpingitis). Differences in diagnostic criteria may have increased the frequency of the diagnosis among IUD users. Patients with lower abdominal pain and only minimal or no elevation in temperature may have been given the diagnosis of PID more often when an IUD was in the uterus.

A second problem is the evidence that use of OCs, condoms, and diaphragms provides protection against development of PID. The data from numerous studies indicate that the incidence of both febrile and nonfebrile PID is about half as much in women using OCs and barrier methods as in women using no method of contraception. In the Oxford Family Planning Association study, the rates of PID requiring hospitalization were similar with these two types of contraception.[39] Most sexually active women use contraception, mainly OCs, barriers, or the IUD. The increased risk of infection with the IUD is due in large part to the protective effect of the other contraceptives.

A third problem is that in most of the studies performed in the 1970s, a high percentage of IUD wearers were using the shield. This device is more likely than the other types to have a causal relationship to PID. Investigators carefully examined the sheaths of the appendages of both new shields in their sterile packages and shields removed from patients.[31] They found that 9% of the new shields and 34% of the used shields had breaks in the sheath around the knot attaching it to the device. These breaks would allow bacteria continuous access from the vagina to the endometrial cavity and thus increase the risk of upper genital tract infection.

Finally, none of these studies differentiated between episodes of PID developing in the first few months after IUD insertion (previously shown to be related to the insertion itself) and episodes developing later. Recently, CDC investigators reported results from a multicenter case-control study of the relationship of the IUD and PID.[44] They found the overall risk of PID in IUD users versus noncontraceptive users to be

Table 38-8
Risk of pelvic inflammatory disease in IUD users
(excluding Dalkon Shield users)
by duration of use

Duration of use of current IUD (months)*	Women with PID†	Controls†	Relative risk‡
≤1	27	17	3.8 (2.1–6.8)
2–4	22	32	1.7 (1.1–3.1)
5–12	33	90	1.1 (0.7–1.7)
13–24	32	81	1.2 (0.7–1.8)
25–60	23	62	1.2 (0.7–2.0)
>60	13	40	1.4 (0.7–2.7)
No method	250	763	1 (referent)

*IUD used in the 3 months before interview.

†Limited to women who reported no past history of PID.

‡Relative risk adjusted for age, marital status, and number of sexual partners within the previous 6 months; 95% confidence intervals in parentheses.

From Lee NC, Rubin GL, Ory HW, et al: Type of intrauterine device and the risk of pelvic inflammatory disease. Obstet Gynecol 62:1, 1983.

1.9. The risk in shield users was 8.3; in other IUD users, it was only 1.6. When the risk of PID in IUD users (other than shield users) was correlated with duration of use, it was found that a significantly increased risk of PID with the loop and copper 7 was present only during the first 4 months after insertion (Table 38-8). After that, there was no significantly increased risk in IUD users other than those with shields. Thus, this report is in agreement with our 1966 study[37] and the 1970 summary of 23,977 IUD users[1] mentioned above. It indicates that PID occurring more than a few months following insertion of loop or copper devices is due to a sexually transmitted disease and not related to the IUD.

The populations at high risk for PID include those with a prior history of PID, nulliparous women under 25 years of age, and women with multiple sexual partners. The FDA has recommended that women with these characteristics be especially advised about the risks of developing PID during IUD use and the possibility of subsequent loss of fertility. They should be told to watch for the early symptoms of PID, so that treatment can be started before complications occur. These data, as well as those of two recent studies showing an increased risk of tubal causes of infertility in nulliparous women who had used an IUD,[45,46] indicate that the clinician should avoid using IUDs in nulliparous women who may want to conceive in the future. The increased risk of impairment of future fertility from PID in the first few months after IUD insertion, as well as the possibility of ectopic pregnancy, must be considered when deciding whether to use an IUD in a nulliparous woman.

Symptomatic PID can usually be successfully treated with antibiotics without removing the IUD until the patient becomes symptom-free. In patients with clinical evidence of a tuboovarian abscess or with a shield in place, the IUD should be removed only after a therapeutic serum level of appropriate parenteral antibiotics has been reached, and preferably after a clinical response has been observed. An alternative method of contraception should be substituted in patients who develop PID with an IUD in place (or in those with a past history of PID).

There is evidence that IUD users may have an increased risk for colonizing actinomycosis organisms in the upper genital tract. The relationship of actinomycosis to PID is unclear; however, at present it would appear best to try to identify these organisms on the routine annual cytologic smear. If they are present, the IUD should be removed and should not be reinserted until the organisms disappear. The use of antibiotics in asymptomatic women with actinomycosis is probably unnecessary.

Overall safety

Several long-term studies have indicated that the IUD is not associated with an increased incidence of endometrial or cervical carcinoma. One author estimated a mortality rate of three to five deaths per million IUD users annually, due mainly to infection.[47] He demonstrated, however, that as far as mortality is concerned, the IUD is at least as safe as other methods of contraception, including sterilization, and safer than using no contraception at all at any age. Nevertheless, the IUD does produce morbidity that may result in hospitalization. The main causes of hospitalization among IUD users are complications of pregnancy, uterine perforation, and hemorrhage, as well as pelvic infection.[48] Despite the increased morbidity with IUDs, the actual incidence of these problems is low and is probably even lower now that the shield is no longer used and physicians are aware of the potential complications associated with IUDs in pregnancy. The IUD is a particularly useful method of contraception for women who have completed their families and do not wish to undergo sterilization, as well as for older women in whom the risks of taking steroid contraceptives may be increased.

References

1. Tietze C, Lewit S: Evaluation of intrauterine devices: Ninth progress report of the Cooperative Statistical Program. *Stud Fam Plan* 1:55, 1970

2. Moyer DL, Mishell DR Jr: Reactions of human endometrium to the intrauterine foreign body. II. Long-term effects on the endometrial histology and cytology. *Am J Obstet Gynecol* 111:66, 1971

3. Tredway DR, Umezaki CU, Mishell DR Jr: Effect of intrauterine devices on sperm transport in the human being: Preliminary report. *Am J Obstet Gynecol* 123:734, 1975

4. Croxatto H: personal communication, 1985

5. Vessey MP, Lawless M, McPherson K, et al: Fertility after stopping use of intrauterine contraceptive device. *Br Med J* 286:106, 1983

6. World Health Organization [WHO]: *Special Programme of Research Development and Research Training in Human Reproduction.* Eleventh Annual Report. Geneva, WHO, November 1982, p 159

7. White MK, Ory HW, Rooks JB, et al: Intrauterine device termination rates and the menstrual cycle day of insertion. *Obstet Gynecol* 55:220, 1980

8. Mishell DR Jr, Roy S: Copper intrauterine contraceptive device event rates following insertion 4 to 8 weeks postpartum. *Am J Obstet Gynecol* 143:29, 1982

9. Luukkainen T, Allonen H, Nielsen NC, et al: Five years' experience of intrauterine contraception with the Nova-T and Copper-T-200. *Am J Obstet Gynecol* 147:885, 1983

10. Sivin I, Tatum HJ: Four years of experience with the T Cu 380A intrauterine contraceptive device. *Fertil Steril* 36:159, 1981

11. Mishell DR Jr: The clinical factor in evaluating IUDs. In Hefnawi F, Segal S (eds): *Analysis of Intrauterine Contraception.* Proceedings of the Third International Symposium on IUDs, Cairo, Egypt, December 1974. New York, American Elsevier, 1975, p 27

12. Brenner PF, Mishell DR Jr: Progesterone and estradiol patterns in women using an intrauterine contraceptive device. *Obstet Gynecol* 46:456, 1975

13. Guillebaud J, Bonnar J: Longer though lighter menstrual and intermenstrual bleeding with copper as compared to inert intrauterine devices. *Br J Obstet Gynaecol* 85:707, 1978

14. Guillebaud J, Bonnar J, Morehead J, et al: Menstrual blood-loss with intrauterine devices. *Lancet* 1:387, 1976

15. Hefnawi F, Askalani H, Zaki K: Menstrual blood loss with copper intrauterine devices. *Contraception* 9:133, 1974

16. Larsson B, Hamberger L, Rybo G: Influence of copper intrauterine devices (Cu-7-IUD) on the menstrual blood-loss. *Acta Obstet Gynecol Scand* 54:315, 1975

17. Liedholm P, Rybo G, Sjöberg N-O, et al: Copper IUD—Influence on menstrual blood loss and iron deficiency. *Contraception* 12:317, 1975

18. Rybo G: The IUD and endometrial bleeding. *J Reprod Med* 20:175, 1978

19. Malmqvist R, Petersohn L, Bengtsson LP: Menstrual bleeding with copper-covered intrauterine contraceptive devices. *Contraception* 9:627, 1974

20. Guillebaud J, Barnett MD, Gordon YB: Plasma ferritin levels as an index of iron deficiency in women using intrauterine devices. *Br J Obstet Gynaecol* 86:51, 1979

21. Heikkilä M, Nylander P, Luukkainen T: Body iron stores and patterns of bleeding after insertion of a levonorgestrel- or a copper-releasing intrauterine contraceptive device. *Contraception* 26:465, 1982

22. Piedras J, Córdova MS, Pérez-Toral MC, et al: Predictive value of serum ferritin in anemia development after insertion of T Cu 220 intrauterine device. *Contraception* 27:289, 1983

23. Anderson ABM, Haynes PJ, Guillebaud J, et al: Reduction of menstrual blood loss by prostaglandin synthetase inhibitors. *Lancet* 1:774, 1976

24. Millen A, Austin F, Bernstein GS: Analysis of 100 cases of missing IUD strings. *Contraception* 18:485, 1978

25. Poland B: Conception control and embryonic development. *Am J Obstet Gynecol* 106:365, 1970

26. Tatum HJ, Schmidt FH, Jain AK: Management and outcome of pregnancies associated with the Copper T intrauterine contraceptive device. *Am J Obstet Gynecol* 126:869, 1976

27. Guillebaud J: Copper IUCDs and pregnancy. [Letter] *Br J Fam Plan* 7:88, 1981

28. Vessey MP, Johnson B, Doll R, et al: Outcome of pregnancy in women using an intrauterine device. *Lancet* 1:495, 1974

29. Lewit SL: Outcome of pregnancies with intrauterine devices. *Contraception* 2:47, 1970

30. Alvior GT Jr: Pregnancy outcome with removal of intrauterine device. *Obstet Gynecol* 41:894, 1973

31. Tatum HJ, Schmidt FH, Phillips DM, et al: The Dalkon shield controversy, structural and bacteriologic studies of IUD tails. *JAMA* 231:711, 1975

32. Williams P, Johnson B, Vessey M: Septic abortion in women using intrauterine devices. *Br Med J* 4:253, 1975

33. Lehfeldt H, Tietze C, Gorstein F: Ovarian pregnancy and the intrauterine device. *Am J Obstet Gynecol* 108:1005, 1970

34. Sivin I: Copper T IUD use and ectopic pregnancy rates in the United States. *Contraception* 19:151, 1979

35. Gibor Y, Pharris B: Grossesse extra-utérine et DIU [Extrauterine pregnancies and IUD use]. *Contraception, Fertilité, Sexualité* 8:109, 1980

36. Ory HW: Ectopic pregnancy and intrauterine contraceptive devices: New perspectives. The Women's Health Study. *Obstet Gynecol* 57:137, 1981

37. Mishell DR Jr, Bell JH, Good RG, et al: The intrauterine device: A bacteriologic study of the endometrial cavity. *Am J Obstet Gynecol* 96:119, 1966

38. Faulkner WL, Ory HW: Intrauterine devices and acute pelvic inflammatory disease. *JAMA* 235:1851, 1976

39. Vessey MP, Doll R, Peto R, et al: A long-term follow-up study of women using different methods of contraception. An interim report. *J Biosoc Sci* 8:373, 1976

40. Weström L, Bengtsson LP, Mardh PA: The risk of pelvic inflammatory disease in women using intrauterine contraceptive devices as compared to non-users. *Lancet* 2:221, 1976

41. Ory HW: A review of the association between intrauterine devices and acute pelvic inflammatory disease. *J Reprod Med* 20:200, 1978

42. Eschenbach DA, Harnisch JP, Holmes KK: Pathogenesis of acute pelvic inflammatory disease: Role of contraception and other risk factors. *Am J Obstet Gynecol* 128:838, 1977

43. Kaufman DW, Watson J, Rosenberg L, et al: The effect of different types of intrauterine devices on the risk of pelvic inflammatory disease. *JAMA* 250:759, 1983

44. Lee NC, Rubin GL, Ory HW, et al: Type of intrauterine device and the risk of pelvic inflammatory disease. *Obstet Gynecol* 62:1, 1983

45. Daling JR, Weiss NS, Metch BJ, et al: Primary tubal infertility in relation to use of an intrauterine device. *N Engl J Med* 312:937, 1985

46. Cramer DW, Schiff I, Schoenbaum SC, et al: Tubal infertility and the intrauterine device. *N Engl J Med* 312:941, 1985

47. Jain AK: Safety and effectiveness of intrauterine devices. *Contraception* 11:243, 1975

48. Kahn HS, Tyler CW Jr: IUD-related hospitalizations: United States and Puerto Rico, 1973. *JAMA* 234:53, 1975

Index

Childhood, 172-173
Chlamydia, 534-535
Chloasma, and OC use, 604
Chlorpromazine, 15
Cholelithiasis, and OC use, 604
Cholesterol
    luteinizing hormone action and, 37
    and OC use, 609, 611, 614
    steroid biosynthesis, 46, 48
Cholesterol esterase, 37
Chromophobe adenomas, 266
Chromosomes
    fertilization and, 109
    gonadal development and, 205-207
    gonadal disorders and, 208-214
    male pseudohermaphroditism and,
        216
    oocytes and, 105-106
    recurrent abortion and, 540-542
    See also Genetics
Chronic endometritis, 341
Cigarette smoking
    heart disease and, 196
    menopause and, 180
    OC use and, 605, 609, 610, 611, 612
Circulatory disease, and OC use, 610,
    611
Cirrhosis, 342
Climacteric, 179
    See also Menopause
Clomiphene citrate
    human menopausal gonadotropin
        combination regimens, 404-405
    in vitro fertilization, 566-567
    luteal phase defects, 561
    ovulation induction, 389-398
Clonidine, 184
CMPT test (postcoital testing), 414
Coagulation defects, 341-342
Coital technique, 418
Colorimetry, 62
Condom
    contraceptive use, 589-590
    and PID, 654

therapeutic use, 528
Congenital adrenal hyperplasia (CAH)
    female pseudohermaphroditism and,
        214
    therapy for, 315
Congenital anomalies
    and IUD use, 649
    after OC use, 609, 612
Contraception
    cervical cap, 589
    condom, 589-590, 654
    contraceptive steroids. See
        Contraceptive steroids
    defined, 583
    diaphragm, 588-589
    effectiveness of, 584-588, 630, 632,
        633, 636, 640, 645
    fertility after discontinuance of, 607,
        627, 640, 641, 651
    interception, 636-637
    IUD. See Intrauterine devices
    oral. See Oral steroid contraceptives
    postcoital, 636-637
    rhythm method, 590
    spermicides, 588
    use of, 583-584
Contraceptive steroids
    CVRs. See Contraceptive vaginal rings
    injectable. See Injectable contraceptive
        steroids
    long-acting, 623-636
    subdural implants, 630-633
    oral. See Oral steroid contraceptives
Contraceptive vaginal rings (CVRs),
    633-636
Copper 7, 640, 642, 647, 655
Copper T, 640, 642, 646, 647, 650, 651
Corpus lutem
    human chorionic gonadotropin and,
        113, 126
    hypothalamic-pituitary ovarian
        regulation, 74
    luteal phase defects, 553-564
    luteinizing hormone action on, 37

Depression, and OC use, 612
DES. *See* Diethylstilbestrol
17, 20 Desmolase deficiency, 248
Desquamation, 96
Dexamethasone suppression test
    Cushing's syndrome, 309-310
    testing dynamics, 367-369
DHEA. *See* Dehydroepiandrosterone
DHEA-S. *See* Dehydroepiandrosterone
    sulfate
DHT. *See* Dihydrotestosterone
Diabetes
    human placental lactogen, 127
    and OC use, 609, 611, 612, 615
    polycystic ovary syndrome, 332
    puberty and, 165
    secondary amenorrhea and, 253
Diaphragm, 586, 588-589
    fertility after stopping use of, 627, 641
    and PID, 654
Didelphic uterus, 471
Diethylstilbestrol (DES)
    exposure to, and OC use, 611
    in interception, 636
    recurrent abortion and, 542
    uterine anomalies and, 476-477
Dihydrotestosterone (DHT)
    fetal sex differentiation, 169
    genitalia development, 207-208
    male pseudohermaphroditism, 217, 218
    testes and, 424
Dihydroxyphenylacetic acid (DOPAC), 10
Dihydroxyprogesterone acetophenide, 628
Dilatation and curettage (D & C)
    dysfunctional uterine bleeding, 349
    uterine synechiae, 270
Distal tubal disease, 482-486
DMPA. *See* Depo-medroxyprogesterone
    acetate
DNA
    estrogen therapy and, 199

gonadal development and, 208
    progestins and, 200-201
    steroid actions and, 42
DOPAC. *See* Dihydroxyphenylacetic
    acid
Dopamine
    β-endorphin and, 17
    gonadotropin-releasing hormone
        pulse activity and, 76
    hyperprolactinemia and, 282
    hypothalamus and, 8-10
    pharmacologic effects on, 15
    polycystic ovary syndrome and, 329-330
    prolactin and, 22, 275, 276, 278
Dysfunctional uterine bleeding. *See*
    Uterine bleeding, dysfunctional
Dysmenorrhea
    OC use and, 618
    secondary, 499

E

Ectopic pregnancy, 492-495
    with IUD in situ, 651, 655
    and OC use, 620-621
Ejaculation, 426, 428
Electroencephalography, 229
ELISA. *See* Enzyme-linked
    immunosorbent assay
Embryo
    gonadal development, 206
    in vitro fertilization, 572-573, 575-577
Embryo transport, 109-110
Empty sella syndrome, 285-288
Endocrinology, defined, 3
Endometrial cancer (carcinoma), 183, 198-199
    DMPA treatment for, 623, 627
    and IUD, 655
    and OC use, 606, 612, 616-617
Endometrial ground substance, 103
Endometrial hyperplasia, 200
    and OC use, 616
Endometriosis. *See* Pelvic endometriosis

dopamine and, 9-10
dysfunctional uterine bleeding and,
  344
endometrium and, 97, 98
fetal sex differentiation, 169
follicle development, 107
fracture prevention and, 192-194
gonadotropin-releasing hormone
  and, 21
gonadotropin secretion and, 27
granulosa cells and, 38
hepatic thyroxine-binding globulin,
  117
hot flushes, 182-183
in injectable contraceptives, 628, 630
lactation, 158-162, 277
menopause, 180, 181, 182
menopause treatment, 185-186, 194-
  201
menstrual cycle and, 95, 101-102
in OCs, 593-595
osteoporosis and, 189-191, 192-194
ovulation induction, 405
pelvic endometriosis, 505-506
peptide steroid-receptor interactions,
  43
primary amenorrhea, 238-239
progesterone and, 42-43
side effects with high dose therapy,
  636
pseudoisosexual precocious puberty,
  231
puberty and, 166, 175
quantitative menstrual effects, 81
synthetic, 594-595, 600
Estrone, 616
fetoplacental production of, 132-133
luteal phase defects, 560
menopause and, 181
steroid biosynthesis, 49
Ethynodiol diacetate, in OCs, 594, 595
Ethinylestradiol
in interception, 636, 637
in OCs, 595, 599, 600, 613

E_2. *See* Estradiol

F
Factor VII, and OC use, 604
Fallopian tube
  fertilization and, 109
  lesions, 457-458
  See also Tubal surgery
Female precocious puberty. *See*
    Precocious puberty (female)
Female pseudohermaphroditism, 214-
  216
Femtogram, 61
Ferritin, and IUD, 647
Fertility (conception)
  after discontinuance of
    contraceptives, 607, 627, 640, 641,
    651
  future, and IUD in nulliparous
    women, 655
Fertilization
  abnormal, 111
  oocyte and, 109-111
  vitelline membrane and, 108-109
  zona pellucida and, 108
  See also In vitro fertilization
Fetal growth retardation, 128
Fetoplacental steroid hormones, 129-
  134
  estradiol/estrone production, 132-133
  estriol production, 133-134
  placental androgen metabolism, 131-
    132
  placental progesterone production,
    129-131
Fetoplacental-unit steroidogenesis, 126
Fetus
  endocrine disorders in, 214-219
  endocrinology of, 135-137
  genitalia development in, 207-208
  gonadal development in, 207
  masculinizing effect of gestagens on,
    612
  progesterone metabolism in, 130

menopause, 179
polycystic ovary syndrome, 329
primary amenorrhea, 240-243, 245-246
puberty, 165
recurrent abortion, 542
uterine agenesis, 247-248
uterine anomalies, 471-475
See also Chromosomes
Genital infection infertility, occult, 531-537
chlamydia, 534-535
mycoplasmas, 531-534
organisms in, 535-536
Gestagens
androgenic effects, 604
and breast cancer, 605-606
in CVRs, 633
masculinizing effect of, on female fetuses, 612
structures of, 594
synthetic, 594-595
Gestation. *See* Pregnancy
Gestational age, 542
GH. *See* Growth hormones
GHRF. *See* Growth hormone-releasing factor
GHRH. *See* Growth hormone-releasing hormone
Globulins, effect of OCs on, 600-601
Glucocorticoid hormones, 309
Glucose metabolism, and OC use, 604
Glucose tolerance, and CVRs, 634
Glycogen
endometrium and, 99, 102
menstrual cycle and, 97-98
β_1-Glycoprotein, 128-129
GnRH. *See* Gonadotropin-releasing hormone
Gonadal dysgenesis, 211-212, 243
Gonadostat
childhood, 173
infancy, 171
Gonadotropin-releasing hormone (GnRH)

anorexia nervosa and, 261
childhood, 173
complete isosexual precocious puberty, 228
dopamine and, 9
dysfunctional uterine bleeding, 339
β-endorphin and, 18
fetal sex differentiation, 169
follicle development and, 69
gonadotropins and, 22-24
hyperprolactinemia and, 279-280
hypothalamic-pituitary ovarian regulation, 74-81
lactation and, 154, 157
norepinephrine and, 10
OC use and, 598, 599, 600, 601
ovulation induction, 407-409
pelvic endometriosis, 508
pituitary hormones and, 19-21
polycystic ovary syndrome, 321
precocious puberty diagnosis, 232, 233
premature thelarche, 225-226
primary amenorrhea, 237-239, 240
prostaglandins and, 16
puberty, 165, 173-174, 176
secondary amenorrhea, 254, 259, 262-263
testes and, 424
testing dynamics, 369-370
thyrotropin-releasing hormone and, 21
transport of, 4-5
Gonadotropins
childhood, 172-173
dopamine and, 9
feedback mechanism, 77-78
fetal endocrinology, 135-136
fetal sex differentiation, 168, 169
follicle development and, 69, 106, 108
gonadotropin-releasing hormone pulses and, 76
infancy, 171
IUDs and, 646

MI. *See* Myocardial infarction

Microagglutination tests, 527

Micromicrograms, 61

Micropenis, 136

Milk production. *See* Lactation

Millimicrogram, 61

Miscarriage. *See* Recurrent abortion; Spontaneous abortion

Monoclonal antibodies, 64

"Morning after pill," 636-637

Mosaicism, 243

Müllerian duct
  normal development of, 207
  recurrent abortion and, 542

Müllerian inhibiting factor, 245-246

Multiple gestations, 396, 399

Mycoplasmas, 531-534

Myocardial infarction, OC use and, 196, 605, 609, 610, 611, 612, 614, 615

Myomectomy
  hysteroscopy, 478-479
  secondary amenorrhea, 270

N

NAD$^+$-dependent 15-hydroxyprostaglandin dehydrogenase (PGDH), 104

Naloxone, 184

Nanogram, 61

Nausea, and OC use, 614

Neoplastic effects, of OCs, 605-608, 618

NET-EN. *See* Norethindrone enanthate

Neural input pathways, 5

Neural output pathways, 4-5

Neurobiology, 3

Neuroendocrinology, 3

Neurohypophysis
  anatomy of, 5-6
  blood supply, 7

Neuromodulators
  hypothalamus and, 15-19
  See also entries under names of specific neuromodulators

Neurophysin, 3

Neurosecretion, 3

Neurotransmitters
  hypothalamus and, 8-15
  mechanism of action of, 15
  pharmacologic agents effects on, 15
  See also entries under specific neurotransmitters

Nicotinamide adenine dinucleotide phosphate (NADPH), 37

Nonsteroidal anti-inflammatory drugs (NSAIDs), 346-348

Norepinephrine
  gonadotropin-releasing hormone pulse activity and, 76
  hypothalamus and, 10
  menstrual cycle and, 279
  pharmacologic effects on, 15
  polycystic ovary syndrome, 330

Norethindrone, in OCs, 594, 595, 600

Norethindrone enanthate (NET-EN), 628, 629
  termination rates, 630

Norethynodrel, in OCs, 594

Norgestrel
  in OCs, 594, 595, 596, 597
  in interception, 637

Normal values calculation, 67-68

19-Nortestosterone, 594

Nova T, 646

Nursing, *See* Breast-feeding; Lactation

Nutrition
  osteoporosis and, 194
  premenstrual syndrome and, 357-358
  puberty and, 165, 166

O

Obesity
  polycystic ovary syndrome, 319, 331-332
  postcoital testing and, 418
  puberty and, 166
  See also Body weight; *entries under* Weight

OCs. *See* Oral steroid contraceptives

Prostacyclin, 139
Prostaglandins
    hypothalamus and, 15-16
    and IUDs, 646-647
    labor initiation, 139
    luteinizing hormone action and, 39
    menstrual cycle and, 103-104
    premenstrual syndrome and, 356-357
Protein hormone receptors, 31
Protein hormones, 41
Protein kinase, 34-36
Protein-receptor binding, 32
Prothrombin deficiency, 341
Protirelin (TRH), 375-376
Proximal tubal blockage, 487-491
Pseudohermaphroditism
    female, 214-216
    male, 213-214, 216-219
Pseudoisosexual precocious puberty,
    231-232
Psychological factors
    complete isosexual precocious
        puberty, 229
    lactation, 148
    menopause, 184-185
    premenstrual syndrome, 353-364
Psychological stress. *See* Stress
Pubarche, premature, 226-227
Puberty, 163-178
    breast and, 144
    breast/pubic hair development in,
        163-165
    endocrine events in, 173-176
    Klinefelter's syndrome, 210
    menarche, 165-167
    normal, 223
    prepubertal endocrine events, 168-
        173
    primary amenorrhea, 237
    skeletal change in, 167-168
    See also Precocious puberty (female);
        Precocious puberty (male)
Pubic hair
    premature pubarche, 226-227

primary amenorrhea, 245, 246
puberty, 163-165, 223
Puerperium, 150-158

R
Radiation therapy, 298
Radioimmunoassay (RIA), 61
    follicle-stimulating
        hormone/luteinizing hormone
        measurement, 77
    gonadotropin-releasing hormone
        measurement, 75
    hormone measurement, 62-63
    human chorionic gonadotropin
        (hCG), 121-122
    menstrual cycle and, 95
    primary amenorrhea diagnosis, 244
Radiology
    androgen excess, 313
    hyperprolactinemia and, 292-293
    hysterosalpingography and, 449-459
Radioreceptor assay (RRA), 66
Reanastomosis
    adjunctive therapy, 496
    end-to-end, 489
    tubal-cornual, 490
    See also Tubal surgery
Receptors, 31
Recurrent abortion, 539-551
    defined, 539
    etiology of, 540-547
    luteal phase defects, 553
    management of, 547-550
    occurrence of, 539-540
Relaxin, 139
Renin-angiotensin mechanism, 116, 117
Reserpine, 15
Resin uptake, 117
Retina, 5
Rheumatoid arthritis, and OC use, 619,
    621
Rhythm method, 590
Rifampicin, and OCs, 615
RNA

prolactin and, 276
pubertal endocrine activity during, 174-175, 228
Slide test, 413
Smoking. *See* Cigarette smoking
Socioeconomic factors, 166
Sodium valproate, 14
Somatostatin
  effect of, 22
  secretion of, 4, 5
Sperm
  antibody localization in, 524
  autoimmunity and, 524-525
  female sperm-agglutinating antibodies, 525
  female sperm-immobilizing antibodies, 525-526
  fertilization and, 109-111
  immunological tests, 526-527
  in vitro fertilization, 574-575
  Klinefelter's syndrome, 210-211
  polyspermia, 111
  postcoital testing and, 418, 420-422
  semen analysis, 429-434
  zona pellucida and, 108
  See also Semen; Semen analysis
Spermatogenesis, 425-426
Spermatozoan antigens, 521-522
Spermicides, 588
Sperm transport, 95
Spontaneous abortion
  early prediction of, 123, 125
  hysteroscopy and, 467
  with IUD in situ, 649-650
  after OC use, 609
  ovulation induction and, 396, 399
  See also Recurrent abortion
Standard preparations (hormone measurement), 66-67
Sterility
  infertility contrasted, 381
  menopause, 181
  See also Infertility; Infertility evaluation

Sterilization
  frequency of, 583, 584
  reversal procedure (tubal), 491-492
Steroid hormone receptors, 31
Steroid hormones, 45-59
  actions of, 40-42
  adrenal, 52-58
  biosynthesis, 46-49
  calcium and, 189
  childhood and, 172-173
  dynamics of, 58
  gonadotropins and, 86-87
  growth and, 167
  hypothalamus and, 5
  infancy and, 171
  ovarian, 49-51, 69-70
  premenstrual syndrome and, 358-360
  puberty and, 173-176
  structure and classification of, 45-46, 47
  testicular, 52, 53
  See also Contraceptive steroids; Oral steroid contraceptives
Steroid-receptor binding, 32
Steroid-receptor interactions, 42-43
Stratum basale, 96-97
Stratum compactum, 95-96
Stratum spongiosum, 95-96
Stress
  polycystic ovary syndrome, 331
  puberty and, 166-167
  secondary amenorrhea and, 258-260
Stroke, and OCs, 604-605, 611, 612, 613
Stromal cells
  endometrium and, 95, 96-97, 98-99
  menopause and, 181
Stromal hyperthecosis, 314
Subdermal implants, steroid
  insertion, 630-631
  and IUD, 632
  removal, 632
  termination rates, 632, 633
Submucous leiomyomas, 542
Sulfonamides, and OCs, 615

transport of, 4, 5
Thyroxine, 143-144
Thyroxine-binding globulin, 117
Transcortin. *See* Corticosteroid-binding globulin
TRH. *See* Thyrotropin-releasing hormone
Tricyclic antidepressants, 15
Trophoblast
    human chorionic gonadotropin and, 120
    human placental lactogen, 127
    steroid hormones, 129
Trophoblastic plate, 109
True hermaphroditism. *See* Hermaphroditism
Tryptophan, 11, 601
TSH. *See* Thyroid-stimulating hormone
Tubal-cornual reanastomosis, 490
Tubal surgery, 481-498
    adjunctive therapy, 496-497
    distal tubal disease, 482-486
    ectopic pregnancy, 492-495
    hysterosalpingography, 481-482
    laparoscopy, 482
    proximal tubal blockage, 487-491
    sterilization reversal, 491-492
Tuberculosis, 482
Turner's syndrome, 212, 240-243
Tyrosine, 8

U

Ultrasound
    abortion prediction and, 123
    human menopausal gonadotropin ovulation treatment, 402
    in vitro fertilization, 571
Unicornuate uterus, 471
Urethra, 182
Urinary bladder
    ejaculation and, 426, 428
    menopause, 182
Urinary sex steroid, 61- 62

Urine pregnancy tests, 123, 124
    See also Pregnancy tests
Urogenital tract, 181-182
Uterine agenesis, 245-250
Uterine anomaly, 454-455
Uterine bleeding, dysfunctional (DUB), 337-351
    cancer and, 341
    and CVRs, 635-636
    described, 337
    differential diagnosis of, 341-342
    and DMPA, 625, 626
    estradiol and, 339
    etiology of, 338-341
    evaluation of, 342-343
    hypothyroidism and, 342
    hysterectomy and, 349
    hysterosalpingography and, 343
    injectable steroids and, 625, 626, 628, 630, 631, 632
    IUDs and, 646-647
    menarche and, 337, 338-339
    and normal menstrual cycle compared, 338
    OCs and, 342, 345, 604
    and ovary, 341
    pharmacology and, 342, 343-350
    therapy for, 343-350
Uterine defects, 542-544
Uterine lesions, 450-454
Uterus
    antibodies in, 523
    congenital absence of, 245-247
    diethylstilbestrol-related anomalies, 476-477
    hysteroscopy of, 461-480
    implantation and, 109-110
    intrauterine adhesions, 462-464
    lactation suppression and, 160
    leiomyomata uteri, 477-478
    myomectomy, 478-479
    oxytocin and, 146
    secondary amenorrhea, 270
    structural defects, 471-475

V

Vagina
    dysfunctional uterine bleeding and, 341
    menopause, 181-182, 185-186
    postcoital testing and, 418
    progestogen treatment and, 183
Vaginal atrophy, 265
Vaginal foams, 588
Vaginitis
    infertility and, 535-536
    menopause and, 182
Vanillylmandelic acid (VMA), 10
Vascular disease, and OC use, 611, 615
Vasoactive intestinal polypeptide (VIP), 14
Vasopressin, 3, 4
VIP. *See* Vasoactive intestinal polypeptide
Virilization, 309
    androgen excess, 308
    female fetus, 131-132
    female pseudohermaphroditism and 214-216
    hirsutism contrasted, 303
    male pseudohermaphroditism and, 216-219

pregnancy, 312
    See also Hirsutism
Vitamin D
    osteoporosis and, 189
    pregnancy and, 118
Vitamin supplements, and OC use, 611
Vitelline membrane, 108-109
VMA. *See* Vanillylmandelic acid
von Willebrand's disease, 341

W

Weight
    gain, 355
    loss, 260-262
    See also Body weight; Obesity
Wolffian duct development, 207

X

X-ray. *See* Radiology

Z

Zona pellucida
    endometrium and, 95
    fertilization and, 109
    follicular development and, 108